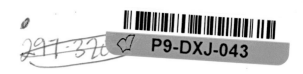
Seattle University
Student Health Center
1111 E. Columbia St.
Seattle, WA 98122
Tel: 206-296-6300
Fax: 206-296-6089

Orthopaedics in Primary Care

THIRD EDITION

Orthopaedics in Primary Care

THIRD EDITION

EDITED BY

GERALD G. STEINBERG, M.D.
Professor of Orthopedics
Department of Orthopedics
UMASS Memorial Medical Center
Worcester, Massachusetts

CARLTON M. AKINS, M.D.
Associate Professor of Orthopedics
Department of Orthopedics
UMASS Memorial Medical Center
Worcester, Massachusetts

DANIEL T. BARAN, M.D.
Professor of Orthopedics, Medicine, and Cell Biology
Department of Orthopedics
UMASS Memorial Medical Center
Worcester, Massachusetts

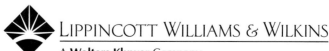

LIPPINCOTT WILLIAMS & WILKINS
A **Wolters Kluwer** Company

Philadelphia • Baltimore • New York • London
Buenos Aires • Hong Kong • Sydney • Tokyo

Editor: Timothy Hiscock
Managing Editor: Fran Klass
Marketing Manager: Meg White
Project Editor: Paula C. Williams

351 West Camden Street
Baltimore, Maryland 21201-2436 USA

227 East Washington Square
Philadelphia, PA 19106

Printed in the United States of America

First Edition, 1992
Second Edition, 1998

Library of Congress Cataloging-in-Publication Data

Orthopaedics in primary care. — 3rd ed. / edited by Gerald G. Steinberg, Carlton M. Akins,
    Daniel T. Baran.
    p. cm.
    Rev. ed. of: Ramamurti's orthopaedics in primary care / edited by Gerald G. Steinberg,
    Carlton M. Akins, Daniel T. Baran. 2nd ed. © 1992.
    Includes bibliographical references and index.
    ISBN 0-683-30258-2
    1. Orthopedics. 2. Primary care (Medicine) I. Steinberg, Gerald G. II. Akins, Carlton M. III. Baran,
    Daniel T. IV. Ramamurti's orthopaedics in primary care.
    [DNLM: 1. Orthopedics. 2. Primary Health Care. WE 168076279 1999]
    RD732.0779 1999
    616.7—dc21
    DNLM/DLC
    for Library of Congress   98-41147
                                                                                                    CIP

To purchase additional copies of this book, call our customer service department at **(800) 638-3030** or fax orders to **(301) 824-7390**. International customers should call (301) 714-2324.

98 99 00 01 02
1 2 3 4 5 6 7 8 9 10

Contributors

Carlton M. Akins, M.D.
Associate Professor of Orthopedics
Department of Orthopedics and Physical
Rehabilitation
UMASS Memorial Medical Center
Worcester, Massachusetts

Daniel T. Baran, M.D.
Professor of Orthopedics, Medicine, and Cell
Biology
Department of Orthopedics and Physical
Rehabilitation
UMASS Memorial Medical Center
Worcester, Massachusetts

James C. Bayley, M.D.
Associate Professor of Orthopedic Surgery
Chief, Section of Spine Surgery
Department of Orthopedics and Physical
Rehabilitation
UMASS Memorial Medical Center
Worcester, Massachusetts

Thomas F. Breen, M.D.
Associate Professor of Orthopedics and
Rehabilitation
Department of Orthopedics and Physical
Rehabilitation
UMASS Memorial Medical Center
Worcester, Massachusetts

Henry DeGroot III, M.D.
Assistant Professor
Chief, Orthopedic Oncology Service
Department of Orthopedics and Physical
Rehabilitation
UMASS Memorial Medical Center
Worcester, Massachusetts

W. Thomas Edwards, Ph.D., M.D.
Professor of Anesthesiology
Pain Relief Services
Harborview Medical Center
Seattle, Washington

Dudley A. Ferrari, M.D.
Assistant Professor of Orthopedic Surgery
Department of Orthopedics and Physical
Rehabilitation
UMASS Memorial Medical Center
Worcester, Massachusetts

Nelson M. Gantz, M.D., F.A.C.P.
Chairman, Department of Medicine
Chief, Division of Infectious Diseases
Clinical Professor of Medicine, Allegheny
University of the Health Sciences
Clinical Professor of Medicine, Pennsylvania
State University School of Medicine

David F. Giansiracusa, M.D.
Professor of Medicine
Vice Chair, Department of Medicine
University of Massachusetts Medical School
Staff Rheumatologist, Division of Rheumatology
UMASS Memorial Medical Center
Worcester, Massachusetts

Thomas P. Goss, M.D.
Professor of Orthopedic Surgery
Department of Orthopedics and Physical
Rehabilitation
UMASS Memorial Medical Center
Worcester, Massachusetts

Walter J. Leclair, M.D.
Assistant Professor of Orthopedic Surgery
Department of Orthopedics and Physical
Rehabilitation
UMASS Memorial Medical Center
Worcester, Massachusetts

John J. Monahan, M.D.
Professor, Department of Orthopedics and
Physical Rehabilitation
UMASS Memorial Medical Center
Worcester, Massachusetts

William J. Morgan, M.D.
Professor of Orthopedic Surgery
Chief, Upper Extremity Service
Department of Orthopedics and Physical
Rehabilitation
UMASS Memorial Medical Center
Worcester, Massachusetts

Errol Mortimer, M.D., F.R.C.S.I.
Assistant Professor of Orthopedic Surgery
Department of Orthopedics and Physical
Rehabilitation
UMASS Memorial Medical Center
Worcester, Massachusetts

Eric A. Seybold, M.D.
Spine Fellow
SUNY HSC Syracuse
Department of Orthopedics
Syracuse, New York

Yvonne A. Shelton, M.D.
Assistant Professor
Department of Orthopedics and Physical
Rehabilitation
UMASS Memorial Medical Center
Worcester, Massachusetts

Gerald G. Steinberg, M.D.
Professor of Orthopedics
Department of Orthopedics and Physical
Rehabilitation
UMASS Memorial Medical Center
Worcester, Massachusetts

Steven L. Strongwater, M.D.
Associate Dean for Clinical Affairs
Medical Director and Chief of Staff
University of Connecticut Health Center
Farmington, Connecticut

Thom A. Tarquinio, M.D.
Associate Professor
Department of Orthopedic Surgery and
Rehabilitation
University of Mississippi Medical Center
Jackson, Mississippi

Anthony K. Teebagy, M.D.
Assistant Professor of Orthopedics
Department of Orthopedics and Physical
Rehabilitation
UMASS Memorial Medical Center
Worcester, Massachusetts

Lisa S. Tkatch, M.D.
Clinical Assistant Professor of Medicine,
Allegheny University of the Health Sciences
Clinical Assistant Professor of Medicine,
Pennsylvania State University School of
Medicine

Richard J. Waite, M.D.
Associate Professor
Department of Radiology
UMASS Memorial Medical Center
Worcester, Massachusetts

Foreword

Approximately 25% of patients seen in the primary care office present with complaints related to the musculoskeletal system.

General knowledge of the musculoskeletal system is important for timely diagnosis and comprehensive treatment of patients, either by the primary care physician or in conjunction with an orthopaedist. This knowledge enhances patient care and keeps the primary care physician informed and involved.

The editors have kept this goal of improved patient care foremost in mind in this third edition of *Orthopaedics in Primary Care.* Their expertise and commitment to the field of orthopaedics is reflected in the contents of this edition, which is thorough and covers a wide range of issues related to orthopaedics.

This text will benefit the readers of the previous editions, as well as the primary care physician, nurse practitioner, physical assistant, and all health care professionals.

Arthur M. Pappas, M.D.

Preface

Although the evaluation and treatment of musculoskeletal problems typically comprise nearly 25% of primary care practice, there are few texts of adequate scope and depth dedicated to this subject. This text is offered as an easily accessible reference for the primary care or emergency room practice dealing with musculoskeletal problems. This third edition of *Orthopaedics in Primary Care* is organized by anatomic region. Each of the regional chapters contains a review of the essential anatomy, pertinent physical examinations, and a discussion of the common nontraumatic and traumatic conditions of the region. Chapter 16 specifically deals with principles of pediatric problems, and Chapters 10 through 15 deal with more general topics. Although the chapters have different authors, we have maintained consistent organization and presentation of the material.

Like the second edition, each of the chapters in this edition has been contributed by authors with subspecialty expertise. Care has been taken, however, to keep the scope and depth of discussion appropriate for the primary care setting. The authors have made a special effort to make specific recommendations regarding the need for referral versus definitive treatment by the primary care provider. It is hoped that the information in this text will allow the interested primary care provider to proceed with definitive treatment or appropriate referral. To the extent that we meet that objective, we will meet our overriding goal: the improved care of the patients we all serve.

CARLTON M. AKINS, M.D.
DANIEL T. BARAN, M.D.
GERALD G. STEINBERG, M.D.

Acknowledgments

The editors would like to gratefully acknowledge the following individuals for their committed work in the preparation of *Orthopaedics in Primary Care, Third Edition:*

The contributing authors for their expertise and devotion to the field of orthopaedics.

Caroline Kuzia for manuscript coordination and word processing.

Joy D. Marlowe for her excellent line drawings, interpretations of the authors' descriptions, and finesse in accommodating the contributors' schedules.

Charlene Baron for her biomedical artwork, photography, and technical assistance.

Contents

Cervical Spine

John J. Monahan, M.D., and Richard J. Waite, M.D.

ESSENTIAL ANATOMY

FUNCTIONAL UNITS OF THE CERVICAL SPINE (Fig. 1.1)

A functional unit of the spine consists of any two adjacent vertebrae and their articulations with one another. The cervical spine (C-spine) contains eight functional units, five of which are alike, and three of which (the first, second, and last) are unique.

The first functional unit is the articulation between the occiput and the first cervical vertebra (the atlantooccipital joint, Fig. 1.2). This unit is controlled primarily by short, deep muscles anteriorly and posteriorly that extend only the width of the segment. Its movement allows for about one-third of full flexion and extension and for about 50% of lateral bending of the head and neck.

The second functional unit is the articulation between the first and second cervical vertebrae (the atlantoaxial joint, Fig. 1.3). It too is controlled primarily by short, deep muscles anteriorly and posteriorly that extend across only the second unit and the first two units. The movement of the second unit allows for 50% of the rotational range of motion of the head and neck.

Weight is borne across each of the first two units of the spine on the broad surfaces of the facet joints.

The next five functional units are the articulations between the second through the seventh cervical vertebrae (Fig. 1.4). These units are controlled by long and short deep muscles anteriorly and posteriorly, the scalenus muscles at middle depth, and the sternocleidomastoid and trapezius muscles superficially. Their

movement allows for approximately two-thirds of full flexion and extension, approximately 50% of rotation, and approximately 50% of lateral bending. In contrast to the first two units, these five units bear weight on three broad surfaces—the two facets and the vertebral bodies. The facet articulations are synovial joints, and the body articulations are fibrocartilaginous joints (the intervertebral discs). The facet articulations are in the same plane as the intervertebral disc. The posterolateral margins of the bodies project slightly beyond the disc to form bony pseudoarthroses, the uncovertebral joints, across each functional unit. The uncovertebral joints are vulnerable to wear and tear and frequently develop degenerative osteophytes.

The cervical nerve roots exit through the foramen formed by the uncovertebral joint anteriorly and the facet joint posteriorly. Thus, the roots are vulnerable to acute impingement during subluxation of any of the units and to compression caused by posterolateral herniation of disc material or protrusion of bony spurs from the uncovertebral and facet joints (Fig. 1.4). The movements of the cervical spine allow for the most severe injuries and greatest wear and tear across the units between C-4 and C-7. The nerve roots passing through the intervertebral foramina of these units are the fifth, sixth, and seventh respectively.

The last functional unit is the articulation between C-7 and T-1 (Fig. 1.5). The C-7 vertebra is unique in two respects: its upward-directed facets are cervical-like, its downward-directed facets are thoracic-like, and its body is nearly of thoracic dimension. (The body of each lower cervical vertebra from C-3 to C-7

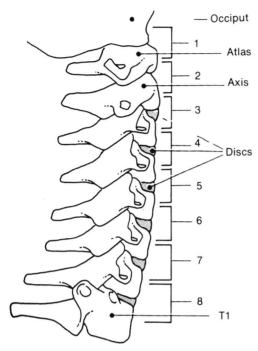

Figure 1.1. The eight functional units.

is slightly larger than its superior neighbor.) These unique characteristics make the last functional unit of the cervical spine similar to a thoracic unit, in that the larger vertebral bodies of C-7 and T-1 bear the bulk of the weight across the unit, and the facet articulations are nearly at right angles to the intervertebral disc. These near-perpendicular articular surfaces allow the unit limited movement in flexion, extension, and rotation. Severe injury or wear and tear across this unit is unusual.

SOFT TISSUES OF THE CERVICAL SPINE

The soft tissues of the cervical spine include the deep fascia, many layers of muscle, the thick ligaments, the synovia of the facet joints, and the intervertebral disc.

Deep Fascia (Fig. 1.6)

The deep fascia consists of three layers of dense connective tissue that separate the neck into compartments. The superficial layer lies beneath the platysma and surrounds all the deeper structures of the neck. The superficial layer splits to invest the sternocleidomastoid and strap muscles anteriorly and the trapezius posteriorly. The prevertebral layer surrounds the cervical spine and the deep muscles that cling to the spine anteriorly and posteriorly. The pretracheal layer surrounds the trachea, esophagus, thyroid, and parathyroid. All three layers fuse to form the carotid sheath that surrounds the carotid artery, the internal jugular vein, and the vagus nerve.

Muscles (Fig. 1.7)

The muscles of the neck accessible to physical examination anteriorly are the accessory muscles of the pharynx and larynx, which in aggregate are often called the strap muscles and the sternocleidomastoid muscle. Muscles that are accessible posteriorly and laterally are the trapezius and parts of the splenius capitis and cervicis, the levator scapulae, and the scalene muscles. The diagnosis of muscular injury depends on the discovery of tenderness in these muscles. Although deeper muscles that surround and lie on the cervical spine are affected in painful processes, the effect cannot be isolated by physical examination.

Ligaments (Fig. 1.8)

The ligamentum nuchae is the most superficial ligament. It represents a thin extension of the supraspinous and interspinous ligaments outward between the trapezius muscles. The supraspinous and interspinous ligaments are distinct entities in the dorsal and lumbar spine; however, in the neck they merge and lose their identities in the ligamentum nuchae. With the neck in full flexion, the ligamentum nuchae can be palpated distinctly as it extends from the spine of the seventh cervical vertebra to the prominence of the occiput. The ligamentum nuchae is the only ligament that can be distinguished as such by palpation.

The capsular ligaments of the facet joints surround each facet joint, extending between the margins of the two articular surfaces. Palpation through the scalene and splenius muscles allows the examiner to detect the facet column. The joints cannot be distinguished

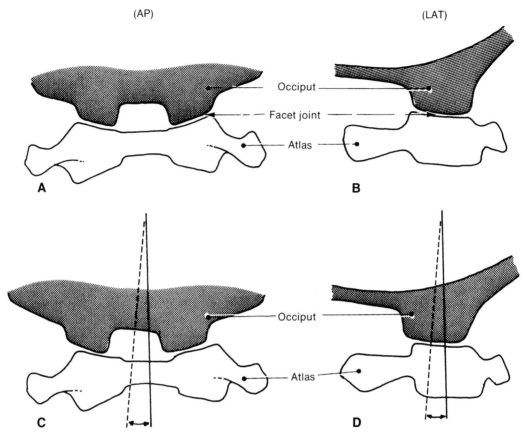

Figure 1.2.   The first functional unit: the atlanto-occipital joint. *A* and *B*, neutral. *C*, lateral bending. *D*, nodding.

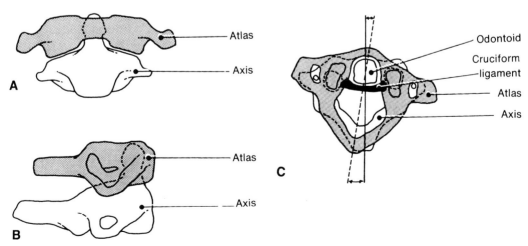

Figure 1.3.   The second functional unit: the atlanto-axial joint. *A*, anteroposterior, neutral. *B*, lateral. *C*, superior, rotated.

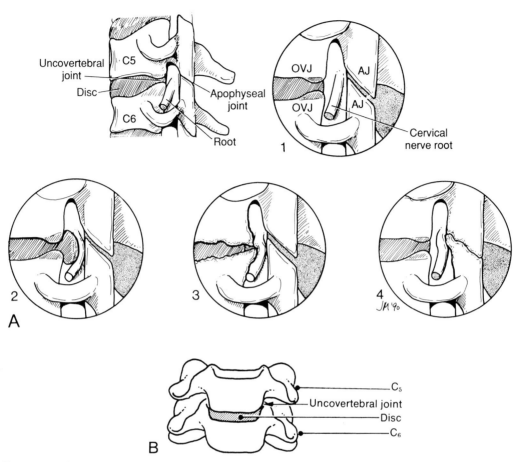

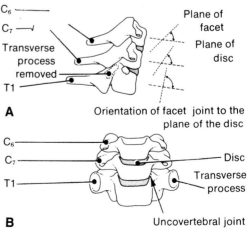

Figure 1.4. *A*, normal and abnormal relationships of a cervical nerve root passing from the spinal canal through the foramen. *1*, normal. *2*, disc protrusion. *3*, uncovertebral osteophyte. *4*, apophyseal osteophyte. *B*, the five similar functional units: articulations between the 2nd and 7th cervical vertebrae.

by palpation, and tenderness of the ligaments cannot be distinguished from tenderness of the overlying muscles. Localized tenderness does, however, indicate a potential injury of the superficial or deep soft tissues.

The posterior longitudinal ligament passes the length of the spinal column, lying against the posterior walls of the vertebral bodies and discs. The anterior longitudinal ligament passes the length of the spinal column, lying against the anterior walls of the vertebral bodies and discs. The ligamenta flava are a series of short ligaments that pass between the lamina of the posterior arches of each functional unit along the length of the spine.

All of these ligaments are pain sensitive.

Figure 1.5. The unique structure of the 7th cervical vertebra.

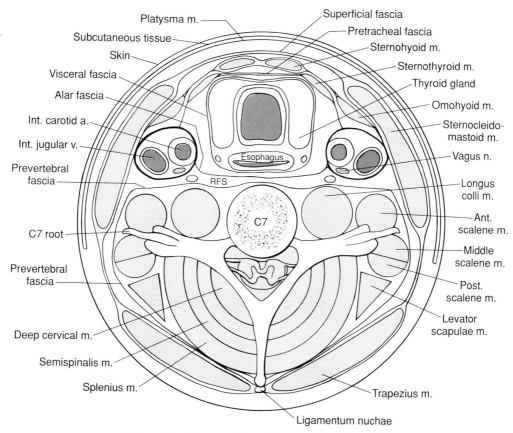

Platysma m.

Subcutaneous tissue

Skin

Visceral fascia

Alar fascia

Int. carotid a.

Int. jugular v.

Prevertebral fascia

C7 root

Prevertebral fascia

Deep cervical m.

Semispinalis m.

Splenius m.

Superficial fascia

Pretracheal fascia

Sternohyoid m.

Sternothyroid m.

Thyroid gland

Omohyoid m.

Sternocleido-mastoid m.

Vagus n.

Longus colli m.

Ant. scalene m.

Middle scalene m.

Post. scalene m.

Levator scapulae m.

Trapezius m.

Ligamentum nuchae

C7

Esophagus

RFS

Figure 1.6.   Cross section of the cervical spine at C-7.

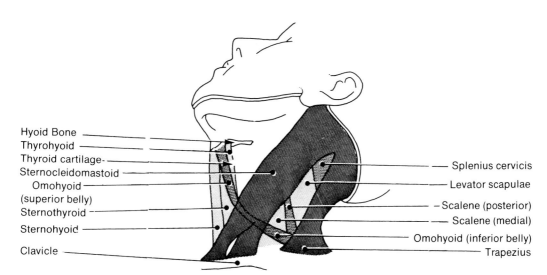

Hyoid Bone

Thyrohyoid

Thyroid cartilage

Sternocleidomastoid

Omohyoid (superior belly)

Sternothyroid

Sternohyoid

Clavicle

Splenius cervicis

Levator scapulae

Scalene (posterior)

Scalene (medial)

Omohyoid (inferior belly)

Trapezius

Figure 1.7.   The muscles accessible to physical examination.

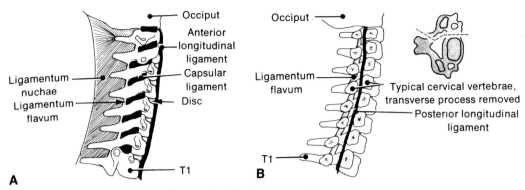

Figure 1.8. The ligaments of the neck.

Synovia of the Facet Joints (Fig. 1.8)

A synovial membrane lies beneath the capsular ligaments and invests and lubricates the articulations of the facets. It may be stretched along with the capsule when the facet joints are subluxed, and it has been postulated that it may be pinched between facet surfaces when they move on one another in slight malalignment. As may be true of all synovial joints, local degenerative and various "systemic" events may cause an inflammation within the synovium. All these processes result in a painful synovitis.

Intervertebral Disc (Fig. 1.8)

The disc consists of two parts, a springy outer ring of interwoven fibrocartilaginous bands called the anulus, and a "hydroelastic," gelatinous inner core called the nucleus pulposus. Young discs are thick, malleable, and elastic, whereas old discs are thin, rigid, and brittle. Thus, greater forces are required to injure young discs than old. The forces that injure discs may injure the anterior and/or posterior longitudinal ligaments as well. Disc material displaced against the posterior longitudinal ligament also may protrude far enough to compress the adjacent nerve root, producing radicular pain and dysfunction. The disc anulus also contains pain-sensitive nerve endings. Therefore, the pain directly attributable to a disc injury is the pain from the disc, injured nerve root (radiculopathy), injured spinal cord (myelopathy), and/or injured anterior or posterior longitudinal ligament.

EVALUATION OF THE PATIENT WITH NECK SYMPTOMS

HISTORY

Since the neck is a complex structure made up of multiple organ systems, a meticulous history is necessary to define the specific system or systems involved. The pathologic process may be local or referred from the upper abdomen, thorax, upper extremities, scalp, temporomandibular joint, or teeth. The clinical characteristics include pain, abnormal posture or range of motion, and neurologic or vascular dysfunction. The history of the present illness should include the how, what, when, and where of the onset of symptoms; details of possible congenital, infectious, inflammatory, traumatic, endocrine, metabolic, or tumor processes; description of pain pattern; description of any deformity; and description of muscle weakness and/or associated disturbance of sensory function or bowel and bladder sphincter control.

PHYSICAL EXAMINATION

The techniques and emphasis of the physical examination of the neck vary with the etiology of neck symptoms: nontraumatic or traumatic.

Inspection

The patient with a traumatic C-spine injury should have been immobilized in a neck brace at the scene of the injury. In addition, the patient should be attached to a spine board. The neck should be in the neutral or least deformed position possible without using undue force or causing pain. Inspection of the patient with a suspected spinal injury must be carried out in the brace with the patient's neck in a neutral or near-neutral position. The primary physician should look for obvious swelling, asymmetry, discoloration, tracheal deviation, respiratory distress, or malalignment of the cervical spine. The patient's neck should not be moved until fracture, dislocation, or unstable ligament injury has been ruled out. The patient with complete cord injury is usually able to identify pain at the site of injury, but the observer notes anesthesia below this level. The sensory loss may mask visceral injuries involving the chest or the abdominal cavity. Suspicion of injury above C-5 should trigger concern for possible respiratory compromise (the diaphragm is innervated by C-3 through C-5).

In the nontraumatic case, the patient is inspected as he or she walks into the examining room and undresses to the waist. The examiner notes abnormal posture or motion (splinting or guarding) and diminished range of motion. Local or diffuse swelling, rashes, discoloration, or scars of the neck and upper extremities are observed. The chest, upper abdomen, scalp, temporomandibular joint, and teeth may need to be inspected.

Palpation

In both traumatic and nontraumatic cases, palpation may reveal areas of tenderness, swelling, induration, asymmetry, or malalignment in the bony and soft tissues of the neck. Anterior bony landmarks include the hyoid bone at the C-3 level, thyroid cartilage at the C-4/C-5 level, and first cricoid ring at the C-6 level. Posteriorly, the occiput, inion, superior nuchal line, mastoid process, spinous processes, and apophyseal joints are examined. The examination of the anterior soft tissues includes the sternocleidomastoid muscles, strap muscles, scalenus muscles, lymph nodes, thyroid gland, carotid pulses, and supraclavicular fossa (e.g., clavicle fractures, cervical ribs,

or superior sulcus tumors). Posteriorly, the trapezius and paraspinous muscles, lymph nodes, greater occipital nerve, and superior nuchal ligament (which extends from the occiput to the C-7 spinous process) are examined.

In traumatic cases, active or passive range of motion should not be tested until appropriate radiographic studies rule out fracture or dislocation.

Range of Motion

The range of motion of the C-spine is age dependent, in that it tends to diminish with aging. The normal painless range of motion of the cervical spine in a young adult is approximately 45° of flexion (the patient is able to touch chin to chest), approximately 45 to 60° of extension, and approximately 90° of rotation (the patient is able to rotate the head from side to side so that the chin is almost in line with the shoulder). Lateral bending, in which the patient tries to touch the ear to the shoulder, should be approximately 45° toward each shoulder.

NEUROLOGIC EXAMINATION

Neurologic Anatomy

There are eight cervical nerves. The individual spinal cord segments correspond to the vertebral segments. One through seven exit on top of their respective vertebrae; the eighth exits between C-7 and T-1. T-1 exits below the T-1 vertebra. The brachial plexus is composed of nerves emanating from C-5 to T-1. As the individual roots travel from the spine to the upper extremity, they form specific trunks, divisions, cords, and peripheral nerves at specific anatomic levels. Impingement of these specific structures produces characteristic signs and symptoms.

Sensory Distribution

From C-2 to T-1, each root supplies sensation to a portion of the extremity in a succession of dermatomes around the extremity. These dermatomal distributions are variable, but the following autonomous zones for each root are useful, though approximate, clinical indices. C-2 supplies the area 2 inches below the tip of the ear; C-3, the base of the neck; C-4, the top of the shoulder; C-5, the lateral arm at the shoulder; C-6, the lateral aspect of the forearm and tip of the thumb; C-7, the tip of the middle finger; C-8, the medial border of the hand; and T-1, the medial aspect of the lower arm.

Motor Distribution and Deep Tendon Reflexes

Roots C-3/C-5 via the phrenic nerve innervate the diaphragm; respiratory paralysis may be present and assisted ventilation necessary with injuries proximal to C-4. C-5 innervates the deltoid and biceps muscles and is responsible for the biceps deep tendon reflex. C-6 supplies the wrist extensors (extensor carpi radialis longus and brevis) and abductor and extensors of the thumb and is responsible for the brachioradialis reflex. C-7 innervates the triceps, wrist flexors, and finger extensors and controls the triceps reflex. C-8 supplies innervation to the finger flexors and has no deep tendon reflex. T-1 innervates the intrinsic muscles of the hand, which include the dorsal interossei and the abductor digiti quinti; there is no definable reflex.

The examiner should also test the function of the intrinsic neck muscles in flexion, extension, lateral rotation, and lateral bending. The primary flexor is the sternocleidomastoid, innervated by the spinal accessory or the 11th cranial nerve. Secondary flexors are the scalenus and paravertebral muscles. Primary extensors are the splenius, semispinalis, capitis (paravertebral extensor mass), and trapezius, innervated by the spinal accessory or the 11th cranial nerve. The sternocleidomastoid muscle is responsible for lateral rotation. Primary muscles acting in lateral bending are the scalenus anticus, medius, and posticus, innervated by the anterior primary divisions of the lower cervical nerves.

Special Tests

Distraction Test

The distraction test is performed by cupping the patient's chin and occiput and gently lifting the head. Distraction opens up the foramen, intervertebral space, and apophyseal and uncovertebral joints. This relieves pressure on the nerve root exiting through the foramen and sensitive para-articular tissues, protruding discs, inflamed synovia, or degenerative osteophytes of the adjacent synovial joints. A positive test (i.e., pain relief) indicates a disorder within the vertebral complex.

Compression Test

The compression test is the opposite of the distraction test. It is performed by gently pushing directly down on the patient's head. The axial loading precipitates or aggravates the pain when the foramen and its contained nerve root, intervertebral space, and degenerated synovial joints are compressed.

Valsalva Test

The patient bears down as if moving the bowels. The examiner notes aggravation of pain as the intrathecal pressure increases. Space-occupying lesions in the cervical canal, such as herniated discs or tumors, cause local and/or radicular pain corresponding to the level of C-spine pathology.

Swallowing Test

Dysphagia or pain on swallowing may be caused by a cervical spine disorder, such as bony protuberances, osteophytes, or soft tissue swelling.

Adson's Test

(See section on "Thoracic Outlet Syndrome.") The Adson's test is used to determine compression of the brachial plexus and/or subclavian artery.

RADIOLOGIC EXAMINATION

Diagnostic Studies

In trauma cases, a lateral cervical spine x-ray should be taken early in the course of the examination, usually during the primary survey immediately after the life-threatening problems are identified and controlled. The

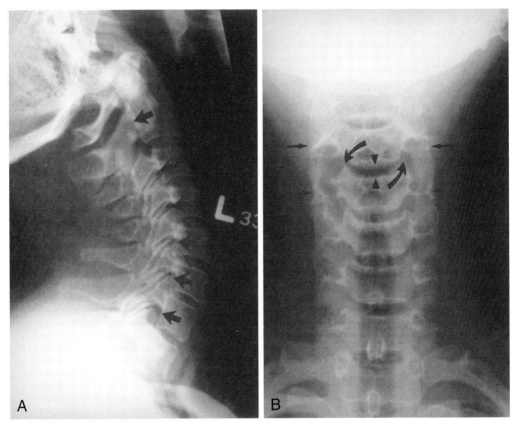

Figure 1.9. Normal: *A,* lateral; *B,* AP; *C,* oblique; and *D,* odontoid views of the cervical spine. *A,* normal lateral shows smooth cervical lordosis with maintained body heights (arrow heads), disk spaces (curved arrows), and vertebral body alignment (arrows) reflected by the posterior longitudinal line. *B,* AP view of the cervical spine shows orthogonal projection relative to *A.* Shown are disk spaces (arrow heads), lateral margins of the lateral masses (arrows), and uncovertebral joints (curved arrows). The central portion of each spinous process forms a vertical column (small arrows).

lateral x-ray (Fig. 1.9A) should be taken with the neck in a neutral position in a nonradiopaque cervical brace. All seven cervical vertebrae must be identified. If C-7 and T-1 cannot be seen, the attending physician should pull the patient's shoulders down gently while the x-ray is being taken. If C-7 and T-1 cannot be seen in the routine lateral view, a lateral swimmer's view, which is a slightly oblique lateral view of the cervical spine, is obtained. This allows the physician to assess spinal injuries and determine the need for further spine x-rays. Once the patient is stable, the full C-spine x-ray series is completed, including anteroposterior (AP) (Fig. 1.9B), oblique cervical (Fig. 1.9C), and open-mouth odontoid views (Fig. 1.9D). Tomography and/or computed tomography (CT) may be necessary to make a radiologic diagnosis. After studies have ruled out fracture or dislocation, stress films should be taken if stability of the C-spine is in question. The study should be performed with caution and supervised by the physician. It includes two lateral x-rays of the cervical spine with the neck moved actively with guidance into the maximum flexed and maximum extended positions within the limits of pain.

X-ray Review

In trauma cases, x-rays should be examined for the alignment of the vertebral bodies and any displacement of bone fragments into the

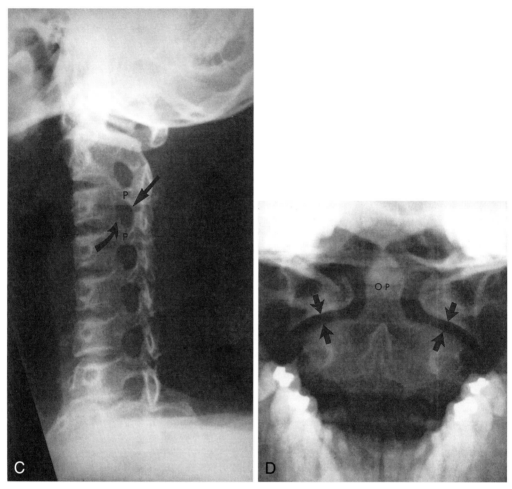

Figure 1.9. (*continued*) *C,* oblique view demonstrates well the intervertebral foramina demarcated by the pedicles superiorly and inferiorly (P), the uncovertebral articulation anteroinferiorly (curved arrow), and the facet joint posterosuperiorly (arrow). *D,* open mouth odontoid view shows the atlanto-occipital joint between C1 and C2 (arrows) pivoting about the odontoid process (OP).

spinal canal. The segments of the vertebral complex involved in the fractures (Fig. 1.10) should be identified. For the evaluation of stability, the spine may be divided into three segments. The first segment includes the anterior longitudinal ligament and anterior two-thirds of the vertebral body; the second segment is composed of the posterior third of the vertebral body, including the posterior longitudinal ligament; and the third segment is composed of the posterior elements (facet joints, neural arch and processes) of the vertebral complex (Fig. 1.10). If a fracture or liga-

mentous disruption involves two or more of the three segments of the vertebral complex, the injury is considered unstable. When assessing the lateral spine, the distance between the pharynx and the anterior-inferior border of C-3 is measured. The prevertebral soft tissue thickness at this level should be less than or equal to 5 mm. An increase in this area of density suggests a vertebral fracture because it could represent a hematoma secondary to the fracture. Any angulation of two adjacent vertebrae greater than 11° more than the angulation between each of those vertebrae and

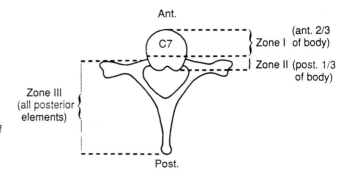

Ant.

C7

(ant. 2/3 of body) } Zone I

Zone II (post. 1/3 of body)

Zone III (all posterior elements)

Post.

Figure 1.10. Structural segments of a cervical vertebra. Fractures involving more than one segment are usually unstable.

their adjacent normal vertebrae indicates instability of the cervical spine. Translation of one vertebra upon another, either anterior, posterior, lateral, or combinations thereof, greater than 3.5 mm also indicates instability. Any evidence of instability requires orthopaedic and/or neurosurgical referral. While waiting for the consultant, the cervical spine should continue to be immobilized.

In nontraumatic cases of neck pain, routine C-spine x-rays may be taken when indicated, (i.e., AP, lateral, both obliques, and odontoid views). In addition to the interpretive criteria described for traumatic cases, evidence of destruction (lytic lesion) or increased bone production (blastic lesion) are sought, as well as narrowing or hypertrophic changes of the disc or apophyseal joints, calcific deposition within the disc space, and associated soft tissue changes. Additional studies, such as tomography, CT scan, magnetic resonance imaging (MRI), and bone scan, are often indicated for further evaluation, but this is usually a decision made after orthopaedic referral.

NONTRAUMATIC CONDITIONS IN ADULTHOOD

DEGENERATIVE DISEASE

As in the thoracic and lumbosacral spine, a theoretical scheme of spinal degeneration provides a good perspective for the primary care physician in evaluating patients with degenerative conditions of the cervical spine. This theory proposes that facet joint synovitis, hypermobility, and progressive degeneration

are "natural" consequences of aging and the repetitive trauma of "normal" activity. The facet joint changes occur along with degenerative changes in the intervertebral disc, which begin with marginal tears of the anulus and progress to radial tears and disc herniation. Subluxation of the facet joints with enlargement of the articular processes occur in parallel with disc resorption and spinal osteophyte formation. In the cervical spine, the uncovertebral joints may be severely involved in this process. In the early phases of this degenerative process, patients may be identified as having "facet joint syndrome," or after relatively minor trauma, the patient may develop an "acute disc herniation." It is important to recognize that the facet joint and the discs are each one part of the motion segment, and it is unlikely that there is isolated trauma or inflammation in one part of the spinal unit without associated abnormalities in the complementary parts.

Acute Disc Herniation

Acute disc herniation in the cervical spine is less common than in the lumbar region. The syndrome may be triggered by an acute injury to the disc, with or without underlying degenerative changes. It may also present with little or no remembered trauma and is frequently associated with degenerative changes of the intervertebral disc. With herniation of the disc, there may be irritation of an associated nerve root or other nerve endings in the disc complex, i.e., anulus fibrosus or posterior longitudinal ligament. A disc herniation, consequently, may cause true radicular pain or nonradicular referred pain felt in the upper extremity. In true radicular pain, the signs and symptoms vary with the level of nerve root irritation.

Clinical Characteristics

C-4/C-5 (fifth root) causes neck, shoulder, and lateral arm pain and motor weakness of the deltoid and biceps. Sensation is diminished over the lateral upper arm, with an autonomous zone over the lateral deltoid. The biceps reflex may be diminished.

C-5/C-6 (sixth root) causes neck pain, with variable radiation into the occiput and/or interscapular area, posterolateral aspect of the shoulder, lateral aspect of the upper arm and forearm, and the thumb and index finger. Sensory dysfunction in the lateral forearm, thumb, and index finger may be noted. There may be weakness of the biceps, long abductor and extensor of the thumb, and wrist extensors. The brachioradialis reflex is usually diminished.

C-6/C-7 (seventh root) causes neck pain, with variable radiation into the occiput and shoulder or interscapular region, lateral aspect of the upper arm and forearm, and, occasionally, the volar aspect of the forearm, ulnar aspect of the hand, and fourth and fifth fingers. Sensory loss involves the fourth and fifth fingers. Muscle weakness is evident in the triceps, wrist flexors, and finger extensors. The triceps reflex is usually diminished.

C-7/T-1 (eighth root) causes neck pain, with variable radiation into the occiput, interscapular region, medial aspect of the upper arm, and forearm. Motor weakness involves the deep and superficial finger flexors. Sensory dysfunction occurs along the C-8 dermatome on the ulnar aspect of the distal forearm and hand.

T-1/T-2 (T-1 root) pain involves the neck, with variable referral to the occiput and interscapular region. Usually, pain is felt in the medial aspect of the arm. Sensory deficits are noted in the medial side of the proximal half of the forearm and distal half of the upper arm. Motor weakness involves the finger abductors.

No deep tendon reflex is associated with the T-1 root.

Pain from an acute disc herniation is usually aggravated by coughing, sneezing, straining, and activities involving prolonged abnormal positioning, especially fixed flexion or extension with rotation. Lifting, pushing, and pulling may trigger pain. There is tenderness to palpation over the posterior elements of the spinous process of the involved root or over the facet joints. Gentle manual traction tends to relieve pain, while compression of the spine increases pain. Further physical findings include pain on active or passive motion of the C-spine, with an overall diminished range of motion. There may be abnormal posture of the C-spine, with flattening of lordosis or development of torticollis. The pain is relieved somewhat by bringing the patient's ipsilateral hand up behind the neck. Pain is aggravated by hyperextension and rotation of the neck to the involved side. There is usually associated muscle spasm of the paravertebral muscles and, occasionally, the more anterior muscle groups. Trigger points may be in the interscapular region.

X-ray studies may be normal or may reveal degenerative changes or disc space narrowing. If there is no response to initial conservative treatment, orthopaedic referral is indicated. CT scan, MRI studies (Fig. 1.11), myelogram, or bone scan may be indicated to further evaluate the patient. Electromyography (EMG) and nerve conduction studies are useful in delineating a specific radiculopathy.

Treatment

Conservative treatment is recommended for acute disc herniation. The keystone is rest. Rest may be defined as limiting the patient's activities of daily living to a point where he or she is comfortable. If the patient is having severe pain, especially when associated with neurologic dysfunction, strict bedrest is indicated (bathroom privileges are allowed). A position of comfort, utilizing soft (not foam rubber) pillows, elevation of the head of the bed, and a soft cervical collar (Fig. 1.12) when

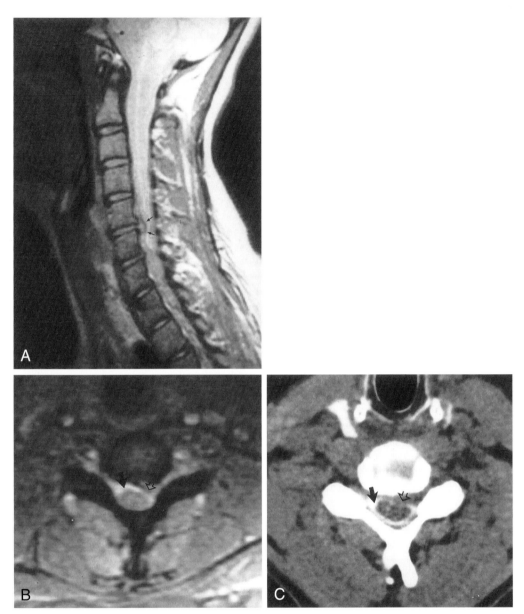

Figure 1.11. Imaging of herniated nucleus pulposus. *A,* sagittal MR proton density scan (TR 2118, TE 30) demonstrates posterior extrusion of disk material at C4-C5 (arrows). *B,* axial gradient echo image (TR 733, TE 18, flip angle = 13°) demonstrates high signal (white) to the normal cerebrospinal fluid (CSF) (solid arrow). Extruded disk material anterolaterally on the left (open arrow) effaces the CSF in this area and noninvasively clarifies the patient's cervical radiculopathy. *C,* axial CT-myelogram in a different patient with a similar herniated disc. The CSF shows high density (white) reflecting the instilled contrast material (solid arrow). This somewhat invasive study (myelogram) shows a similar pattern of anterior CSF effacement and cord distortion (arrows) compared with B.

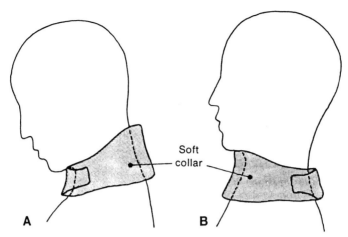

Figure 1.12. Applications of the soft collar. *A*, flexion. *B*, extension.

necessary, is recommended. Bedrest is continued, with the neck protected in a cervical collar until the patient can sit, stand, and walk comfortably in the collar. At this point, ambulatory activity is allowed as tolerated. The period of bedrest is usually 2 to 10 days. While on bedrest, the patient may maintain muscle tone in the trunk and lower extremities by an isometric exercise regimen.

If the signs and symptoms are moderate, relative rest is indicated, utilizing a firm or soft cervical collar to provide comfort and support to the cervical spine. Limited activities are permitted as tolerated, using pain as the limiting factor.

The rest regimen may be supplemented by intermittent cervical traction, unless this makes the patient more uncomfortable. Careful positioning for traction is essential (Fig. 1.13). Traction should begin with the neck in a comfortable position, usually slight flexion. The neck should be well supported, with the halter applying a distractive force posteriorly below the occiput. Traction for 20 minutes four times a day should begin with light weight, i.e., 5 to 7 pounds, with the patient supine in bed, or 10 to 12 pounds, with the patient sitting. Weight should be increased gradually as tolerated for as long as the traction affords relief, up to a maximum of 10 to 15 pounds, with the patient supine in bed, or 20 to 25 pounds, with the patient sitting. Before traction, moist heat should be applied to the neck for 15 to 20 minutes, with gentle massage of the area as tolerated.

Medications may include nonsteroidal anti-inflammatory drugs, muscle relaxants, and analgesics.

If the patient does not respond to these conservative measures within 2 to 3 weeks, additional studies as well as orthopaedic or neurosurgical consultation are indicated. If the patient demonstrates progressive weakness, sensory loss, or loss of bowel or bladder control at any point in the program, immediate consultations should be obtained.

If the patient has improved on the conservative program (i.e., the patient is comfortable under rest conditions, and range of motion and motor strength of the neck are improving without precipitating pain), rehabilitative measures are indicated. These measures involve a physical therapy program to gain full functional range of motion and strength of the C-spine and the affected extremity. The program begins with active range of motion exercises and isometric exercises and progresses to isotonic exercises of the neck and involved upper extremity, while maintaining a mobilizing and strengthening program for the trunk and lower extremities. During the rehabilitation period, patients should be encouraged to perform activities of daily living as tolerated to lessen the overall period of disability and hasten full recovery.

Rehabilitation also involves weaning the patient from the restrictions imposed during the acute phase. The patient should be weaned from bedrest by initiating progressive periods of ambulation over the day. Initially, the neck is protected by a cervical collar. The three or four periods out of bed each day are gradually lengthened. The patient is taught to avoid pain, or better, to recognize the warnings that precede pain (e.g., fatigue, dull burning ache) and indicate that the patient is proceeding too quickly.

The cervical collar is gradually discontinued. The progressive isometric and isotonic exercises are continued three to five times a day for 5 to 7 minutes each session, while the periods out of the collar are gradually extended in 20- to 30-minute increments, beginning with 15 to 20 minutes every 2 to 3 hours.

Pain should be avoided while reducing time in the collar.

The author suggests that the weaning process be carefully monitored over 2 to 3 weeks to avoid prolonged immobilization and its attendant chronic pain syndrome with persistent pain, muscle atrophy, stiffness, depression, and disability.

The patient should be guided back to full activity when he or she is out of the collar and comfortable with the physical therapy program. A general aerobic exercise program should be prescribed. Walking is excellent. Swimming is equally beneficial, but occasionally causes recurrent pain and spasm with specific strokes that stress the neck improperly.

The patient should avoid lifting, pushing, pulling, or using the hands above shoulder level. Malpositioning should be discouraged, i.e., prolonged neck flexion while typing or the

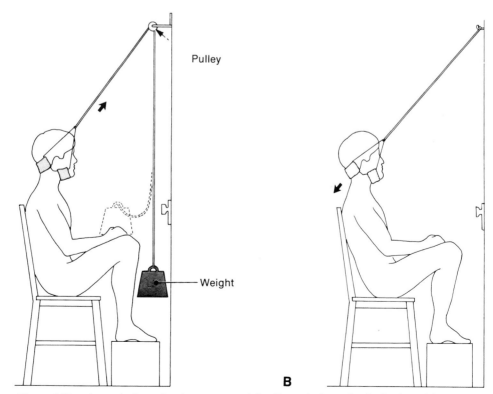

Figure 1.13.   *A,* cervical traction by counterweight. *B,* cervical traction by body weight.

extension/rotation that occurs when falling asleep while sitting with the head unsupported. An early return to rigorous sports is discouraged, and contact sports are contraindicated. Most patients can return to sedentary occupations in 2 to 4 weeks, whereas manual laborers may require 6 to 8 weeks or longer.

Chronic Degenerative Disease of the Cervical Spine, Cervical Spondylosis, Osteoarthritis

The constellation of symptoms grouped under these diagnostic categories occur in an older population, usually over age 45. The underlying pathology of the intervertebral disc, facet and uncovertebral joints, and ligaments has been described. While these conditions are often more benign in their clinical presentation than an acute cervical disc syndrome, they are frequently associated with true radiculopathy because of the relationship of the nerve root to the surrounding structures, as demonstrated in Figure 1.4A.

Clinical Characteristics

Pain may be limited to the involved facet joints but is more often a generalized ache in the cervical spine without a radicular component. Referred, nonradicular shoulder and arm pain may occur. If the nerve root is involved, true radiculitis or radiculopathy may be noted with sensory and motor dysfunction. The pattern of symptoms depends on the nerve root involved, as discussed above. Symptoms may occur because of the loss of mobility in the cervical spine from minor trauma (see Fig. 1.14).

Treatment

Symptoms usually respond to the traction program as described previously. Further treatment is the same as that described under "Acute Disc Herniation." A more recent alternative to relieving root pain is "epidural steroids" (Fig. 1.15), and an alternative for lessening facet joint pain is with facet joint injection with steroids (Fig. 1.16).

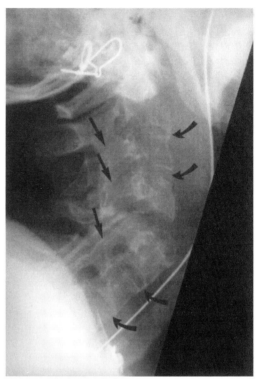

Figure 1.14. Fracture-dislocation of the cervical spine in a 32-year-old male with ankylosing spondylitis. There is disruption of the C4-C5 disk space extending posteriorly through the ankylosed posterior elements with diastasis, retrolisthesis, and acute kyphosis. Syndesmophytes (curved arrows) and ankylosed facet joints (arrows) are seen. This patient suffered this severe cervical spine injury with resultant paraplegia after relatively minimal trauma, highlighting the increased risk in a spine with limited mobility (Courtesy of Dr. Richard Waite, Department of Radiology, University of Massachusetts Medical Center, Worcester, MA).

Acute Cervical Myalgia (Muscular Wryneck)

Wryneck is a symptom complex; its etiology is unclear. It appears to be some type of soft tissue inflammation or irritation, either in the muscles, ligaments, or facet joints (synovia).

Clinical Characteristics

Onset is gradual, usually without history of significant trauma. Onset may be associated with exposure to cold, tension or anxiety, or repetitive motion or prolonged positioning of the C-spine. Pain is felt in one of the posterior cervical triangles. Occasionally, pain may be referred into the ipsilateral shoulder, interscapular region, and occiput. Range of motion is usually diminished. The greatest restriction is in those directions that stretch the affected muscle groups. A tender focus is often discovered by careful palpation of the trapezius, splenius capitis, and levator scapulae on the painful side (Fig. 1.7). This area is often indurated and exhibits crepitus on deep palpation. Palpation over the spinous processes has no effect on pain. X-rays are within normal limits.

Treatment

Acute cervical myalgia is treated as a mild cervical sprain (see section on "Cervical Sprains and Strains"), except that the exercise regimen is initiated as early as possible and emphasizes movements that stretch the tender muscle. The condition tends to clear spontaneously in 7 to 10 days, with no significant sequelae.

Rheumatoid Arthritis

Rheumatoid arthritis may involve the cervical spine, as it does other parts of the axial and appendicular synovial joints. (Refer to Chapter 12 for a discussion of the underlying pathology.) Cervical instability is the most serious and potentially life-threatening sequela of rheumatoid arthritis of the cervical spine.

Clinical Characteristics

The history and physical findings include neck pain with occipital and lower cervical

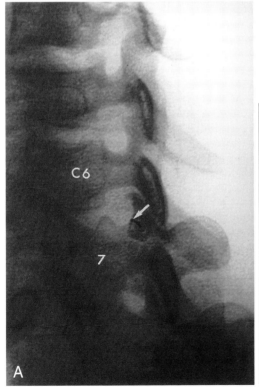
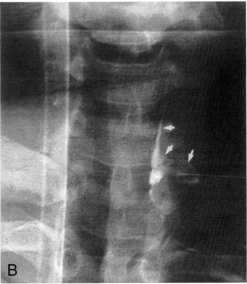

Figure 1.15. Fluoroscopic-guided transforaminal perineural and local epidural Medrol injection at the left C7 level. *A*, oblique view demonstrates needle advancement along the posterior margin of the C6-C7 neural foramen. *B*, AP view of lower cervical spine after the injection of 0.5 mL of nonionic contrast demonstrates central perineural flow with extension into the local epidural space, confirming positioning for therapeutic cortisone injection.

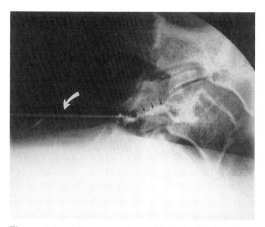

Figure 1.16. Fluoroscopic-guided C3-C4 facet injection using a posterior approach in a patient with symptomatic degenerative facet arthropathy for instillation of local anesthetic and corticosteroids. Needle (curved arrow) extends to the posterior margin of the facet joint, which is opacified by high-density contrast, confirming intra-articular location (arrows).

Surgical treatment must be considered in instances in which the disease has progressed to produce joint instability. There are three basic types of instability: atlantoaxial impaction (platybasia), C-1/C-2 subluxation, and subluxations of the lower cervical vertebrae, which is most common at the C-3/C-4 level. The reported incidence of instability in rheumatoid arthritis ranges from 43 to 86%. These lesions are expected to progress. Lateral cervical spine films in neutral, flexion, and extension are useful for evaluating the degree of instability and platybasia. Initially, cervical bracing is a reasonable treatment. If neurologic signs of cord or root entrapment are present or if there is evidence of instability on x-ray, orthopaedic referral is indicated for possible decompression and/or stabilization. An incidence of neurologic deficits of 7 to

radiculopathy, neck crepitus, variable signs of cervical myelopathy, and generalized signs and symptoms of the disease process. Significant laboratory abnormalities include elevated erythrocyte sedimentation rate and the presence of rheumatoid factors. X-rays (Fig. 1.17 reveal osteopenia, joint space narrowing, soft tissue swelling around involved joints, bone erosions near the capsular attachments of involved joints, and joint malalignment and subluxation.

Treatment

General treatment of C-spine rheumatoid arthritis consists of rest, gentle massage, a soft cervical collar, isometric neck exercises within pain tolerance, and intermittent heat, i.e., 15 minutes three times a day (a hot shower in the morning to "loosen up" is an excellent technique). Medications begin with salicylates. If these do not provide adequate pain control, nonsteroidal anti-inflammatory drugs are used. Diagnostic and therapeutic epidural or facet injections can be useful (Figs. 1.15 and 1.16). Rheumatologic consultation determines the role of further pharmacologic therapy.

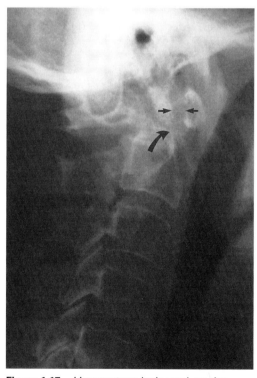

Figure 1.17. Ligamentous laxity and erosive disease in a 71-year-old male with rheumatoid arthritis. There is widening of the atlanto-dens interval (arrows) with areas of erosion to the odontoid (curved arrow).

34% and sudden death of 10% have been reported.

FIBROMYALGIA (MYOFASCIAL PAIN SYNDROME, EXTRA-ARTICULAR RHEUMATISM, FIBROSITIS)

Fibromyalgia affects musculoskeletal tissues other than joints, including muscle, tendon, fascia, bursa, ligament, and synovial sheath. There may be a psychologic overlay.

Clinical Characteristics

These entities present a spectrum of signs and symptoms. A common form is characterized by multiple localized sites of deep tenderness in the trapezius, rhomboids, and levator scapulae. These are considered trigger points. Diffuse aching of more than 3 months duration and sleep disturbances in a patient of less than 50 years of age are characteristic of this disorder. Physical findings include normal C-spine range of motion, normal motor strength, and exquisitely tender "trigger points" in the above-mentioned muscle groups. The EEG is usually abnormal and indicative of sleep disturbance. X-rays are within normal limits.

Treatment

Treatment should include reassurance, psychotherapy, and physical therapy, i.e., intermittent heat, massage, gentle active range of motion exercises, and isometric programs. Vacation or rest is recommended to relieve stress. Medications include amitriptyline, salicylates, nonsteroidal anti-inflammatory drugs, and occasional local injection of trigger points with lidocaine with or without corticosteroids. Addictive drugs should be avoided. Prognosis is poor with chronic relapses.

OSTEOPOROSIS

This generalized disease of bone affects the cervical spine as it does other parts of the axial and appendicular skeleton (see Chapter 14 for full discussion).

THORACIC OUTLET SYNDROME

The thoracic outlet syndrome presents as neck and shoulder pain with radicular or nonradicular referred pain into the upper extremity with variable neurovascular signs and symptoms. It results from compression of the brachial plexus and the subclavian vessels, usually at one of three sites as they pass through the neck and superior thoracic outlet toward the axilla: (a) supraclavicular, (b) costoclavicular, and (c) infraclavicular (Fig. 1.18). These anatomic zones define the three subgroups that comprise the thoracic outlet syndrome.

Essential Anatomy and Pathomechanics

As the plexus descends toward the first rib (Fig. 1.18), it passes through the first zone of potential entrapment (supraclavicular), which is a triangular area bounded by the anterior scalene muscle, the middle scalene muscle, and the first rib. Distally in this zone, the plexus is joined by the subclavian artery and vein from below. This segment of the neurovascular bundle may be compressed by (a) an enlargement of the transverse process of C-7 (cervical rib); (b) a fibrous band that extends from the C-7 transverse process of C-7 to the first rib (pseudocervical rib); (c) degenerative arthritis of the first costovertebral joint; (d) hypertrophy or spasm of the anterior and/or medial scalene muscles; or (e) any process that causes traction on the neurovascular bundle as it crosses the first rib, such as poor posture, kyphosis, muscle weakness, heavy breasts, or obesity.

The second point of potential compression is the costoclavicular area (Fig. 1.18), which involves impingement of the neurovascular bundle as it exits the subclavicular zone and enters a rigid narrow space formed by the clavicle superiorly and the first rib inferiorly. This space may be further narrowed by abnormal configuration of the first rib or clavicle caused by trauma, tumor, or inflammation; elevation of the first rib; or drooping of the shoulder girdle from backpacking or weightlifting.

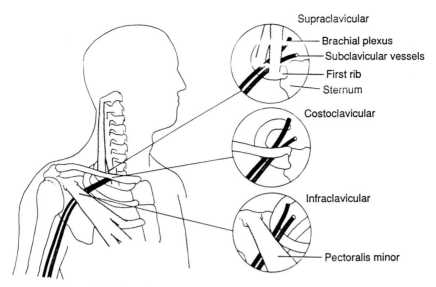

Figure 1.18.   Point of neurovascular compression in the thoracic outlet.

The third point of compression is at the coracoid process (subcoracoid zone) (Fig. 1.18). The neurovascular bundle is trapped between the pectoralis minor and the rib cage, where the bundle is sharply angulated during hyperabduction and extension of the shoulders. Symptoms develop when patients work for prolonged periods with the arms stretched overhead or sleep with the shoulders hyperabducted.

Clinical Characteristics

The essential picture of the thoracic outlet syndrome, whether supraclavicular, costoclavicular, or infraclavicular, is similar since it usually involves compression of the inferior trunk of the brachial plexus, which makes up the ulnar nerve. The pain pattern usually extends from the neck or shoulders into the ulnar aspect of the arm, forearm, and ring and little fingers. Occasionally, it involves the entire hand. Depending on the relative involvement of the neurovascular elements, there is a spectrum of either nonradicular referred pain associated with deep, diffuse, ill-defined aching, heaviness, weakness, burning, edema, discoloration, temperature changes, and painful throbbing of the fingers; or a more defined radicular referred pain pattern with associated specific motor, sensory, and deep tendon reflex aberrations. A positive Adson maneuver (Fig. 1.19) (producing a diminished radial pulse and/or precipitation or aggravation of the patient's symptoms in the involved extremity) is often a useful confirmatory test for the syndrome. X-rays of the neck, chest, and shoulder should be obtained. Other studies may be deferred to the time of referral if symptoms do not respond to treatment.

Differential Diagnosis

The thoracic outlet syndrome must be differentiated from the subclavian steal syndrome, in which blood is diverted from the cerebral circulation, causing CNS neurologic symptoms and signs with the upper extremity symptoms of the thoracic outlet syndrome. Subclavian steal syndrome is not usually precipitated by the Adson maneuver and is differentiated by a subclavian arteriogram (Fig. 1.20), which shows blockage of the subclavian artery proximal to the origin of the vertebral artery.

Other entities to be included in differential diagnosis are cervical disc syndrome, cervical spondylosis, Pancoast tumor, carpal tunnel syndrome, or entrapment of the ulnar nerve at the elbow or wrist. Conditions to be excluded are reflex sympathetic dystrophy, occlusions of the axillary and brachial artery or vein, and brachial neuritis.

Treatment

The first choice in management is a conservative program. Treatment goals for the three types of thoracic outlet syndrome are the same, i.e., increase the space of the thoracic outlet and lessen pressure on the neurovascular elements. The program includes correction of faulty posture and body mechanics; manual stretching to increase mobility of the neck, shoulder girdle, and first and second ribs; and a specific home program. At home, the patient performs deep diaphragmatic breathing for relaxation, cervical-dorsal glide to stretch the neck, and strengthening

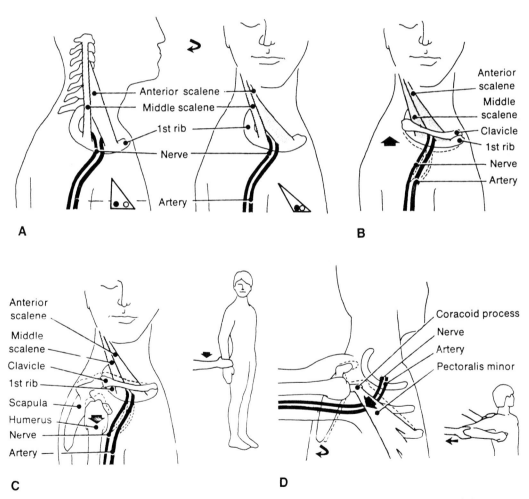

Figure 1.19. Mechanisms of the Adson maneuvers. *A*, rotation of the head and neck toward the affected side compresses the neurovascular structures between the anterior and middle scalene muscles. *B*, a full inspiration elevates the first rib, which thus stretches out the neurovascular structures and also further narrows their passage between the first rib and the middle and anterior scalene muscles. *C*, downward traction on the arm stretches out the neurovascular structures and also narrows their passage between the first rib and the clavicle. *D*, abduction and extension of the shoulder stretches out the neurovascular structures and retracts the scapula, thereby stretching the pectoralis minor tightly over the ribs, narrowing the neurovascular passage between the pectoralis minor and the ribs.

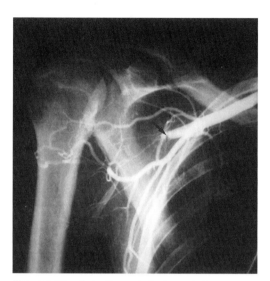

Figure 1.20. Selective subclavian arteriogram centered at the right shoulder in a 29-year-old professional baseball pitcher, demonstrating acute thrombosis of the axillary artery. Abrupt termination is seen at the proximal axillary artery (arrow) related to intimal injury created by repetitive trauma secondary to compression caused by throwing-related thoracic outlet syndrome.

TRAUMATIC CONDITIONS IN ADULTHOOD

CERVICAL SPRAINS AND STRAINS

The exact nature of injury to the cervical spine depends on many variables. The intensity of the injuring force, the degree of protective muscle tone at the time of impact, the underlying strength of the bone and soft tissue, the position of the head and neck at the time of impact, and the presence of a protective support are all significant. Injury may involve the muscular tissue, the anterior and posterior longitudinal ligaments, the capsular ligaments of the facet joints, the intervertebral disc, the bony elements, the cervical nerve roots, and the spinal cord. There also may be injury to the temporomandibular joint, cervical sympathetic chain, and brain stem. Because of the numerous structures potentially involved, the symptoms following cervical injury may be numerous and complex, with an often confusing pattern of localized, referred, and radicular pain.

Most cervical injuries represent a combination of sprain and strain. These injuries are usually the result of hyperflexion and/or hyperextension injuries with or without a rotational component. The injuries are most often sustained in motor vehicle accidents or in sporting activities. The severity of the sprain is determined by a knowledge of the injuring force applied, the severity of symptoms, the physical findings, and careful analysis of x-rays.

Clinical Characteristics

Most patients recall the mechanism of injury, describing it variably as hyperextension, hyperflexion, rotation, or a combination. There may be a history of transient confusion or unconsciousness. Many patients do not note immediate pain, but after several minutes or hours they begin to develop pain and a sense of tightness in the neck. Some patients also complain of nausea.

With mild injuries, initial physical examination usually reveals little in the way of

exercises for the neck and shoulder girdle. The patient also must work to correct faulty sleeping or occupational habits. Patients must avoid slumped positions, round shoulders, and carrying heavy objects in the hands or over the shoulders. Patients must minimize over-head activity and support their arms when sitting. They are instructed to avoid over-exertion. Patients must avoid prone sleeping with the head rotated and extended and shoulders hyperextended or hyperabducted. Having a physical therapist manage the exercise and postural program may be beneficial.

Continuing conservative treatment is reasonable as long as the patient responds. If the signs and symptoms do not improve or if they increase, the patient should be referred to a surgeon for further evaluation and possible surgical intervention. This may involve resecting the constricting structure, e.g., the cervical rib and its fibrous attachments, a portion of the scalenus anterior and medius muscles, or the first rib.

abnormal findings. There may be some tenderness or mild restriction of motion, but often there is no tenderness or significant limitation of motion. After several hours or days, however, findings are usually more significant. Muscle tenderness, swelling, and spasm may develop. The symptom complex may include pain referred to the interscapular area, shoulders, or upper extremities. The patient may sense vague numbness, tingling, or heaviness in a nonradicular pattern, or there may be true radicular numbness and muscle weakness. Headaches, dizziness, and visual disturbances may be noted.

With moderate injuries, radicular pain may develop into one or both extremities. Spinal cord injury produces a myelopathy, and the patient may complain of a deep, aching, ill-defined pain about the shoulder girdle and/or pelvis associated with a feeling of weakness and instability in the lower extremities. Nerve root injury causes a radicular pattern of motor, sensory, and reflex signs and symptoms. Injury to the disc complex may cause local and radicular signs and symptoms.

Diagnostic work-up should include routine x-rays of the cervical spine. Normal static x-rays support the diagnosis of a mild to moderate soft tissue injury without instability. Plain x-rays also rule out fracture or dislocation. It is important to evaluate the plain films carefully. X-ray demonstration of prevertebral soft tissue widening, particularly in the upper cervical spine, indicates significant injury with hemorrhage and edema. The prevertebral space anterior to C-1 in the normal adult should not exceed 10 mm; at the C-2/C-3 level it should not exceed 5 to 7 mm. The relationship between vertebral bodies must also be assessed. Any anterior or posterior translation greater than 3.5 mm indicates potentially significant soft tissue injury and instability. Any angulation between two vertebrae that is 11° greater than the angulation between adjacent vertebrae also indicates possible instability. It is also important to be aware of any sharp reversal in the normal cervical curve. For the patient who has had a significant injury, stress views (flexion, extension, and possibly traction) should be obtained if stability is at all uncertain.

Treatment of the Stable Cervical Sprain-Strain

The patient who has a neurologic deficit or evidence of an unstable cervical spine injury should be referred promptly for orthopaedic evaluation and treatment. Fortunately, most patients do not have an unstable injury. These patients are treated with rest in a position of comfort, which is maintained by a soft cervical collar, for 1 to 2 days. For patients with moderate or severe symptoms, bedrest may be necessary. After 3 to 5 days, pain usually lessens, and by 2 weeks, most patients have improved significantly. The soft cervical collar should be used symptomatically in the initial days after the injury. Subsequently, as symptoms resolve and healing occurs, the patient should be encouraged to wean out of the collar to avoid habitual use. Application of cold packs is usually more effective initially than heat. Cold packs are applied for 15 minutes, four to six times daily for the first 2 days. After this, moist heat may be used if symptomatically helpful. Analgesics and muscle relaxants may be used on a symptomatic basis and are helpful, particularly for nighttime pain and spasm that interfere with sleep.

As symptoms subside and healing occurs, exercises to gently stretch muscles and increase motion are encouraged within the limits of comfort. Early motion of a stable C-spine injury (proved by negative stress films) brings about a better result than prolonged immobilization. Gentle active range of motion and isometric exercises are recommended (Fig. 1.21). Isometric neck exercises are simple to perform and can be done independently. Exercises are first performed in the collar, which limits the range of motion. As long as the patient is pain free, the exercises should be performed for 5 minutes, three times a day. Should pain occur, the duration but not frequency of the exercises should be decreased. A physical therapist may be helpful in guiding the patient.

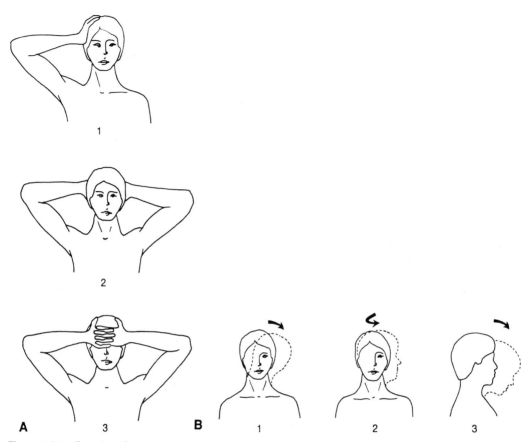

Figure 1.21. Exercises for cervical pain syndromes. *A*, isometric exercises. *1*, press head sideways against the heel of the hand (place the heel of the hand just above the ear), tense, relax, repeat. *2*, clasp hands behind head (over large bony prominence), tense head backward with chin tucked in, relax, repeat. *3*, press forehead against clasped hands, tense muscles without moving head, relax, repeat. *B*, range of motion exercises. Sit in a comfortable chair and take a moment to relax. Shrug shoulders in all directions, both together and alternately, until you relax. Shrug shoulders between exercises if you need to relax more. *1*, tip ear toward shoulder, turn to midposition, relax, tip to opposite side, relax, repeat. *2*, turn head and chin toward shoulder, return to midposition, relax, turn toward opposite shoulder, return to midposition, relax, repeat. *3*, tip head forward, return to erect position, relax, repeat.

After 2 to 3 weeks of gradual mobilization of the neck, the patient is weaned from the collar and the exercise program is expanded appropriately to include isotonic exercises. Once again, care is taken to avoid pain by not overtaxing the healing tissues.

Manipulative treatment is contraindicated in the acute phase of moderate sprain-strains since it may cause additional injury. Cervical halter traction (steady or intermittent) (Fig. 1.13), as described under "Acute Disc Herniation," may assist in mobilizing the spine in patients with stable injuries in the subacute or chronic phase who present with persistent cervical pain, stiffness, tenderness, and muscle atrophy. If traction produces more discomfort, it should be discontinued immediately.

If severe pain persists or symptoms progress after 1 week, the patient should be reevaluated, and repeat x-ray should be considered. If the patient does not improve, orthopaedic referral should be made.

Many patients with stable soft tissue neck injuries recover satisfactorily over a 4- to 6-week period, whereas a significant percentage continue to have varying degrees of symptoms several months or years after injury. As would be expected, patients with more severe symptoms initially, x-ray abnormalities (including degenerative disease and sharp cervical curve reversal), and neurologic involvement have a poorer prognosis.

Treatment of the Unstable Cervical Sprain-Strain

These patients should be promptly placed under the care of an orthopaedic and/or neurosurgeon. The injuries frequently require surgical stabilization or prolonged bracing with a halo brace or halo cast apparatus. In the acute phase, the patient's cervical spine must be immobilized as described earlier in this chapter.

Burner's Syndrome

Burner's syndrome is a variant of the sprain-strain syndrome that occurs in athletes. A ballplayer complains of a transient burning pain in the neck, arm, and possibly hand following an injury that occurs while tackling or blocking an opponent, i.e., when the involved shoulder is depressed and the neck is bent to the opposite side on contact. This may produce injuries to the spinal cord, cervical roots, and supporting tissues of the neck and shoulder, and traction on elements of the brachial plexus. Variable degrees of pain, weakness, paresthesia, and sensory and reflex changes are noted on physical examination. Pain, tenderness, and limited motion of the cervical spine and, occasionally, the shoulder are present. This is treated as a moderate or severe cervical sprain-strain. Further evaluation is necessary to rule out fracture, dislocation, subluxation, and associated injuries to the cervical disc and root complex at the level of injury, and injury to the brachial plexus. The symptoms usually resolve within a few minutes, but the player should not resume play and should be evaluated by an orthopaedic surgeon.

CERVICAL FRACTURE, DISLOCATION, SUBLUXATION

As with soft tissue injury, the mechanisms of injury causing fracture and/or dislocation of the cervical spine include excessive flexion, extension, bending, rotation, compression, and distraction, alone or, more commonly, in some combination. A compressive force may produce a burst or explosion type fracture of the vertebral body, with ruptures of the anterior and/or posterior longitudinal ligaments. Extension forces produce fractures of the posterior bony elements, with disruption of the anterior longitudinal ligament. Flexion injuries disrupt the posterior longitudinal ligament and compress the vertebral bodies; there may be injury to the facet joint capsule and

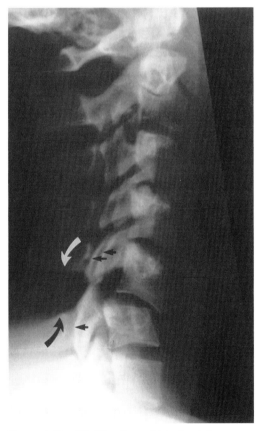

Figure 1.22. C5-C6 unilateral interfacetal malalignment in a 20-year-old male who dove into the shallow end of a swimming pool. There is anterior subluxation at C5-C6, which is approximately 25% of the AP diameter of C5 associated with abrupt kyphosis, anterior subluxation of the facet joints (arrows), and splaying of the spinous processes (curved arrows). Rotation is indicated by the abrupt loss of overlap of the lateral masses comparing C5 with C6 (short arrows).

intervertebral disc. Rotational injuries cause disruption of the ligaments, with fracture or dislocation of the facet joints. The vertebral body also may be injured. Injuries that are the result of a combination of forces tend to be more severe and more unstable.

The classification of a fracture-dislocation as stable or unstable is not always a simple judgement; however, the three-segment concept is helpful. As described previously (Fig. 1.10), if two of the three segments of the spine are disrupted, the fracture-dislocation is considered unstable. An unstable injury cannot withstand normal physiologic forces without abnormal deformity, and jeopardizes the underlying spinal cord and/or nerve roots. Such instability may be acute or chronic as a result of late bony deformity. It must also be noted that in the cervical spine, cord injury has been documented in the presence of what appears to be a stable fracture.

Whenever a fracture-dislocation of the cervical spine is noted, the primary care physician's role is to stabilize the spine until orthopaedic and/or neurosurgical care can be instituted. In addition, initial treatment of a patient with a documented spinal cord injury should include the administration of high-dose methylprednisolone. Recent studies indicate that a dose of methylprednisolone, 30 mg/kg of body weight, administered within 8 hours of injury has a positive effect on neurologic recovery. After this initial bolus, a dose of methylprednisolone, 5.4 mg/kg of body weight per hour, should be administered for 23 hours.

Following is a brief description of the common fractures and dislocations of the cervical spine.

Fractures of C-1 (atlas) are caused by axial loading that compresses and explodes the atlas; they are usually not associated with cord

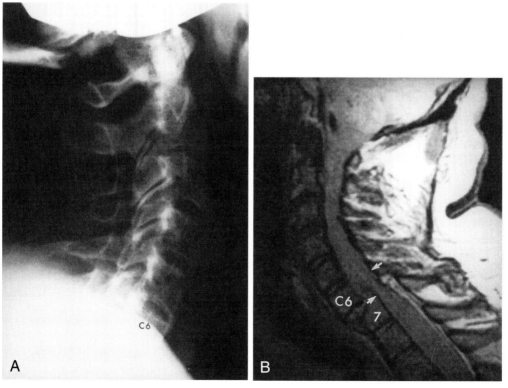

Figure 1.23.   Fracture-dislocation at C6-C7 in a 39-year-old male involved in a motor vehicle accident. *A,* initial portable lateral that was interpreted as unremarkable is inadequate since visualization is seen only to the mid C6 level. *B,* sagittal MR proton density scan (TR 2000, TE 30) through the cervical spine demonstrates gross disruption at C6-C7 with marked encroachment upon the neural canal (arrows).

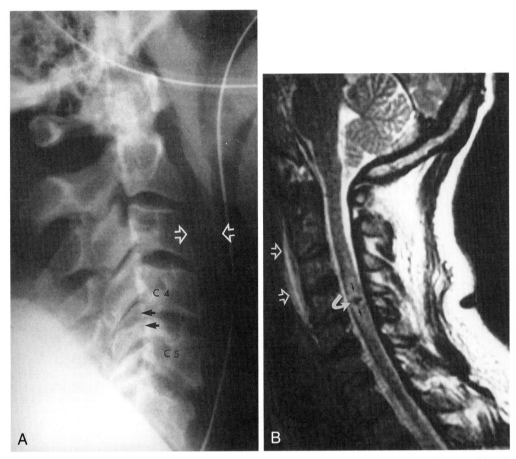

Figure 1.24. Hyperextension ligamentous injury with hemorrhagic cord contusion in a 39-year-old male involved in a motor vehicle accident. *A*, lateral view of the cervical spine shows subtle retrolisthesis at C4-C5 (solid arrow). *B*, sagittal MR T2-weighted (TR 2100, TE 112) shows bulbus enlargement of the cervical cord, centered at C4-C5, related to a broad area of cervical contusion manifested as high signal (white arrows). Focal area of low signal (curved arrow) indicates subacute hemorrhage and qualifies the cord contusion as a hemorrhagic contusion, which has a more ominous prognosis. Associated prevertebral hematoma shows high signal (open arrows).

injuries. However, they are unstable and should be treated initially with a rigid neck brace. A neurosurgeon or orthopaedic surgeon should be consulted. Definitive treatment is usually with a halo jacket or halo vest for at least 8 weeks, followed by a cervical orthosis.

C-2 fractures usually involve fracture of the odontoid. The success rate for healing depends on the degree of displacement, the age of the patient, and the location of the fracture. Most of these injuries are treated with a halo body jacket, although some injuries with a poor prognosis should be stabilized immedi-

ately. Fractures associated with spinal cord injury at this level are often fatal.

In addition to fractures through the odontoid, C-2 fractures also may be through the pedicles. This is the so-called "hangman's" fracture. These injuries usually unite well when treated with a halo brace.

Fractures of C-3 through C-7 may involve all possible combinations of forces. One of the most severe is the injury caused by combined axial compression force with flexion. This is the common diving accident where the head strikes a solid object. This produces a comminuted fracture of the vertebral body with retropulsion into the spinal canal and injury to the cord. Many of these patients need surgical stabilization.

The common dislocations of the cervical spine usually occur between C-3 and C-7 (Fig. 1.22). These involve unilateral or bilateral facet dislocations. The injury is indicated on the lateral cervical spine x-ray by varying degrees of displacement of the superior vertebra anteriorly on the adjoining inferior vertebra. In unilateral facet dislocation, there is approximately a 25% anterior listhesis of the superior on inferior vertebra. In bilateral dislocation, this is usually in the 50% range. In addition to the listhesis, careful review of the x-ray shows the abnormal relationship of the facet joints (Fig. 1.23). An MRI is useful to define cord injury (Fig. 1.24).

Occipital/C-1 dislocations are rare and almost always fatal. If the patient does not die as a result of his injury, halo immobilization is indicated, followed by surgical stabilization.

C-1/C-2 dislocations or subluxations may occur with or without odontoid fracture. One type of C-1/C-2 dislocation is the "adult rotatory subluxation of the atlantoaxial joint," which presents with the same characteristics as the childhood variant but is related to significant injury. This injury occurs when a rotational force is applied to the head, causing the inferior facet of C-1 to slip forward on the superior facet of C-2. If the articulation becomes fixed in this position, there is marked limitation of motion, and a painful post-traumatic torticollis develops. Neurologic deficits often occur. X-rays demonstrate an asymmetry in the position of the odontoid. The odontoid is deviated to one side and remains deviated (i.e., fixed subluxation), even with rotation of the head and repeat x-ray. CT scan is helpful in evaluating this.

INJURY TO THE CERVICAL DISC

Acute cervical disc injuries occur in decreasing frequency between units C-5/C-6, C-6/C-7, and C-7/T-1 (Fig. 1.1). Injury to the disc–annular ligament–posterior ligament complex may result in protrusion or hernia-

tion of the nucleus pulposus, with subsequent radicular pain patterns, depending on the level of injury. Mechanisms of injury are similar to those producing fracture, dislocation, or subluxation. Clinical features and treatment are described in the section "Acute Disc Herniation."

SUGGESTED READINGS

Anderson JE. Grant's Atlas of Anatomy. 8th ed. Baltimore: Williams and Wilkins, 1983.

Bracken MB, Shepard MJ, Collins WF, et al. A randomized, controlled trial of methylprednisolone or naloxone in the treatment of acute spinal-cord injury. N Engl J Med 1990;322(20):1405–1411.

Bracken MB, Shepard MJ, Holford TR, et al. Administration of methylprednisolone for 24 or 48 hours or tirilazad mesylate for 48 hours in the treatment of acute spinal cord injury. Results of the Third National Acute Spinal Cord Injury Randomized Controlled Trial. JAMA 1997; 277:1597–1604.

Cervical Spine Research Society Editorial Committee. The Cervical Spine. 2nd ed. Philadelphia: JB Lippincott Co., 1989.

Committee on Trauma. Advanced Trauma Life Support Course Instructor Manual. Chicago: American College of Surgeons, 1990.

Daffner RH, ed. Imaging of Vertebral Trauma. Rockville, MD: Aspen Publishers, 1988.

Edmonson AS. Spinal anatomy and surgical approaches. In: Crenshaw AH, ed. Campbell's Operative Orthopaedics. 8th ed. St. Louis: Mosby Yearbook, 1991.

Evarts C McC, Mayer PJ. Complications. In: Rockwood CA Jr, Green DP, Bucholz RW, eds. Fractures in adults. 3rd ed. Philadelphia: JB Lippincott Co., 1991.

Freeman BL III. Fractures, dislocations, and fracture-dislocations of spine. In: Crenshaw AH, ed. Campbell's Operative Orthopaedics. 8th ed. St. Louis: The Mosby Yearbook, 1991.

Grant JCB, Basmajian JV. Grant's Method of Anatomy by Regions, Descriptive and Deductive. 8th ed. Baltimore: Williams and Wilkins, 1971.

Harris JH Jr, Mirvis SE, eds. The radiology of acute cervical spine trauma. 3rd ed. Baltimore: Williams and Wilkins, 1996.

Hollinshead WH. Anatomy for Surgeons, Vol 3: The Back and Limbs. 2nd ed. New York: Harper and Row, 1969.

Hoppenfeld S. Physical Examination of the Spine and Extremities. Norwalk, CT: Appleton-Century-Crofts, 1976:105–132.

Iverson LD, Swiontkowski MF. Manual of Acute Orthopaedic Therapeutics. 4th ed. Boston: Little, Brown and Co., 1994.

Keats TE. Atlas of Normal Roentgen Variants That May Simulate Disease. 6th ed. St. Louis: Mosby, 1996.

Novelline RA, ed. Squire's Fundamentals of Radiology. 5th ed. Cambridge, MA: Harvard University Press, 1997.

Pappas AM. Muscles, joints, and ligaments. In: Southmayd W, Hoffman M. Sports Health: The Complete Book of Athletic Injuries. New York: Quick Fox, 1981:70–85.

Rodnan GP, Schumacher R, Zvaifler NJ, eds. Rheumatoid arthritis. In: Primer on the Rheumatic Diseases. 8th ed. Atlanta, GA: Arthritis Foundation, 1983:38–48.

Salter RB. Textbook of Disorders and Injuries of the Musculoskeletal System: An Introduction to Orthopaedics, Fractures and Joint Injuries, Rheumatology, Metabolic Bone Disease and Rehabilitation. 2nd ed. Baltimore: Williams and Wilkins, 1983.

Sculco TP. Neck pain. In: Beary JF III, Christian CL, Johanson NA, eds. Manual of Rheumatology and Outpatient Orthopedic Disorders: Diagnosis and Therapy. 2nd ed. Boston: Little, Brown and Co., 1987:77–80.

Simeone FA, Rothman RH. Cervical disc disease. In: Rothman RH, Simeone FA, eds. The Spine. 2nd ed. Philadelphia: WB Saunders Co., 1982:440–499.

Stauffer ES. Fractures and dislocations of the spine. Part I: the cervical spine. In: Rockwood CA Jr, Green DP, Bucholz RW, eds. Fractures in Adults. 3rd ed. Philadelphia: JB Lippincott Co., 1991.

Wood GW. Infections of spine. In: Crenshaw AH, ed. Campbell's Operative Orthopaedics. 8th ed. St. Louis: Mosby Yearbook, 1991.

Wood GW. Other disorders of spine. In: Crenshaw AH, ed. Campbell's Operative Orthopaedics. 8th ed. St. Louis: Mosby Yearbook, 1991.

Shoulder and Upper Arm

Thomas P. Goss, M.D.

ESSENTIAL ANATOMY

The shoulder is a complex comprised of three bones (the clavicle, the scapula, and the proximal humerus) and four articulations (the glenohumeral joint, the acromioclavicular joint, the sternoclavicular joint, and the scapulothoracic articulation). The shoulder is designed for maximal mobility, allowing the hand to be placed in the wide variety of positions necessary for optimal upper extremity function.

GLENOHUMERAL JOINT

The glenohumeral joint can be thought of as a "soft tissue articulation," since bony restraint is minimal. Only one-fourth of the articular surface of the proximal humerus is in contact with the small, shallow glenoid at any one time. The surrounding soft tissues must fulfill the somewhat contradictory roles of providing stability while allowing considerable mobility. The glenohumeral joint is the most mobile articulation in the body and also the one most prone to symptomatic instability when the peri-articular soft tissues are damaged. The glenohumeral joint is also a "distractive articulation," as opposed to the "compressive joints" of the lower extremities. This makes the glenohumeral joint much less prone to degenerative joint disease. The joint space is defined by the synovial membrane and the fibrous capsule, which are attached to the bony glenoid via the glenoid labrum, a fibrocartilaginous structure that surrounds its periphery. Ligamentous restraint is minimal posteriorly; however, the glenohumeral joint is stabilized by the superior, middle, and inferior glenohumeral ligaments anteriorly.

One layer more superficial is the musculotendinous (rotator) cuff. (The deltoid muscle and the rotator cuff are the most important and second most important dynamic structures in the shoulder complex, respectively.) The rotator cuff is the confluence of the tendons of four muscles: the subscapularis (upper and lower subscapular nerves), the supraspinatus (suprascapular nerve), the infraspinatus (suprascapular nerve), and the teres minor (axillary nerve). The supraspinatus, infraspinatus, and teres minor muscles arise over the dorsal aspect of the scapula and insert on the greater tuberosity of the proximal humerus. The subscapularis muscle arises over the ventral aspect of the scapula and inserts on the lesser tuberosity of the proximal humerus (Fig. 2.1). The rotator cuff has four functions: (*a*) it serves as a soft tissue "shock absorber" between the superior aspect of the proximal humerus and the undersurface of the acromion; (*b*) it lends passive stability to the glenohumeral joint; (*c*) it allows each of the four muscles to perform its own particular dynamic function(s); and (*d*) it firmly seats the humeral head within the glenoid cavity so that stronger, more superficial muscles such as the deltoid can optimally move the arm. The blood supply for the articular segment of the proximal humerus comes from branches of the circumflex humeral vessels that enter via the greater and lesser tuberosities.

Between the tuberosities is the bicipital groove, which contains the long head of the biceps tendon as it passes from its origin at the superior margin of the glenoid to its junction with the short head to form the belly of the biceps muscle (musculocutaneous nerve). The short head of the biceps tendon originates

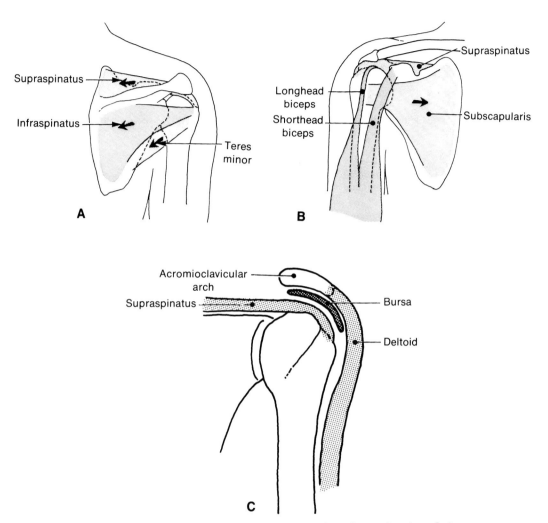

Figure 2.1. *A* and *B*, the musculotendinous cuff. *A*, posterior view; *B*, anterior view. *C*, the acromioclavicular arch and the subacromial bursa.

at the tip of the coracoid process (Fig. 2.1). The coracoid process is also the origin of the coracobrachialis muscle (musculocutaneous nerve), which lies over the anteromedial aspect of the upper arm, deep to the biceps. Posterior to the glenohumeral joint is the teres major muscle (lower subscapular nerve), which originates over the inferior angle of the scapula and inserts on the anterior aspect of the proximal humerus. The long head of the triceps muscle originates along the inferior aspect of the glenoid and joins the lateral and medial heads distally to form the belly of the triceps muscle (radial nerve).

The acromial process of the scapula is a bony arch that overhangs the proximal humerus. The subacromial bursa lies between the bony acromion and the rotator cuff (Fig. 2.1). The coracoacromial ligament runs from the coracoid process to the anterior margin of the acromion.

The deltoid muscle (axillary nerve) lies just beneath the skin and subcutaneous tissue. It arises over the distal third of the clavicle (anterior deltoid), the acromion (middle deltoid), and the spine of the scapula (posterior deltoid) and inserts along the lateral aspect of the humeral shaft. Finally, within the axilla medial

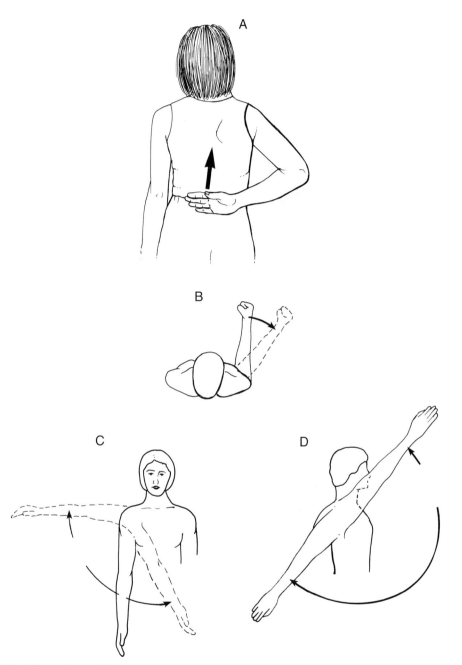

Figure 2.2. The motions of the glenohumeral joint and the positions of the arm at the glenohumeral joint. *A*, internal rotation up the back. *B*, external rotation. *C*, abduction-adduction. *D*, forward flexion-extension.

to the glenohumeral joint lie the brachial plexus and axillary vessels.

The arcs of motion of the glenohumeral joint are shown in Figure 2.2. The prime muscles that control these movements are the following: forward flexion—anterior deltoid, pectoralis major; abduction—middle deltoid, supraspinatus; adduction—pectoralis major, latissimus dorsi, teres major; extension—latissimus dorsi, posterior deltoid; internal rotation—subscapularis; external rotation—infraspinatus, teres minor. As bipedal animals, we clearly benefit from this "global range of motion."

SCAPULOTHORACIC ARTICULATION

The scapulothoracic articulation is not a true joint. Considerable movement, however, is provided to the shoulder complex as the scapula glides over the posterior rib cage.

The scapula is a thin, triangular-shaped bone with three processes: the spine of the scapula arises over its dorsal aspect and extends laterally to become the acromial process; the glenoid process serves as the socket for the glenohumeral joint; and the coracoid process protrudes anteriorly and provides a point of attachment for a variety of musculotendinous and ligamentous structures. Stability depends on the soft tissues that surround the scapula and the clavicle. The clavicle (via the acromioclavicular joint laterally and the sternoclavicular joint medially) is the only bony connection between the shoulder complex/upper extremity and the axial skeleton. Posteriorly, the levator scapulae (deep branches of the cervical plexus), the rhomboideus minor (dorsal scapular nerve), and the rhomboideus major (dorsal scapular nerve) muscles originate over the cervical and thoracic vertebrae and insert onto the upper, middle, and inferior thirds of the medial margin of the scapula, respectively. The serratus anterior muscle (long thoracic nerve) originates over the anterior aspect of the upper 8th-9th ribs and inserts on the inferior angle of the scapula. More superficially, the trapezius muscle (spinal accessory nerve and several cervical nerves) arises from the

spinous processes of the cervical and thoracic vertebrae, and inserts on the spine and acromial process of the scapula. The latissimus dorsi muscle (thoracodorsal nerve) arises from the lower half of the vertebral spine and iliac crest, and inserts on the anterior aspect of the upper third of the humeral shaft. Anteriorly, the scapula is controlled by the pectoralis major (medial and lateral pectoral nerves) and pectoralis minor (medial pectoral nerve) muscles, which originate over the anterior thoracic cage and insert on the proximal humeral shaft and coracoid process, respectively. The six scapular movements and their prime controllers are illustrated in Figure 2.3.

ACROMIOCLAVICULAR JOINT (FIG. 2.4)

The lateral end of the clavicle articulates with the acromial process of the scapula to form the acromioclavicular (AC) joint. Its capsule is reinforced by the superior and inferior acromioclavicular ligaments, and a fibrocartilaginous disc is contained within the articulation. Additional stability is provided by the coracoclavicular ligaments, which run from the coracoid process of the scapula to the undersurface of the distal clavicle.

STERNOCLAVICULAR JOINT (FIG. 2.5)

The medial end of the clavicle articulates with the sternum to form the sternoclavicular (SC) joint. Its capsule is reinforced by the anterior and posterior sternoclavicular ligaments, and a fibrocartilaginous disc lies within the articulation. Additional stability is provided by the costoclavicular ligament, which runs from the medial end of the clavicle to the first rib.

Scapulothoracic movement is accompanied by corresponding movement through the AC and SC joints.

UPPER ARM

The structural scaffolding of the upper arm is the humeral shaft. The biceps, coracobrachialis, and brachialis (musculocutaneous nerve) muscles reside within the anterior portion of

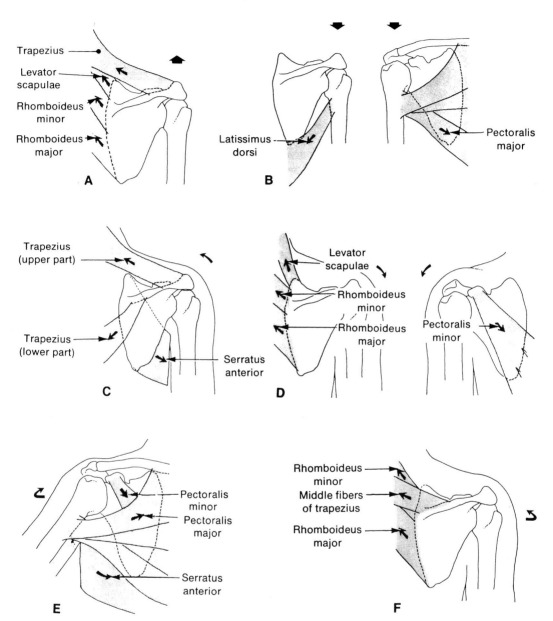

Figure 2.3. The motions of the scapulothoracic joint and their controlling muscles. *A,* elevation, posterior view. *B,* depression; *left,* posterior view; *right,* anterior view. *C,* upward rotation, posterior view. *D,* downward rotation; *left,* posterior view; *right,* anterior view. *E,* protraction, anterior view. *F,* retraction, posterior view.

the upper arm, while the triceps muscle lies posteriorly. The coracobrachialis muscle inserts, while the brachialis muscle originates over the anterior portion of the humerus. The medial and lateral heads of the triceps muscle originate along the posterior aspect of the humeral shaft (Fig. 2.6). The deltoid muscle inserts over the lateral aspect of the upper third of the humerus (Fig. 2.7).

The radial nerve enters the upper arm via the axilla, posterior to the humerus, and then spirals distally (medially to laterally), adjacent to the shaft of the humerus and deep to the medial and lateral heads of the triceps muscle, which it innervates. The nerve is especially vulnerable to injury at two points: (*a*) as it curves around the midshaft of the humerus posterolaterally and (*b*) as it enters the forearm between the brachioradialis and biceps muscles. The ulnar nerve courses posterior to the brachial artery along the medial aspect of the upper arm. Proximally, the ulnar nerve lies within the anterior compartment. At the middle third of the upper arm, it pierces the medial intermuscular septum to enter the posterior compartment. The median nerve runs anterior to the brachial artery along the medial aspect of the upper arm. The musculocutaneous nerve lies between the biceps and brachialis muscles and innervates the biceps, brachialis, and coracobrachialis muscles. The axillary nerve curves around the upper arm (posteromedially to anterolaterally) along the undersurface of the deltoid muscle, which it innervates. The brachial artery courses with the median and ulnar nerves along the medial

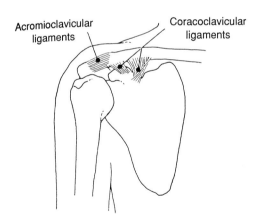

Figure 2.4.   The acromioclavicular joint and its ligaments.

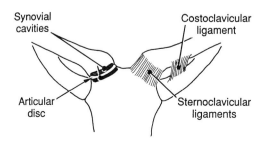

Figure 2.5.   The sternoclavicular joint: its synovial cavities, disc, and ligaments.

aspect of the upper arm, separated from the humerus by the brachialis and the medial head of the triceps muscles.

EVALUATION OF THE PATIENT WITH SHOULDER SYMPTOMS

The shoulder region and upper arm are susceptible to a wide variety of disorders, both traumatic and nontraumatic. In evaluating the individual with symptoms in these areas, the initial step is to obtain a good history. Questions should first be general. The second group of questions is directed toward specific clinical entities suggested by the patient's responses to the general questions.

The second step is the physical examination. This should begin with a gross visual inspection of the shoulder and/or upper arm from all aspects, looking for deformities, asymmetry, discoloration, and muscle atrophy. The region is then palpated for masses, defects, deformities, and areas of tenderness. One should be familiar with the surface anatomy as well as palpable anatomic landmarks: the coracoid process, the biceps tendon, the impingement interval, the SC joint, the AC joint, the trapezius and deltoid muscles, the supraspinatus and infraspinatus fossae, the clavicle, the spine of the scapula, the scapular body, the greater tuberosity, the acromial process, the humeral shaft, and the biceps and triceps muscles. The examiner should then put the shoulder through a gentle passive circular range of motion, followed by having the patient perform the same maneuver actively. The patient is asked to localize any pain that is elicited. The examiner notes any restriction of motion and keeps one hand on the shoulder, feeling for associated fine crepitus (highly suggestive of an underlying full thickness rotator cuff tear). The shoulder is then put through a full passive and active range of motion (forward flexion, abduction, adduction, extension, internal rotation up the back, and external rotation). The examiner notes any associated fine crepitus and its general location; any associated pain, its location, and the position of the shoulder when it occurs; any asymmetry of glenohumeral-scapulothoracic motion; and

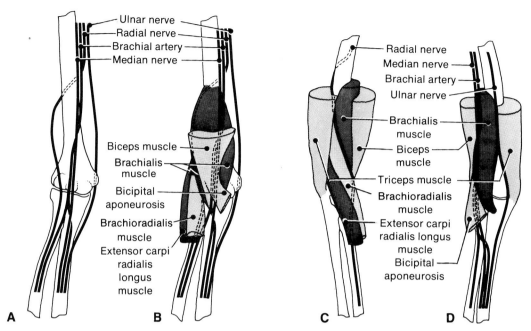

Figure 2.6.   Relationships of the muscles and neurovascular structures in the upper arm. *A*, anterior view, neurovascular structures alone. *B*, anterior view with muscles added. *C*, lateral view. *D*, medial view.

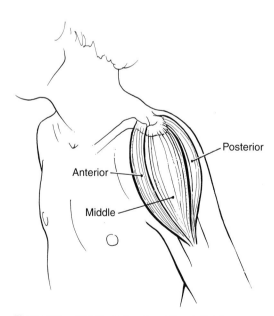

Figure 2.7.   The three heads of the deltoid muscle and their insertion over the lateral aspect of the humeral shaft: anterior deltoid (forward flexor), middle deltoid (abductor), posterior deltoid (extensor).

any loss/restriction of motion. Decreased passive range of motion may be caused by pain or a mechanical block; loss of active motion when passive movement is normal suggests neuromuscular pathology.

A basic neurovascular evaluation should be included. One should test the active function of the musculature about the shoulder and upper arm, including the trapezius, rhomboids, serratus anterior, deltoid, biceps, triceps, and rotator cuff. Median, ulnar, musculocutaneous, and radial nerve function should be evaluated. Distal pulses should be palpated to determine both their presence and symmetry. If glenohumeral instability is suggested by the patient's history, apprehension and stress testing should be performed (Fig. 2.8). If degenerative disease of the AC joint is suspected, the arm is brought across the chest and the articulation manually compressed to see if pain is elicited (Fig. 2.9).

A brief examination of the cervical spine and ipsilateral elbow, forearm, wrist, and hand should also be performed to make sure that "shoulder/upper arm symptoms" are not originating from these areas. Finally,

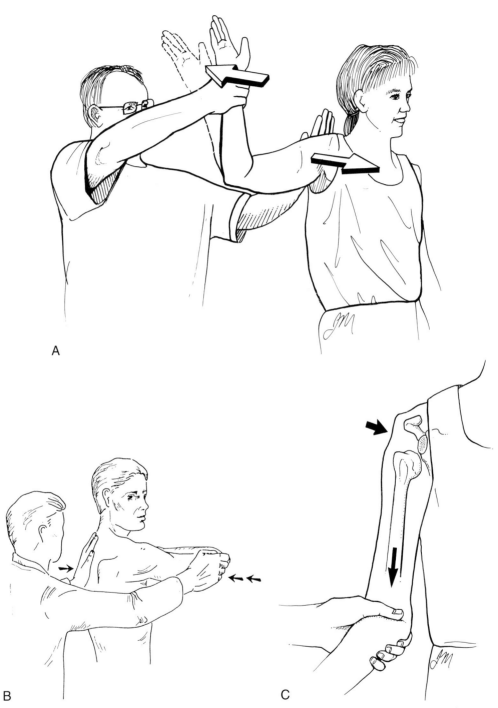

Figure 2.8.   Stress testing of the glenohumeral joint to detect instability. *A*, anterior stress testing. *B*, posterior stress testing. *C*, inferior stress testing.

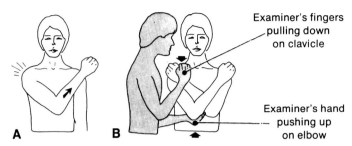

Examiner's fingers pulling down on clavicle

Examiner's hand pushing up on elbow

Figure 2.9. Tests for acromioclavicular pain. *A*, cross-chest maneuver designed to compress the AC joint. *B*, technique used to stress the AC joint in the vertical plane.

one should remember that "shoulder/upper arm symptoms" can be referred from the respiratory, cardiovascular, and gastrointestinal systems.

The third step in evaluating the patient is the radiologic examination. The basic shoulder series includes true anteroposterior (AP) (with the arm in neutral rotation) and axillary views of the glenohumeral joint. Figure 2.10 demonstrates these projections with accompanying line drawings showing the major bony landmarks. One must be familiar with the normal appearance of each projection to recognize the presence of an abnormality. One must also be able to mentally convert each two-dimensional x-ray into a three-dimensional anatomic region. Supplementary radiographs include the tangential or lateral scapular view (Fig. 2.10), the transthoracic lateral view, and AP projections of the shoulder with the arm in internal and external rotation. If one is concerned about the integrity of the linkage between the clavicle and scapula via the coracoclavicular ligaments and the AC joint, an AP view of the shoulder with weights hung from the patient's wrists should be obtained (Fig. 2.11). The radiologic evaluation of the upper arm consists simply of AP and lateral projections. Other and more sophisticated diagnostic studies are available if warranted by the specific clinical situation.

SHOULDER PHYSIOTHERAPY AND REHABILITATION

For any shoulder disorder, whether traumatic or nontraumatic, maintaining and re-

gaining range of motion, flexibility, and strength are critical to achieving a successful functional result. Consequently, physiotherapy and rehabilitation are extremely important. The specifics of the program vary with the nature of the disorder. There are, however, a few basic principles that should be observed, and a general program can be outlined.

BASIC PRINCIPLES

One works for shoulder range of motion, flexibility, and strength in six directions: forward flexion (most important), abduction, adduction, extension, internal rotation up the back (most important), and external rotation (most important). Multiple short exercise sessions are more productive than a few lengthy sessions and are less likely to irritate, damage, or overtax the peri-articular soft tissues. Each exercise session should be preceded by local application of moist heat, followed by local application of ice. Range of motion and strengthening exercises are performed initially with the patient lying supine (gravity-assisted). Then the patient is gradually advanced to standing techniques (against gravity) as symptoms and strength allow. The patient should strive for gentle, relaxed motion without excessive pain, and should not overdo. Exercises causing lingering pain are temporarily omitted. Formal sessions with the therapist become less frequent as the patient demonstrates knowledge of his or her program. With steady progress, the therapist's role changes from a "doer" to an instructor.

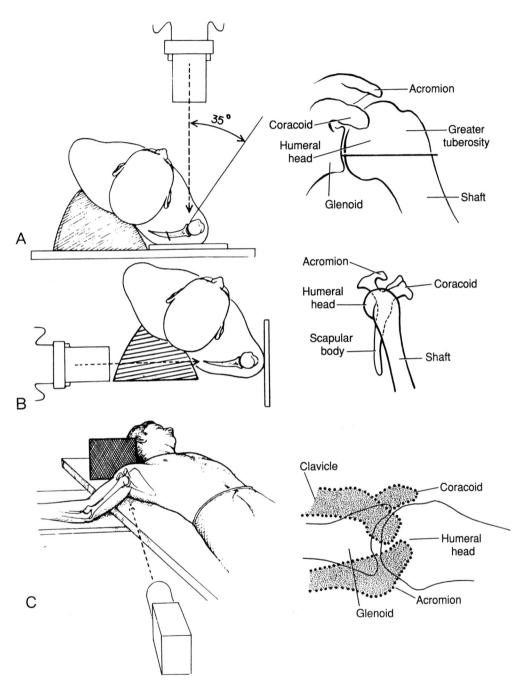

Figure 2.10. Standard radiologic views of the glenohumeral joint. *A,* true AP view of the glenohumeral joint with the arm in neutral rotation. (Reprinted with permission from Rockwood CA, Green DP, eds. Fractures; vol. 1. 2nd ed. Philadelphia: JB Lippincott Company, 1984:679,821.) *B,* true lateral projection of the glenohumeral joint. (Reprinted with permission from Rockwood CA, Green DP, eds. Fractures; vol. 1. 2nd ed. Philadelphia: JB Lippincott Company, 1984:679.) *C,* true axillary view of the glenohumeral joint. (Reprinted with permission from Neer CS. Displaced proximal humeral fractures: I. classification and evaluation. J Bone Joint Surg [Am] 1970;52A:1077–1089.)

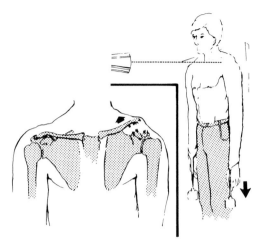

Figure 2.11. Technique for obtaining stress films of the acromioclavicular joint (used to detect injury to the acromioclavicular and coracoclavicular ligaments). (Reprinted with permission from Rockwood CA, Green DP, eds. Fractures; vol. 1. 2nd ed. Philadelphia: JB Lippincott Company, 1984:877.)

GENERAL PROGRAM (FIG. 2.12)

The shoulder should be immobilized until judged sufficiently stable or healed to begin physiotherapy. The simplest exercise consists of dependent circular and pendulum range of motion techniques. When healing is sufficient, the patient begins progressive passive/active assistive exercises to maintain or regain range of motion and flexibility (in all directions but especially forward flexion, internal rotation up the back, and external rotation). When healing, range of motion, and flexibility are satisfactory, the patient can begin active exercises to maintain or regain strength. When healing, range of motion, flexibility, and strength are satisfactory, aggressive stretching and strengthening techniques are prescribed if deficiencies exist. As range of motion, flexibility, and strength improve, the functional capabilities of the shoulder increase accordingly. The patient should continue his or her rehabilitation program until range of motion, flexibility, and strength are maximized.

NONTRAUMATIC DISORDERS

GLENOHUMERAL JOINT DISEASE

Degenerative disease of the glenohumeral joint can occur as the result of a number of different processes, including primary osteo-

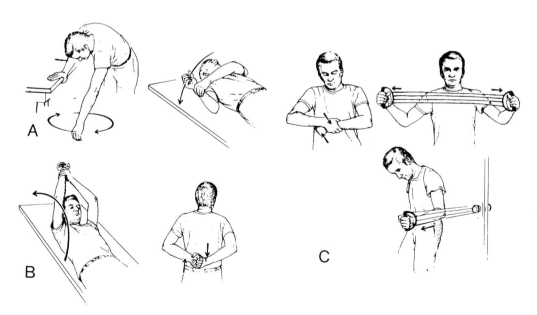

Figure 2.12. Shoulder physiotherapy and rehabilitation. *A*, dependent circular range of motion exercises. *B*, active-assistive range of motion exercises for forward flexion, internal rotation up the back, and external rotation. *C*, active strengthening exercises. (Reprinted with permission from Rockwood CA, Green DP, eds. Fractures; vol. 1. 1st ed. Philadelphia: JB Lippincott Company,1975:595)

arthritis, posttraumatic degenerative joint disease, posttraumatic and nontraumatic avascular necrosis, a variety of inflammatory arthritides including rheumatoid arthritis, and others (Chapter 12). The humeral articular surface, the glenoid articular surface, or both may be involved. Clinical characteristics include the following: shoulder pain (particularly posteriorly) that is worse with motion; palpable "hard" crepitus on gentle range of motion; restriction of glenohumeral movement secondary to pain or mechanical block; and radiologic evidence of degenerative joint disease, including subchondral cysts, sclerosis, joint space narrowing, marginal osteophytes, and irregularity of the articular surfaces.

If disruption of the humeral articular surface is present, but the glenohumeral joint space and glenoid appear relatively normal, referral to an orthopaedist is indicated for consideration of a prosthetic replacement of the humeral articular segment. In addition to alleviating the patient's symptoms, the prosthetic replacement protects the glenoid articular surface from secondary damage and avoids a later total shoulder replacement. If both sides of the articulation are involved, a trial of nonoperative treatment is recommended. This consists of avoidance of aggravating positions and activities, rest, application of moist heat, nonsteroidal anti-inflammatory medications, and analgesics. Intra-articular steroid injections may be helpful. Should pain or disability become unacceptable, referral to an orthopaedist is indicated for consideration of a shoulder arthroplasty, or in some cases, a shoulder arthrodesis.

DEGENERATIVE DISEASE OF THE AC AND SC JOINTS

Degenerative disease of the AC and SC articulations may be caused by a variety of processes, including primary osteoarthritis, rheumatoid disease, posttraumatic degenerative joint disease, and others. Clinical characteristics include the following: discomfort localized to the AC or SC articulation, worsened by shoulder movement and palpation; crepitus over the affected articulation on range of mo-

tion; localized swelling; and palpable marginal irregularity (the cross-chest maneuver will generally cause increased AC joint discomfort) (Fig. 2.9). The radiologic examination may show subchondral sclerosis or cyst formation, narrowing of the joint space, marginal osteophytes, and irregularity of the articular surfaces.

Initial treatment is nonoperative and includes avoidance of aggravating positions and activities, moist heat, and analgesic medications for discomfort. Anti-inflammatory medications and intra-articular steroid injections may be helpful. If nonoperative treatment is ineffective, referral to an orthopaedist is indicated for consideration of surgical resection of the clavicular portion of the affected articulation.

CHRONIC INSTABILITY OF THE GLENOHUMERAL JOINT

Chronic instability of the glenohumeral joint presents the greatest diagnostic and therapeutic challenge of any of the disorders that affect the shoulder region. The three types of chronic instability are dislocation, subluxation, and functional instability (Fig. 2.13). Dislocation is an instability in which an applied force causes the apex of the humeral head circumference to move beyond the rim of the glenoid cavity. Subluxation is an instability in which an applied force causes the humeral head to move excessively relative to the glenoid but is short of an actual dislocation. Functional instability refers to situations in which a piece of tissue (a displaced labral fragment, a loose osseous body, a loose cartilaginous body, etc.) becomes intermittently interposed between the glenohumeral articular surfaces, causing the shoulder to catch, slip, or lock (symptoms similar to that of a torn knee meniscus). In addition, one must determine whether the articulation is unstable anteriorly, posteriorly, inferiorly, or in multiple directions (Fig. 2.14).

Chronic (Recurrent) Dislocation

Characteristic clinical features include the following. The patient usually remembers a clear initiating event followed by multiple

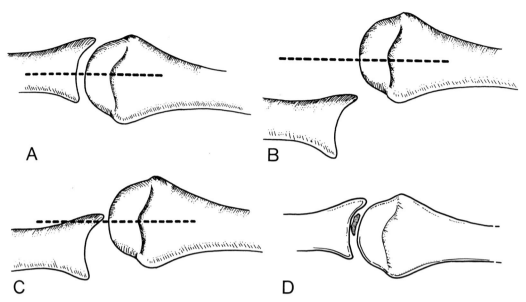

Figure 2.13. Types of chronic glenohumeral instability. *A*, normal relationship. *B*, dislocation (note the apex of the humeral head circumference moves beyond the rim of the glenoid fossa). *C*, subluxation (note the apex of the humeral head circumference moves out to, but not beyond, the rim of the glenoid fossa). (*B* and *C* from Goss TP. Factors to consider in chronic symptomatic shoulder instability. Orthop Rev 1985;XIV(10):27–32. *D*, functional instability (note the fragment of tissue interposed between the glenohumeral articulating surfaces).

recurrences. When the shoulder dislocates, the patient feels that the humeral head is "caught out of joint" for a variable period, and the patient or someone else must manipulate the shoulder back into place. Each recurrence requires less trauma and each relocation becomes easier. The patient can often relate the dislocation to a specific position of the arm: extension-abduction above the horizontal-external rotation for anterior instability and forward flexion-adduction-internal rotation for posterior instability. Apprehension and stress testing in the direction of instability are generally positive. X-rays of the glenohumeral joint often show an impression defect over the humeral head or a fracture, erosion, or ectopic calcification along the glenoid rim. Obviously, x-rays showing the articulation dislocated confirm the diagnosis. If the diagnosis is in question, arthro CT scanning will usually show soft tissue as well as bony changes consistent with prior events. Once the diagnosis is made or suspected, referral to an orthopaedist is in order since sur-

gical repair of the damaged retaining structures is generally indicated to restore stability.

Chronic (Recurrent) Subluxation

This clinical entity is much more difficult to diagnose than chronic (recurrent) dislocation, since this is a milder form of glenohumeral instability. Signs and symptoms are similar to those of chronic dislocation but more subtle. There has usually been no actual dislocation of the shoulder requiring a reduction by the patient or a companion. The individual may describe the shoulder as catching, slipping, or going out of place. They may say their arm transiently "goes dead" or may only state that their shoulder bothers them intermittently. Apprehension and stress testing are often equivocal, and x-rays are generally unremarkable.

Many if not most individuals with chronic glenohumeral subluxation will respond to a nonoperative therapeutic program consisting of avoidance of aggravating positions, and activities and exercises designed to strengthen

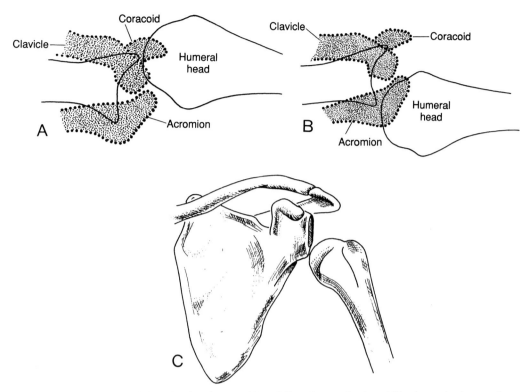

Figure 2.14. Directions of chronic glenohumeral instability. *A*, anterior instability (note the humeral head moves excessively relative to the glenoid toward the coracoid process). *B*, posterior instability (note the humeral head moves excessively relative to the glenoid toward the acromion process). *C*, inferior instability (note the humeral head moves excessively inferiorly relative to the glenoid). (From Goss TP. Factors to consider in chronic symptomatic shoulder instability. Orthop Rev 1985;XIV(10):27–32.)

the muscles that control the glenohumeral articulation. Referral to an orthopaedist is indicated if one suspects the diagnosis but is uncertain, or if the diagnosis is made and nonoperative therapeutic modalities are ineffective. For those individuals who are unresponsive to nonoperative care, surgery designed to repair damaged retaining structures is considered.

Functional Instability

This clinical entity is particularly difficult to diagnose because signs and symptoms may be even more subtle than those of chronic subluxation. The patient may or may not be able to remember a primary initiating event. Individuals may describe the shoulder as catching, slipping, clicking, locking, or may simply say

their shoulder is bothering them. The patient may or may not be able to relate his or her symptoms to certain shoulder positions. Apprehension and stress testing are negative. Routine radiographs are unremarkable unless the cause of the patient's symptomatology is an intermittently interposed intra-articular osseous body. Sophisticated radiographic studies (glenohumeral arthro CT scanning or MRI imaging) or glenohumeral arthroscopy are often necessary to reveal the intra-articular lesion responsible for the patient's symptomatology.

Once the diagnosis is confirmed or suspected, referral to an orthopaedist is indicated. Definitive treatment involves removal (frequently arthroscopically) of the intra-articular pathology responsible for the patient's symptomatology.

IMPINGEMENT SYNDROME

Impingement syndrome is an extremely common shoulder disorder. The space between the undersurface of the anterior acromion and the superior aspect of the proximal humerus is called the "impingement interval." This space is normally narrow and is maximally narrow when the arm is raised from 60 to 120° of elevation. Several soft tissue structures reside within this interval: the subacromial bursa, the long head of the biceps tendon, and the rotator cuff (Fig. 2.15). Any condition that further narrows this space (a calcium deposit, swelling of the soft tissues, excessive overhang of the anterior acromion, etc.) can cause the soft tissues to become "impinged upon." If impingement involves the subacromial bursa, a bursitis occurs; if the long head of the biceps tendon is involved, a bicipital tendinitis results; and if the rotator cuff is affected, a rotator cuff tendinitis occurs. These familiar clinical entities are all included under the designation, "impingement syndrome."

There are three stages of impingement that can be classified as age-related. Stage I is essentially an inflammation of the soft tissues within the impingement space. This may occur at any age but is particularly common in younger adults. Stage II is most frequently seen in individuals between 25 and 40 years of age. The soft tissues within the impingement interval are inflamed, but because these patients by definition have had multiple episodes in the past, some permanent scarring, thickening, or fibrosis is also present. Stage III is almost invariably seen in individuals over 40 years of age who have had previous episodes of impingement. There is inflammation of the soft tissues within the subacromial space and permanent fibrosis, scarring, or thickening. In addition, either a complete thickness tear of the rotator cuff or a ruptured long head of the biceps tendon is present as well as associated bony changes.

Clinical Characteristics

Pain is noted over the anterior aspect of the shoulder and may radiate down to, but

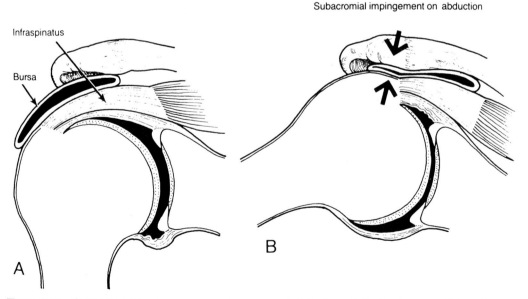

Figure 2.15. Subacromial impingement on glenohumeral abduction. *A,* the impingement interval and associated structures with the arm in neutral position. *B,* subacromial impingement on abduction. (Reprinted with permission from Rowe CR, Leffert RD. Subacromial syndromes. In: Rowe CR, ed. The Shoulder. New York: Churchill Livingstone, Inc., 1988:106.)

not below, the elbow. Discomfort is elicited by palpation over the impingement interval. Pain is maximal when the arm is raised from 60 to 120° of elevation (the so-called "painful arc") (Fig. 2.16), and especially if the shoulder is internally rotated. If one injects the impingement interval with lidocaine (without epinephrine), the patient's symptoms are transiently relieved (Fig. 2.17). X-rays of the shoulder may show bone spurs along the anteroinferior aspect of the acromion or the inferior surface of the clavicle; cysts, irregularity, or sclerosis over the greater tuberosity; and calcific deposits within the subacromial space.

If bicipital tendinitis is present, maximal discomfort is elicited when one palpates over the bicipital groove and rolls the biceps tendon under the examining finger. Elevation of the arm is more painful when the elbow is

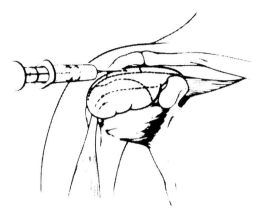

Figure 2.17. The impingement injection test. (Lidocaine, 5 mL, is injected into the subacromial space. If the patient's symptoms on glenohumeral abduction are relieved, the diagnosis of impingement is highly likely.) (Reprinted with permission from Neer CS II. Impingement lesions. Clin Orthop 1983;173:70–77.)

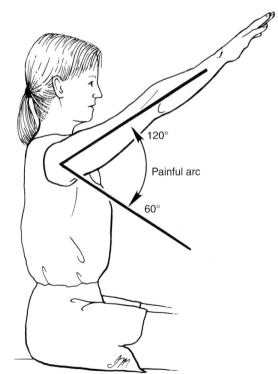

Figure 2.16. The "painful arc." Patients with impingement syndrome frequently have maximal discomfort as they raise their arm from 60 to 120° of elevation—worse when the shoulder is internally rotated and less when the shoulder is externally rotated.

extended and the forearm supinated, and less painful when the elbow is flexed and the forearm pronated. With the forearm in supination, flexion of the elbow against resistance will often cause pain over the anterior aspect of the shoulder.

Acute subacromial bursitis often has an abrupt onset and pain can be severe. Intense tenderness to palpation is frequently present, and glenohumeral motion may be extremely uncomfortable. Erythema, edema, and visible swelling over the anterior aspect of the shoulder may be present. The patient's body temperature and erythrocyte sedimentation rate are often elevated.

Characteristic clinical features associated with rotator cuff involvement and rupture of the long head of the biceps tendon will be discussed later in this chapter ("Musculocutaneous [Rotator] Cuff Syndrome" and "Acute Rupture of the Long Head of the Biceps Tendon").

Treatment

Stage I Impingement

When symptoms are acute, management includes avoidance of aggravating positions and activities (particularly raising the arm from 60 to 120° of elevation), ice packs applied to the anterior aspect of the shoulder, and analgesics. Anti-inflammatory medications are also helpful. Patients should, however, put their shoulder through a full range of motion at least two to three times a day to prevent adhesive capsulitis. Resting and protecting the arm in a sling may be necessary if the patient's symptoms are particularly severe. Occasionally, a subacromial injection of cortisone is required if other modalities are not particularly successful. As the patient's symptoms improve, sling protection can be discontinued gradually and increased functional use of the shoulder allowed. When the patient is pain free, physiotherapy is instituted and has both a therapeutic and prophylactic function. The patient works initially on regaining shoulder range of motion followed by strength. Most individuals improve fairly rapidly with a good prognosis.

Stage II Impingement

These patients tend to be more refractory to treatment. Initial management, however, is the same as that for Stage I impingement. If unsuccessful, the subacromial bursa can be injected with a corticosteroid (Fig. 2.17). The author's preference is to use 2 mg of methylprednisolone and 2 mL of 1% lidocaine without epinephrine. Care should be taken to avoid injecting directly into the biceps tendon or the rotator cuff. The injection has both a diagnostic and a therapeutic function. If the lidocaine alleviates discomfort during the first hour after the procedure, the diagnosis of impingement is confirmed. The cortisone may provide lasting relief. Corticosteroids may cause degenerative changes within the local soft tissues, however, so no one area should be injected more than twice in a year.

Once symptoms have subsided, therapeutic physiotherapy is prescribed to help the individual regain normal shoulder range of motion, flexibility, and strength. These individuals should be informed that the condition can be chronic and that recurrences are common. Activities that require forceful or repetitive

elevation of the arm through the painful arc are likely to cause symptoms to recur. Prophylactically, patients are encouraged to perform muscle strengthening exercises (with emphasis on the rotator cuff musculature) on a regular basis to prevent upriding of the proximal humerus and open up the subacromial space.

If impingement symptoms persist, referral to an orthopaedist is indicated for consideration of operative intervention. Surgical treatment consists of either an open or an arthroscopic procedure designed to decompress or enlarge the impingement interval. Patients over 40 years of age whose symptoms are refractory to nonoperative care may have a full thickness rotator cuff tear and should therefore be considered for an arthrographic examination.

Stage III Impingement

These individuals have sustained either a rupture of the long head of the biceps tendon or a full thickness tear of the rotator cuff. These clinical entities will be discussed later in this chapter ("Acute Rupture of the Long Head of the Biceps Tendon" and "Stage III Rotator Cuff Syndrome").

MUSCULOTENDINOUS (ROTATOR) CUFF SYNDROME

Lying within the impingement interval, the rotator cuff and particularly the supraspinatus tendon are prone to attritional disease. The same three stages occur as described in the section on "Impingement Syndrome."

Stage I Rotator Cuff Syndrome

This is generally seen in younger adults and is simply a rotator cuff tendinitis secondary to forceful or repetitive use of the shoulder (particularly elevation of the arm through the horizontal). Signs and symptoms are the same as those described for impingement syndrome, and treatment is identical to that outlined for Stage I impingement disorders. Improvement is usually rapid and the prognosis is good.

Stage II Rotator Cuff Syndrome

This is a Stage II impingement lesion and is most commonly seen in individuals 25 to 40 years of age who have had multiple previous episodes. In addition to inflammation of the rotator cuff, some permanent fibrosis, thickening, scarring, or partial tearing is present. Impingement signs and symptoms are evident. Calcific deposits may be noted within the rotator cuff on x-ray. Treatment is the same as that described for Stage II impingement syndrome. If simple nonoperative modalities such as rest, ice followed by heat, analgesics, and oral anti-inflammatory medications are ineffective, the impingement interval may be injected with a steroid and lidocaine. If symptoms persist or return quickly, referral to an orthopaedist is indicated for consideration of a surgical decompression and debridement. Individuals over the age of 40 whose symptoms are refractory to nonoperative care but who do not wish to consider surgical management should be considered for an arthrographic examination to make sure a full thickness rotator cuff tear is not present.

Stage III Rotator Cuff Syndrome (Fig. 2.18)

This is a Stage III impingement lesion—a complete thickness tear of the rotator cuff. These individuals are almost invariably 40 years of age or older and have had multiple episodes of impingement in the past. The rotator cuff gradually degenerates until it finally tears through. The process may be insidious, or a precipitating traumatic event of variable severity may be recalled. Once a complete thickness tear occurs, the involved tendons begin to retract and the defect becomes increasingly larger. In addition to the usual impingement symptoms, patients describe increasing shoulder pain and crepitus as the proximal humerus begins to rub against the undersurface of the acromion. These individuals also note increasing weakness when trying to elevate and externally rotate their arm. On physical examination, fine subacromial crepitus is usually palpable during passive and active range of motion of the shoulder. Once the diagnosis is suspected (particularly if the individual is over 40 years of age and does not respond to nonoperative management of impingement symptoms), a shoulder arthrogram should be obtained. If a full thickness rotator cuff tear is present, dye injected into the glenohumeral joint space escapes through the defect into the more superficial soft tissues (Fig. 2.19).

These individuals should be referred to an orthopaedist for subsequent care. Assuming the patient is amenable and medically fit, full thickness rotator cuff tears should be surgically repaired and the impingement interval decompressed/debrided as soon as possible. As time passes, the tear gradually becomes larger and the patient's signs and symptoms worsen. In addition, the surgical repair becomes increasingly difficult, the postoperative rehabilitation program more prolonged, and the postoperative result less satisfactory.

ACUTE RUPTURE OF THE LONG HEAD OF THE BICEPS TENDON

The long head of the biceps tendon passes through the shoulder impingement interval and is therefore prone to degenerative/attritional disease. In individuals under the age of 40, this results in episodes of bicipital tendinitis (Stage I and Stage II impingement) (see section on "Impingement Syndrome"), and in older individuals a complete rupture of the tendon may occur (Stage III impingement) (Fig. 2.20).

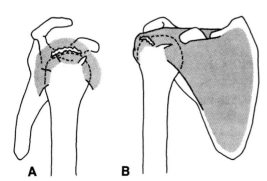

A   **B**

Figure 2.18. A musculotendinous cuff tear. *A*, lateral view. *B*, anterior view.

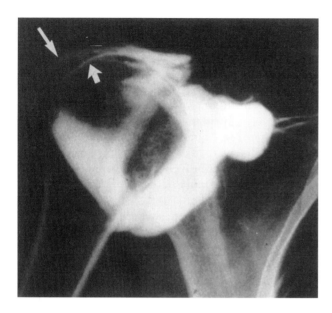

Figure 2.19. A shoulder arthrogram confirming the presence of a full thickness rotator cuff tear. Radio-opaque dye within the glenohumeral joint (thick arrow) extrudes through the tear and layers out over the superficial surface of the rotator cuff (thin arrow) creating the "double crescent sign."

Clinical Characteristics

The individual is usually 40 years of age or older and has had episodes of impingement in the past. The patient reports a sudden and usually painful "popping" sensation over the anterior aspect of the upper arm/shoulder during a lifting effort. The retracted belly of the biceps muscle bulges over the anterior aspect of the distal arm, and a concavity is visible over the anterior aspect of the proximal arm. This bulge is particularly prominent when the elbow is flexed against resistance. The upper arm is painful and tender to palpa-

tion for several days after the rupture. Active use of the shoulder and elbow usually increases the discomfort. Ecchymosis appears over the distal arm and elbow several days after the event. As the acute soft tissue irritation subsides, pain diminishes and upper extremity function improves.

Treatment

Referral to an orthopaedist is indicated. If diagnosed within 5 to 7 days, surgical repair of the biceps tendon is considered as well as a subacromial decompression/debridement to

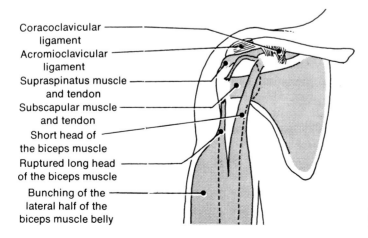

Coracoclavicular ligament
Acromioclavicular ligament
Supraspinatus muscle and tendon
Subscapular muscle and tendon
Short head of the biceps muscle
Ruptured long head of the biceps muscle
Bunching of the lateral half of the biceps muscle belly

Figure 2.20. Rupture of the long head of the biceps tendon.

prevent continued impingement. After 7 days, the ruptured tendon is usually too contracted to allow repair. Fortunately, these individuals do well despite the altered cosmetic appearance of their upper arm and the loss of approximately 5 to 10% of elbow flexion/forearm supination strength. If shoulder discomfort persists, an arthrogram should be obtained to make sure a full thickness rotator cuff tear has not occurred as well.

ADHESIVE CAPSULITIS (FROZEN SHOULDER)

The glenohumeral joint is particularly prone to symptomatic stiffness. This is formally known as adhesive capsulitis, but commonly referred to as a frozen shoulder. Anything that causes shoulder discomfort, such as intrinsic disorders (fractures, impingement syndrome, etc.) or pain referred from another area (left shoulder discomfort secondary to angina pectoris or myocardial infarction, etc.) can be the initiating event. The patient consciously or subconsciously limits the use of the shoulder because of pain, and soft tissue tightness or stiffness develop in one or more directions. Discomfort then occurs when the patient moves the arm and the contracted soft tissues are stretched. As the individual limits motion even more, further stiffness occurs, and a vicious cycle ensues. The patient eventually seeks medical care (usually 2 to 3 months after onset) because of increasing shoulder discomfort and decreasing glenohumeral range of motion.

Clinical Characteristics

The shoulder is comfortable when at rest. Shoulder movement is limited in one or more directions, with pain occurring at the limits of motion. The physical examination is otherwise rather unremarkable. Usually no local pain or abnormalities to palpation are found. Routine radiographs are usually unremarkable, although diffuse osteoporosis secondary to chronic disuse may be noted. The diagnosis is essentially one of exclusion.

Treatment

Treatment consists of breaking up the adhesions and stretching out the contracted soft tissues responsible for the condition. Daily intensive sessions with a physiotherapist for 3 weeks are prescribed, focusing on manually stretching the shoulder in the direction(s) of limited mobility. The patient is instructed to perform the same exercises four times a day at home at evenly spaced intervals. The patient is also told that this is a "no pain, no gain" proposition. The stretching exercises are uncomfortable, but as motion returns, pain gradually subsides and overall function of the shoulder improves. Judicious use of analgesic and anti-inflammatory medications are often helpful in allowing the individual to perform the stretching exercises optimally. The patient's progress is noted by the physician at 3 week intervals. Physiotherapy should continue until either full range of motion is achieved or until the patient's improvement plateaus. If the individual's range of motion plateaus short of normal, the patient and the physician must decide whether residual symptoms or shoulder mobility are acceptable. If not, referral to an orthopaedist is indicated for consideration of a manipulation of the shoulder under anesthesia.

GRADE I SPRAINS, GRADE I STRAINS, CONTUSIONS, AND OVERUSE SYNDROME

The most common injuries to the shoulder and upper arm are minor sprains, minor strains, contusions, and overuse syndrome.

Grade I Sprain

This is a minor injury to a ligamentous structure caused by an indirectly applied force. The tissues are merely stretched—neither partially torn nor ruptured.

Grade I Strain

This is a minor injury to a musculotendinous structure caused by an indirectly applied force. The tissues are merely stretched—neither partially torn nor ruptured.

Contusion

This is a minor injury to a bony or soft tissue structure caused by a directly applied force.

Overuse Syndrome

This is a minor injury to a bony or soft structure caused by the application of stresses to which the tissues are not accustomed. In general, symptoms do not occur during the activity but develop gradually over the ensuing 24 to 48 hours.

These injuries share similar clinical features. The individual may or may not be able to remember a specific initiating event and may or may not be able to precisely localize his or her symptoms. Swelling, discoloration, or both may be present over the involved area. Localized pain to palpation is generally present, and movements that stress or require use of the involved tissues elicit pain. X-rays are unremarkable. The diagnosis is generally one of exclusion: one rules out more significant clinical entities.

Treatment is similar for each of these injuries. The patient is advised to rest the shoulder/upper arm (avoid aggravating positions and activities) to allow healing of the involved tissues. Local application of ice during the first 48 hours after injury is helpful, followed by local moist heat thereafter. Over-the-counter analgesics are usually sufficient and anti-inflammatory medications may be useful. Sling immobilization may be necessary initially for discomfort, but the individual should put his or her shoulder through a full range of motion two to three times a day to prevent adhesive capsulitis. Occasionally, an injection of cortisone into an area of particularly localized pain will be helpful. The patient should be encouraged to gradually increase the functional use of the shoulder/upper arm as symptoms resolve. Physiotherapy to regain shoulder range of motion, flexibility, and strength may be necessary. These individuals generally improve fairly rapidly, although symptoms may persist for 4 to 6 weeks. A full functional recovery can be anticipated.

RADIAL NERVE ("SATURDAY NIGHT") PALSY

The radial nerve is vulnerable to a compression neuropathy commonly referred to as a "Saturday Night Palsy." This is caused by prolonged pressure over the nerve at any point along its course down the upper arm. (Individuals acutely intoxicated by a Saturday night binge may fall deeply asleep and remain motionless for a significant period of time with the posterior aspect of their upper arm resting against an object, causing compression of the radial nerve. The individual later awakens with a radial nerve palsy, hence the origin of the name.) These patients either have difficulty actively extending their wrist or metacarpophalangeal joints, or are unable to do so. They also note diminished or absent sensation over the first dorsal web space. Referral to an orthopaedist for subsequent care is indicated. Treatment consists primarily of reassurance that nerve function will return. The individual is told to avoid positions that apply pressure over the nerve. A removable volar splint is made to hold the wrist and metacarpophalangeal joints in an extended position. The radial neuropathy gradually resolves over time.

DELTOID TENDINITIS

A variety of mechanisms may result in inflammation of the tendinous insertion of the deltoid muscle. This clinical entity is fairly common.

Clinical Characteristics

Middle-aged adults are the most commonly affected. The individual may relate the onset of symptoms to a direct blow over the area, a sudden abduction strain, or an activity that involved prolonged or repetitive abduction of the arm. Pain is maximal over the lateral aspect of the upper arm at the junction of its proximal and middle thirds. Passive range of motion of the shoulder is usually full, although uncomfortable. Pain is especially acute when the arm is actively abducted against resistance. The patient is tender to palpation directly over the deltoid insertion. X-rays are usually unremarkable.

Treatment

The patient should avoid aggravating positions and activities. Use of an arm sling may be helpful. The individual is instructed, however, to remove the sling and put his or her shoulder through a full range of motion two to three times a day to prevent adhesive capsulitis. The patient is encouraged to gradually increase the use of his or her arm as symptoms subside. Nonprescription analgesics are sufficient and anti-inflammatory medications may be helpful. Local application of ice during the first 48 hours after onset of symptoms is recommended. Thereafter, application of moist heat to the symptomatic area is helpful. In severe or persistent cases, an injection of corticosteroid plus 1% lidocaine adjacent to but not within the affected tendon can result in rapid and complete alleviation of symptoms.

TRAUMATIC DISORDERS OF THE SHOULDER AND UPPER ARM

SPRAINS OF THE ACROMIOCLAVICULAR JOINT

A sprain is an injury to the ligamentous structure(s) that stabilizes an articulation. Three grades of AC joint sprains may occur (Fig. 2.21): Grade I, Grade II (subluxation of the AC joint), and Grade III (dislocation of the AC joint) injuries. The mechanism is usually a fall on the superior aspect of the acromial process that forces the scapula down and applies stress to the acromioclavicular and coracoclavicular ligaments.

Grade I Sprains of the Acromioclavicular Joint

In this injury, the acromioclavicular ligaments are significantly stressed (stretched or partially torn but not ruptured). The coracoclavicular ligaments are either uninvolved or simply stretched. A traumatic event has oc-

curred, and the patient notes discomfort over the AC joint. The articulation is tender to local palpation and painful on attempted shoulder motion. The area may be slightly swollen. AP x-rays of the AC joint obtained with the patient standing and 10-lb weights hung from both wrists show a normal relationship between the affected acromion and the clavicle.

Treatment

A sling and swathe dressing is initially prescribed for comfort. Gradually increasing use of the shoulder is encouraged as symptoms subside. Local application of ice is helpful during the first 48 hours, followed by moist heat thereafter. Over-the-counter pain medications should be sufficient and anti-inflammatory medications may be useful. Physiotherapy for pain control and restoration of normal function is occasionally necessary as is an injection of a corticosteroid into the articulation if symptoms are refractory to lesser modalities. Symptoms usually resolve within 4 to 6 weeks. Approximately 5 to 10% of patients note persistent or recurring discomfort over the AC joint. If the discomfort is sufficiently bothersome, referral to an orthopaedist is indicated for consideration of a distal clavicle resection.

Grade II Sprains of the Acromioclavicular Joint (Subluxation)

This injury represents a complete tear of the acromioclavicular ligaments and either a stretching or a partial tearing of the coracoclavicular ligaments. The patient describes a traumatic event and notes discomfort over the AC joint. The articulation is locally tender to palpation and painful on shoulder range of motion. Swelling may be present over the AC joint, and the outer end of the clavicle may protrude superiorly. AP x-rays of the AC joint obtained with the patient standing with 10-lb weights attached to both wrists reveal the inferior margin of the distal clavicle to lie above the inferior margin but below the superior margin of the acromion.

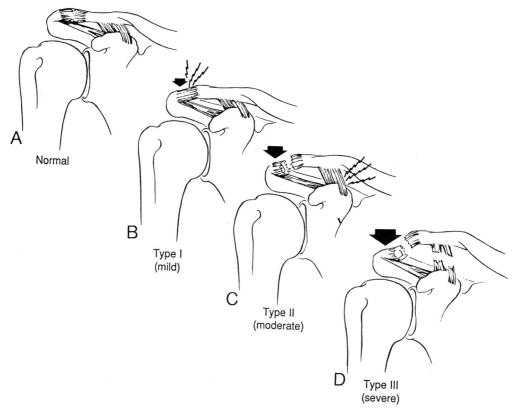

Figure 2.21. Schematic drawing illustrating the three types of ligamentous injuries that can occur at the acromioclavicular joint. *A*, normal. *B*, type I: stretched acromioclavicular ligaments. *C*, type II: torn acromioclavicular ligaments and stretched coracoclavicular ligaments, allowing partial displacement of the acromioclavicular joint. *D*, type III: torn acromioclavicular and coracoclavicular ligaments, allowing complete displacement of the acromioclavicular joint. (Reprinted with permission from Allman FL Jr. Fractures and ligamentous injuries of the clavicle and its articulation. J Bone Joint Surg [Am] 1967;49A:774–784.)

Treatment

The vast majority of orthopaedists treat this injury in the same manner as that described for Grade I acromioclavicular sprains. The end result is usually satisfactory, although the outer end of the clavicle will remain somewhat prominent, some loss of shoulder strength usually occurs, and approximately 10 to 25% of patients develop persistent or recurring AC joint discomfort. Referral to an orthopaedist is therefore indicated so that the injury can be fully discussed and evaluated. Should the AC joint remain unacceptably symptomatic despite nonoperative therapeutic modalities, a distal clavicle resection is the surgical procedure of choice.

Grade III Sprains of the Acromioclavicular Joint (Dislocation)

Grade III sprains of the AC joint represent a complete disruption of the acromioclavicular and coracoclavicular ligaments. This injury permits the sternocleidomastoid muscle to pull the clavicle superiorly, while the weight of the extremity draws the scapula inferiorly. A clear traumatic event has occurred, followed by discomfort over the AC joint. The articulation is significantly tender to local palpation and painful on shoulder range of motion. Swelling is present over the AC joint, and the outer end of the clavicle is usually prominent superiorly. AP x-rays obtained with the patient standing with 10-lb weights attached to both wrists reveal significant inferior displacement of the acromion relative to the clavicle (the inferior margin of the distal clavicle lies at or above the superior margin of the adjacent acromion).

Treatment

Controversy exists regarding the management of these injuries. The majority of orthopaedists, including the author, believe that most Grade III sprains can and should be treated in the same manner as Grade I and II sprains. The patient should be made aware, however, that there will be a permanent prominence of the distal clavicle, and approximately 5 to 10% loss of shoulder strength is likely as well as muscle fatigue discomfort with prolonged or aggressive use. In addition, some individuals develop impingement or neurovascular symptoms from anteroinferior displacement of the scapula. Consequently, as with Grade II sprains of the AC joint, referral to an orthopaedist is indicated so that operative versus nonoperative treatment can be fully discussed as well as the potential adverse sequelae. Individuals who perform heavy, manual work and those that require optimal upper extremity function may benefit from an acute surgical repair. Those treated nonoperatively, who go on to develop persistent and unacceptable symptoms, are candidates for a surgical reconstruction of the acromioclavicular articulation.

SPRAINS OF THE STERNOCLAVICULAR JOINT

Sprains of the SC joint are uncommon injuries resulting from strong and unusually directed forces applied to the stabilizing ligaments. Three grades can occur, depending on the severity of the force involved (Fig. 2.22).

Grade I and II (Subluxation) Sprains of the SC Joint

A Grade I sprain represents a stretching or a partial tearing of the sternoclavicular ligaments. The costoclavicular ligament is either uninvolved or simply stretched. A Grade II sprain (subluxation) represents a complete tear of the sternoclavicular ligaments accompanied by a stretching or a partial tearing of the costoclavicular ligament. The individual presents with pain (increased by shoulder motion), tenderness, and swelling over the involved articulation. A radiographic evaluation is indicated, and with Grade II injuries, subluxation of the proximal clavicle relative to the sternum is present. Treatment is symptomatic. Sling or figure-of-eight splintage may be prescribed for comfort, but gradually increasing functional use of the extremity is permitted and encouraged as symptoms allow. Ice is applied to the involved area during the first 48 hours after injury, followed by local moist heat thereafter. Analgesic medications may be necessary and anti-inflammatories are frequently helpful. Symptoms generally resolve within 4 to 6 weeks. Adverse long-term sequelae rarely occur—symptomatic instability or degenerative disease of the sternoclavicular joint are extremely uncommon.

Grade III Sprains (Dislocation) of the SC Joint

In this injury, the costoclavicular ligament as well as the sternoclavicular ligaments are completely torn, allowing the articulation to dislocate either anteriorly or posteriorly.

Clinical Characteristics

Anterior Dislocation Severe pain and tenderness are present over the SC joint. Any movement of the shoulder causes increased pain and discomfort. Pain is maximal when the patient is supine—the individual prefers to be in the sitting position, supporting the arm on the injured side. The anteriorly displaced medial end of the clavicle is generally visible.

Posterior Dislocation Severe pain and tenderness are present over the SC joint. Any movement of the shoulder causes increased discomfort. Pain is maximal when the patient is supine—the individual prefers to be in the

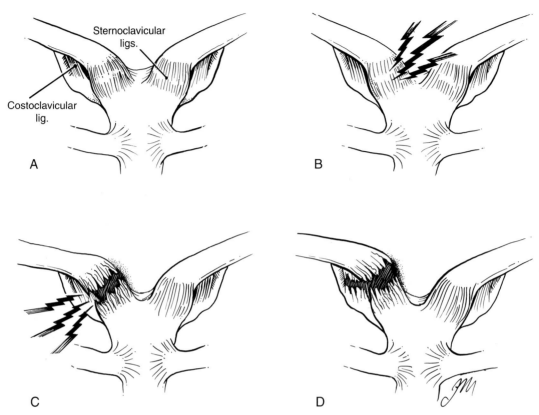

Figure 2.22.   Schematic drawing illustrating the three types of ligamentous injuries that can occur at the sternoclavicular joint. *A*, normal. *B*, type I: stretched sternoclavicular ligaments. *C*, type II: torn sternoclavicular ligaments and stretched costoclavicular ligament, allowing partial displacement of the sternoclavicular joint. *D*, type III: torn sternoclavicular and costoclavicular ligaments, allowing complete displacement of the sternoclavicular joint.

sitting position, supporting the arm on the injured side. The usually prominent medial end of the clavicle is not visible or palpable because of its posterior displacement. A posterior dislocation of the SC joint may cause pressure on the great vessels, the trachea, or the esophagus. Either the dislocation itself or associated injuries to the chest may result in a pneumothorax. As a result, the patient may display venous congestion in the neck, a partial or complete airway obstruction, and difficulty swallowing, and/or signs and symptoms consistent with a pneumothorax.

X-ray is necessary to confirm the presence of a sternoclavicular dislocation (Fig. 2.23). Oblique radiographs are often helpful, because standard AP projections are frequently difficult to interpret. Even more definitive and frequently necessary is a CT scan of the articulation (Fig. 2.24).

Treatment (Fig. 2.25)

Anterior Dislocation   At least one attempt at a closed reduction is reasonable. Intravenous sedation is usually adequate, but occasionally general anesthesia is necessary. The patient is positioned supine at the edge of a table with a sandbag beneath the scapula. The injured arm is abducted 90° and extended to the point of resistance (approximately 15°). While traction is being applied to the injured extremity, the medial end of the clavicle is pushed posteriorly. Reduction is usually easy

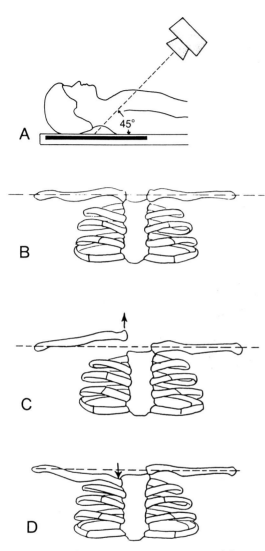

Figure 2.23. Cephalic tilt roentgenogram of the sternoclavicular joint. *A,* positioning of the patient. *B,* normal appearance at the sternoclavicular joint. *C,* when the clavicle is dislocated anteriorly, it is projected above the horizontal plane. *D,* when the clavicle is dislocated posteriorly, it is projected below the horizontal plane. (*B–D* Reprinted with permission from DePalma AF. Surgery of the Shoulder. 3rd ed. Philadelphia: JB Lippincott Company, 1983:452.)

but generally unstable. If the reduction is unstable and the anterior dislocation recurs, the patient is treated symptomatically. If the reduction is stable, a figure-of-eight bandage is applied, and the arm is placed in a sling for support. Both are worn for 6 weeks, while strenuous activities are prohibited for an additional 2 weeks. If the dislocation cannot be reduced or the reduction cannot be maintained, an orthopaedist should be consulted. Whether or not the articulation heals in anatomic position, satisfactory painless function usually results.

Posterior Dislocation An immediate orthopaedic consultation should be requested. The dislocated clavicle must be reduced, which becomes an emergency if pressure on the great vessels or the trachea poses a threat to life. (Appropriate management of an accompanying pneumothorax is obviously a priority as well.) Unless the patient is in extremis, general anesthesia or intravenous sedation is used. The patient is positioned supine at the edge of a table with a sandbag beneath the scapula, and the arm is abducted 90° and extended to the point of resistance (approximately 15°). As traction is applied to the extremity, reduction of the dislocation may occur. However, it may be necessary to pull the medial end of the clavicle anteriorly either manually or with a towel clip. In most cases, the clavicle will reduce with a notable "pop." Again, reduction *must* be achieved and operative intervention may occasionally be necessary. Once obtained, the articulation is generally stable. A figure-of-eight bandage is then applied, and the arm is placed in a sling for support. Both are worn for 6 weeks, and strenuous activities are prohibited for an additional 2 weeks. Satisfactory painless function can be anticipated.

ACUTE DISLOCATIONS OF THE GLENOHUMERAL JOINT

The glenohumeral joint is the most mobile articulation in the body but also the most prone to symptomatic instability. Acute (happening for the first time) dislocations are usually the result of indirect (occasionally direct) forces and are most commonly seen in vigorous young adults. The shoulder can dislocate either anteriorly or posteriorly—the former

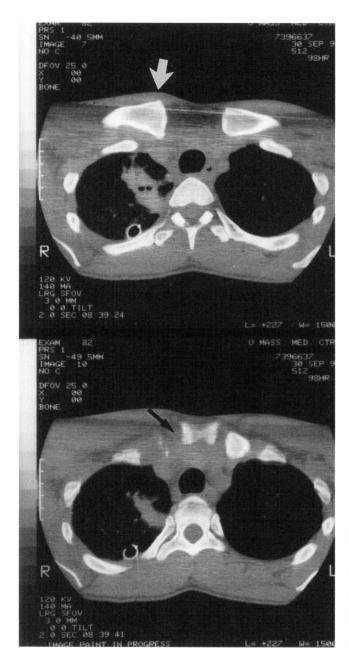

Figure 2.24. Axial CT images confirming the presence of an anterior dislocation of the sternoclavicular joint. Note the anterior soft tissue prominence over the sternoclavicular joint (white arrow) and the failure of the clavicle to articulate with the sternum as compared with the opposite side (black arrow).

comprise approximately 95% of such injuries, whereas the latter make up the remaining 5%.

Acute Anterior Dislocation of the Glenohumeral Joint (Fig. 2.26)

This injury usually occurs when the arm is abducted, extended, and externally rotated with considerable violence. The humeral head is forced out of the glenoid cavity anteriorly and comes to rest beneath the coracoid process, the clavicle, or the glenoid process.

Clinical Characteristics

The arm is held close to the body, slightly abducted and internally rotated. The patient

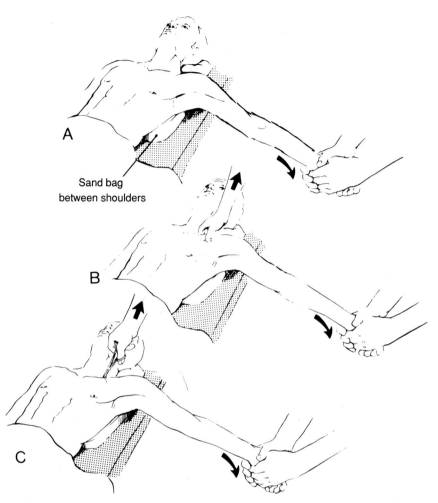

Sand bag
between shoulders

Figure 2.25.   Technique for closed reduction of the sternoclavicular joint. *A*, positioning the patient and application of longitudinal traction with the arm in abduction and slight extension. In anterior dislocations, direct anterior pressure may be required to replace the medial end of the clavicle. *B*, in posterior dislocations of the sternoclavicular joint, in addition to traction, it may be necessary to lift the clavicle from behind the manubrium with the fingers. *C*, in difficult cases of posterior dislocation of the sternoclavicular joint, a sterile towel clip may be used to grasp the medial end of the clavicle to lift it laterally and anteriorly. (Reprinted with permission from Rockwood CA, Green DP, eds. Fractures, vol. 1. 2nd ed. Philadelphia: JB Lippincott Company, 1984:929.)

is usually in significant distress, and any attempt to move the shoulder accentuates his or her pain. The shoulder appears flattened laterally and unusually prominent anteriorly. X-rays taken in two planes at 90° to each other (ideally an AP with the arm in neutral rotation and a true axillary view; occasionally supplemented by lateral scapular and transthoracic lateral projections) should be obtained and will confirm the diagnosis.

The physician should consider and look for associated injuries including fractures of the proximal humerus, scapula, and clavicle (see appropriate sections); avulsion of the rotator cuff (see section on "Musculotendinous [Rotator Cuff] Syndrome"); and involvement of adjacent neurovascular structures. Vascular injuries and full thickness tears of the rotator cuff may occur in individuals over the age of 40, the frequency increasing with age. Injury

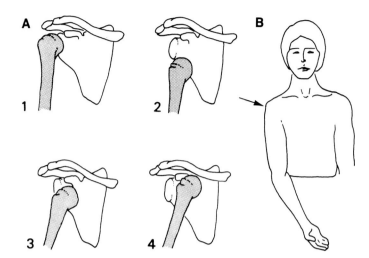

Figure 2.26. Acute anterior dislocation of the glenohumeral joint. *A,* the positions: *1,* normal; *2,* subglenoid; *3,* subcoracoid; *4,* subclavicular. *B,* anterior view of the patient's appearance. The round prominence of the shoulder has shifted anteriorly, leaving the lateral salient flat (arrow).

to the axillary vessels is rare, but when it occurs the consequences can be catastrophic. Neurologically, involvement of the axillary nerve is most common. These individuals are unable to actively contract their deltoid muscle and note a small area of decreased sensation over the lateral aspect of the shoulder. The injury is usually a neurapraxia, and function gradually returns to normal (several weeks may be required) once the shoulder is reduced. Other nerves in the area are rarely involved. A repeat neurovascular examination should be performed after reduction of the dislocation as well.

Treatment

Glenohumeral dislocations should be reduced expeditiously. Many maneuvers have been described, but two basic principles must be observed: (1) the patient should be completely relaxed, and (2) the maneuver should be performed gently to avoid further damage to the articulation. The author presently uses intravenous diazepam for sedation. The patient is positioned supine on the examining table, with the injured arm abducted as far as possible and the elbow flexed to 90°. An assistant standing at the opposite side of the table stabilizes the individual by holding onto a sheet passed around his or her torso. The physician ties another sheet in a loop, then stands inside and places it around the patient's

injured arm (Fig. 2.27). As the physician gradually leans back against the looped sheet, this progressive pull down the long axis of the humerus, combined with gentle anterior pressure over the shoulder and slight internal rotation usually affects the reduction quickly, easily, and gently. X-rays are then obtained in two planes (an AP with the arm in neutral rotation and an axillary view of the glenohumeral joint) to be certain that the humeral head lies concentrically within the glenoid cavity and that any associated fracture(s) has been recognized and is in acceptable position. If the dislocation is irreducible or if associated fractures fail to reduce satisfactorily, referral to an orthopaedist is indicated. One should also involve an orthopaedist and not attempt a reduction if the dislocation is accompanied by a fracture through the anatomic or surgical neck region of the proximal humerus, because the maneuver may distract the fracture site and damage the adjacent soft tissues. (The anatomic neck is the area between the articular segment and the tuberosities, whereas the surgical neck is the region between the tuberosities and the humeral shaft.)

After the dislocation is reduced, the patient's arm is immobilized in a sling and swathe dressing (Fig. 2.28). Individuals over the age of 40 are protected for 7 to 10 days and then encouraged to gradually increase the functional use of their shoulder as symptoms

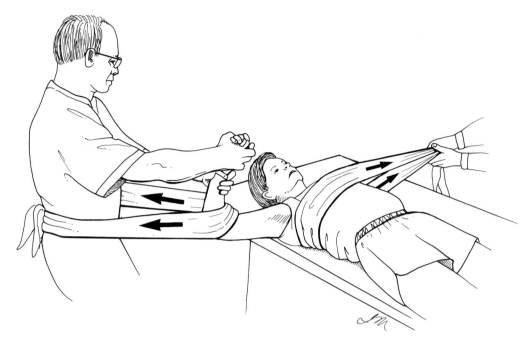

Figure 2.27. Closed reduction of a dislocated glenohumeral joint using the "double-looped sheet" method.

allow. (An arthrogram to rule out an associated full thickness rotator cuff tear should be obtained in those who note persistent shoulder discomfort.) Individuals under the age of 40 are at significant risk for redislocation (the younger they are at the time of the initial event, the higher the risk). Consequently, the author recommends a full 6 weeks of sling and swathe immobilization to promote healing of the damaged retaining tissues. After the period of immobilization, an intensive physiotherapy program is initiated that is designed to help the patient regain shoulder range of motion initially. Strengthening exercises for all muscle groups are then added to restore normal function and lessen the chances of redislocation.

Acute Posterior Dislocation of the Glenohumeral Joint (Fig. 2.29)

Posterior dislocation of the glenohumeral joint is relatively uncommon and, unfortunately, frequently missed on the initial evaluation. This dislocation may be the result of either a direct or an indirect force applied to the proximal humerus/humeral head. Posterior dislocations are frequently seen in individuals who have experienced a convulsion or sustained an electric shock as a result of the severe associated contraction of the glenohumeral internal rotators.

Clinical Characteristics

The patient is in considerable distress and resists any attempt to move his or her shoulder. The arm is kept in a position of adduction and internal rotation. The coracoid process may seem to protrude anteriorly, while the humeral head may be unusually prominent and/or palpable posteriorly. Three abnormalities are often noted on a routine AP x-ray projection: (1) the smooth, curved lateral contour of the greater tuberosity is absent because of internal rotation of the humerus; (2) the parallelism between the humeral articular surface and the anterior glenoid rim is lost; and (3) the dislocated humeral head is displaced upward relative to the glenoid cavity. The AP

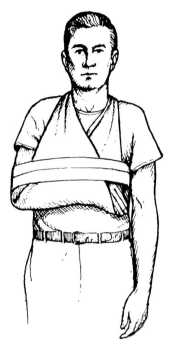

Figure 2.28. The conventional sling and swathe dressing for immobilization of the shoulder. (Reprinted with permission from Rockwood CA, Green DP, eds. Fractures, vol. 1. 2nd ed. Philadelphia: JB Lippincott Company, 1984:684.)

radiograph may, however, appear normal, making it *absolutely mandatory* that one obtain either a true axillary view of the glenohumeral joint or a true lateral view of the scapula (less ideal) in any shoulder that has been injured. Obtaining two radiographic projections at 90° to each other (particularly if one is a true axillary view of the glenohumeral joint) will confirm the presence of a posterior dislocation and ensure that one never misses the diagnosis. As discussed in the section "Acute Anterior Dislocation of the Glenohumeral Joint," one should also look for associated fractures, injuries to adjacent soft tissues, and neurovascular involvement.

Treatment

The therapeutic principles described in the section "Acute Anterior Dislocation of the Glenohumeral Joint" should be followed, and the "looped sheet reduction maneuver" can be used. Once again, one must make sure that neither a fracture of the anatomic neck nor of the surgical neck region of the proximal humerus is present. As traction is applied, the

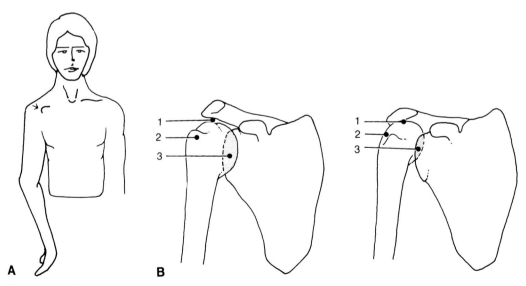

Figure 2.29. Posterior dislocation of the glenohumeral joint. *A,* patient's appearance (note that the shoulder is flat and the coracoid process protrudes) (arrow). *B,* three diagnostic features on the AP x-ray projection. *Left,* normal. *1,* upper border of the head of the humerus in normal position. *2,* normal contour reveals the greater tuberosity. *3,* half moon crescent of projected overlap. *Right,* posterior dislocation. *1,* head of the humerus after dislocation, superior to normal position. *2,* internal rotation hides the greater tuberosity. *3,* half moon crescent of the projected overlap no longer apparent.

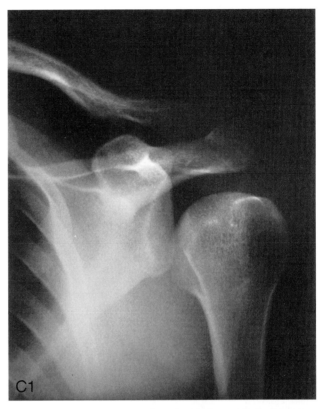

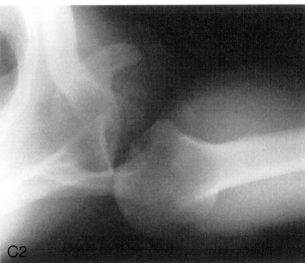

Figure 2.29. (*continued*) *C*, radiographs of an individual with a posterior dislocation of the glenohumeral joint. *1*, a "suggestive" AP x-ray projection. *2*, an unequivocal axillary x-ray projection.

shoulder is gradually rotated externally and the humeral head pushed forward. X-rays in the AP and axillary planes should then be obtained to confirm that the dislocation has been reduced and to make sure that any associated fractures have been recognized and are in acceptable position. A repeat neurovascular examination should be performed. A shoulder spica cast holding the arm in 20° of external rotation is then applied (Fig. 2.30). Conse-

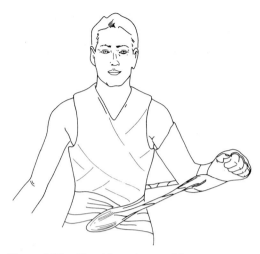

Figure 2.30. Shoulder spica used for immobilization after reduction of a posterior glenohumeral dislocation. Note that the shoulder is held in abduction and external rotation. (From Goss TP. Factors to consider in chronic symptomatic shoulder instability. Orthop Rev 1985;XIV(10):27–32.)

quently, an orthopaedic referral for initial treatment and subsequent care is usually most practical. (Obviously, if the shoulder is irreducible or if an associated fracture does not reduce satisfactorily, referral to an orthopaedist is clearly indicated.) As with acute anterior dislocations, patients over 40 years of age are immobilized 7 to 10 days, whereas those under 40 are kept in a spica cast for 6 weeks. When immobilization is discontinued, an intensive physiotherapy program is instituted to help the patient regain shoulder range of motion initially. Strengthening exercises for all muscle groups are then added to restore normal function and lessen the chances of redislocation.

FRACTURES OF THE CLAVICLE

Fractures of the Middle Third of the Clavicle

Clavicle fractures comprise 10% of all fractures, and the majority (85%) involve the middle third. The medial or proximal fragment usually is displaced superiorly and posteriorly by the pull of the sternocleidomastoid muscle, whereas the lateral or distal fragment usually

is drawn inferiorly and anteriorly by the weight of the arm (Fig. 2.31A). Neurovascular injury is uncommon. A traumatic event has occurred and signs and symptoms are very localized. Diagnosis is ultimately radiographic, and a routine AP projection usually will reveal the injury clearly.

The figure-of-eight bandage (Fig. 2.31B) is the traditional method of treatment and is primarily intended to reduce motion at the fracture site, thereby lessening the patient's discomfort. Some reduction of the fracture usually is obtained as well. During the first 7 to 10 days after injury, a sling may be added to support the weight of the arm to provide further pain relief. Although anatomic reduction of the fracture is seldom obtained, these injuries almost always heal with full restoration of shoulder function and an acceptable cosmetic deformity. If a significant gap is present at the fracture site after application of the figure-of-eight bandage, referral to an orthopaedist is indicated.

The figure-of-eight bandage is worn constantly for a period of at least 6 weeks. The patient is allowed to use his or her arm for light activities as symptoms allow. The fracture is judged to be healed at any time after 6 weeks when adequate callous is visible on x-ray examination, when palpation of the fracture site is painless, and when the patient can move his or her arm fully without discomfort at the fracture site. Following removal of the figure-of-eight bandage, the patient is encouraged to gradually increase the functional use of the affected extremity, but no strenuous activities are allowed (sports, etc.) for at least an additional 6 weeks. If one feels that union is not proceeding satisfactorily, referral to an orthopaedist is indicated.

Fractures of the Lateral Third of the Clavicle

These injuries comprise 10% of all clavicular fractures. Three types have been described in the adult age group (Fig. 2.32). These injuries are the result of a traumatic event, and signs and symptoms are localized. Diagnosis is radiographic and *must* include an AP view

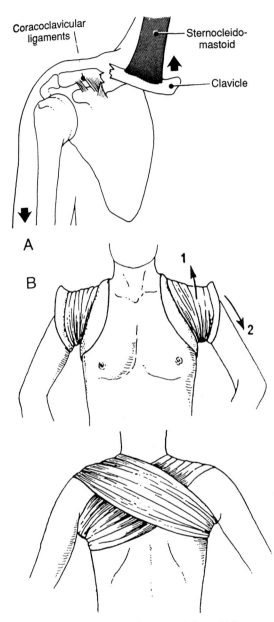

Coracoclavicular ligaments

Sternocleido-mastoid

Clavicle

A

B

Figure 2.31. A complete fracture of the middle third of the clavicle. *A,* forces causing displacement. *B,* the figure-of-eight bandage used for immobilization (Reprinted with permission from DePalma AF. Surgery of the Shoulder. 3rd ed. Philadelphia: JB Lippincott Company, 1983:351).

of the shoulder with the patient standing with 10-lb weights hung from both wrists (a "weightbearing" radiograph).

In Type I injuries, the coracoclavicular ligaments remain attached to the proximal fragment. Consequently, displacement at the fracture site is usually within acceptable limits. Treatment consists of figure-of-eight bandage immobilization. Therapeutic principles are the same as those described for fractures of the middle third of the clavicle.

In Type II injuries, the coracoclavicular ligaments are detached from the proximal fragment. This allows the proximal fragment to be drawn superiorly and posteriorly by the unopposed pull of the trapezius and sternocleidomastoid muscles, while the distal fragment is displaced inferiorly and anteriorly by the weight of the arm and a significant gap at the fracture site may result. If the separation is moderate, the fracture will be slow to heal; if it is severe, a nonunion can occur. Consequently, if displacement at the fracture site is significant, referral to an orthopaedist is indicated, because a surgical open reduction and internal fixation may be necessary to ensure healing and restoration of normal function.

In Type III injuries, the articular surface of the distal clavicle is violated. These fractures are managed symptomatically with a figure-of-eight bandage or sling immobilization for comfort and gradual increase in functional use of the extremity as symptoms allow. (If a large fracture fragment is present and significantly displaced, a surgical open reduction and internal fixation can be considered, but this is rare.) Union generally occurs within 6 weeks. Symptomatic degenerative disease of the AC joint may occur at a later date. If the area is sufficiently painful and disabling, and nonoperative modalities are ineffective, surgical excision of the distal half-inch of the clavicle is the treatment of choice.

Fractures of the Medial Third of the Clavicle

These injuries comprise 5% of all clavicular fractures and are caused by severe traumatic

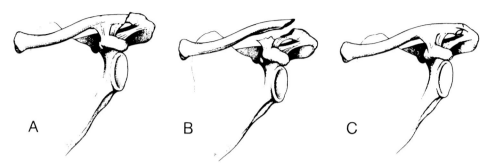

Figure 2.32. Classification of fractures of the distal clavicle. *A*, type I (minimal displacement and intact ligaments). *B*, type II (significant displacement due to ruptured coracoclavicular ligaments). *C*, type III (intra-articular fracture). (Reprinted with permission from Rockwood CA, Green DP, eds. Fractures, vol. 1. 2nd ed. Philadelphia: JB Lippincott Company, 1984:708.)

forces. Signs and symptoms are localized. AP and oblique radiographs of the area may be diagnostic; however, CT scanning may be necessary. One must consider and rule out associated injuries to adjacent vital structures. Treatment is essentially symptomatic (figure-of-eight bandage or sling and swathe immobilization initially; gradual increase in functional use of the extremity as symptoms allow; local application of ice followed by moist heat, analgesic and anti-inflammatory medications as needed, etc.), and healing occurs reliably in 6 weeks.

Epiphyseal Fracture/Separations of the Clavicle (Fig. 2.33)

The ossific nuclei at the lateral and medial ends of the clavicle do not appear and unite with the shaft until the ages of 16 and 25,

respectively. These areas are relatively weak, and as a result, traumatic injuries to individuals in these age groups that appear to be AC joint and SC joint sprains are almost invariably epiphyseal fracture separations. Treatment is symptomatic (use of a figure-of-eight bandage or sling and swathe immobilization initially, gradual increase in functional use of the extremity as symptoms allow, local application of ice followed by moist heat, etc.), and healing time is in the order of 3 weeks.

FRACTURES OF THE PROXIMAL HUMERUS

Fractures of the proximal humerus comprise 4 to 5% of fractures in general and are seen more commonly in older individuals.

Clinical Characteristics

A significant force has been applied either directly or indirectly to the shoulder region,

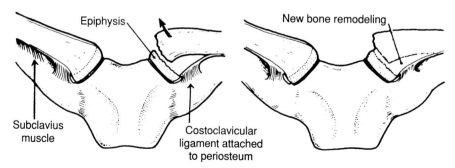

Figure 2.33. Epiphyseal separation at the sternal end of the clavicle. (Reprinted with permission from Rowe CR. Acromioclavicular and sternoclavicular joints. In: Rowe CR, ed. The Shoulder. New York: Churchill Livingstone, Inc., 1988:317.)

and the patient localizes discomfort to the area. The shoulder is usually swollen, ecchymotic, and diffusely tender. Any attempt to move the shoulder causes increased pain. An AP radiograph with the arm in neutral rotation as well as a true axillary view of the glenohumeral joint, supplemented as needed by transthoracic lateral and lateral scapular views of the shoulder, demonstrate the fracture. CT scanning, however, may be necessary to accurately define the injury and determine the degree of displacement of the bony fragment(s).

Treatment

The proximal humerus is composed of four major segments: the articular segment, the greater tuberosity, the lesser tuberosity, and the humeral shaft (Fig. 2.34A). Eighty percent of proximal humeral fractures are minimally displaced, i.e., none of the four major segments is displaced greater than or equal to 1 cm nor rotated greater than or equal to 45°. Treatment consists of protection of the arm in a sling and swathe bandage for 6 weeks. When the humerus moves as a unit (approxi-

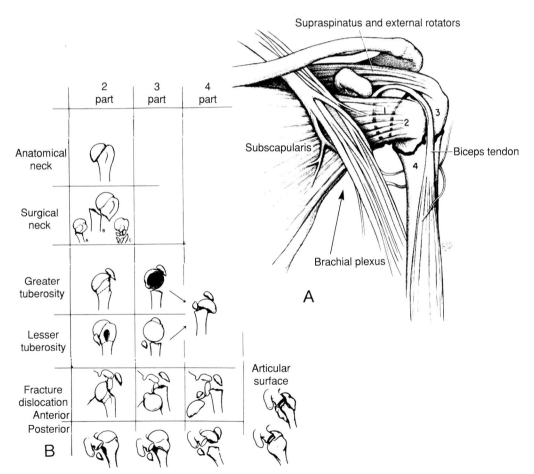

Figure 2.34. Fractures of the proximal humerus. *A*, the four major segments of the proximal humerus: *1*, articular segment; *2*, lesser tuberosity; *3*, greater tuberosity; *4*, humeral shaft (Reprinted with permission from Neer CS. Displaced proximal humeral fractures: I. classification and evaluation. J Bone Joint Surg [Am] 1970;52A:1077–1089). *B*, the various types of significantly displaced fractures that can occur (Reprinted with permission from Neer CS. Displaced proximal humeral fractures: I. classification and evaluation. J Bone Joint Surg [Am] 1970;52A:1077–1089).

mately 14 days), gentle dependent circular and pendulum range of motion exercises plus external rotation to but not past neutral are begun. Moving as a unit means that when the arm is gently internally and externally rotated, one can feel the humeral head rotate correspondingly. At 4 weeks, progressive passive/active assistive shoulder range of motion exercises (especially forward flexion, internal rotation up the back, and external rotation) are instituted. At 6 weeks, union is generally complete, sling and swathe protection is discontinued, and active use of the shoulder is allowed and encouraged. Physiotherapy, however, continues on a regular basis until the patient regains maximal range of motion followed by strength. Referral to an orthopaedist is indicated if one is unsure whether the position of the fracture fragment(s) is acceptable.

Twenty percent of proximal humeral fractures involve significant displacement of one or more of the four major segments. If a major segment is displaced greater than or equal to 1 cm or rotated greater than or equal to 45°, it is called a "part"; therefore, a variety of 2-, 3-, and 4-part fractures are possible as well as fractures of the articular surface of the proximal humerus and fracture dislocations (Fig. 2.34B). Referral to an orthopaedist is indicated because surgery usually is necessary. The blood supply to the articular segment comes in via the tuberosities. Consequently, if the articular segment is separated significantly from the tuberosities or vice versa, the articular segment has a 90% risk of undergoing avascular necrosis with subsequent collapse and degenerative joint disease. Therefore, a primary prosthetic replacement is usually the treatment of choice. The rotator cuff inserts on the greater and lesser tuberosities. Consequently, if a fractured tuberosity is displaced significantly, a complete tear of the rotator cuff is present by definition. In addition, a significantly displaced tuberosity may fail to heal or may interfere with glenohumeral range of motion. Therefore, a significantly displaced tuberosity should be surgically reduced anatomically and internally fixed, and the rotator cuff should be repaired. Finally, significant

displacement at a surgical neck fracture site can result in a failure of the fracture to heal (a nonunion) or a healed fracture in abnormal position (a malunion) with resulting pain, cosmetic deformity, or limitation of glenohumeral range of motion in one or more directions. Here again, surgery may be required to avoid such an outcome.

Fractures involving the articular surface of the proximal humerus should be referred to an orthopaedist as well. If the articular surface is disrupted significantly, an open reduction and internal fixation or even a primary prosthetic replacement may be indicated to prevent later symptomatic joint disease or glenohumeral instability.

Fracture—Dislocations of the Proximal Humerus

Fractures of the tuberosities may accompany dislocations of the glenohumeral joint (a fractured greater tuberosity with anterior dislocations and a fractured lesser tuberosity with posterior dislocations) but often return to normal position after reduction of the dislocation. If not, and for those injuries that include a fracture of the anatomic or surgical neck of the proximal humerus (see "Acute Dislocations of the Glenohumeral Joint"), referral to an orthopaedist is indicated. Surgical treatment usually is indicated and entails reduction of the dislocated humeral head followed by reduction and stabilization of the associated fracture(s). On occasion, a primary prosthetic replacement is necessary if the articular surface is badly damaged or if its blood supply is interrupted.

FRACTURES OF THE SHAFT OF THE HUMERUS

Fractures of the shaft of the humerus may be transverse, oblique, or spiral, as well as complete, incomplete, or comminuted. They may also be closed or open. Alignment and apposition are often satisfactory when the arm is dependent, but occasionally displacement or angulation are unacceptable. Associated neurovascular injury is not uncommon. The radial nerve is particularly vulnerable because of its proximity to the humeral shaft (Fig. 2.35).

Clinical Characteristics

The injury is caused by a significant direct or indirect force applied to the humeral shaft. The arm is visibly swollen, frequently deformed, and extremely painful. When the fracture is complete, the arm is mobile, and bony crepitus is felt with any manipulation of the arm. The area is exquisitely tender to local palpation. A few days after injury, ecchymosis and edema are visible over the dependent elbow and forearm areas. Anteroposterior and lateral x-rays of the arm (which should include the shoulder joint above and the elbow articulation below) confirm the presence of the fracture and define its configuration and position.

Treatment

Open fractures should be referred immediately to an orthopaedist for definitive care. Regarding closed fractures, the presence of a strong radial pulse should be confirmed; if absent, the arm should be splinted and an orthopaedic consultation should be obtained. Radial, ulnar, and median nerve function should be assessed; if evidence of peripheral nerve dysfunction is noted, the fracture should be splinted and an orthopaedist consulted. The fracture is immobilized with two well-padded plaster splints (Fig. 2.36). The first is applied over the lateral aspect of the shoulder and upper arm, under the flexed elbow, and up the inner aspect of the upper arm to the axilla. A posterior splint is then added, running over the posterior aspect of the shoulder and upper arm, under the elbow, and along the ulnar aspect of the forearm to the metacarpal-phalangeal portion of the hand. The two splints are held in place with Ace bandages applied from the hand to the axillary aspect of the upper arm. The splints are allowed to set with the elbow in 90° of flexion and the forearm in neutral rotation. The arm is then allowed to hang dependently with either a sling or a collar and cuff for support. Usually the weight of the arm and the splints hanging

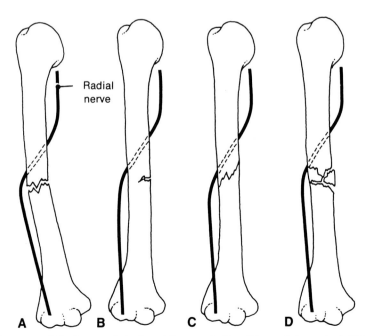

Figure 2.35. Fractures of the humeral shaft and the proximity of the radial nerve. *A*, transverse complete. *B*, transverse incomplete. *C*, oblique undisplaced. *D*, comminuted.

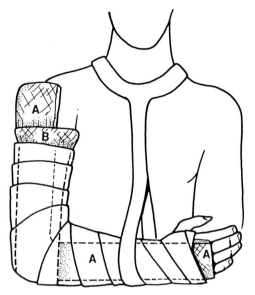

Figure 2.36. Immobilization of humeral shaft fractures using one long-arm posterior splint (*A*) and one medial-lateral splint (*B*). The arm is further supported by a sling or a collar and cuff dressing, and allowed to hang dependently.

in a dependent mode will affect an adequate reduction of the fracture. Postsplinting x-rays of the fracture site in the AP and lateral planes should be obtained, and if the position is unsatisfactory (unacceptable displacement, distraction or angulation), an orthopaedic consultation should be obtained. If the reduction is satisfactory, referral to an orthopaedist should be arranged for subsequent care.

If neurovascular and, in particular, radial nerve function are lost following the reduction of the fracture and splint immobilization, an orthopaedic consultation is clearly indicated. It is possible that the radial nerve is impaled by or caught between the fracture fragments during the maneuver, in which case immediate surgical exploration must be considered. Average healing time for these fractures is 8 weeks; however, delayed union and nonunion are not uncommon.

FRACTURES OF THE SCAPULA (FIG. 2.37)

Fractures of the scapula account for only 1% of all fractures. The vast majority (90+%)

are insignificantly displaced and are managed symptomatically (a sling for comfort, local ice followed by moist heat, analgesic medications, gradual increase in use of the shoulder as symptoms allow, etc.). Bony union is complete by 6 weeks and a good to excellent functional result can be expected. Scapular fractures, however, are usually the result of high-energy (usually direct but occasionally indirect) trauma and therefore have an 80 to 95% incidence of associated osseous and soft tissue injuries (local and distant) that can be major, multiple, or even life-threatening. These individuals should be carefully evaluated when they present in the emergency room, and appropriate supportive care must be rendered.

Localized signs and symptoms may direct one's attention to the area. However, most scapular fractures are detected incidentally on the patient's admission chest radiograph. A "scapular trauma series" consisting of true AP and lateral views of the scapula as well as a true axillary projection of the glenohumeral joint (supplemented by a weightbearing

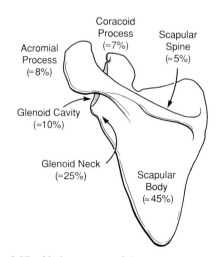

Figure 2.37. Various areas of the scapula that may be fractured and their relative frequency: scapular body, approximately 45%; glenoid process, approximately 35% (glenoid neck, approximately 25%; glenoid rim and fossa, approximately 10%); acromial process, approximately 8%; coracoid process, approximately 7%; scapular spine, approximately 5%.

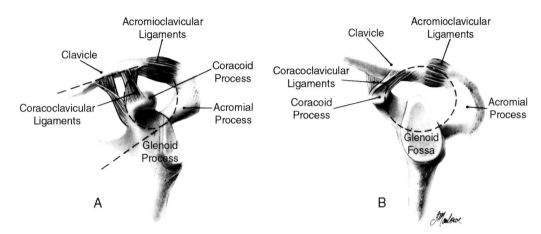

Figure 2.38. The superior shoulder suspensory complex. *A,* its appearance in the AP plane and *B,* its appearance laterally.

AP of the shoulder if a disruption of the clavicular-scapular linkage is suspected) should be obtained. Because of the complex bony anatomy in the area, however, CT scanning may be necessary to accurately define the injury. One must be able to visualize and evaluate the scapular body and the glenoid, coracoid, and acromial processes. (One should look for and aggressively treat serious associated injuries such as multiple rib fractures resulting in a flail chest; hemothorax and/or pneumothorax; myocardial contusion; aortic tears; etc.).

Fractures of the scapular body and spine comprise 50% of such injuries. Although multiple fracture lines with varying degrees of displacement may be present, these injuries are invariably treated nonoperatively/symptomatically as outlined in preceding text. Fractures of the glenoid process usually are managed nonoperatively as well. However, significantly displaced fractures of the glenoid fossa, the glenoid rim, or the glenoid neck may require surgical management to ensure union, avoid posttraumatic degenerative joint disease or glenohumeral instability, and restore normal shoulder biomechanics. If one is uncertain, evaluation by an orthopaedist is indicated. Isolated fractures of the coracoid and acromial processes are usually minimally displaced and managed nonoperatively/symptomatically as discussed previously. Significant displacement, however, may occur if there is a second disruption of the superior shoulder suspensory complex (Fig. 2.38). If this occurs, referral to an orthopaedist is indicated, because surgical reduction and stabilization of one or both disruption sites are necessary.

SUGGESTED READINGS

Bateman JE. The Shoulder and Neck. 2nd ed. Philadelphia: WB Saunders, 1978.
Crenshaw AH, ed. Campbell's Operative Orthopedics. 8th ed. St. Louis: Mosby Yearbook, 1992.
DePalma AF. Surgery of the Shoulder. 3rd ed. Philadelphia: Lippincott and Co., 1983.
Evarts CM, ed. Surgery of the Musculoskeletal System. 2nd ed. New York: Churchill Livingstone, 1990.
Neer CS II. Shoulder Reconstruction. Philadelphia: WB Saunders, 1990.
Post, M. The Shoulder. 2nd ed. Philadelphia: Lea & Febiger, 1988.
Rockwood CA Jr, Green DP, eds. Fractures. 4th ed. Philadelphia: JB Lippincott, 1996.
Rockwood CA Jr, Matsen FA III, eds. The Shoulder. Philadelphia: WB Saunders, 1990.
Rowe CR, ed. The Shoulder. New York: Churchill and Livingstone, 1987.
Tachdjian MO. Pediatric Orthopedics. 2nd ed. Philadelphia: WB Saunders, 1990.

Elbow and Forearm

William J. Morgan, M.D.

ESSENTIAL ANATOMY

SKELETAL ANATOMY

The distal end of the humerus forms a complex articulation with the proximal radius and ulna to form the elbow joint (Fig. 3.1). The capitellum and trochlea form the lateral and medial articulating condyles of the humerus respectively. These articulating condyles are rotated 30° anteriorly with respect to the long axis of the humerus. The capitellum is sphere shaped, providing axial rotation in its articulation with the radius. The trochlea has a grooved surface into which the proximal ulna fits to provide flexion and extension.

Located just above the articular surface of the trochlea are the anterior coronoid fossa and the posterior olecranon fossa. These accommodate the coronoid in full flexion and the olecranon in full extension. The coronoid and olecranon fossae are bordered medially and laterally by the supracondylar bony columns, which end as the lateral and medial epicondyles.

There is approximately a 6 to 8° valgus tilt of the distal humeral articular surface. The long axis of the ulna is in valgus with respect to the long axis of the humerus. This angulation is called the carrying angle and shows some variation with respect to age and sex. The "normal" carrying angle is approximately 15°.

The proximal radius is a concave articular disc with articular cartilage covering approximately 240° of the outside circumference of the radial head. This provides articulation with the capitellum and the proximal ulna in rotation. Distal to the radial head and proxi-mal to the shaft of the radius is a narrowed portion called the neck of the radius. This area is stabilized by the annular ligament in rotation (Fig. 3.2). The radial tuberosity is the distal landmark for the neck of the radius and is the site of attachment of the biceps tendon. The radial tuberosity also provides a valuable landmark in aligning midshaft fractures of the radius. Distally, the radius flares to form articulations with the carpus and the distal ulna. The radiocarpal joint is comprised of the scaphoid fossa adjacent to the radial styloid and the lunate fossa located distally and ulnarly. On the distal ulnar surface of the radius is the concave semilunar facet, which provides rotation about the ulna at the distal radioulnar joint (Fig. 3.3). The proximal ulnar articulating surface is known as the sigmoid notch, which articulates with the trochlea of the humerus and is bordered posteriorly by the olecranon and anteriorly by the coronoid process. Just lateral to the sigmoid notch is a concave articulation of approximately 70° known as the lesser sigmoid notch. This forms the articulation of the circumference of the radial head in rotation. The lesser sigmoid notch is positioned perpendicular to the greater sigmoid notch.

The shaft of the ulna is somewhat narrowed compared with the proximal ulna, but distally flares to form the head of the ulna. This is comprised of the ulnar styloid and the convex distal ulna, which is covered with articular cartilage for 270° of its total circumference (Fig. 3.3). This articulation with the sigmoid notch of the distal radius allows rotation of the distal radius around the ulnar head.

In full supination the radius and ulna are aligned in a somewhat parallel position and

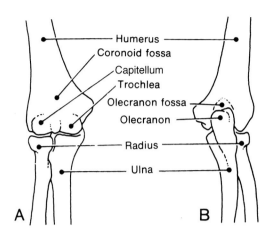

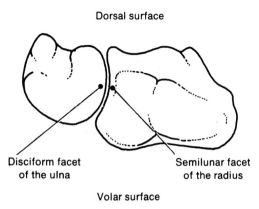

Dorsal surface

Disciform facet of the ulna

Semilunar facet of the radius

Volar surface

Figure 3.3. Distal end of the radioulnar joint—forearm in midrotation.

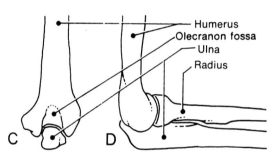

Figure 3.1. The elbow joint. *A*, anterior view. *B*, posterior view *C*, posterior view, 90° flexion. *D*, lateral view.

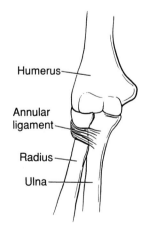

Figure 3.2. Annular ligament.

form a rectangle with respect to their proximal and distal articulations. In full pronation, the distal radius rotates around the distal ulnar head, causing the radial shaft to cross over the anterior immobile ulnar shaft (Fig. 3.4).

LIGAMENTOUS AND CAPSULAR ANATOMY

The joint capsule makes its proximal attachments along the superior margin of the coronoid fossa anteriorly and along the superior margin of the olecranon fossa posteriorly (Fig. 3.5). The anterior capsule is thin and renders little stability to the elbow. The anterior capsule then makes its distal attachments along the articular margin of the trochlea medially and along the radial neck, blending into the annular ligament laterally. Posteriorly, the capsule makes its distal attachments to the medial and lateral margins of the trochlea.

The ligaments of the elbow are specialized thickenings of the capsule. The medial collateral ligament complex consists of three parts: the anterior bundle, posterior bundle, and transverse ligament (Fig. 3.5B). The anterior bundle makes up the major portion of the medial ligament complex and takes its origin just inferior to the medial apophysis and inserts into the medial aspect of the coronoid process. The lateral ligament complex is made up of the radial collateral ligament and the lateral ulnar collateral ligament (Fig. 3.5C). The lateral ligament complex is not so well defined as the medial complex and appears to be more of a capsular blend. It takes its origin from the lateral epicondyle apophysis and attaches to the annular ligament of the radius distally. The annular ligament has its origin and insertion on the anterior and posterior

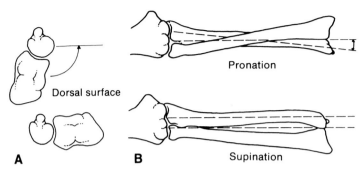

Figure 3.4.   Movement of the radius and ulna during rotation of the forearm. *A*, semilunar facet of the distal end of the radius slides around the disciform facet of the distal end of the ulna. *B*, the ulna diverges 8 to 9° away from the longitudinal axis of the forearm during rotation from full supination to full pronation.

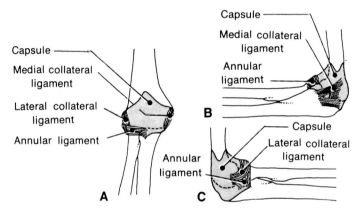

Figure 3.5.   Articular capsule of the elbow joint. *A*, anterior view. *B*, medial view. *C*, lateral view.

margins of the lesser sigmoid notch. It contains the radial head adjacent to the ulna, prevents anterior-posterior subluxation, and stabilizes the rotation of the radius on the capitellum (Fig. 3.2).

The distal radioulnar joint is stabilized by the proximal aspect of the triangular fibrocartilage complex. This complex arises from the ulnar aspect of the lunate fossa of the distal radius and extends ulnarward to the base of the ulnar styloid. The dorsal and volar portions of the triangular fibrocartilage complex are thickened and form the poorly defined dorsal and volar radioulnar ligaments. The carpus is then stabilized to the distal radioulnar joint by the strong volar and weak dorsal perpendicular arms of the triangular fibrocartilage complex.

BURSAE AND MUSCLES

Twelve bursae have been reported to occur about the elbow joint, with three showing consistent clinical significance (Fig. 3.6). The olecranon bursa is situated posteriorly between the skin and the olecranon, allowing smooth gliding of the skin on the triceps tendon. The bicipitoradial bursa lies in the angle between the radial tuberosity and the insertion of the biceps tendon, allowing smooth gliding of the tendon on the surface of the bone. The radiohumeral bursa lies deep to the common extensor tendon attachments to the lateral epicondyle, inferior to the extensor carpi radialis brevis, and superficial to the radiocapitellar joint capsule. This allows gliding of the extensor origin over the radiocapitellar capsule.

Many muscles take their origin and insertion about the elbow and forearm. On the anterior aspect of the elbow (Fig. 3.7), the deepest elbow flexor is the brachialis muscle. This muscle crosses the anterior capsule, with some fibers inserting into the capsule and the final insertion of the brachialis tendon into the coronoid process. The biceps muscle overlies the brachialis and has two insertions. The bicipital aponeurosis, the lacertus fibrosis, inserts into the anterior medial muscle fascia of the proximal forearm. The distal biceps tendon then attaches to the posterior aspect of the radial tuberosity,

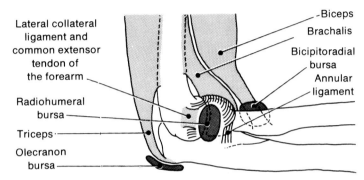

Lateral collateral ligament and common extensor tendon of the forearm

Radiohumeral bursa

Triceps

Olecranon bursa

Biceps

Brachalis

Bicipitoradial bursa

Annular ligament

Figure 3.6. Three elbow bursae. The lateral collateral ligament and common extensor tendon have been reflected away to expose the radiohumeral bursa.

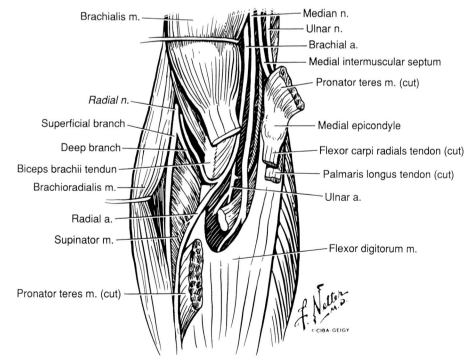

Brachialis m.

Radial n.

Superficial branch

Deep branch

Biceps brachii tendun

Brachioradialis m.

Radial a.

Supinator m.

Pronator teres m. (cut)

Median n.

Ulnar n.

Brachial a.

Medial intermuscular septum

Pronator teres m. (cut)

Medial epicondyle

Flexor carpi radials tendon (cut)

Palmaris longus tendon (cut)

Ulnar a.

Flexor digitorum m.

Figure 3.7. Anatomy of anterior elbow. (Copyright 1987 CIBA-GEIGY Corporation. Adapted with permission from the Ciba Collection of medical illustrations by Frank Netter, M.D. All rights reserved.)

acting as an elbow flexor and forearm supinator. Both the brachialis and biceps muscles are innervated by the musculocutaneous nerve. Also acting as an elbow flexor is the brachioradialis, which takes its origin along the lateral supracondylar region of the distal humerus and goes on to insert into the radial styloid. The extensor carpi radialis longus (ECRL) and brevis (ECRB) also take their origins from the lateral supracondylar ridge of the distal humerus, with the ECRB finding origin on the inferior surface of the lateral epicondyle. The ECRB is covered by the extensor carpi radialis longus at the level just distal to the lateral epicondyle. The brachioradialis, ECRL, and ECRB make up the "mobile wad of Henry" and are innervated by the radial nerve proximal to its bifurcation.

The extensor digitorum communis originates from the lateral epicondyle and is innervated by the deep branch of the radial nerve. The extensor carpi ulnaris originates from two heads—the lateral epicondyle and the aponeurosis of the anconeus muscle. Also, the extensor carpi ulnaris is innervated by the deep branch of the radial nerve. The supinator muscle is an important forearm rotator that is a rhomboid-shaped muscle originating from the lateral aspect of the lateral epicondyle, the lateral collateral ligament, and the proximal ulna. This muscle then runs obliquely to insert in the proximal one-third of the radius along its dorsal surface. Its innervation is derived from the posterior interosseous nerve as the nerve traverses through the substance of the muscle.

The triceps muscle originates from three separate heads, two of which arise from the posterior aspect of the humerus. The long head has its origin in the infraglenoid tuberosity of the scapula. The three heads then form a common expansion that inserts into the olecranon, thus acting as the primary elbow extensor. The triceps is innervated by the radial nerve. The anconeus muscle is a small oblique muscle running from the lateral epicondyle into the lateral aspect of the olecranon; its function has been debated, but it appears to act as a joint stabilizer.

The flexor pronator muscle group consists of the pronator teres, flexor carpi radialis, palmaris longus, flexor carpi ulnaris, and flexor digitorum superficialis (Fig. 3.7). This muscle group originates from the medial epicondyle and the proximal ulna. The pronator teres inserts into the radius beneath the brachioradialis muscle at the junction of the proximal and middle thirds of the radius, thus acting as a strong pronator of the forearm. The pronator teres, flexor carpi radialis, palmaris longus, and flexor digitorum superficialis are innervated by the median nerve, whereas the flexor carpi ulnaris muscle is innervated by the ulnar nerve. The flexor digitorum profundus muscle originates from the proximal ulna and does not cross the elbow joint. The muscle bellies contributing to the flexor digitorum profundus tendons to the index and long fingers are innervated by the median nerve, and those contributing to the ring and small fingers are innervated by the ulnar nerve.

INNERVATION AND BLOOD SUPPLY

The brachial artery enters the antecubital fossa medial to the brachialis muscle anteriorly and medial to the biceps tendon distally. This artery is crossed in the antecubital fossa by the median nerve and comes to lie lateral to the nerve. At the level of the radial head, the brachial artery bifurcates into the radial and ulnar arteries (Fig. 3.7). The radial artery then emerges from the antecubital space between the brachioradialis and pronator teres muscles and continues down the forearm under the brachioradialis muscle. The ulnar artery emerges between the two heads of the pronator teres and runs distally down the forearm beneath the flexor carpi ulnaris muscle.

The median nerve accompanies the brachial artery into the antecubital fossa, after crossing to a position medial to the artery. At this point, the median nerve passes under the bicipital aponeurosis and between the humeral and ulnar heads of the pronator teres muscle. Before diving beneath the flexor digitorum superficialis arch, the median nerve gives off the branch of the anterior interosseous nerve and then runs distally in the forearm beneath the flexor digitorum superficialis muscle belly. The radial nerve emerges from the lateral intermuscular septum at the junction of the middle and distal thirds of the humerus. At the lateral elbow, the radial nerve lies between the brachialis muscle and the brachioradialis, ECRL, and ECRB muscle bellies. At the level of the radial head, the nerve bifurcates, with the superficial branch continuing on down the forearm beneath the brachioradialis muscle belly. This branch supplies sensation to the dorsoradial aspect of the hand. At the bifurcation, the deep branch, or the posterior interosseous nerve, dives beneath the arcade of the Frohse into the supinator muscle belly from which it emerges distally. This deep branch then branches to innervate the extensor muscles of the fingers and thumb.

The ulnar nerve emerges from the medial intermuscular septum and runs along the muscle belly of the triceps and into the cubital tunnel, which lies just posterior to the medial epicondyle. This nerve splits the two proximal heads of the flexor carpi ulnaris muscle and runs distally in the forearm between the flexor digitorum profundus and the flexor carpi ulnaris muscle bellies. The ulnar nerve's entrance into Guyon's canal is described in Chapter 4, "Wrist and Hand."

INFLAMMATORY AND OVERUSE DISORDERS OF THE ELBOW AND FOREARM

LATERAL EPICONDYLITIS

Lateral epicondylitis is an overuse syndrome of the upper extremity. Although called "tennis elbow," it is seen in many competitive athletes who use the upper extremity (e.g., tennis, baseball, and golf players). Tennis elbow is also a common complaint from individuals whose occupations require repetitious extension of the wrist or rotation of the forearm (e.g., carpenters, electricians, etc.).

Although the exact cause of lateral epicondylitis is unclear, it presents as an inflammatory process at the extensor origin at the lateral epicondyle, most specifically at the origin of the extensor carpi radialis brevis.

Clinical Characteristics

The patient with lateral epicondylitis presents with pain, generally felt at the lateral epicondyle; but if the problem is chronic, referred pain to the extensor surface of the forearm may be noted (Fig. 3.8). This pain is intensified by palpation over the lateral epicondyle, particularly along the anterior edge at the origin of the extensor carpi radialis brevis. There is full range of motion of the elbow and wrist without weakness, but the pain is exacerbated by resisted extension of the wrist or fingers with the elbow in extension. Pain also may be exacerbated by passively flexing the fingers and wrist with the elbow fully extended. In advanced cases, swelling and erythema may be present about the lateral epicondyle. X-rays are usually normal and are not routinely recommended. Calcific deposits may be noted adjacent to the lateral epicondyle in chronic cases.

Radial tunnel syndrome or posterior interosseous nerve syndrome is frequently misdiagnosed as lateral epicondylitis. Radial nerve entrapment also may occur coincident with lateral epicondylitis. The pain caused by radial tunnel syndrome can generally be produced

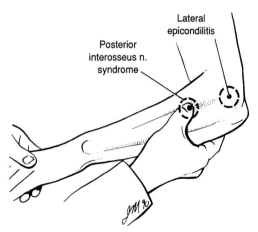

Figure 3.8. Areas of palpation to differentiate lateral epicondylitis from posterior interosseous nerve syndrome.

by forearm supination with the elbow flexed. In radial tunnel syndrome, there is also pain to palpation in the area between the mobile wad and the extensor digitorum communis just distal to the radial head (the area where the posterior interosseous nerve enters the supinator). Electromyographic studies usually are not helpful in the differentiation because there is a high incidence of false-negative results in radial tunnel syndrome. Other entities that may show similar presentations must be ruled out, including cervical spondylosis with cervical root compression and intra-articular abnormalities of the elbow.

Treatment

Treatment of lateral epicondylitis is related to the severity and chronicity of the problem at the time of presentation. In the acute onset with mild to moderate pain, nonsteroidal anti-inflammatory medications are recommended in conjunction with rest of the extremity and avoidance of aggravating activities. A counterforce brace about the proximal forearm may decrease the force absorbed at the lateral epicondyle. Immobilization of the wrist in a volar splint is helpful in alleviating repetitious flexion and extension activities of the wrist.

Physical therapy may be helpful in the early stages of lateral epicondylitis with the use of stretching, heat modalities, and activity modification. Steroid phonophoresis and steroid iontophoresis may be helpful modalities in the treatment of lateral epicondylitis, but their efficiency has not been proven.

If physical therapy treatment is ineffective, a cortisone injection using 1 mL of 1% Xylocaine and 20 mg of triamcinolone is appropriate. This is injected in the area just anterior to the lateral epicondyle below the origin of the extensor brevis muscle. Care must be taken to avoid intradermal injections, and the patient must be warned of subcutaneous atrophy or pigmentation changes after injection of cortisone. No more than three injections are advisable.

Once the acute inflammatory response has been controlled and the patient's pain has been relieved, a rehabilitation program should be in-

stituted. The patient should be protected in the early parts of rehabilitation with a counterforce brace, a canvas or Velcro strap that fits around the proximal forearm. A graduated exercise program is instituted, which includes specific rehabilitation exercises and the gradual resumption of the patient's usual activities. This exercise program is done in conjunction with stretching exercises (Fig. 3.9). In cases of lateral epicondylitis related to sports activities, alterations in technique or equipment may be helpful in preventing recurrences. If the patient's symptoms are recalcitrant to the above treatment or if symptoms recur with resumption of the patient's usual activities, referral should be made to an orthopaedist for potential surgical treatment.

MEDIAL EPICONDYLITIS

Clinical Characteristics

Many athletes and laborers note the onset of pain on the medial aspect of the elbow overlying the medial epicondyle, similar to the onset of lateral epicondylitis. This appears to arise from repeated flexion activities of the wrist and fingers, thus initiating increased stresses at the flexor pronator origin.

In the physical evaluation, one must differentiate medial epicondylitis from cubital tunnel syndrome, i.e., ulnar nerve entrapment at the elbow. In medial epicondylitis, pain is elicited by direct palpation of the bony prominence of the medial epicondyle and anterior to the medial epicondyle at the flexor pronator origin. Pain is exacerbated by resisted flexion of the fingers and swelling and erythema may occur at the medial epicondyle. In a like manner, patients with cubital tunnel syndrome may present with medial elbow and forearm pain. In contrast to medial epicondylitis, there is a positive Tinel sign over the ulnar nerve. The nerve may be subluxable. Paresthesias of the ulnar nerve may be elicited by prolonged elbow flexion in cubital tunnel syndrome. Electromyography may help in problematic clinical cases.

Treatment

The treatment for medial epicondylitis is similar to that for lateral epicondylitis, starting

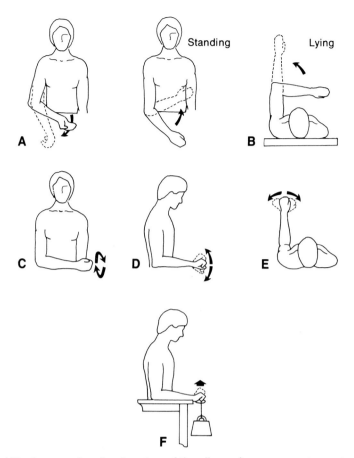

Figure 3.9. Rehabilitation exercises for disorders of the elbow. *A*, common extensor tendon stretching for mild tennis elbow. *B*, acute flexion/extension with and against gravity. *C*, unopposed forearm rotation. *D* and *E*, range of motion exercises for the wrist. *F*, common extensor strengthening exercise.

with rest and anti-inflammatory medication, then proceeding to steroid phonophoresis, local steroid installation (great care must be taken to avoid injection into the adjacent ulnar nerve), and orthopaedic referral in recalcitrant cases.

BURSITIS

Many deep bursae about the elbow have been described, and these were reviewed in the "Essential Anatomy" section. Although any one of these bursae has the potential of becoming inflamed, by far, the most common presentation is olecranon bursitis.

Olecranon Bursitis

Olecranon bursitis is the most common superficial bursitis presenting about the elbow. The treatment of olecranon bursitis depends on its etiology, pathology, and chronicity.

Clinical Characteristics.

The onset of painless swelling of the olecranon bursa is usually the result of direct or indirect trauma, namely repetitive stresses such as "student's elbow" or "miner's elbow" or direct contact as in football players who play on artificial surfaces. Full range of motion of the elbow is usually present, but with a very swollen bursa, flexion may be limited as a result of pain from compression of the distended bursa.

In patients presenting with a painful olecranon bursitis, differentiation between inflammatory and septic causes must be made. Systemic inflammatory processes associated with olecranon bursitis include gout, hydroxyapatite crystal deposition, chondrocalcinosis, and rheumatoid arthritis. In cases of rheumatoid arthritis, there may be a direct communication of the elbow joint with the bursa. To further make this differentiation, it is imperative that painful swelling of the olecranon bursa, particularly when associated with erythema, be aspirated. This should be done under sterile conditions as noted previously. Diagnosis can be made by analyzing the fluid for leukocyte count, Gram stain, and culture and sensitivity testing. The fluid should also be analyzed for crystals in those cases where a crystalline inflammatory process is suspected.

Treatment

Treatment of aseptic bursitis consists of taking anti-inflammatory medication, resting the elbow in a splint, and using compressive elastic wraps. Aspiration may be combined with the above treatment protocol for very swollen bursae. After sterile preparation, an 18-gauge needle is inserted into the olecranon bursa laterally (Fig. 3.10). A direct approach into the tip of the elbow may lead to a chronic sinus tract. Upon completion of the aspiration, a compressive dressing should be applied and the extremity rested in a splint. In traumatic olecranon bursitis, the future use of el-

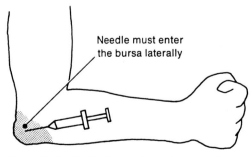

Figure 3.10. Aspiration and/or irrigation of the olecranon bursa space.

Needle must enter the bursa laterally

bow pads may be helpful. Recurrences are treated as described above. In recalcitrant cases, referral should be made to an orthopaedist for possible excision.

The treatment of olecranon bursitis associated with a systemic inflammatory process is directed at control of the underlying disease.

In cases of septic bursitis, treatment is initiated by aspiration and systemic antibiotics. Initial antibiotic treatment should be directed by the result of the Gram stain of the aspirate. Begin treatment with a broad-spectrum antibiotic. When the culture results are available, appropriate antibiotic modifications are made. Aspiration and irrigation are repeated upon re-accumulation of the fluid. In cases that do not respond to aspiration, irrigation, and systemic antibiotics, referral to an orthopaedist should be made for incision, drainage, and possible bursectomy.

INTERSECTION SYNDROME

Encountering an inflammatory tenosynovitis in the forearm is unusual, because there are no discrete tenosynovial compartments noted. One exception is the entity known as "intersection syndrome."

Clinical Characteristics

Intersection syndrome presents as pain and swelling over the dorsoradial aspect of the distal forearm in the area where the abductor pollicis longus and extensor pollicis brevis muscle bellies cross the extensor carpi radialis brevis and longus tendons. In advanced cases, intersection syndrome may be associated with erythema and crepitus. It may also be associated with tenosynovitis of the second dorsal compartment. Care must be taken to differentiate intersection syndrome from de Quervain tenosynovitis (described in Chapter 4).

Treatment

The initial conservative treatment consists of rest by immobilizing the wrist in a cock-up splint in approximately 15° of extension. Anti-inflammatory medication is useful, and in more advanced cases, steroid phonophoresis or corticosteroid injection into the area of tenderness may be helpful. In more advanced cases or those resistant to conservative therapy, referral to an orthopaedist for surgical decompression may be necessary.

ENTRAPMENT NEUROPATHIES

Most entrapment and compression neuropathies about the elbow and forearm manifest themselves as pain and paresthesias in the hand. Some will also present as localized pain about the forearm and elbow itself. The following will be a review of radial and ulnar neuropathies about the elbow. Median nerve entrapment syndromes occur about the elbow and will be discussed in Chapter 4, "Wrist and Hand," with carpal tunnel syndrome.

CUBITAL TUNNEL SYNDROME

Entrapment of the ulnar nerve may occur in the cubital tunnel posterior to the medial epicondyle, more proximally at the intramuscular septum or more distally between the two heads of the flexor carpi ulnaris muscle belly (Fig. 3.11).

Clinical Characteristics

Ulnar nerve entrapment about the elbow generally presents as pain in the proximal ulnar aspect of the forearm and dysesthesias about the small and ulnar half of the ring fingers. Diagnosis is often made by palpation of the ulnar nerve at the medial epicondyle. Subluxation of the ulnar nerve over the medial epicondyle may exist associated with pain and paresthesias. A positive Tinel sign may be found at the cubital tunnel, proximally at the intramuscular septum or more distally at the entrance of the ulnar nerve into the flexor carpi ulnaris muscle. Decreased sensation in the ulnar nerve distribution may be found and should be evaluated by the moving two-point discrimination testing.

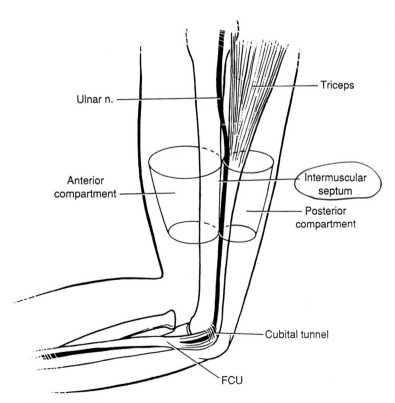

Figure 3.11.   Potential areas of ulna nerve entrapment around the elbow include the following: intermuscular septum, cubital tunnel, and two heads of flexor carpi ulnaris muscle belly.

In more severe cases, intrinsic wasting of the hand may be present, and first dorsal interosseous atrophy and a positive Froment sign may be apparent. The Froment sign is a manifestation of weakness of the adductor pollicis and the first dorsal interosseous muscle (innervated by the ulnar nerve). When asked to pinch a piece of paper between the thumb and index finger (key pinch), the patient with an ulnar neuropathy will attempt to compensate by use of the flexor pollicis longus muscle (innervated by the median nerve). This will result in hyperflexion of the thumb interphalangeal joint (Fig. 3.12).

The paresthesias of cubital tunnel syndrome may be elicited or exacerbated by elbow flexion; this is a helpful diagnostic maneuver. Electromyography and nerve conduction studies are also helpful diagnosing cubital tunnel syndrome.

Treatment

Conservative treatment of cubital tunnel syndrome consists of rest of the elbow, avoidance of compression of the ulna nerve (with an elbow pad), and avoidance of elbow hyperflexion. Treatment should be done in conjunction with nonsteroidal anti-inflammatory drugs (NSAIDs). Persistent pain, paresthesias, and evidence of intrinsic muscle wasting indicate prompt orthopaedic referral for surgical decompression.

RADIAL TUNNEL SYNDROME

Radial tunnel syndrome is most frequently caused by a compression neuropathy of the posterior interosseous nerve at the arcade of Frohse as it enters the proximal border of the supinator muscle.

Clinical Characteristics

The clinical presentation of this syndrome is most commonly aching pain along the extensor surface of the forearm and hand, as well as pain about the elbow at the site of the posterior interosseous nerve entrapment. This proximal location often makes it difficult to differentiate it from the pain of tennis elbow. If fascicles of the superficial branch of the radial nerve are involved, there may be dysesthesias or decreased sensation along the dorsoradial aspect of the wrist and hand.

Diagnosis is often difficult to make and must be differentiated from tennis elbow or a cervical radiculopathy. Deep palpation approximately 4 cm distal to the lateral epicondyle between the heads of the extensor digitorum communis and extensor carpi radialis brevis muscle bellies elicits pain and paresthesias duplicating the patient's clinical presentation (Fig. 3.13). This pain should be out of proportion to palpation of the contralateral limb. Resisted supination from a fully pronated position may also duplicate the presenting pain. Injection of 0.25% Sensorcaine into the area of the posterior interosseous nerve and arcade of Frohse may be diagnostic if the patient has relief of symptoms for a few hours postinjection. In severe cases of posterior interosseous nerve entrapment, weakness of finger extensors may be present and is diagnostic. Electromyography and nerve

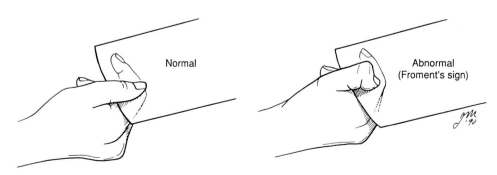

Figure 3.12.   Normal key pinch versus Froment's sign.

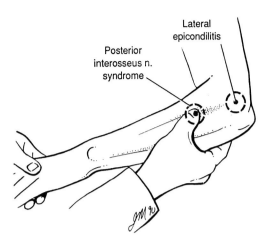

Figure 3.13. Areas of palpation to differentiate lateral epicondylitis from posterior interosseous nerve syndrome.

conduction studies have not been helpful in the diagnosis of radial tunnel syndrome because false-negative results occur frequently.

Treatment

Conservative treatment of radial tunnel syndrome involves avoidance of overuse activities. For example, excessive supination and pronation, as seen with use of a screwdriver, may elicit these symptoms. Anti-inflammatory medication and short-term rest of the extensor muscles by a wrist splint may be helpful. If the symptoms persist after 2 weeks of conservative therapy or if weakness of the finger extensors is present, orthopaedic referral for probable surgical decompression is necessary.

WARTENBERG SYNDROME (CHEIRALGIA PARESTHETICA)

Wartenberg syndrome (cheiralgia paresthetica) represents an entrapment of the superficial radial nerve in the distal forearm.

Clinical Characteristics

Pain localized to the dorsoradial aspect of the distal forearm with paresthesias in the distribution of the superficial branch of the radial nerve is characteristic of Wartenberg syndrome. The syndrome may be iatrogenic or secondary to injury. Tight watchbands and

bracelets have been associated with this syndrome.

Treatment

Treatment involves relieving any obvious extrinsic compressive devices and short-term wrist immobilization. In cases in which conservative treatment is ineffective, orthopaedic referral is necessary for surgical exploration.

TRAUMATIC DISORDERS OF THE ELBOW AND FOREARM

Fractures and dislocations occurring about the elbow and forearm are common in children and adults. These represent severe and complex injuries and frequently require orthopaedic referral. These injuries are plagued by the potential for severe and deforming complications. In the primary care setting, the initial recognition and treatment of these injuries may determine the outcome of a gratifying recovery or permanent disability. Most nondisplaced fractures about the elbow and forearm can be treated by the primary care physician. In this section, the author will describe most of the injuries and recommend a level of responsibility that the primary physician should assume for each. Potential complications and the steps to avoid complications in the initial treatment will be described.

Understanding the bony anatomy as well as the chronologic occurrence of the ossification centers about the elbow is imperative to the diagnosis and treatment of these injuries. The presence of an ossification center or the irregular appearance of such a center on x-ray may be misinterpreted as a fracture (Fig. 3.14).

FRACTURES OF THE DISTAL HUMERUS

Fractures of the distal humerus in the adult usually represent complex high-energy injuries that are peri- and intra-articular, and are often displaced and therefore not amenable to nonsurgical treatment. These fractures are frequently associated with capitellum fractures, intercondylar fractures, trochlea fractures, or comminuted T condylar fractures with a supracondylar extension (Fig. 3.15).

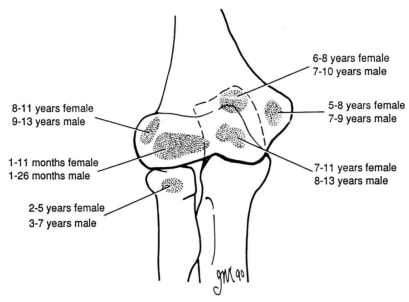

Figure 3.14.   Ossific nuclei about the elbow and age of appearance.

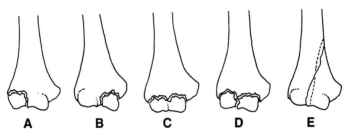

Figure 3.15.   Fractures of the articular surfaces of the condyles, anterior view. *A*, fracture of the capitulum. *B*, fracture of the trochlea. *C*, transverse intercondylar fracture. *D*, T-shaped intercondylar fracture. *E*, spiral fracture.

Clinical Characteristics

These fractures are usually the result of a high-energy injury such as a fall from a significant height or a motor vehicle accident. Most patients will present with clinical deformity of the elbow. Neurovascular examination must be carefully performed, because associated injuries to the brachial artery as well as the median, radial, and ulnar nerves are not uncommon. In nondisplaced fractures about the elbow, radiographic analysis may demonstrate a fat pad sign (Fig. 3.16). The fat pad sign is caused by joint distension from the intra-articular hematoma displacing the fat

that is lining the inner surface of the brachialis muscle anteriorly.

Treatment

Nondisplaced Fractures

The nondisplaced fracture can be treated definitively by the primary care physician by immobilization in a posterior elbow splint at 90° of flexion and the forearm in neutral rotation. Careful neurovascular checks should be made during the first week. If the fracture remains nondisplaced after the first week of immobilization, the patient should be placed in a long-arm circumferential cast with the elbow at 90° of flexion and the forearm in neutral rotation. Cast immobilization should be continued for another 3 to 5 weeks as dictated by radiographic evidence of healing and clinical examination.

Upon removal of the cast, a supportive thermoplastic splint or a bivalve cast should be fabricated to be used while the patient begins rehabilitation. Active and active-assisted range of motion of elbow flexion, extension, supination, and pronation should be initiated. This range of motion therapy may be facilitated by the use of heat modalities such as hot packs or warm soaks. Gentle passive motion may be needed if active-assisted range of motion fails to regain a full arc of motion. Care must be taken to avoid painful passive stretch because it may exacerbate the formation of heterotopic ossification about the elbow.

Once maximal range of motion has been achieved, the splint may be discontinued and strengthening exercises should be initiated. As the patient's strength approaches that of pre-injury, a return to full activities is allowed.

Displaced Fractures

Displaced distal humerus fractures require anatomic reduction and therefore should be referred to an orthopaedist for operative reduction and, most likely, internal fixation. The patient should be placed in a posterior splint for transport to the orthopaedist.

FRACTURES OF THE MEDIAL EPICONDYLE

These fractures are thought to represent an avulsion injury by the flexor-pronator mass from its origin at the medial epicondyle.

Clinical Characteristics

The patient presents with posttraumatic pain, swelling, and tenderness over the medial aspect of the elbow. Undisplaced or minimally displaced fractures are defined as those displaced less than 1 cm from the anatomic position. Displaced fractures are defined as those displaced greater than 1 cm from the anatomic position or displaced into the joint. Associated neurovascular compromise usually is manifested as an ulnar neuropathy, and the appropriate examination of the ulnar nerve should be performed when confronted with this injury. The degree of instability of the medial elbow must be ascertained. Gross instability may be apparent by a valgus resting posture of the elbow. If not, the elbow should be stressed in valgus by flexing the elbow approximately 20°, stabilizing the lateral elbow with one hand and pulling the forearm in a valgus direction with the other hand. Because the normal ligamentous laxity varies from one individual to another, comparison with the unaffected elbow is necessary.

Treatment

The treatment of the fracture is based on the degree of displacement and the presence of instability.

Undisplaced or Minimally Displaced Fractures

The primary care physician can treat this fracture by immobilization in a splint or cast. As this injury is an avulsion injury by the flexor-pronator mass, it is best held reduced by flexion of the wrist and pronation of the

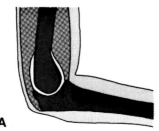   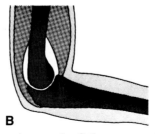

A   **B**

Figure 3.16. Diagrammatic illustration of the fat pad sign. *A*, normal soft tissue x-ray of elbow, lateral projection. *B*, soft tissue x-ray of elbow with fluid in joint, lateral projection.

forearm. During and after application of the immobilization device, frequent neurovascular examinations must be performed.

Displaced Fractures

Those fractures displaced greater than 1 cm or unstable to valgus stress require closed or open reduction. The primary care physician may attempt a closed reduction by manipulation of the medial epicondyle fragment with the elbow flexed, the forearm pronated, and the wrist flexed (Fig. 3.17). Closed reduction is often unsuccessful, and if so, referral to the orthopaedic surgeon should be made.

FRACTURES OF THE RADIAL HEAD

Fractures of the radial head usually occur as a result of a fall onto the outstretched hand with the elbow partially flexed and forearm pronated. This type of fall usually results in a valgus force at the elbow causing compression forces to the radial head. When evaluating a patient with a radial head fracture, it is important to consider more serious associated injur-

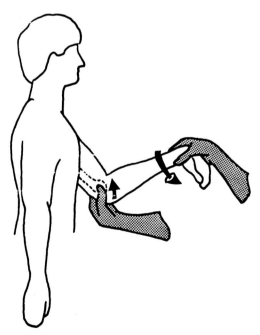

Figure 3.17. Closed reduction of the displaced fracture of the medial epicondyle.

ies such as an elbow dislocation with subsequent relocation, interruption of the interosseous membrane and distal radial ulnar joint (Essex Lopresti fracture complex), and injury to the medial ligamentous complex of the elbow.

Clinical Characteristics

The patient will present with limited motion of the elbow caused by pain and an associated effusion (hemarthrosis) of the elbow. Examination will demonstrate pain to supination and pronation and pain to palpation of the radial head. Further examination should be done to rule out medial elbow injury as well as injury to the distal radioulnar joint.

Radiographs of the elbow may not demonstrate evidence of injury to the radial head. Under these circumstances, one should look for a positive fat pad sign (Figure 3.16), which indicates a hemarthrosis. If positive, a high index of suspicion for a radial head fracture should be noted, and plans for follow-up x-rays within 1 week should be made. Displaced fractures will be seen radiographically, and definitive treatment will be based on these findings.

Treatment

Nondisplaced Fractures

Patients will frequently present with a painful hemarthrosis with minimally displaced or nondisplaced fractures of the radial head. Aspiration of the hemarthrosis under sterile conditions through a posterior lateral portal and in conjunction with instillation of an anesthetic will alleviate significant discomfort and facilitate further examination. Nondisplaced or minimally displaced fractures should be protected in a removable posterior splint or in a sling, depending on the anticipated compliance of the patient. Active elbow and forearm range of motion in the planes of flexion, extension, and supination and pronation is begun immediately to minimize postinjury stiffness of the elbow. The patient is instructed not to lift with that extremity, and no passive range of motion is allowed. Follow-up radiographs should be obtained within 1 week to document that no further displacement has occurred. The elbow should be protected with either a splint or a sling. The patient should avoid any lifting activities for approximately 4 weeks, when early radiographic healing should be evident. At this point, gentle passive exercises may be initiated if necessary, and strengthening can begin as tolerated.

Displaced Intra-Articular Radial Head Fractures

Displaced fractures of the radial head will result in limited motion and degenerative changes of the radiocapitellar joint. These fractures should be referred to an orthopaedist for surgical reduction and fixation.

FRACTURES OF THE OLECRANON

Fractures of the olecranon often are caused by direct trauma to the elbow during a fall. They also may occur with avulsion of the olecranon by the triceps mechanism.

Clinical Characteristics

The patient presents with posttraumatic pain, swelling, and tenderness over the olecranon. Range of motion is usually limited. The ossification center for the olecranon appears at age 10 and is generally fused to the proximal ulna by age 16. Epiphyseal plates of the olecranon can persist into young adulthood. This should not be mistaken for a fracture of the olecranon, particularly in trauma cases. Persistent epiphyseal plates are generally bilateral,

and contralateral elbow films should be obtained if questionable.

Treatment

Treatment by the general practitioner depends on the degree of displacement and the location of the fracture. Undisplaced fractures of the olecranon or avulsion fractures at the tip of the olecranon (Fig. 3.18) with minimal displacement may be treated in a long-arm cast with the elbow flexed 30 to 60°, determined by the patient's comfort. Immobilization should continue for approximately 4 weeks, at which time guided rehabilitation should be instituted. Radiographs should be repeated 1 week after the initial fracture to be sure that displacement has not occurred. In significantly displaced avulsion fractures of the tip of the olecranon or in intra-articular displaced fractures, a posterior splint holding the elbow at 30° should be applied, and orthopaedic referral should be made for open reduction, internal fixation.

FRACTURES OF THE CORONOID PROCESS

Fractures of the coronoid process are generally caused by an avulsion injury by the brachialis muscle at its insertion into the ulna.

Clinical Characteristics

The patient presents with swelling about the elbow and pain in the antecubital fossa. Care must be taken to evaluate the stability of the elbow, because an associated elbow dislocation and relocation must be ruled out. A sudden, strong, resisted contraction of the

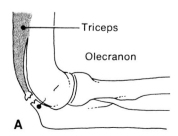 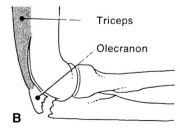

Figure 3.18. Fractures of the olecranon. *A*, lateral view. Avulsion fracture of the tip of the olecranon. *B*, lateral view. Transverse fracture through the body of the olecranon.

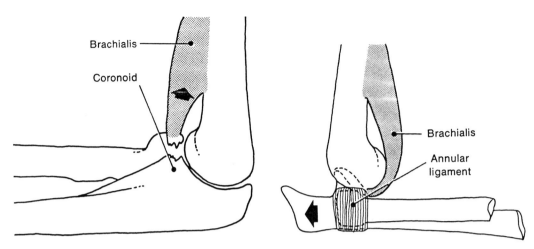

Figure 3.19. Medial view. Avulsion fracture of the tip of the coronoid process.

brachialis muscle may result in avulsion of the coronoid attachment. Radiographically, this fracture appears as a small chip on the lateral view (Fig. 3.19). Avulsion fractures of the coronoid process may be associated with more significant injuries, especially elbow dislocation, which will be reviewed later in this chapter.

Treatment

The elbow is flexed to 90°, and the radial pulse is checked to be sure it is not diminished in flexion. The lateral radiograph is then obtained, and position of the fracture fragment is assessed. Continued displacement of the fracture fragment greater than 5 mm indicates the need for orthopaedic referral. As noted above, this fracture can occur with an elbow dislocation, and the dislocation may have been spontaneously reduced. In addition, on occasion the fracture fragments are not small and might include a significant amount of articular surface. These injuries should also be referred for orthopaedic evaluation and treatment. If the reduction is acceptable, the primary care physician should immobilize the elbow in 90° of flexion and in full supination. Immobilization should continue for 4 weeks, and guarded rehabilitation should be instituted as outlined in the section on "Fractures of the Distal Humerus."

DISLOCATIONS OF THE ELBOW

Dislocation of the humeroradioulnar joint is seen rarely in skeletally immature children and is seen more commonly in young adults. An elbow dislocation generally is the result of a fall onto the outstretched hand with the arm in extension and adduction. Approximately 80 to 90% of elbow dislocations are posterior or posterolateral. Treatment of posterior dislocation will be discussed in this section. Anterior dislocation and divergent radial and ulnar dislocations are rare, and patients with these conditions should have a splint applied and be referred to an orthopaedist. Dislocation of the radial head associated with fractures of the ulna will be discussed later in this chapter.

Clinical Characteristics.

Diagnosis of posterior dislocation of the elbow is obvious by the apparent deformity. The patient presents with significant swelling and pain about the elbow. Gross deformity of the elbow is usually apparent. The normal anatomic triangle, which is palpable posteriorly at the elbow, is made by the medial epicondyle, lateral epicondyle, and olecranon tip. This anatomic triangle is distorted in posterior dislocation (Fig. 3.20). Radiographs should be obtained to rule out associated fractures. Diligent neurovascular examination should be undertaken before and after elbow reduction.

Treatment

Complete muscle relaxation is imperative in achieving a nontraumatic reduction. Depending on the age of the patient, time since dislocation, and degree of muscle spasm, the physician must choose general or regional anesthesia or intravenous sedation.

Many methods of elbow reduction have been described. Those involving countertraction in the axilla by use of a folded towel are not recommended because of the possibility of brachial plexus injury. In most instances, the primary physician will not have the use of an assistant experienced in dislocations and fractures, and therefore the following simple method of reduction is suggested. Once adequate muscle relaxation has been obtained, the patient is placed in the prone position, and the forearm is hung from the side of the stretcher. Gentle downward traction is then applied at the wrist, while the examiner guides the reduction of the olecranon with the thumb. After reduction, the elbow should be flexed and gently extended through a full range of motion to assess the adequacy of reduction and to be sure nothing is blocking motion within the joint. Postreduction x-rays should be obtained to rule out fractures that may not have been seen with the elbow dislocated and to confirm that no bone injury occurred during reduc-

tion, which rarely happens. In addition, the x-ray is necessary to assess the quality of reduction of the elbow and any associated coronoid process fracture. If intra-articular fractures are noted or the coronoid fracture remains displaced, orthopaedic referral is recommended.

If the dislocation is associated with condylar fractures, immediate orthopaedic referral before reduction should be obtained. If associated neurovascular compromise of the elbow is present, and orthopaedic assistance is unavailable, the primary physician should attempt reduction as outlined above. If no neurovascular compromise exists, the elbow should be immobilized by a posterior splint, and the patient should be admitted to the hospital with close neurovascular observation until an orthopaedist is available. If the patient is not hospitalized, frequent neurovascular checks should be described to the family and performed at home. The extremity should be elevated and ice packs applied.

Treatment after reduction depends on the stability noted during range of motion following reduction. In those dislocations that are stable through a full range of motion after reduction, early, guarded, gentle, active range of motion should be encouraged at 3 to 4 days, with splinting intermittently. At 3 weeks, the splints are discarded and more aggressive, active range of motion is encouraged. Passive or forced manipulation following an elbow dislocation should not be performed. If the

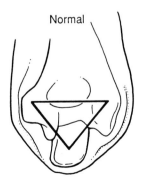
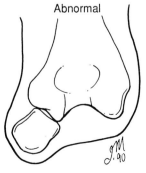

Figure 3.20.   Normally, a triangle is palpable between medial epicondyle, lateral epicondyle, and olecranon.

elbow is unstable after reduction, the patient should be held in a long-arm splint for 3 weeks. After 3 weeks, active-assistive range of motion is begun in a protective splint within which elbow extension can be progressively increased.

The patient should be told at the time of dislocation that full range of motion after healing most likely will not be recovered, especially full extension of the elbow. The potential to develop posttraumatic myositis ossificans also should be discussed.

DISTAL BICEPS TENDON RUPTURE

Rupture of the distal biceps tendon occurs infrequently, but if left unrecognized, may result in loss of strength, particularly in supination. Early recognition is essential because the results of acute repair are much more predictable than with a late reconstruction.

Clinical Characteristics

Rupture of the distal biceps tendon usually occurs as the result of a sudden, powerful eccentric contraction of the biceps muscle against a heavy weight. The patient will usually give a history of hearing a pop at the elbow, with pain radiating into the upper anterior arm and antecubital fossa. Weakness through flexion of the elbow is apparent acutely; however, this diminishes over time. Patients will have persistent weakness to resisted supination of the forearm.

Ecchymosis is apparent in the antecubital fossa, and retraction of the biceps muscle and tendon is manifested by a bulge overlying the antibrachium. A palpable defect may be present in the antecubital fossa.

Treatment

Acute treatment is to place the elbow into a posterior splint at 90° of flexion with the forearm in supination. Nonoperative treatment usually results in mild weakness of elbow flexion and moderate weakness of forearm supination. The results of surgical reattachment are superior to those of nonsurgical treatment, and therefore, referral to an orthopaedist for surgical intervention is recommended.

FRACTURES OF BOTH BONES OF THE FOREARM IN ADULTS

Fractures of both bones of the forearm in adults are usually displaced and almost always require surgical intervention and fixation. Therefore, the vast majority of these fractures in adults should be referred for orthopaedic consultation. In totally nondisplaced fractures of both bones of the forearm in the adult, treatment should be as that delineated in the section "Fractures of Both Bones of the Forearm in Children."

ESSEX LOPRESTI FRACTURE

The Essex Lopresti fracture is a high-energy injury, which results in a fracture of the radial head, disruption of the interosseous membrane, and disruption of the distal radioulnar joint either from a displaced fracture of the ulna styloid or an avulsion of the triangular fibrocartilage complex. The diagnosis of this injury requires a high index of suspicion. When a patient presents with a radial head fracture, an examination of the wrist for associated instability or pain must be undertaken to differentiate an isolated radial head fracture from an Essex Lopresti fracture complex.

Clinical Characteristics

The patient presents with pain at the elbow secondary to a radial head fracture. The patient will have difficulty with pronation and supination because of pain at the elbow. Associated wrist pain frequently is found with palpation of the distal radioulnar joint. Usually, an associated instability of the distal radioulnar joint is found.

Treatment

These injuries are rarely amenable to nonsurgical treatment and should be referred to an orthopaedist.

MONTEGGIA FRACTURES

The Monteggia fracture is a dislocation of the radial head that occurs in combination with fracture of the ulnar metaphysis or diaphysis. Because of the parallelogram, or mechanics of the radius and ulna working through the distal and proximal radial ulnar joints, an isolated fracture of the ulna is often associated with displacement of the radial head. The most common pattern of the Monteggia fracture is anterior dislocation of the radial head with fracture of the ulnar diaphysis or metaphysis. Lateral or anterolateral radial head dislocation also occurs, with posterior radial head dislocation being uncommon.

CLINICAL CHARACTERISTICS

The patient presents with posttraumatic pain, swelling, and deformity of the elbow and forearm. Depending on the type of injury, the tenderness is located in the ulnar metaphysis or diaphysis, and displacement of the radial head may be palpable. Any attempt to rotate the forearm or otherwise move the elbow is painful. Neurologic examination should be performed. Injury to the deep branch of the radial nerve is the most common neurologic injury.

As noted above, the forearm represents a parallelogram with ulna, radius, and distal and proximal radioulnar articulations. Therefore, in an isolated fracture of the ulna, further investigation of the wrist and elbow is imperative to rule out articular disruptions.

Treatment

These injuries should be splinted and referred for orthopaedic evaluation. Closed treatment can be successful in children; however, operative treatment is usually necessary in adults.

GALEAZZI FRACTURES

The Galeazzi fracture is a fracture of the distal shaft of the radius that occurs in combination with dislocation of the distal radioulnar joint. The joint disruption occurs because of the same "parallelogram effect" that operates in the Monteggia fracture that causes radial head dislocation with fracture of the ulna.

Clinical Characteristics

The patient presents with posttraumatic pain, swelling, and deformity of the distal radius and wrist. Subluxation or dislocation of the distal ulna may be evident with prominence of the distal ulna dorsally. Range of motion of the wrist is limited and painful.

X-rays reveal the deformity. The subluxation of the distal ulna is best seen on a true lateral x-ray. Comparison views of the contralateral wrist are often necessary to make a diagnosis with certainty.

Treatment

These injuries require open reduction, internal fixation, and should be splinted and subsequently referred to the orthopaedist.

COMPARTMENT SYNDROME

Compartment syndrome and Volkmann ischemic contracture may be complications of elbow and forearm fractures. In the past, Volkmann ischemic contracture was a far too common, unfortunate result of fractures about the elbow in children, particularly supracondylar fractures. Volkmann ischemic contracture results from prolonged ischemia of the forearm musculature with muscle necrosis, and ultimately replacement by fibrous tissue. This results in a severe deformity of the hand and wrist with paralysis. The key to avoiding Volkmann ischemic contracture is recognizing arterial injury and compartment syndrome early and providing immediate, nonoperative or operative intervention. The primary physician is in the best position to observe the early manifestations of this syndrome, when it is reversible.

Clinical Characteristics

The patient may present with an arterial injury caused by open laceration or arterial disruption secondary to a severely displaced fracture or dislocation. These patients will have a cool, pale extremity with altered pulse. The patient also may present with a closed blunt injury with or without fracture. In these patients, a high index of suspicion must be maintained. Early signs of a compartment syndrome will be manifested by pain on passive stretch of the muscles in that compartment. Tense swelling will also occur. A patient with an impending compartment syndrome of the volar forearm compartment will experience significant pain on passive extension of the fingers. Later (and often too late) findings will include paresthesias, numbness, and muscle weakness. The pathophysiology of compartment syndrome is discussed in more detail in Chapter 8.

Treatment

Effective treatment of ischemia from arterial injury and for compartment syndrome is based on early recognition. Therefore, in supracondylar, elbow, or forearm fractures or dislocation, the following principles should be observed. In acute fractures, meticulous neurovascular examination should be undertaken to ascertain the presence of adequate distal pulses. Nail beds are checked for adequate capillary refill and lack of cyanosis. Neurologic examination should be performed to establish any neurologic injury. Initial immobilization should be in the form of splints, which can accommodate swelling and provide access for further examination. In displaced fractures about the elbow, immediate application of a cylindrical cast is ill-advised. Frequent neurovascular checks should be made in the first 1 to 2 days after the fracture. As stated above, early muscle ischemia is manifest by complaints of pain out of proportion to the underlying injury. The pain is exacerbated by passive stretch of ischemic muscle. Frequent passive manipulation of the fingers both in flexion and extension may indicate an early compartment syndrome if this is associated with extreme pain.

If any of these physical findings are present, immediate relief of external pressures must be provided by splitting dressing and bivalving casts. In the supracondylar fracture, if relief is not achieved by these means, the elbow should be extended. If pain and swelling continue, a compartment syndrome needs to be considered and immediate orthopaedic consultation should be obtained for possible fasciotomies. If arterial injury is diagnosed, orthopaedic or vascular referral should be made immediately.

HETEROTOPIC OSSIFICATION

The formation of heterotopic bone is, unfortunately, a common complication of trauma to the elbow and is most often associated with extensive damage to the brachialis muscle. Formation of heterotopic bone can cause bridging across the elbow joint and frank ankylosis.

Pathogenesis

Many factors have been implicated in the pathogenesis of heterotopic ossificans, but it is primarily a result of the initial soft tissue injury. Excessive force used in reducing a fracture or dislocation about the elbow, leading to increased soft tissue damage, may be contributory. Aggressive rehabilitation, particularly passive stretching exercises, may be another contributory factor.

Prevention

The following recommendations are made to avoid heterotopic ossificans. In the early rehabilitation of elbow fractures, active and active-assisted range of motion exercises that are not painful should be performed. Painful passive stretching should be avoided. A high index of suspicion should be maintained in patients who have prolonged tenderness and pain about the elbow and difficulty in regaining motion. In these patients, a slow rehabilitation program should be maintained with careful radiographic monitoring. More immobilization may be indicated. It is important to note that the radiographic evidence of developing myositis ossificans is not usually present for 3 to 4 weeks after the injury and, consequently, the clinician must have a high index of suspicion based on the clinical presentation. In patients where x-rays show progressive myositis ossificans, it is best to immobilize the elbow in approximately 45° of elbow flexion and refer the patient for further evaluation and treatment to the orthopaedic surgeon. Recently, indomethacin has been used in the prophylaxis of myositis ossificans in severe elbow injuries. The recommended dose is 25 mg TID. This medication is suggested only for those patients who do not have a contraindication to its use.

ELBOW AND FOREARM DISORDERS IN CHILDREN

OSTEOCHONDRITIS DISSECANS AND MEDIAL ELBOW PROBLEMS IN CHILDREN

Articular damage to the radiocapitellar and ulnohumeral joint can occur with repetitive stresses similar to those causing extra-articular disorders. In North America, this articular damage is frequently seen in adolescents involved in overhand throwing activities, particularly Little League pitching.

Clinical Characteristics

The patient with the entity known as "Little Leaguer's elbow" may present with lateral or medial elbow pain or a combination of the two. Little Leaguer's elbow is the result of compressive forces at the radiocapitellar joint and distraction forces in the medial aspect of the elbow. This may result in articular damage to the capitellum, ligamentous instability of the medial elbow ligamentous complex, and tardy ulnar nerve palsy. (Fig. 3.21). In this presentation it is important to examine radiographs, because findings relating to osteochondritis dissecans of the capitellum may be found. Osteochondritis dissecans of the capitellum clinically presents as pain and swelling over the lateral aspect of the elbow. With intra-articular injury, the joint will usually be tender to axial compression or varus/valgus stresses while flexing and extending the joint. In severe cases, the patient may present with locking of the elbow caused by fragmentation of the capitellum, resulting in intra-articular loose bodies. X-ray evaluation will demonstrate apparent resorption and fragmentation of the capitellum.

Treatment of osteochondritis dissecans requires orthopaedic referral. Avoidance of

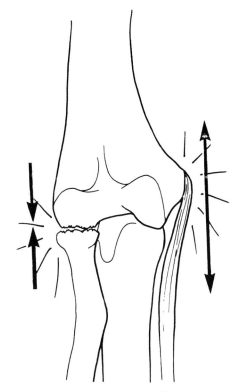

Figure 3.21. Pathogenesis of radiocapitellum articular damage and medial ligamentous laxity in "Little Leaguer's elbow."

stressful activities, e.g., pitching, is recommended in mild cases. In advanced cases, surgical intervention may be necessary.

Panner's disease, or idiopathic avascular necrosis of the capitellum, presents clinically and radiographically as osteochondritis dissecans but without an apparent stressful etiology. Treatment is as delineated above.

Traction injuries caused by overstress may also occur about the elbow of a child. These injuries will often present as pain along the medial elbow, i.e., traction of the medial epicondyle, or pain at the posterior elbow, i.e., traction of the olecranon apophysis. Treatment should be geared to the severity of the injury. In mild cases, immobilization for 3 weeks is recommended, followed by a gradual rehabilitation program. If symptoms persist, the child has severe pain, or abnormalities are present on x-ray, the child should be referred for orthopaedic evaluation and treatment.

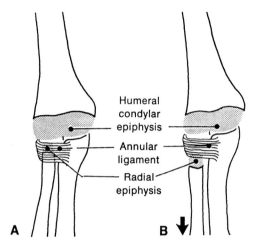

Figure 3.22. Nursemaid's elbow. *A*, normal articulation. *B*, radiohumeral subluxation.

Subluxation of the Head of the Radius

Subluxation of the radial head in children may be subtle in its presentation. This injury is a subluxation of the nonossified radial head from the capitellum and through the annular ligament (Fig. 3.22). Subluxation of the radial head is most common in children between the ages of 2 and 3 years and is caused by abrupt axial forces on the radius, usually associated with a pronating force.

The injury has many common names, including "pulled elbow" and "nursemaid's elbow," which was derived from the frequent occurrence of subluxation of the radial head in children cared for by nursemaids. This injury is thought to result from a sudden jerk on the extended arm of a toddler, such as pulling the child up over an obstruction in its path. The injury may also be caused by a fall while the toddler holds onto a suspending structure with one hand, again duplicating an axial force.

Clinical Characteristics

The history is usually consistent with an axial force on the toddler's arm. The toddler cries immediately and refuses to move the involved extremity, positioning the elbow in extension and the forearm in pronation. The clinical appearance of the arm is normal. The examiner who wins the trust of the child may note that gentle palpation localizes the pain to the radiocapitellar joint. X-rays are generally normal. Some subluxations of the radial head in children are reduced by the radiologic technologist when positioning the child's elbow in flexion and supination for a true lateral x-ray. Although many x-rays are normal, it is important to view an x-ray before attempting reduction to preclude the possibility of displacement of an associated fracture. As radiographic changes in the child's elbow are often subtle, it is recommended that comparison views of the unaffected elbow be obtained.

Treatment

The child is usually more comfortable sitting in the parent's lap. The examiner must gain the child's confidence before attempting an examination and reduction. The examiner approaches the child slowly and face-to-face. The examiner then holds the elbow in one hand with the thumb overlying the head of the radius (Fig. 3.23). The elbow is slowly flexed while the forearm is rotated into full supination. Once the elbow has been flexed

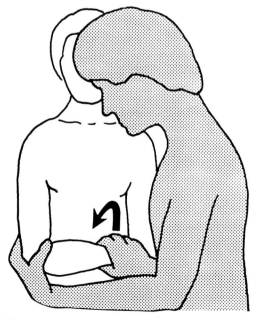

Figure 3.23. Reduction of nursemaid's elbow. Rotate from full pronation to full supination.

and supinated, the examiner may perceive a click at the radiocapitellar joint, signifying reduction. At this point the child no longer attempts to withdraw the arm, and full flexion-extension of the elbow is possible. After reduction, the child is quickly comfortable in resuming normal activities. At this point, reassurance to the parents that no permanent damage has been sustained and a simple explanation of the injury is all that is necessary. The child should not be immobilized or restricted in any way.

Supracondylar Fractures

Supracondylar fractures of the humerus are serious fractures occurring most frequently in children usually between the ages of 5 and 8 years, with a peak at 6-1/2 years. The fracture is frequently associated with neurovascular complications and the possibility of permanent impairment and deformity. In undisplaced supracondylar fractures without evidence of neurovascular compromise, treatment by the primary care physician is indicated. In displaced supracondylar fractures or fractures associated with neurovascular compromise, immediate orthopaedic referral is mandatory. Appropriate splinting while awaiting orthopaedic evaluation will be reviewed. In the event of vascular compromise not controlled by elbow manipulation, further evaluation with arteriogram and vascular consultation must be obtained immediately.

Clinical Characteristics

Extension-type supracondylar fractures are the most common, accounting for 98% of supracondylar fractures (Fig. 3.24). The distal fragment is most often displaced in a posteromedial direction, although posterolateral displacement does occur. Flexion-type supracondylar fractures with anterior displacement are rare.

Consideration of elbow anatomy is helpful in predicting possible neurovascular compromise as well as planning the reduction maneuvers. In extension-type supracondylar fractures, the proximal humeral fragment may impale the anterior joint capsule, placing the median nerve and brachial artery at risk. In posteromedial displacement, the radial nerve is also at risk.

Vascular compromise may manifest as arterial rupture, venous rupture, arterial spasm, or compressive effects caused by hematoma or transudation obstructing venous outflow and, potentially, arterial inflow. Failure to institute immediate treatment may lead to compartment syndrome and, ultimately, Volkmann ischemic contracture. Therefore, in the event of a supracondylar fracture, the following neurovascular examination is imperative.

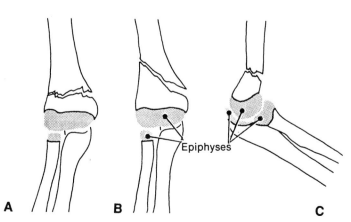

Figure 3.24. Supracondylar fractures of the humerus. *A*, transverse. *B*, oblique. *C*, lateral view, showing most common angulation.

Vascular pulses about the wrist must be palpable. If not immediately palpable and if the elbow is in a flexed position, extension may encourage return of the pulse. If the pulse is not palpable and nail beds are cyanotic, arterial disruption should be presumed and further evaluation and consultation be instituted immediately. If this examination is also associated with significant swelling of the forearm and severe pain on extension of the fingers, associated compartment syndrome may be present and fasciotomy should be performed immediately. The median nerve can be evaluated by sensory check of the index finger and active wrist and finger flexion. If this motion and sensation are lacking, median nerve injury should be presumed. Decreased sensation along the dorsal web of the thumb and inability to extend the fingers at the metacarpophalangeal joints suggests injury to the radial nerve. Decreased sensation to the volar surface of the small finger or inability to actively adduct and abduct the straightened fingers suggests injury to the ulnar nerve.

Evidence of vascular or neural dysfunction requires immediate referral to an orthopaedist.

Treatment

All patients with displaced supracondylar fractures must be admitted to a hospital.

Emergency Treatment Once the patient's neurovascular examination has been completed and found to be acceptable, the patient should be splinted immediately while awaiting referral to an orthopaedist or hospital admission. A posterior splint is applied to the elbow and secured with an elastic bandage that does not cross the antecubital fossa. If there are good pulses and neurologic function is intact, the splint may be simply applied to the arm in the position in which the arm is resting. An area over the radial aspect of the wrist is left open for frequent palpation of the radial pulse. Flexing the elbow to apply this splint may cause obliteration of the pulse. The elbow should be extended until the radial pulse is palpable and the posterior splint should be

applied in that position. A splint applied with the elbow in approximately 30° of flexion is satisfactory until definitive treatment can be instituted (Fig. 3.25).

Reduction Patients with nondisplaced fractures may be treated by the primary care physician, whereas patients with displaced supracondylar fractures should be referred to an orthopaedist. Treatment of the displaced supracondylar fracture in children by skeletal or skin traction was a popular method infrequently used today that involves the insertion of a skeletal traction wire through the olecranon (Fig. 3.26). Overhead traction is preferred to control the swelling of the elbow. Although traction is a safe method of treatment, it requires frequent evaluation and a prolonged hospital stay. Also, while in skeletal traction, the 5- to 8-year-old child is constantly moving about, thus increasing the likelihood of malrotation or angulation of the fracture, frequently resulting in a cubitus varus malunion. The preferred treatment for the displaced supra-

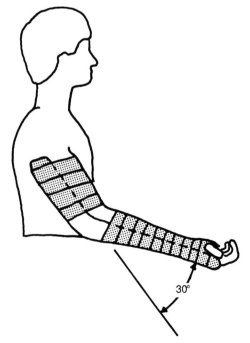

Figure 3.25. Posterior splint for emergency stabilization of elbow fractures and dislocations.

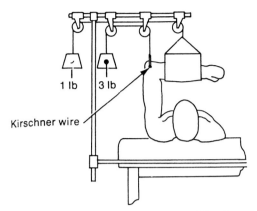

Figure 3.26. Traction reduction/immobilization of supracondylar fractures of the humerus.

condylar fracture in children is reduction under anesthesia and percutaneous pinning. This method assures an anatomic reduction and decreases the hospital costs.

Treatment After the Acute Phase For a nondisplaced fracture or a fracture treated by percutaneous pinning, the patient is maintained in a posterior splint with the elbow in approximately 90° of flexion and the forearm in pronation. During the initial 1 to 2 weeks, frequent neurovascular checks are necessary until all swelling has decreased. Anteroposterior and lateral x-rays are taken weekly through the first 2-1/2 weeks to ensure maintenance of reduction. After 2 weeks, a long-arm cast is applied, holding the elbow in 90° of flexion and the forearm in pronation. Casting is maintained until x-rays demonstrate callus formation, which usually occurs within 6 weeks.

Rehabilitation The goals of rehabilitation should be to restore a functional range of motion that is painless and associated with good strength. After cast removal, range of motion exercises in flexion, extension, supination, and pronation should be undertaken, which can be followed by resistive exercises when motion is obtained. To preclude further injury, the child should be maintained in a removable bivalve cast, except when exercising, until maximal range of motion is obtained. Full range of motion may not return.

A lack of full extension by 10 to 15° is often noted. Passive painful stretching exercises are not indicated, since they may increase the incidence of heterotopic ossification.

Fractures of the Radial Neck

Fractures of the radial neck in children are relatively rare and are usually fractures to the epiphyseal plate of the radial head and into the metaphysis of the radius (Salter II fracture). Associated injuries to the elbow frequently occur with fractures of the radial neck and include the following: fractured olecranon, dislocation of the elbow, avulsion of the medial epicondyle, and injuries to the medial collateral ligament.

Clinical Characteristics

The child will present with loss of motion because of pain as well as the findings of an effusion secondary to a hemarthrosis. There will be pain to palpation of the radial head. Examination of the wrist also should be performed to preclude the findings of any associated injuries.

Treatment

Nondisplaced or Minimally Displaced Fractures Angulation of less than 30° or displacement of less than 2 mm will rarely require reduction. The child may be placed in a long-arm cast with the elbow at 90° of flexion and the forearm in neutral rotation for 3 to 4 weeks. Repeat radiographs should be performed 4 to 5 days after injury to ensure that no further displacement or angulation has occurred. The child should be re-evaluated 3 to 4 weeks postinjury and removed from the cast for repeat radiographs and clinical examination. If healing has occurred at this time, the patient should be placed into a bivalved long-arm cast and started on range of motion exercises. This usually is accomplished in the home, and rarely is structured physical therapy necessary. Follow-up examination in 3 months should be made to ensure that full range of motion has returned and that physeal closure has not occurred.

Displaced Fractures   Displaced fractures, i.e., angulation greater than 30° or displacement greater than 2 mm, should be reduced. In these injuries, closed reduction is preferred over open reduction and should be performed gently and preferably under general anesthesia. If closed reduction is successful, treatment should be continued as delineated above in nondisplaced fractures. If closed reduction is unsuccessful, then referral to an orthopaedist should be made for percutaneous manipulation or open reduction.

FRACTURES OF BOTH BONES OF THE FOREARM IN CHILDREN

The radius and ulna comprise a parallelogram that includes the proximal and distal radioulnar joints. Therefore, a fracture of one bone of the forearm often is associated with disruption of either the distal or proximal radioulnar joint. These have been described in the sections "Monteggia Fractures" and "Galeazzi Fractures."

Clinical Characteristics

The patient usually presents with posttraumatic pain, swelling, and variable deformity depending on the degree of displacement. These injuries are almost always displaced to some extent. The patient has pain with any attempted motion of wrist or elbow. A careful evaluation of the neurologic status and vascular status should be performed.

Treatment

The treatment of fractures of both bones of the forearm is determined by the age of the patient and the location of the fracture (in the proximal, middle, or distal third of the forearm). Displaced fractures of both bones of the forearm in adults should be referred for orthopaedic evaluation and treatment because they usually require open reduction and internal fixation. In children, treatment depends on the age of the child and the location of the fracture. The younger the child and the closer the fracture to the epiphyseal plate, the greater the amount of angulation that is acceptable.

As a general guide, all deformities exceeding 10°, especially in the middle third of the forearm, should be corrected. The greater the residual angulation after healing, the greater the loss of supination and pronation of the forearm.

The position for reduction and the position of maintenance in a long-arm cast after reduction depend on the location of the fracture in the proximal, middle, or distal third of the forearm. Rotation of the proximal radius can be predicted by the position of the bicipital tuberosity on anteroposterior film of the proximal radius. The rotation of the forearm after fracture depends on the relationship of the site of the fracture to the insertion of the two supinators of the forearm, i.e., the supinator and the biceps tendon and the two pronators of the forearm, i.e., the pronator teres and the pronator quadratus.

In fractures of the proximal third of the forearm, the proximal fracture fragment of the radius is controlled only by the supinator and the biceps tendon. The distal fragments are controlled by both the pronator teres and the pronator quadratus. Therefore, many fractures of the proximal third of the forearm are best reduced and held in supination (Fig. 3.27). This must be correlated radiographically by the location of the bicipital tuberosity and the alignment of the fracture.

Fractures of the middle third of the forearm are distal to the insertion of the pronator teres and, therefore, the action of the supinators is offset by the action of the pronator, thus holding the proximal fragments in neutral rotation (Fig. 3.28). These fractures are therefore best held in a long-arm cast in neutral rotation. Once again, postreduction radiographic correlation must be confirmed.

Fractures of the distal third of the forearm are often stabilized by the broad origin and insertion of the pronator quadratus, and rotational deformities are unlikely. In these fractures, the action of the brachioradialis muscle on the radial styloid may contribute to angulation of the distal radial fragment. These fractures should be held in slight pronation, wrist flexion, and ulnar deviation.

nance of reduction. Any displacement or angulation that takes place must be referred for orthopaedic follow-up. If no displacement occurs, the follow-up films should be made at 4 to 6 weeks.

In children, no more than 10° of angulation should be accepted. Some appositional overlap may be accepted if no associated angulation occurs. Once again, rotational alignment of the fragments must be checked appropriately.

Fractures of the distal third of the forearm

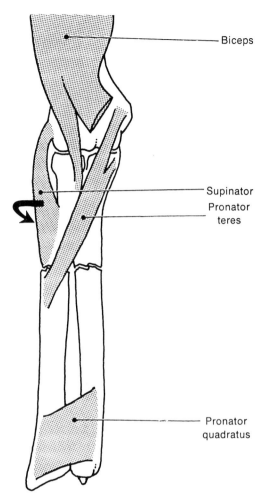

Figure 3.27. Proximal fragment of the radius supinates following fractures through the proximal third of the forearm, as the action of the supinator is unopposed.

Undisplaced fractures of both bones of the forearm should be treated in a well-molded long-arm cast, taking advantage of the interosseous membrane to help hold the reduction (Fig. 3.29). The time of immobilization should be approximately 6 weeks, which is modified based on the evidence of callus formation and clinical stability on follow-up examination. In fractures of the distal third of the radius and ulna, conversion to a short-arm cast can be made at approximately 4 weeks. Repeat radiographs should be made after approximately 3 days and then 1 week to be sure of mainte-

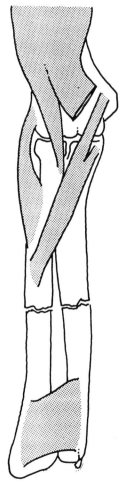

Figure 3.28. Proximal half of the radius remains in the neutral rotation following fractures through the middle third of the forearm, as the action of the pronator teres balances the action of the supinators.

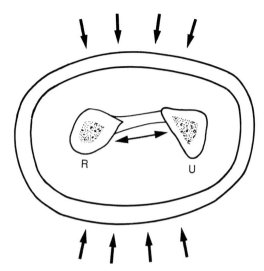

Figure 3.29. Proper A-P mold in cast to help reduce forearm fracture via tension on interosseous membrane.

may be held in slight pronation and wrist flexion, with three-point fixation within the plaster. Reduction of proximal and middle one-third fractures of both bones in children may be obtained by placing the child under anesthesia in finger trap traction to obtain length. Once length has been obtained, rotational control must be obtained and checked by x-ray. Once this is completed, a long-arm cast is applied and molded along the interosseous membrane as described in Figure 3.29. Radiographic follow-up should be obtained at 3 days, 7 days, 2 weeks, and 3 weeks.

GREENSTICK FRACTURES

Greenstick fractures may appear to have only angular deformity, but often have a rotational deformity as well. These should be reduced with gentle counter pressure, taking care to check both angulation and rotational deformities. Once reduction is obtained, a long-arm cast should be applied. Completion of the fracture is unnecessary, and may lead to further loss of rotational stability.

PLASTIC BONE DEFORMATION

Occasionally, a child will present with mild to moderate clinical deformity of the forearm after an injury. Pain is not usually extreme. X-rays reveal deformity of the radius or ulna but no obvious fracture line. These findings represents plastic deformation of the bones. Patients should be referred for orthopaedic treatment.

SUGGESTED READINGS

Bora FW Jr, ed. The Pediatric Upper Extremity. Philadelphia: WB Saunders, 1986.
Green D, ed. Operative Hand Surgery. New York: Churchill Livingstone, 1988.
Stern P, ed. Hand Clinics—Difficult Fractures of the Hand and Wrist. Philadelphia: WB Saunders, 1985.
Strickland J, ed. Hand Clinics—Flexor Tendon Surgery. Philadelphia: WB Saunders, 1985.
Taleisnik J, ed. The Wrist. New York: Churchill Livingstone, 1985.
Zook E, ed. Hand Clinics—The Perionychium. Philadelphia: WB Saunders, 1990.

CHAPTER 4

Wrist and Hand (Including Upper Extremity Nerve Injuries)

Thomas F. Breen, M.D.

This chapter will be devoted to frequently encountered disorders in the hand and wrist as well as compressive neuropathies of the hand and forearm.

ESSENTIAL ANATOMY

X-RAY ANATOMY

Figure 4.1 shows the anteroposterior (AP) radiograph of the hand. These are the basic screening x-rays for the workup of any hand or wrist problems. Specific x-ray views and supplementary imaging studies will be discussed when appropriate in each section.

BONES OF THE WRIST

The wrist is a series of complex joints with multiple bones and articulations including the distal radius and ulna. The anatomic limits of the carpus often are defined as extending from the distal articular surface of the radius to the carpometacarpal joints. Because fractures of the distal radius have such a direct effect on wrist function, the wrist is defined as starting 3 cm proximal to the radiocarpal joint extending distally to the carpometacarpal joint.

The carpus consists of eight bones with multiple concave and convex articular surfaces, allowing complex arcs of motion in multiple planes without sacrificing stability. The radiocarpal joint is a triangular biconcave articular surface with its apex toward the radial styloid. The radiocarpal articulation is composed of two fossae, the radioscaphoid and radiolunate. The joint surface is directed in a palmar and ulnar direction of 11° and 22°, respectively, which is important when treating distal radius fractures and will be discussed later.

The ulnar side of the wrist has no direct bony articulation between the distal ulna and the carpus. Rather, the ulnar side of the carpus is supported in a slinglike fashion by the triangular fibrocartilage complex, which lies interposed between the distal ulna and triquetrum, allowing for an increased arc of pronation and supination of the forearm at the distal radioulnar joint.

The majority of wrist flexion and extension occurs at the radiocarpal joint with a small amount occurring at the midcarpal joint, which is the articulation between the lunate and capitate as well as the triquetrum and hamate. Clinically, this area of the wrist is a common source of wrist ligament instability, degenerative joint disease, and chronic wrist pain.

The carpometacarpal joints have relatively little motion and are not common sites of clinical pathology; however, the thumb metacarpotrapezial joint is the site of frequent fractures, such as Bennett and Rolando fractures, which will be discussed later in this chapter. The thumb metacarpotrapezial joint is the joint in the body that most frequently develops degenerative arthritis because of its high joint reaction forces and wide arc of motion in

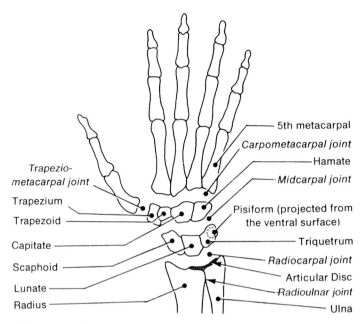

Figure 4.1. Schematic drawing of hand and carpal bony anatomy.

multiple planes. This joint is composed of two orthogonal saddle-shaped bones that permit a wide range of motion, facilitating complex thumb function.

The scaphoid bone is the most important bone in the wrist, providing a stabilizing bridge or link between the proximal carpal row (lunate and triquetrum) and distal carpal row (trapezium-trapezoid-capitate and hamate). The scaphoid bone is also the most frequently fractured bone in the adult wrist. Diagnosis of a scaphoid fracture is sometimes difficult to make; however, an accurate diagnosis is essential for proper treatment, because a precarious blood supply predisposes a scaphoid fracture to develop avascular necrosis or nonunion after fracture.

The lunate has a proximal convex surface that articulates with the lunate fossa of the distal radius and a distal concave articular surface that articulates with the head of the capitate. Radially, the lunate articulates with the scaphoid where trauma to the scapholunate interosseous ligament results in painful radial wrist instability. Ulnarly, the lunate articulates with the triquetrum, which is the site of ulnar-sided wrist pain and carpal instability secondary to attenuation of the lunotriquetral ligament. The lunate, like the scaphoid, has a precarious vascular supply that predisposes it to idiopathic avascular necrosis known as Kienbock's disease.

The triquetrum articulates with the lunate radially, the hamate distally, the pisiform palmarly, and the triangular fibrocartilage complex proximally. Trauma to the triangular fibrocartilage complex is a common cause of ulnar-sided wrist pain.

The hamate is a member of the distal carpal row articulating with the triquetrum, lunate, and the fourth and fifth metacarpals. The hook of the hamate extends in a palmar direction constituting the medial wall of the carpal tunnel. The hook may be fractured, which can be the source of "occult" wrist pain.

The pisiform is the smallest bone of the wrist and is the only carpal bone with a tendon insertion. This bone is a sesamoid bone within the substance of the flexor carpi ulnaris tendon, articulating with the triquetrum dorsally; it is frequently affected by degenerative arthritis.

The trapezoid, in the distal carpal row, is the only bone that articulates with a single metacarpal (index metacarpal). The trapezoid also articulates with the scaphoid, trapezium, and capitate.

The capitate is the center of wrist rotation and articulates with the second, third, and fourth metacarpals distally, the trapezoid radially, and the hamate ulnarly. Proximally, the capitate articulates with the lunate and is the major articulation of the midcarpal joint, where instability and ligamentous disruption commonly occur.

LIGAMENTS OF THE WRIST

The purpose of the wrist ligaments is to provide interosseous stability to an inherently unstable bony arrangement. The ligaments are divided into dorsal and palmar contributions. Key ligaments responsible for stability are the palmar ligaments, which are more stout and morphologically distinct than their dorsal counterparts. Palmarly, the major ligaments are the radiocapitate, radiolunotriquetral, and radioscaphoid (Fig. 4.2).

Distally, the most important palmar intrinsic wrist ligament is the capitotriquetral liga-

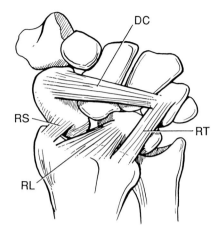

Figure 4.3. Dorsal wrist ligamentous anatomy. *DC,* dorsal complex; *RS,* radioscaphoid; *RL,* radiolunate; *RT,* radiotriquetral.

ment, which is primarily involved with stabilizing the distal to the proximal carpal row. The radial collateral ligament and ulnar collateral ligament are specialized condensations of the wrist capsule and do not appear to be true wrist ligaments.

Dorsally, the ligaments are less strong and less distinct structures. The major dorsal ligaments are the radioscaphoid, radiolunate, and radiotriquetral ligaments (Fig. 4.3). The remaining dorsal ligament is the scapholunate interosseous ligament. This is a short, stout, triangular ligament that is commonly injured in dorsiflexion wrist sprains.

The clinically important ligaments are palmar, which function to stabilize the proximal carpal row to the distal radius. There are fewer ligaments stabilizing the distal to proximal row (midcarpal joint); hence, this joint is a source of symptomatic wrist instability.

BIOMECHANICS OF THE WRIST

The wrist can be thought of as a central flexion-extension link composed of the radius, lunate, and capitate. Since no extrinsic tendons from the forearm musculature insert onto any carpal bone (except the flexor carpi ulnaris on the pisiform), motion across the wrist is initiated at the base of the metacarpals where the tendons insert. Flexion and exten-

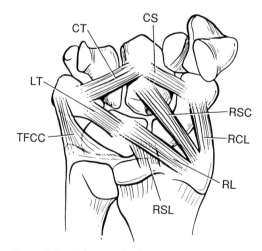

Figure 4.2. Palmar wrist ligamentous anatomy. *RCL,* radiocollateral; *RSC,* radioscaphocapitate; *RL,* radiolunate; *LT,* lunotriquetral; *RSL,* radioscapholunate; *CS,* scaphocapitate; *CT,* capitotriquetral; *TFCC,* triangular fibrocartilage complex.

sion forces are transferred across the inherently unstable proximal and distal carpal bones, which would tend to collapse with any force transferred across them. Stability is afforded by the scaphoid, which bridges these two intercalated segments. As the wrist is dorsiflexed or palmar flexed, the scaphoid moves in a synchronous direction, allowing motion but maintaining a stabilizing bridge across both links of the intercalated chain. With radial and ulnar deviation, similar changes occur between the scaphoid and the proximal and distal links.

CARPAL TUNNEL

This is a common site of hand and wrist pathology. The carpal tunnel is a closed tunnel on four sides with three sides composed of the carpal bones, and the roof (palmar surface) formed by the flexor retinaculum (transverse carpal ligament) extending from the hook of the hamate and pisiform ulnarly to the trapezium and scaphoid radially. The contents of the carpal tunnel are the nine extrinsic flexor tendons (eight flexor profundus and superficialis tendons and one flexor pollicis tendon) and the median nerve. The ulnar nerve and artery, radial artery, flexor carpi ulnaris, flexor carpi radialis, and palmaris longus lie outside the carpal tunnel (Fig. 4.4).

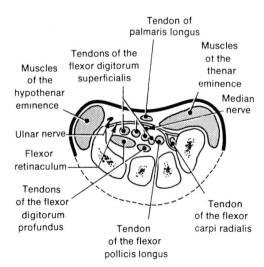

Figure 4.4.   Cross section of carpal tunnel.

FLEXOR TENDON SYSTEM

Wrist flexors (flexor carpi radialis and flexor carpi ulnaris) insert at the base of the index and little metacarpals, respectively. Extrinsic flexor tendons to the digits all course through the carpal tunnel. The flexor pollicis longus tendon, the deepest and most radial tendon within the tunnel, inserts onto the base of the distal phalanx of the thumb. The flexor digitorum superficialis tendons are the most superficial tendons in the carpal tunnel and palm. At the level of the proximal phalanx of each digit, the superficialis tendon divides and splits into two slips that insert along the palmar aspect of the middle phalanx. The flexor digitorum profundus, which lies deep to the flexor digitorum superficialis, emerges between the two slips of the superficialis, inserting at the base of the distal phalanx.

The flexor tendons in each digit travel in a fibro-osseous tunnel between the metacarpal neck and the distal interphalangeal (DIP) joint. This fibro-osseous tunnel serves a dual purpose—providing nutrition to the tendon by synovial diffusion and mechanical stability by a series of pulleys or thickenings of the sheath.

Lying just ulnar to the flexor carpi radialis and radial to the palmaris longus is the median nerve, which courses deep to the transverse carpal ligament. The ulnar nerve lies dorsal to the flexor carpi ulnaris and does not enter the carpal tunnel. The ulnar artery courses radial to the ulnar nerve. The radial artery runs just radial to the flexor carpi radialis tendon, then travels dorsally through the base of the anatomic snuff box.

EXTRINSIC EXTENSOR TENDONS

The extensor tendons pass over the dorsum of the wrist, which is arranged in six separate compartments (Fig. 4.5). In the first dorsal compartment are the abductor pollicis longus (APL) and the extensor pollicis brevis (EPB). The second extensor compartment contains the tendons of the extensor carpi radialis longus (ECRL) and the extensor carpi radialis brevis (ECRB). The third dorsal wrist com-

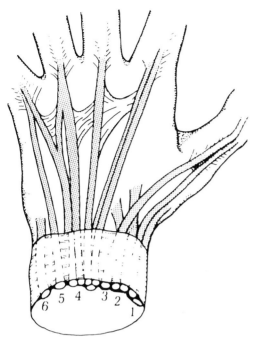

Figure 4.5. Dorsal extensor compartments of the hand.

partment contains the extensor pollicis longus (EPL), which passes around Lister's tubercle of the dorsal distal radius. Contained in the fourth extensor compartment are the four extensor digitorum communis (EDC) tendons to each digit and the extensor indicis proprius (EIP) tendon to the index finger, providing independent extension. The fifth dorsal compartment contains the extensor digiti minimi (EDM) tendon. This tendon provides independent extension to the little finger. The EIP and EDM lie to the ulnar side of their respective EDC tendons. The sixth dorsal compartment contains the tendon of the extensor carpi ulnaris, which inserts at the base of the fifth metacarpal.

INTRINSIC MUSCULATURE OF THE HAND

Unlike the extrinsic muscles, the intrinsic muscles of the hand are defined as those that have both their origins and insertions within the hand. These are the thenar, interosseous, lumbrical, and hypothenar muscles. The thenar muscles lie on the radial palmar side of

the hand covering the thumb metacarpal. The components of the thenar muscle group are the abductor pollicis brevis (APB), opponens pollicis (OP), flexor pollicis brevis (FPB), and adductor pollicis (AdP) muscles. The APB, OP, and FPB pronate and oppose the thumb and are median innervated, while the adductor pollicis adducts the thumb and is innervated by the ulnar nerve.

The lumbrical and interosseous muscles flex the metacarpophalangeal (MCP) joints and extend the interphalangeal (IP) joints of each finger. There are two groups of interosseus muscles, four dorsal and three palmar, both of which are innervated by the ulnar nerve. While each contributes to MCP joint flexion and IP joint extension, the palmar layer adducts and the dorsal layer abducts the digits.

There are four lumbrical muscles, which are unique in that they have no bony origin. They originate from their respective flexor digitorum profundus tendons in the palm, coursing to the radial side of the MCP joints. Like the interosseous muscles, the lumbricals flex the MCP joints and extend the IP joints. In most instances, the radial two lumbrical muscles are innervated by the median nerve and the ulnar two by the ulnar nerve.

The hypothenar muscle group is comprised of the abductor digiti minimi (ADM), flexor digiti minimi (FDM), and opponens digiti minimi (ODM). The ADM originates from the pisiform bone and inserts onto the ulnar side of the proximal phalanx base of the little finger. The FDM arises from the hamate and transverse carpal ligament and inserts with the abductor digiti minimi upon the proximal phalanx. The ODM lies deep to these muscles. The hypothenar muscles abduct and supinate the little finger.

DORSAL EXTENSOR APPARATUS

Special mention is made of the dorsal extensor apparatus of the digit because of its complex anatomy and the many hand problems that are associated with its pathology (Fig. 4.6). The dorsal extensor apparatus of the digit has contributions from both the extrinsic extensors (EDC, EIP, EDQ [extensor digiti quinti]) as well as the intrinsic extensors (lumbricals and interossei). Extension of the MCP joint is through the sagittal band, which is a sling enveloping the MCP joint. Through this sling, the extrinsic extensor extends the MCP joint. The lumbrical and interosseous form the oblique and transverse fibers of the intrinsic apparatus. The transverse fibers act to flex the MCP joint, and the oblique fibers act to extend the IP joint. The central continuation of the extrinsic extensor forms the central slip, which inserts at the base of the middle phalanx and is the extrinsic contributor to PIP joint extension. The lateral bands course distally and fuse to form the terminal extensor tendon, which inserts at the base of the distal phalanx,

functioning as the prime extensor of the DIP joint.

COMPARTMENTS AND SPACES OF THE PALM

Within the palm are distinct compartments and potential spaces. Infections of the hand are common, and knowledge of the compartmental anatomy will aid in detection and treatment.

The three distinct compartments are the hypothenar and thenar compartments, which lie on either side of the central compartment, and the central compartment, which houses the flexor tendons of the digits, common digital nerves, as well as the superficial palmar arch (Fig. 4.7).

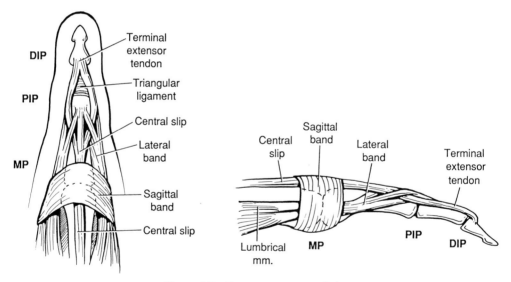

Figure 4.6.   Extensor anatomy digit.

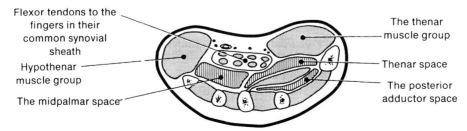

Figure 4.7.   Compartments of the hand.

Infections in the hand usually are confined to one of these three compartments and most often do not violate the compartment boundaries. Infections in the digital flexor tendon sheaths can penetrate into the central compartment. Infections within the sheath of the flexor pollicis longus of the thumb usually are confined to the thenar compartment, which is clinically evident dorsally in the first web space. Most early infections will lie in the subcutaneous fascia and loose connective tissue; however, when inadequately treated or discovered late, these infections can spread into the synovial and deep fascial spaces of the hand.

NONTRAUMATIC CONDITIONS OF THE WRIST AND HAND

MEDIAN NEUROPATHY OF THE FOREARM AND HAND

Carpal Tunnel Syndrome

The anatomy of the carpal tunnel is discussed at the beginning of this chapter. Any process that increases the pressure within the carpal tunnel, such as a tumor, ganglion, synovial proliferation, or simple edema, can result in median nerve dysfunction. The median nerve at the wrist is 94% sensory and only 6% motor. Therefore, dysfunction at the wrist is usually manifested by sensory changes. Chronic or severe median nerve disorders may manifest both sensory and motor changes.

Clinical Characteristics

The carpal tunnel is the most common site in the upper extremity for median nerve compressive neuropathy. Patients will complain of pain, paresthesias, numbness, or a "pins and needles" sensation in the median nerve distribution of the hand, classically described in the thumb, index, middle, and radial aspect of the ring finger. However, symptoms may be isolated to one or two digits. The patients may also experience nocturnal paresthesias and complain that they awaken in the middle of the night with these symptoms and have to "hang the hand over the bed and shake it" to obtain relief. There is an increased incidence of carpal tunnel syndrome in patients with diabetes, thyroid disease, amyloidosis, and rheumatoid arthritis, and also during pregnancy.

Examination will reveal a Tinel's sign, which is performed by percussing the median nerve at the level of the palmar wrist, resulting in an uncomfortable or painful tingling radiating distally into the thumb, index, or middle finger. Maintaining the involved wrist in a palmar-flexed position also will frequently reproduce symptoms. This is known as a Phalen's sign. Phalen's sign is a more specific predictor of carpal tunnel syndrome than is a positive Tinel's sign. The earliest objective sensory finding seen in a patient with carpal tunnel syndrome is diminished vibratory sensation. This can be tested with a 256-cycle tuning fork. More severe median nerve involvement at the carpal tunnel will result in an abnormal two-point sensory discrimination. The examination of the patient with carpal tunnel syndrome should always include motor testing of the median-innervated thenar musculature. Weakness or atrophy is a sign of significant compression and usually warrants decompression without a trial of conservative nonoperative therapy.

The workup of carpal tunnel syndrome also should include electrodiagnostic study. The patient with a prolonged distal motor latency of the median nerve at the wrist on electromyogram (EMG) testing should be suspected of having a carpal tunnel syndrome, although it is certainly possible to have a negative EMG testing in a clinically positive carpal tunnel syndrome. Radiographic examination of the patient with a suspected carpal tunnel syndrome is rarely helpful.

Treatment

Once the diagnosis has been made, the patient without thenar atrophy can be treated initially with conservative therapy. This includes resting splints with the wrist in neutral flexion, which minimizes the carpal tunnel pressure and often gives temporary relief.

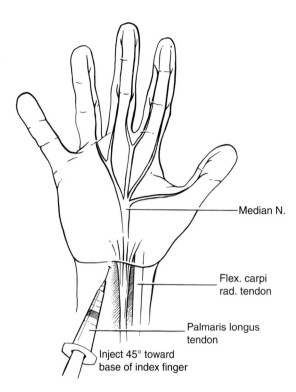

Median N.

Flex. carpi
rad. tendon

Palmaris longus
tendon

Inject 45° toward
base of index finger

Figure 4.8. Carpal tunnel injection
technique.

These splints are most effective at night while sleeping; however, many patients will use them during the day.

If the patient has persistent symptoms even with the splint, and symptoms are less than 6 months old, consideration can be given to injection of the carpal tunnel with 1 mL of soluble steroid such as dexamethasone and 1 mL of 1% Xylocaine without epinephrine. Using a 25-gauge needle, injection is 1 cm proximal to the distal wrist flexion crease just ulnar to the palmaris longus tendon. The needle enters the skin at an angle of 45° and is advanced 1 cm where it pierces the transverse carpal ligament. This is depicted in Figure 4.8. After penetration of the transverse carpal ligament, the needle is then advanced approximately 1 cm further. If at this time the patient describes any median nerve distribution paresthesias, the needle should be withdrawn and redirected in a slightly more superficial angle. Injection is given into the space of the carpal tunnel, not into the nerve. After the patient is injected, the wrist is

splinted in a neutral wrist splint for a few days, and then a gradual increase in activity is allowed.

If the carpal tunnel symptoms progress or do not improve over the span of 4 weeks, surgical referral is indicated for decompression of the carpal tunnel. If upon initial workup there is evidence of thenar muscle weakness or atrophy, conservative therapy is not warranted and immediate referral to an orthopaedic surgeon is indicated.

Pronator and Anterior Interosseous Nerve Syndrome

The workup of a patient with pain and paresthesias in the median nerve distribution should include an examination of the entire median nerve to rule out a more proximal site of compression. Although compression at the carpal tunnel is the most common site for median nerve dysfunction, the nerve may become entrapped in the proximal forearm, closely mimicking carpal tunnel syndrome.

The median nerve can be compressed at the level of the pronator teres along the volar forearm, just distal to the elbow where the median nerve travels between the two heads of the pronator teres. The symptoms are purely sensory and identical to a carpal tunnel syndrome. Suspicion should be directed to the pronator tunnel when the examination and workup do not indicate carpal tunnel syndrome yet symptoms persist. There will often be tenderness over the median nerve at this level as well as a positive Tinel's sign. The workup of a suspected pronator syndrome should include electromyography, asking the neurologist to look specifically for compression more proximally at the pronator tunnel in addition to the carpal tunnel. Treatment of this entity includes intermittent long-arm posterior splinting with the elbow in 90° of flexion and mid-position forearm rotation. Most symptoms will resolve within 4 to 6 weeks. Persistent symptoms or progressive symptoms are an indication for referral for operative decompression.

The anterior interosseous nerve syndrome is a specific compression of the anterior interosseous nerve branch of the median nerve. This occurs just distal to the pronator teres where the nerve branches from the median nerve. The patient will usually present with few sensory changes but will have weakness or paralysis of the flexor pollicis longus or flexor digitorum profundus of the index and middle fingers. Patients will complain of weakness, especially with pinching maneuvers, and have tenderness at the level of the anterior interosseus nerve origin. This lies on the volar aspect of the forearm along the midline, approximately 8 cm distal to the elbow flexion crease where the nerve travels under the proximal muscle origin of the flexor digitorum superficialis. As with the pronator syndrome, the anterior interosseous nerve syndrome can be intermittently splinted in a long-arm posterior splint maintaining the elbow in 90° of flexion and the forearm in neutral rotation. Most of these symptoms will resolve in 4 to 6 weeks. If weakness or paralysis continue, referral should be made for decompression. EMG studies are helpful to document the diagnosis and to serve as a baseline for future studies if indicated.

COMMONLY SEEN SOFT TISSUE AFFLICTIONS OF THE HAND AND WRIST

DeQuervain's Syndrome

DeQuervain's syndrome is a stenosing tenosynovitis of the first dorsal compartment over the radial styloid, which houses the abductor pollicis longus and extensor pollicis brevis tendons. It is commonly seen in patients who use their hands and thumbs in a repetitive fashion. The dorsal sensory branch of the radial nerve passes directly over these inflamed tendons. If the inflammation is severe enough, the dorsal sensory branch of the radial nerve can become irritated and the patients may also complain of pain and a paresthesia-like sensation radiating distally into the thumb and over the dorsum of the hand and index finger.

Clinical Characteristics

On examination, the patients will have tenderness to palpation over the area of the first dorsal compartment, which lies at the radial styloid. They will have a positive Finkelstein test. This maneuver is performed by having the patient make a fist with the thumb tucked underneath the digits, followed by a manual ulnar deviation of this fisted hand. Radiographs should be obtained to rule out fracture of the radial styloid or bony protuberances that may be causing a mechanical irritation of the first dorsal compartment contents.

Treatment

After diagnosis, initial treatment is conservative. This involves injection of the first dorsal compartment with a solution of 1.0 mL of soluble steroid and 1 mL of 1% plain Xylocaine using a 25-gauge needle. The site of injection is depicted in Figure 4.9. After injection, the thumb and wrist are placed in a thumb spica splint made of plaster or thermoplastic. The splint is worn continually for 2 weeks then discontinued. If after this time the patient is still symptomatic, surgical referral should be made for possible decompression of the first dorsal compartment.

Stenosing Tenosynovitis of the Flexor Tendons (Trigger Finger/Trigger Thumb)

The fibro-osseous tunnel and thickenings that constitute the flexor tendon pulley system have been described at the beginning of this chapter. The most proximal portion of the fibro-osseous tunnel (A-1 pulley) is the site commonly seen called trigger finger or trigger thumb.

Clinical Characteristics

Irritation or inflammation of the fibro-osseous tunnel and tendon system may result in a nodule on the flexor digitorum superficialis tendon, which prevents smooth gliding within this fibro-osseous tunnel. As the nodule enlarges and the inflammation and edema increase, the tendon may actually catch on the most proximal portion of this A-1 pulley, causing a locking of the finger in flexion. This catching of the flexor tendon will produce a sensation of snapping and will often elicit pain in the palm at the level of the A-1 pulley, which may radiate along the digit up to the level of the proximal interphalangeal (PIP) joint. Triggering can also occur in the thumb at the level of the thumb A-1 pulley and involves the flexor pollicis longus tendon.

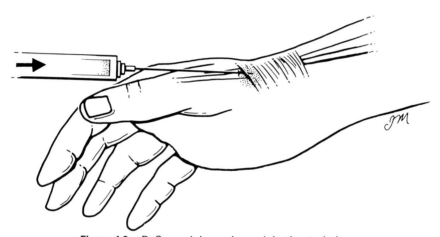

Figure 4.9.   DeQuervain's syndrome injection technique.

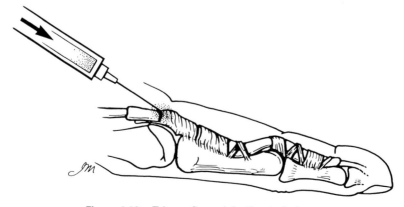

Figure 4.10.   Trigger finger injection technique.

Treatment

If the symptoms have been present for less than 3 months, conservative therapy may be considered. An injection is given into the fibro-osseous sheath at the level of the A-1 pulley using a solution of 0.5 mL of soluble steroid and 1 mL of 1% plain Xylocaine (Fig. 4.10). Injection is into the fibro-osseous tunnel and not the flexor tendon. This local deposition of anti-inflammatory medication may diminish tenderness and synovial edema, allowing for smoother excursion of the flexor tendon. If symptoms persist for 2 weeks after injection, or if symptoms have been present for greater than 3 months, referral should be made for division of the A-1 pulley under local anesthesia.

Congenital Trigger Thumb

Occasionally, a young child or infant will be seen with a congenital trigger thumb. The child will have a small nodule on the palmar surface of the flexor pollicis longus that catches on the proximal edge of the A-1 pulley. The etiology of this is unclear and is usually not amenable to injection therapy. This should be referred to a hand surgeon for definitive operative care consisting of division of the A-1 pulley. This can done as soon as the diagnosis is made in the child. Recovery is quick, and hand function and motor skill development are unaffected.

Ganglion Cyst

Clinical Characteristics

The most common mass seen in the hand is the ganglion cyst, which typically occurs in one of four locations: (*a*) on the dorsal aspect of the wrist, emerging from the scapholunate joint capsule; (*b*) on the radial volar aspect of the wrist, from either the tenosynovium of the radial wrist flexors or the joint capsule of the wrist; (*c*) on the dorsal aspect of the hand, emerging from the sheath of the extensor tendons to the fingers; (*d*) on the palmar aspect of the fingers, usually near the MCP joints. Ganglions in this location often present as hard nodules and may seem bony to the patient. These cysts classically contain a thick, gelatinous material secondary to concentration of the synovial fluid contents. They are often painless, cause no functional limitation, and can simply be observed. If the cysts become large, however, they can be painful, or patients may complain of the appearance. These are relative indications for surgical excision. The size of the ganglion cyst will often wax and wane.

Treatment

If the cyst is small, aspiration of the cyst contents with a large-bore needle is indicated. A small amount of soluble steroid can be injected into the cyst after aspiration to facilitate cyst wall sclerosis. Besides relieving the distention of the cyst and flattening the contour of the hand, the wall of the cyst may scar enough to obliterate the lumen and prevent recurrence. Because of the cyst's long stalk, which usually originates from one of the carpal joints, recurrence is common. If there is pain, a large cyst, or question of etiology, surgical excision should be considered and orthopaedic referral made. Meticulous dissection is needed to fully excise the entire cyst as well as its stalk down to the wrist joint.

Mucous Cysts

Mucous cysts are cysts that occur on the dorsal aspect of the distal phalanx of the digits secondary to mucoid degeneration of the deep fascia, usually associated with osteoarthritic dorsal spurring of the DIP joint.

Clinical Characteristics

The cyst, which is often painful, protrudes between the proximal nail fold and the attachment of the terminal extensor tendon of the DIP joint. Pressure on the germinal matrix of the nail by the cyst may result in abnormal nail production manifested by longitudinal grooving. Unlike the ganglion cyst, mucous cysts usually do not spontaneously remit.

Treatment

Local care of these cysts by percutaneous draining or unroofing and cauterizing, almost always results in a recurrence and, occasionally, infection. Definitive removal requires a meticulous surgical excision and, often, excision of overlying skin that has become attenuated. Because of these surgical considerations, mucous cysts should be referred to a hand surgeon for definitive treatment.

Dupuytren's Contracture

The palmar fascia of the hand may undergo a nodular, hypertrophic degeneration of uncertain etiology that can result in flexion contractures of the MCP and occasionally PIP joints, known as Dupuytren's contracture.

Clinical Characteristics

Degeneration usually begins in the distal palm as a palpable nodularity of dense fascia that often becomes adherent to the overlying skin. This can result in puckering of the skin at the level of the distal palm. As the degenerative process continues, it extends distally into the digit, resulting in contracture of the involved fascia, flexing the MCP joint or PIP joint. This occurs more commonly in the ulnar half of the palm and ring and little fingers. Dupuytren's contracture is more commonly seen in patients of Northern European descent and is associated with Peyronie and lederhosen disease.

Treatment

Treatment of Dupuytren's contracture is surgical. Simple palmar nodularity can be observed and may not progress beyond this point. Developing flexion contracture in the digit should alert the practitioner to the potential need for surgical excision. Flexion contractures beyond 30° at the MCP joint or *any* flexion contracture of the PIP joint is an indication for referral to a hand surgeon for definitive surgical care.

Human and Animal Bites

Human bites most often result in a laceration to the dorsum of the hand secondary to a blow by the fist to the mouth of another individual. This will often result in a laceration at the level of the MCP joint. Because of the mixed flora and virulent anaerobic organisms in the mouth, these injuries should be treated as emergencies. It is common to have associated intra-articular penetration by the tooth, resulting in a deep inoculation of microbes. Extensor tendon lacerations frequently occur with these injuries.

Human bite injuries should be treated with aggressive surgical debridement and vigorous irrigation. The wounds should be left open and dressed. The hand should be splinted and the patient treated with intravenous antibiotics covering *Streptococcus, Staphylococcus,* and anaerobic organisms, especially *Eikenella corrodens.* The antibiotic coverage should be a penicillin and a broad-spectrum cephalosporin. These injuries are best treated on an inpatient basis for wound care and intravenous antibiotic therapy. Duration of hospital care depends on the magnitude of the wound. Intravenous antibiotic prophylaxis for 48 hours followed by a 2-week course of oral antibiotics will usually suffice. Evidence of intra-articular involvement or signs of infection should be cause for immediate transfer to an orthopaedic surgeon. It is important to splint and elevate the involved hand. This can be done with a palmar forearm-based splint, maintaining the wrist in neutral position with the MCP joints flexed to 70° and the IP joints in extension (Fig. 4.11). If there is any doubt regarding the severity of a human bite injury to the hand, prompt referral should be made.

Domestic animal bites can produce rapidly developing cellulitis and lymphangitis. The usual pathogens are *Pasteurella multocida* (a Gram-negative coccus), *Staphylococcus,* and anaerobes. The antibiotics of choice are penicillin and a cephalosporin. Recommendations regarding irrigation, debridement, splinting, elevation, and the need for intravenous antibiotics are the same as those for human bite wounds.

These wounds should not be sutured primarily. They should be left open and loosely packed to facilitate any drainage. All wounds

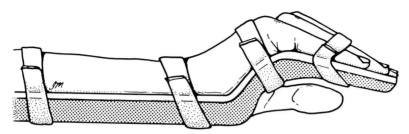

Figure 4.11. Forearm-based resting splint.

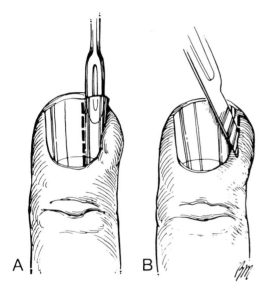

Figure 4.12. Paronychial infection drainage incisions. *A*, elevation and removal of lateral one-third of nail plate. *B*, longitudinal incision of abscess.

should be cultured for both aerobic and anaerobic organisms at the time of presentation.

ACUTE INFECTIONS

Paronychia

A paronychia is the most common infection seen in the hand and involves the soft tissue fold around the finger nail (Fig. 4.12). The infection is usually secondary to the introduction of *Staphylococcus aureus* into the paronychial tissues by either a hang nail, manicure instrument, or tooth.

Clinical Characteristics

This infection causes exquisite tenderness. During the early stages, the presentation is usually a tender cellulitis with no obvious abscess formation.

Treatment

If seen in the early stages, a paronychia can be treated with warm saline soaks, oral antibiotics (a first-generation cephalosporin), splinting, and elevation of the affected digit. If an abscess is present and is superficial, it can be treated by opening the thin layer of tissue over the abscess with a sharp blade. This can often be done without anesthesia; however, if anesthesia is necessary, a routine digital block will suffice.

If larger, more extensive lesions are found, such as a large abscess or one that has traveled to the other side of the nail, referral should be made for surgical care. This involves a complete unroofing of the paronychia and occasional removal of a portion of the nail. The wound is then cultured, irrigated, and packed with plain gauze to facilitate drainage, followed by primary IV antibiotic therapy. The packing is removed 2 to 3 days later, and warm saline soaks are started, which will often be adequate to eradicate the infection. It is critical when unroofing the abscess that the blade be directed away from the nail bed to keep from damaging the nail-producing matrix underneath the nail plate (Fig. 4.12).

Felon

A felon is a subcutaneous abscess involving the distal pulp of the digit. Because of the dense collection of fibrous septa that are normally found in the pulp, the infection is particularly resistant if inadequately treated. The multiple septa divide the pulp into many small compartments, and unless drainage is meticulous and complete, there will often be a residual focus of infection left behind.

Clinical Characteristics

A felon usually will present as a swollen, cellulitic, exquisitely tender mass on the palmar aspect of the fingertip, involving the entire pulp. The progression of the infection is rapid, and the patient will present early because of the exquisite tenderness and pain. The abscess can break down the vertical septa within the pulp and extend to the distal phalanx, producing an osteomyelitis, or it can penetrate the skin superficially. Untreated felons can also involve the neurovascular bundles and obliterate the terminal portions of the digital vessels, resulting in a slough of the distal portion of the finger. Extension can also progress to the flexor tendon sheath or the DIP joint.

Treatment

Because of all of these potential sequelae, prompt care of the felon is essential. The sole treatment for a felon is surgical drainage, which usually can be done in the emergency department by the primary treating physician using distal block anesthesia. There is usually a palpable and clinically apparent fluctuation in the pulp within 48 hours of onset. The incisions for drainage are depicted in Figure 4.13. Whatever the choice of incision, it is imperative to avoid injury to the digital nerve and vessels. The flexor sheath should not be violated. To ensure adequate drainage, all vertical septa should be divided. The cavity is then irrigated with 2 liters of normal saline using a 50-mL syringe with an 18-gauge flexible catheter on the end. After irrigating the wound, a loose, plain gauze pack is placed in the cavity and the hand placed in a compressive bulky dressing with a plaster splint to rest the extremity. After 36 hours, the packing is removed and warm soaks can be started. The wound is never sutured closed and is allowed to heal by secondary intention. After initial cultures have been obtained, the patient is started on IV cephalosporin antibiotic therapy

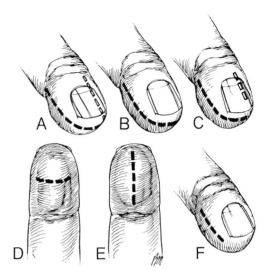

Figure 4.13. Felon infection drainage incisions. *A–F*, accepted incisions for drainage of felon abscess. *D–E*, should be avoided because of sensitive scar potential.

for 48 hours followed by 2 weeks of oral antibiotic therapy.

Herpes Simplex Whitlow

Special mention is made of this critically important entity. The primary care physician must make the differential diagnosis between a bacterial paronychia, felon, and the herpetic whitlow. The herpetic whitlow is a viral infection caused by the herpes simplex virus. It is seen frequently in small children and dental or medical personnel. The recognition of this infection is important because it is treated nonoperatively, unlike the surgical drainage necessary for routine pyogenic infections.

Clinical Characteristics

The affected finger is painful with secondary erythema, vesicles, or bullae present, but overall the tenderness is less than with pyogenic infections. Fluid in the vesicles may be clear or turbid but not purulent. Over time, the lesions become encrusted and the superficial epidermis can desquamate.

Treatment

The process is usually self-limiting and usually resolves in 3 to 4 weeks. The vesicles can be cultured if seen early. The diagnosis is made on clinical impression and a high index of suspicion. When a patient presents with symptomatic erythema and swelling of the distal digits along with small vesicles or bullae, it is extremely important to consider the diagnosis of herpes simplex whitlow. Incising this aseptic (nonpyogenic) area is contraindicated because of the possibility of secondary bacterial infection. Showering of virions to the blood stream with secondary viral encephalitis has been described. If there is any question of the diagnosis of distal fingertip infection, whether a pyogenic infection or herpetic whitlow, prompt referral to a hand surgeon is appropriate.

TRAUMATIC DISORDERS OF THE WRIST AND HAND

LIGAMENTOUS SPRAINS TO THE WRIST AND CARPAL INSTABILITY

These injuries can range from a mild sprain treatable with simple immobilization for 2 weeks to severe ligamentous disruption of the wrist with concomitant fracture, nerve dysfunction, or compartment syndrome. Although low-grade ligament sprains of the wrist are relatively common and can usually be treated conservatively, it is important to understand the pathomechanics of these injuries so that the pathologic anatomy can be appreciated and proper treatment instituted. Unrecognized ligamentous injuries can lead to chronic carpal instability. The treatment is more difficult and less predictable than the proper primary treatment of the acute injury.

Most severe wrist ligament injuries can be categorized as some form of perilunate disassociation. A dorsiflexion injury to the wrist with ligamentous disruption will generally force the carpal bones dorsally out of their normal relationship to the radius and ulna, leaving only the lunate normally articulated with the radius (Fig. 4.14). As shown in Figure 4.15, these injuries occur in a predictable fashion about the lunate, hence the term perilun-

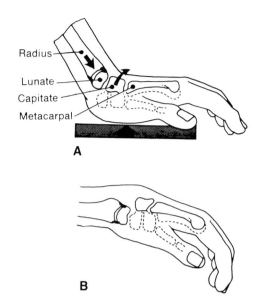

Figure 4.14. Perilunate dissociation mechanism of injury. *A*, fall on outstretched extended wrist. *B*, resultant dorsal subluxation of carpals with lunate remaining collinear with radius.

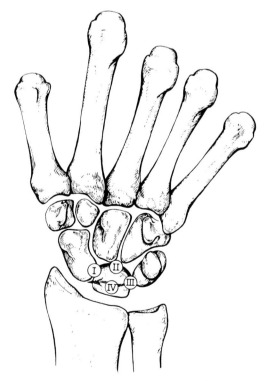

Figure 4.15. Clockwise sequential perilunate ligamentous disruption.

ate disassociation. The most common injuries are to the ligaments stabilizing the lunate and scaphoid, causing an abnormal relationship between these two bones. As the severity of the injury increases, the pathology proceeds in a clockwise direction around the lunate, causing disassociation not only between the lunate and scaphoid but also the lunate and capitate, and lunate and triquetrum. The most severe of these injuries is a complete lunate dislocation where the lunate dislocates into the carpal tunnel. Many ligamentous injuries seen in the emergency department will be some variation of the perilunate disassociation.

When working up the patient with acute wrist pain, it is critically important to obtain good AP and lateral radiographs of the hand and wrist in neutral position, i.e., without any ulnar-radial deviation or palmar dorsiflexion of the hand or wrist. This procedure may require supervision.

Several measurements should be made on these radiographs and compared with accepted normal values and with the contralateral wrist if outside the normal range. The first measurement is the scapholunate angle seen on the lateral x-ray, depicted schematically in Figure 4.16. The normal range is from 40 to 60°. With a dorsiflexion wrist ligamentous injury (perilunate dissociation) the ligamentous pathology will allow the scaphoid to palmar flex, assuming a more vertical position.

This would result in an increased scapholunate angle. The second important angle on the lateral x-ray is the radiolunate angle. The longitudinal axes of both of these bones should be colinear (with the accepted norm from 0 to 11°, as depicted in Fig. 4.16). Thirdly, the angle between the lunate and capitate should be measured. Again, this should be collinear. When these angles fall outside the normal range, it should alert the practitioner to possible ligamentous disruption. On the AP radiograph, the scapholunate interosseous space should be measured. The accepted amount of space between the scapholunate is 2 to 3 mm. Distances greater than this should alert the practitioner to possible ligamentous injury. If the above abnormalities are noted, referral to an orthopaedist is indicated. Surgical treatment may include closed reduction and percutaneous pinning or open reconstruction.

The x-ray evidence of carpal instability may be subtle. When the instabilities occur in association with fractures of the distal radius or carpus, it is common to focus on the fractures and miss an associated ligamentous injury. Consequently, it is essential to carefully assess x-rays for any evidence of wrist instability, which is most commonly seen in association with fractures of the scaphoid, triquetrum, radial styloid, and distal radius.

ASSOCIATED MEDIAN NERVE INJURIES

It is important to recognize the potential for median nerve injury with fractures and dislocations of the wrist. This presents with pain and paresthesias in the median nerve distribution associated with an acute injury. Although usually transient, it needs to be addressed promptly with reduction and stabilization of the bony pathology. Median nerve symptoms occur more frequently with severe ligamentous disruptions in the wrist and should alert the practitioner to the potential severity of the injury. Once these injuries have been recognized, simple splinting with a palmar-based plaster splint maintaining the wrist at neutral, combined with elevation to

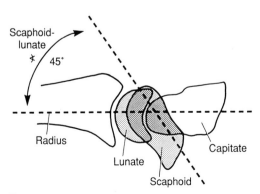

Figure 4.16. Critical radiographic angles assessing perilunate instability.

minimize swelling, are necessary before referral. This referral should be made immediately because of the difficulty in treating these injuries after swelling occurs.

One particular ligamentous injury to the wrist mentioned earlier is the lunate dislocation. It is readily recognized on the lateral x-ray as a dislocated lunate lying palmarly in the carpal tunnel. This dislocation occurs with extremely high energy force to the dorsiflexed wrist. The median nerve is often contused and rarely disrupted. The patient will present with extreme pain in the wrist and a palpable mass on the palmar aspect of the wrist. Examination of AP and lateral radiographs of the wrist will reveal the palmarly dislocated lunate.

This severe injury is an indication for primary reduction by an orthopaedic surgeon or, if none is available, the primary care practitioner. Reduction without delay will minimize swelling, relieve the pressure on the median nerve, and make transport to the orthopaedic surgeon much easier for the patient. Reduction should be done with intravenous regional anesthesia (Bier method). There are many techniques to reduce the palmar dislocation of the lunate; however, the easiest is with the hand suspended in finger traps. The initial maneuver is to dorsiflex the wrist to its maximal extent. With the patient's wrist dorsiflexed, push distally and dorsally on the lunate as the wrist is flexed. With the wrist distracted, the lunate can be manipulated over the palmar edge of the radius and can be felt to engage this articulation. Once this is felt, the hand and wrist are palmar flexed while continuing to apply thumb pressure on the lunate. The reduction occurs with an audible snap. After the reduction has been accomplished, the wrist should be splinted in a long-arm posterior splint, maintaining the elbow at 90° with the wrist in neutral rotation. Radiographs should be obtained to document relocation, and the patient should immediately be referred to an orthopaedic surgeon. Before the referral, median nerve function should be reassessed and documented.

FLEXOR AND EXTENSOR TENDON INJURIES

Injuries to the Flexor Tendons and Neurovascular Bundles

Diagnosis

All flexor tendon lacerations in the hand should be referred immediately to a hand surgeon for primary repair. Referral should be prompt because of the necessity for primary repair within the first few days. The challenge for the primary care practitioner is to recognize the injury and make the proper diagnosis. In examining for lacerations of the flexor digitorum superficialis (FDS), flexor digitorum profundus (FDP), and flexor pollicis longus (FPL), it is important to systematically assess all flexor tendons in the hand, as well as the overall posture of the resting hand. Specific examination for the FDS, FDP, and FPL are illustrated in Figures 4.17, 4.18, and 4.19. The presenting resting posture of the hand often will give a clue as to which tendons are disrupted. The normal cascade of the digits is depicted in Figure 4.20. Lacerations of the FDP or FDS tendons will alter this normal cascade and should be compared with the contralateral hand. It is always critical to examine each suspected tendon in addition to assessing the presenting cascade.

Frequently, lacerated flexor tendons are associated with injuries to the digital nerves and arteries. It is important to assess the overall neurovascular integrity of the digit. A digit that is avascular distal to the laceration is an acute emergency, and the patient should be referred to an orthopaedic surgeon or emergency room immediately. The involved finger should be examined closely for digital nerve involvement. This is best done by testing for two-point discrimination at the tip of the finger. The normal two-point discrimination at the tip of the finger should be 4 to 5 mm on either side of the fingertip and should be compared with the uninvolved fingers. An abnormal two-point discrimination should alert the practitioner to possible digital nerve in

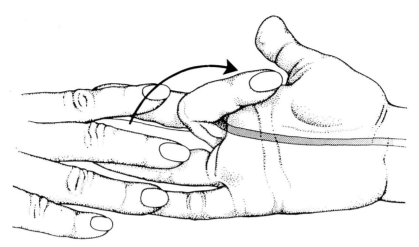

Figure 4.17.   Examining for flexor digitorum superficialis integrity.

jury. Because of the close relationship of the nerve and the artery in the digit (artery is dorsal to the nerve in the digital vascular bundle), digital artery disruption usually is accompanied by digital nerve laceration. Excessive bleeding from the laceration may indicate a digital artery injury. No attempt should be made to insert clamps into the wound to control the bleeding. Prolonged digital pressure with a compressive bandage over the site usually will alleviate most bleeding problems while waiting for surgical consultation.

Consideration also should be given to possible partial flexor tendon lacerations. A partial laceration often will not exhibit an abnormal cascade of the resting hand. Although function of the suspected flexor tendon will be intact grossly, there will be considerable discomfort when the patient is asked to flex the involved DIP or PIP joint. There will also be tenderness at the site of the partial laceration. Partial flexor tendon lacerations should be treated by the practitioner as complete lacerations and referred to a hand surgeon.

Treatment

After the pathology has been well delineated, the skin laceration can be sutured primarily after wound irrigation and installation of either 1% plain Xylocaine digital block or local anesthetic at the site of the wound.

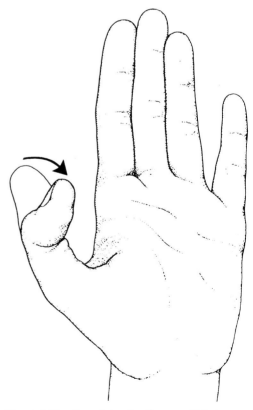

Figure 4.18.   Examining for flexor pollicis longus integrity.

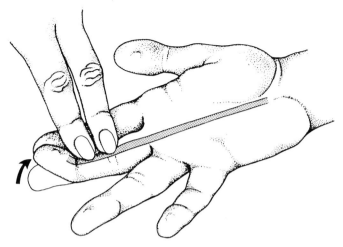

Figure 4.19. Examining for flexor digitorum profundus integrity.

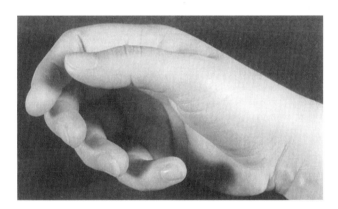

Figure 4.20. Normal cascade of digits.

It is important to perform the examination of the hand before local anesthesia. After the wound is closed with 4-0 nylon simple sutures, the hand should be placed in a dry sterile dressing, protected with a dorsal splint maintaining the wrist in 25° of palmar flexion, with the MCP joints of the involved digits at 70° of flexion and the IP joints extended at 0° to protect the hand until seen by the surgeon.

Extensor Tendon Injuries

Unlike flexor tendon injuries, extensor tendon injuries may be amenable to treatment by the primary care practitioner. All extensor tendon lacerations need to be surgically repaired. However, because of the extensor tendon's superficial location on the dorsum of the hand combined with little retraction of lacerated ends, the tendon stumps are often visible within the laceration. If there has been retraction of the tendon ends, exploration is needed to locate them, and this is an indication for referral to an orthopaedist. If the extensor tendon ends are exposed in the wound, however, primary repair can be performed in the emergency department using nonabsorbable sutures such as 4-0 prolene or nylon. This can be performed using a modified Kessler stitch as outlined in Figure 4.21. After repair, the wrist should be immobilized in 25° of dorsiflexion. This will enable the MCP joints to be placed in 70° of palmar flexion with the IP joints extended, reducing postoperative joint

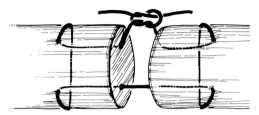

Figure 4.21. Modified Kessler tendon core suture.

stiffness while still protecting the repair (Fig. 4.11).

There is never an indication for splinting the wrist in neutral and the MCP and PIP joints in extension. Extensor tendon repairs should be protected for 4 weeks. After 4 weeks of immobilization, the splint can be removed and therapy started with active and active-assistive range of motion of the wrist, MCP, and IP joints. Extensor tendon injuries distal to the MCP joint should be referred to a hand surgeon for definitive repair. If a laceration of a portion of the extensor tendon over the MCP joint or dorsal digit is suspected, the skin laceration can be sutured primarily after adequate local or digit block anesthesia, then splinted, and referred. Tendon avulsions on both the flexor and extensor side will be discussed in the next section.

LIGAMENTOUS INJURIES AND TENDON AVULSIONS IN THE DIGIT

Mallet Finger

The mallet finger is a common avulsion injury of the terminal extensor tendon of the DIP joint.

Clinical Characteristics

This injury occurs when there is an acute, forceful passive flexion of the DIP joint during concomitant active extension of the joint. This disruption of the terminal extensor tendon results in a droop or extension lag of the DIP joint (Fig. 4.22). The abnormal posture of the digit will be obvious to the examiner. There will be tenderness over the dorsum of the DIP joint and no active extension of the joint. Ra-

diographic examination is essential to rule out a bony avulsion, which is best seen in the lateral view.

Treatment

It is critical to assess any degree of subluxation of the DIP joint on the lateral radiograph, which may accompany bony avulsion. Subluxation of the joint, usually in a palmar direction, is an indication for prompt referral for operative treatment. Most mallet fingers, however, are amenable to closed nonoperative treatment, including those that are associated with bony avulsion. Conservative treatment consists of maintaining the DIP joint in extension for 6 weeks while bony union occurs or a midsubstance disruption heals. It is important to reinforce the need for *continuous* splinting of the DIP joint in extension. A variety of splints can be placed either on the dorsal or palmar aspect. Commercially available plastic splints that come in a variety of sizes can be used. These splint the finger on the palmar aspect, maintaining the DIP joint in extension. In splinting the mallet finger, it is important to keep the PIP joint unrestricted. Motion of the MCP and PIP joints of the involved digit is encouraged, which will help maintain a supple finger. Any extension lag after 6 weeks of splinting should be resplinted for an additional 4 weeks. If after that time there is still an extension lag, the patient should be referred

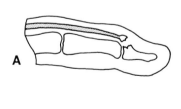

A

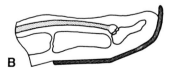

B

Figure 4.22. Mallet finger deformity. *A*, bony avulsion of terminal extensor tendon. *B*, reapproximation of bony fragment using extension splint.

to a hand surgeon for possible operative intervention.

Boutonniere Deformity

The boutonniere deformity of the digit is second only to the mallet finger in the incidence of tendon disruptions in the digit.

Clinical Characteristics

The posture of the boutonniere deformity, depicted in Figure 4.23, is flexion of the PIP joint combined with a hyperextension deformity of the DIP joint. This injury is usually secondary to a blow to the end of the finger, resulting in a rupture of the central slip at the dorsal base of the middle phalanx. Also disrupted is the triangular ligament, the dorsal stabilizer of the lateral bands, resulting in palmar subluxation of the lateral bands, which converts these structures from extensors of the PIP joint to flexors of the PIP joint. This results in a loss of extensor power at the PIP joint and a relative increase in tension force at the DIP joint, creating a secondary hyperextension deformity. When these injuries are seen acutely, there is tenderness at the central slip insertion and an inability to extend the PIP joint, with a loss of active flexion at the DIP joint.

Treatment

Treatment should consist of splinting the PIP joint in extension while leaving the MCP joint and DIP joint unsplinted (Fig. 4.24). The splint should be worn for 6 weeks. As with the mallet finger, this is not a part-time splinting regimen and should be worn continuously.

Chronic untreated mallet and boutonniere deformities often have secondary stiff PIP and DIP joints. Because these deformities are not usually fully passively correctable, they are not amenable to splinting regimens. Chronic mallet and boutonniere deformities should be referred to a hand surgeon for more specific dynamic splinting and possible surgical correction. These deformities are also seen as sequelae of rheumatoid arthritis. Although the pathologic anatomy is similar, there are some subtle differences. The indications for primary surgery are greater when associated with rheumatoid arthritis, thus the patient should be referred initially to a hand surgeon for definitive care.

Swan-Neck Deformity

Swan-neck deformity (Fig. 4.25) occasionally is seen as an acute injury; however, it is more commonly seen as a late sequela of a chronic untreated mallet finger or in the patient with rheumatoid arthritis. This deformity also is seen in the digit with a chronic posttraumatic absence of the flexor digitorum superficialis tendon. The deformity is a hyperextension deformity at the PIP joint with an extension lag or flexion contracture of the DIP

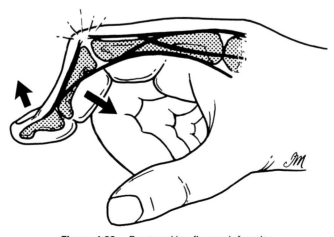

Figure 4.23. Boutonniére finger deformity.

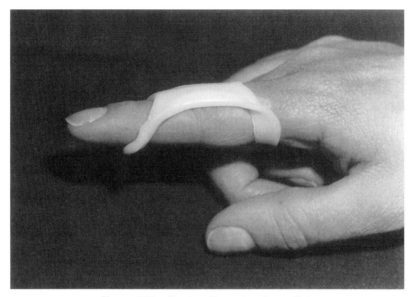

Figure 4.24. Boutonniére extension splint.

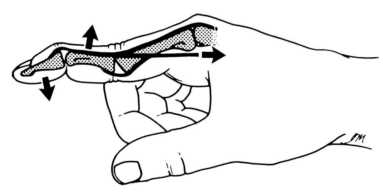

Figure 4.25. Swan-neck deformity anatomy.

joint. Unlike the mallet or boutonniere deformity, the swan-neck deformity is an indication for primary referral to a hand surgeon.

Gamekeeper's Thumb

Gamekeeper's thumb (often called skier's thumb) is a traumatic disruption to the ulnar collateral ligament complex of the thumb MCP joint.

Clinical Characteristics

This injury often occurs after a fall on the thumb with a hyperextension and hyperabduction force, which results in ulnar laxity of the MCP joint and often dorsal subluxation of the joint secondary to palmar plate involvement. Ulnar collateral ligament integrity is essential for a strong pinch, and if chronically lax, the patient will complain of weakness in activities such as opening a car door, a jar, or turning a key. In the acute setting, the patient will have swelling, ecchymosis, and tenderness along the MCP joint. Of all ligamentous injuries to the MCP joint of the thumb, 95% are to the ulnar collateral ligament and 5% to the radial collateral ligament. Radiographic examination is essential. If the ligamentous injury is through the midsubstance of the ligament, the x-rays will show only soft tissue swelling and possible joint subluxation. Frequently, however, there is bony avulsion of the ulnar collateral ligament insertion at the base of the proximal phalanx.

Treatment

If the bony fragment is more than 1 mm displaced or involves greater than 10% of the articular surface, operative repair may be indicated and referral should be made to a hand surgeon. If, however, the fragment is anatomically aligned or displaced less than 1 mm (Fig. 4.26), this can be treated nonsurgically with a well-molded short-arm thumb spica cast for 6 weeks.

If radiographs show no bony involvement, the degree of laxity should be assessed with thumb MCP joint stress radiographs, which

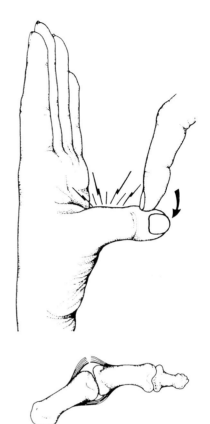

Figure 4.27. Midsubstance tear of ulnar collateral ligament from metacarpophalangeal joint of thumb.

are critical in determining whether or not operative intervention is indicated (Fig. 4.27). Laxity of the ulnar collateral ligament of the thumb greater than 35° on an AP radiograph, or laxity greater than 15° relative to the contralateral thumb are indications for surgery and referral. If the laxity falls within these limits, the injury can be treated with a thumb spica cast for 6 weeks and followed up by the orthopaedist.

Avulsion of the Flexor Digitorum Profundus Tendon

Avulsion of the distal osseous insertion of the flexor digitorum profundus tendon at the base of the distal phalanx is a common injury seen in sporting activities. This occurs most often in the ring finger and is secondary to a

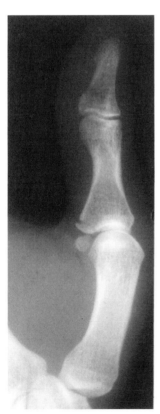

Figure 4.26. Ulnar collateral ligament avulsion from metacarpophalangeal joint of thumb (gamekeeper).

player catching his or her fingertip in the jersey of an opposing player. There is a sudden hyperextension force of the DIP joint against the actively flexed DIP joint, resulting in an avulsion of the FDP insertion from the base of the distal phalanx.

Clinical Characteristics

The patient will present with an inability to actively flex the DIP joint and will have considerable discomfort over the area of the FDP insertion. Depending on the degree of retraction of the tendon, the tenderness over the stump may range from the level of the distal digital crease proximally to the palm. With a midsubstance rupture of the tendon, retraction of the proximal stump can occur to the level of the palm. Radiographs are essential in assessing this injury, because often the avulsion will have a bony component and the fleck of bone will be seen on the lateral x-ray.

Treatment

These injuries should be treated like flexor tendon lacerations: splinted as described and referred to a hand surgeon for definitive surgical treatment.

FINGERTIP INJURIES

Injuries to the fingertip are among the most common hand injuries that the primary care practitioner will see. Often, there is injury to the nail bed and associated distal phalanx fracture. As with any injury to the digit, examination requires a systematic evaluation of the flexor and extensor tendons and the radial and ulnar neurovascular bundles, and an overall assessment of the viability of the tip. Most of these injuries occur distal to the nail fold, which would preclude any surgical revascularization or reimplantation.

Digital Tip Amputations

Fortunately, the majority of these injuries do not cause a devascularization of the tip. The main concerns are (a) soft tissue coverage of the tip, (b) bony stabilization, and (c) repair of nail bed injuries. Treatment consists of suture repair of pulp and nail bed lacerations. If there is soft tissue loss to the fingertip, the configuration of the remaining tip often will dictate suitable options for closure. Fingertip amputations with soft tissue loss can be divided into three different configurations, as depicted in Figure 4.28. Figure 4.28B shows a vertical loss of soft tissue. Without shortening the distal phalanx, these are difficult to close primarily and often are treated with dressing changes and allowed to granulate in secondarily. If consideration is given to restoring the length and contour of the fingertip, the patient should be referred to a hand surgeon. The configuration in Fig. 4.28A shows greater soft tissue loss on the dorsum than on the palmar side. As one can visualize, with this type of configuration, closure will be easier than with the vertical loss. Closure can be accomplished with various palmar-based flaps brought up to the dorsum or it can be treated in a closed nonoperative fashion. At this level there is often exposed bone, and bone shortening will be necessary to facilitate soft tissue closure. The configuration depicted in 4.28C shows

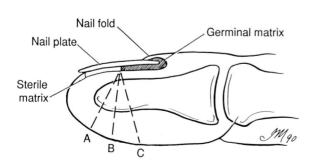

Figure 4.28.   Nail anatomy. *A-C*, see text.

that there is more soft tissue loss on the palmar side. Palmar based flaps obviously will not be suitable in this particular situation, and other options such as thenar flaps or flaps from distant sites would be necessary to gain primary soft tissue closure.

With fingertip amputations, a smooth and well-padded tip is desired for good functional restoration. In addition, inadequate soft tissue support of the nail bed will lead to abnormal nail growth around the tip, known as a parrot beak deformity. Therefore, it is important to maintain soft tissue support as much as possible. Soft tissue loss of 1 cm^2 or less will heal well by secondary intention if no local flap coverage or primary suture repair is possible. If this course of treatment is followed, simple dressing changes will suffice. This is an especially useful strategy when treating minor soft tissue loss of the digital tip in children. Considerable contouring of the tip can be expected in the pediatric setting.

Digital Tip Crush Injuries

The majority of fingertip injuries are not amputations of the tip but rather lacerations or crush injuries. Most of these soft tissue lacerations can be sutured primarily. Often, the tip injury will be distressing for the patient because of the less than acceptable *initial* cosmetic appearance. However, with healing and maturation, fingertip injuries tend to contour nicely and most often will end up with a good cosmetic result.

When a fingertip crush injury is seen in the emergency department, close inspection should be made of the nail bed. The nail bed can be divided into two parts, the germinal matrix and the sterile matrix, as shown in Figure 4.28. Lacerations of the germinal or sterile matrix should be recognized and sutured primarily with 6-0 absorbable suture, enhancing chances for a normal nail growth. Severe crush injury to the fingertip with an intact nail plate should not lead the examiner to assume that there is no nail bed injury. A significant crush injury to the fingertip requires nail plate removal to inspect the germinal and sterile matrix. After inspection and repair of any matrix

lacerations, the nail plate should be replaced into its original bed underneath the proximal nail fold to prevent adhesion formation. Small holes can be made in the nail plate with a portable cautery or heated paper clip to facilitate any drainage from the subungual area. If the nail plate is unavailable, a substitute can be inserted in its place in the form of a nonadherent dressing or piece of foil from a suture pack.

Few fractures of the distal phalanx need to be internally fixed. With sutured soft tissue and an intact nail bed or repaired nail bed, the fracture will often be adequately supported, and only external splinting will be necessary. Splinting for fingertip injuries is necessary more for soft tissue support and protection than for bony immobilization. These injuries are painful, and splinting will give some protection against the inevitable bumping of the tip during healing. Virtually all fingertip injuries can be treated with digital block anesthesia utilizing 1% plain Xylocaine.

Pediatric Fingertip Injuries

Although the adult guidelines for treatment of fingertip crush injuries apply to children, the treatment of fingertip amputations varies somewhat. Soft tissue loss to the fingertip in children almost always can be treated conservatively without flap coverage or skin grafting. Children do well with regeneration, granulation, and ultimate contouring of the finger with loss not exceeding 1 cm^2. Not infrequently, a small child will be brought in with a tip amputation secondary to various home accidents. If the tip is brought in, it can be sutured on primarily as a composite graft after cleansing and may do well. Activity and discontinuance of splinting should depend on the extent of soft tissue healing and the lack of pain, not the x-ray appearance, because x-rays often will show little healing of the distal phalanx fracture. If the injury is isolated to the fingertip, it is important to mobilize the remaining joints of the hand to minimize stiffness during recovery. Splinting for protection is confined to the DIP joint and soft tissue tip. If the loss of tissue is greater than 1 cm^2, referral to a hand surgeon should be considered. Because of the extensive nature of these injuries, these patients, both adults and children, should be covered prophylactically with a first-generation cephalosporin for 1 week.

GUIDELINES FOR THE CARE OF AMPUTATION OF DIGITS OR THE HAND

The success of digital and hand replantation has increased dramatically in recent years with the improvements in microvascular techniques. Consequently, any patient with an amputated thumb, digit, or multiple digits should be considered as a candidate for possible replantation.

After the overall stability of the patient has been secured, treatment of the amputated part as well as the stump is undertaken. One of the most important factors in the success or failure of replantation is the warm ischemia time of the amputated part—this must be minimized. The amputated part should be kept cold to reduce the metabolic demands of the part and slow cell necrosis. It is critical, however, not to freeze the part because cells and fluid will crystallize and preclude a successful revascularization. The simplest way to maintain the digit cold is to place the amputated part in a cellophane bag filled with normal saline. Direct submergence within the saline for a period of time will not have an adverse effect on the soft tissues. This bag containing the amputated part is placed in an ice chest to provide rapid cooling without inadvertent freezing (Fig. 4.29). This setup can be transported with the patient to a medical center that is equipped to perform microvascular surgery.

The finger or hand stump should be wrapped in sterile gauze dressings with compression as necessary to slow any bleeding. Arterial bleeding usually can be easily controlled with a compressive dressing. If the bleeding is uncontrollable, a tourniquet can be applied as long as it is diligently monitored by a physician. The tourniquet should be released every 15 minutes to ensure that the extremity remains well perfused.

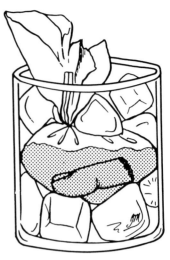

Figure 4.29.   Amputated part—preservation and transport.

The ultimate decision regarding suitability of the patient and amputated part for replantation should be made by the microvascular team.

FRACTURES OF THE HAND AND WRIST

Fractures of the hand and wrist are the most common hand problems seen by the primary care practitioner. This section will cover the most commonly seen fractures in the hand and wrist, including intra- and extra-articular fractures of the distal radius.

Although some fractures are amenable to initial and definitive care by the primary practitioner, certain fractures should be referred directly to the orthopaedic surgeon. Emphasis over the last 15 years has been on a more aggressive surgical approach to many of these fractures, providing accurate fracture healing and early motion that facilitate rehabilitation and functional recovery.

Extra-Articular Distal Radius Fractures

Colles' Fracture

Extra-articular distal radius fractures are the most commonly seen fractures of the wrist and hand, occurring secondary to falls on the outstretched arm and hand. The fracture configuration depends on the position of the hand at the time of impact. The most common mechanism of injury is a fall on the dorsiflexed hand, resulting in a Colles' fracture of the distal radius. This fracture is seen most often in the elderly and osteoporotic patient. By definition, a Colles' fracture is extra-articular and occurs 2.5 to 3 cm proximal to the articular surface of the distal radius (Fig. 4.30).

Clinical Characteristics   Because this fracture occurs with the hand dorsiflexed, the distal fracture fragment is angulated dorsally and may be displaced dorsally and radially as well. The ulnar styloid may or may not be fractured. The displacement produced by this fracture has been called a "silver fork" deformity because of the gross appearance of the hand and wrist. The patient presents with swelling and often ecchymosis if some time has passed since the injury occurred. Because of the nature of the injury as well as the angulation and displacement of the proximal fragment in the volar direction, careful examination should be made of the integrity of the median nerve because it can be injured secondary to bony fragments or traumatic swelling around the carpal tunnel.

X-ray Appearance   Routine AP and lateral radiographs will show the characteristic fracture through the metaphysis of the distal radius. There is dorsal displacement of the distal fragment with frequent comminution and intra-articular extension. The fracture fragments can be impacted, adding to the difficulty of an adequate reduction. Anteroposterior and lateral tomograms can be obtained to more accurately delineate the fracture configuration.

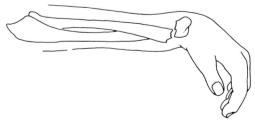

Figure 4.30. Colles' fracture of distal radius.

Treatment   Although the majority of Colles' fractures can be treated conservatively with closed reduction and casting, there are indications for more aggressive intervention. When the fracture has extensive comminution or impaction that cannot be reduced and controlled adequately with closed methods, open reduction and internal fixation or external fixation may be indicated. These techniques permit more precise fracture fragment alignment, increased stability, and early functional rehabilitation of the hand and elbow.

The mildly comminuted extra-articular distal radius fracture with dorsal angulation usually can be treated with closed reduction and casting. These fractures can be handled in the office or emergency department setting with adequate anesthesia using either a hematoma or regional (Bier) block. Although some practitioners use intravenous analgesia and sedation with agents such as meperidine and diazepam, it is risky in the elderly patient and not always as effective as either of the above methods. A hematoma block can be given easily using 1 or 2% Xylocaine injected into the hematoma around the fracture site. Precise location can be documented by aspiration of the syringe, noting the withdrawal of blood from the fracture site. Injection of 5 mL of local anesthetic into the hematoma will give adequate anesthesia for most of these fractures. Frequently, muscle relaxation of the extremity is necessary for an adequate closed manipulation. This can be achieved with an IV regional block. When performed correctly, it is a safe and effective anesthesia. The specific technique is discussed in Chapter 11.

Once the arm is anesthetized, the reduction is performed by one of two methods—either manual traction and manipulation or manipulation following weighted hand suspension using finger traps. With both techniques, the critical factor is distraction of the fracture fragments followed by precise manual manipulation.

The most commonly used technique is counter traction of the proximal forearm to disimpact the fragments as shown in Figure 4.31. Counter traction is followed by an exag-

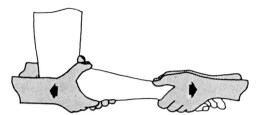

Figure 4.31. Colles' fracture reduction technique, with initial counter traction.

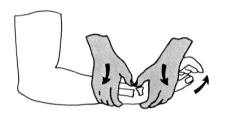

Figure 4.32. Colles' fracture reduction technique, with exaggeration of the dorsal angulation.

geration of the dorsal angulation (Fig. 4.32). After adequate distraction and exaggeration of the deformity, the distal fragment is reduced in a dorsal and ulnar direction as shown in Figure 4.33. Traction is necessary to distract and disimpact the fracture fragments. While the reduced fracture is held in position, a short-arm cast is applied, leaving the MCP joints free. The reduction is then checked with an x-ray in the cast.

When using finger traps and counterweights, as shown in Figure 4.34, adequate anesthesia and relaxation are necessary for patient tolerance. The patient is instructed to lie supine on a bed or stretcher with the shoulder and affected arm just at the edge. The shoulder should be abducted 90° and the elbow flexed 90°. The forearm is then suspended by finger traps attached to the thumb and index finger. Leave the middle, ring, and little fingers free to facilitate an ulnar deviating force to the hand and wrist that results in a more anatomic realignment of the fracture fragments. Depending on the degree of impaction, counterweights can be used with a sling over the proximal arm; however, this is often unnecessary. When counterweights are used, weights ranging from 5 to 10 lb will

suffice. After suspending the arm for approximately 10 minutes, the fracture is reduced in the same fashion as depicted in Figures 4.31 and 4.32. After reducing the fracture, a plaster short-arm cast is applied, leaving the MCP joints free. The arm can then be removed from the traps and radiographs obtained to document the reduction.

As with all fractures of the distal radius, three radiographic criteria should be reviewed to assess the adequacy of reduction. These are the radial styloid height and inclination (Fig. 4.35), both seen on AP film, and distal radius articular tilt (Fig. 4.35), seen on the lateral film. The most critical of these parameters is the articular tilt seen on the lateral view. The normal tilt is 11°

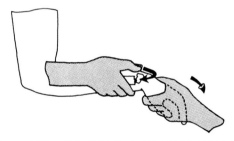

Figure 4.33. Colles' fracture reduction technique, with manipulation into final reduction.

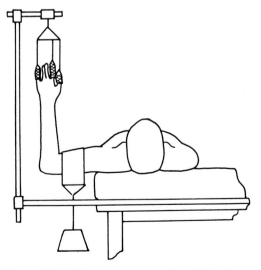

Figure 4.34. Finger trap suspension of distal radius fracture.

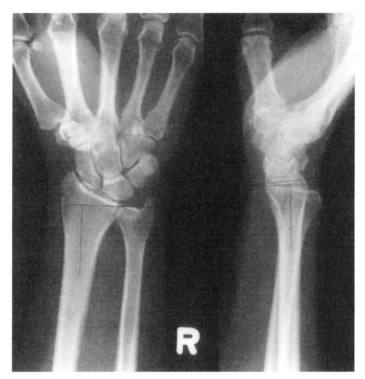

Figure 4.35. Radiographic parameters of reduction adequacy.

palmar. Any tilt less than neutral, i.e., any dorsal tilt, should not be accepted and is an indication for referral.

The duration of immobilization is usually 5 to 8 weeks. Removing the cast as soon as the fracture is stable is beneficial, minimizing the almost invariable loss of some wrist motion that will occur after these fractures. Because the fractures occur more commonly in the elderly, hand therapy will often be necessary after the cast is removed to maximize motion and function.

There has been some debate regarding the benefits of a short-arm vs. long-arm cast for adequate immobilization of this fracture. In the elderly, a long-arm cast can be debilitating, and most fractures can be treated with a short-arm cast. If the reduced fracture cannot be stabilized with a short-arm cast, then more aggressive intervention such as external fixation may be indicated to maintain reduction while allowing mobilization of both the hand and elbow.

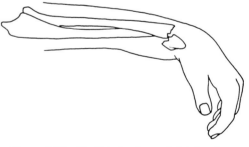

Figure 4.36. Smith's fracture of distal radius.

Smith's Fracture

This fracture, less common than the Colles' fracture, is often called a reverse Colles' fracture. Smith's fracture occurs when an individual falls on the outstretched arm while the wrist is palmar flexed (Fig. 4.36), resulting in a palmar-angulated distal fragment. Like the Colles' fracture, it is a fracture of adults, especially in the elderly and osteoporotic patient.

Clinical Characteristics The patient presents with swelling, pain, and tenderness at the wrist. Ecchymosis may be present. The hand appears to be displaced in a palmar direction relative to the forearm. There may be prominence of the distal ulna.

X-ray Appearance   Routine AP and lateral radiographs of the wrist will show the characteristic volar displacement of the distal metaphyseal fragment with the characteristic fracture through the distal radial metaphysis. The angulation and displacement are essentially the opposite of the more commonly seen Colles' fracture, which is often comminuted and impacted. Anteroposterior and lateral tomograms are helpful in delineating the details of the fracture if not clear on the plain radiographs.

Treatment   The anesthesia and distraction techniques are the same as those described for the Colles' fracture. Because the mechanism of injury is different, the reduction technique is the opposite of the Colles' fracture. The reduction is accomplished by manipulating the distal fragment posteriorly and the proximal fragment anteriorly. The wrist is then immobilized in a neutral position in a well-molded long-arm cast. Radiographic examination is necessary after the fracture reduction, and the same criteria for acceptable reduction as the Colles' fracture are used. The indications for orthopaedic referral are also the same as for the Colles' fracture.

Barton's Fracture

The Barton's fracture, depicted in Figure 4.37, has the same pathomechanics as the Smith's fracture. Unlike the Colles' or Smith's fracture, however, the Barton's fracture is intra-articular with a large palmar fragment. Hence, the reduction must be anatomic, often requiring open reduction and internal fixation for accurate realignment and fixation. Displaced Barton's fractures should be referred after splinting to an orthopaedist for definitive care.

Although the Colles', Smith's, and Barton's fractures are most often seen in the middle-aged and elderly patient, comminuted intra-articular distal radius fractures are increasingly seen in the young active patient. These fractures should not be confused with the Colles', Smith's, or Barton's fractures. Intra-articular distal radius fractures in young individuals are the result of high-energy trauma often secondary to motor vehicle accidents or falls from heights. These fractures, which have a concomitant large zone of injury to the perifracture soft tissues and marked displacement, are treated with open reduction and internal fixation, bone grafting, or external fixation. Nondisplaced fractures can be managed with a long-arm cast by the primary care physician. Many of these fractures will appear relatively anatomically aligned on plain radiographs. These radiographs should be viewed critically, and tomograms should be used if there is any question as to the degree of joint incongruity, impaction, or displacement.

Carpal Fractures

Fractures of the carpal bones, unlike the extra-articular distal radius fractures in the elderly, are more commonly seen in the adolescent and young adult, occurring secondary to a fall on the dorsiflexed hand and wrist. Radiographs initially may be negative, but if the clinical suspicion is sufficient, follow-up x-rays are mandatory to definitively rule out a fracture that may become radiographically evident after a short time (approximately 2 weeks) because of early resorption or subsequent displacement at the site. With any fracture workup within the carpus, wrist instability or subluxation or dislocation of neighboring carpal bones must be ruled out. Because of the potential morbidity of carpal fractures and associated carpal instabilities, early follow-up

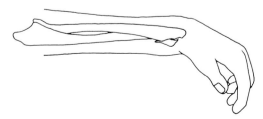

Figure 4.37.   Barton's fracture of distal radius.

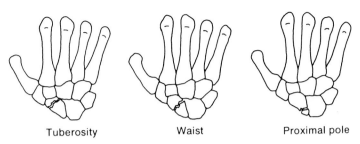

Figure 4.38. Scaphoid fracture (as labeled in text).

with an orthopaedist is warranted. Surgery is frequently required to restore proper alignment and stability.

Scaphoid Fractures

The scaphoid is the most frequently fractured carpal bone. This usually occurs secondary to a fall on the outstretched, dorsiflexed hand and wrist. The scaphoid may be fractured at one of three points: the tuberosity, waist, or proximal pole (Fig. 4.38). Because of the precarious vascular supply to the scaphoid, avascular necrosis or nonunion of the fracture always should be anticipated and discussed with the patient. Although this is a recognized problem with scaphoid fractures, approximately 90% of these fractures will heal well when properly treated. The more proximal the fracture, the greater the incidence of vascular compromise to the scaphoid and, thus, potential for nonunion or avascular necrosis of the proximal fragment. Because of these complications, it is essential that the fracture fragments be aligned adequately.

Clinical Characteristics   The history will include the patient falling on the extended arm with the wrist dorsiflexed with subsequent severe wrist pain, particularly on the radial side. The entire wrist may be somewhat tender, but the anatomic snuff box (the region of the wrist on the radial aspect delineated by the extensor pollicis longus and extensor pollicis brevis tendons) will be exquisitely tender. Anteroposterior, lateral, and oblique x-rays of the wrist should be obtained. The oblique or scaphoid view may show a fracture line not always visible on the AP and lateral views. Not infrequently, fractures of the scaphoid will be undetectable during the first few days after injury. Therefore, when a scaphoid fracture is clinically suspected, and initial x-rays fail to confirm the diagnosis, the patient should be treated as if he or she did have a fracture and immobilized for 2 weeks with repeat x-rays obtained at the end of the 2-week period. If the x-rays at that time are still inconclusive, and the patient clinically is still suspected of having a scaphoid fracture, then a bone scan or MRI study can be obtained to definitively rule out this fracture.

Treatment   The natural tendency is for the distal fragment to become palmar flexed. This is seen on the AP film as a foreshortened scaphoid and the classic "humpback" deformity with volar angulation on the lateral x-ray. If the fracture is allowed to heal with this deformity, posttraumatic arthritis and carpal instability may result. Consequently, adequate reduction is necessary. A palmar-to-dorsal pressure on the distal pole of the scaphoid reduces the distal fragment on the proximal fragment. The wrist is then immobilized in a short-arm thumb spica cast to the tip of the thumb, immobilizing the MCP as well as IP joint. If displacement is more than 1 mm on either the AP or lateral postreduction x-ray, the patient should be referred to an orthopaedist for possible open reduction and internal fixation. This fracture requires meticulous follow-up care with serial x-rays. Adequate alignment of the fracture fragments will most often lead to a satisfactory result; however, acceptance of a less than satisfactory reduction will predispose the patient to developing a nonunion or malunion with potential debilitating sequelae.

Because these fractures heal slowly, the treating physician should counsel the patient that prolonged immobilization for 10 to 12 weeks may be necessary to obtain union. If after 10 weeks of immobilization there is still a lack of adequate radiographic evidence for union, the fracture may be considered a delayed union but not necessarily a nonunion. At this point the patient should be referred to an orthopaedist for further care, which may necessitate continued immobilization or surgical intervention including bone grafting or internal fixation.

Hamate Fractures

Although not as serious an injury as the scaphoid fracture, fractures of the hamate can be debilitating.

Clinical Characteristics   Fractures of the hamate, especially the hook that protrudes into the palm, can cause considerable pain. This fracture is most often secondary to racquet sports, construction injuries using a jack hammer, or falls on the outstretched wrist. The patient will present with pinpoint tenderness over the hook in the palm. Radiographic examination, including AP and lateral views, will often be inconclusive, but the fracture usually can be delineated with a carpal tunnel view, CT scan, or bone scan if the diagnosis is uncertain.

Treatment   If a fracture of the hamate is documented, simple immobilization with a short-arm cast for 4 to 6 weeks usually will heal the fracture. Occasionally, the fracture will fail to heal and will develop a painful nonunion. If this happens, the patient should be referred to an orthopaedist for excision of the fracture fragment, which usually relieves the symptoms.

Metacarpal and Phalangeal Fractures

Fractures of the metacarpals and phalanges are common injuries. They can be the result of blunt trauma or twisting or torquing forces and often are associated with dislocations of the MCP or PIP joints. Most of these fractures go on to primary union without difficulty. However, because of intrinsic and extrinsic muscle forces, these fractures may be displaced, angulated, or malrotated, resulting in malunions that may adversely affect hand function. Because of this, more emphasis has recently been given to surgical treatment of displaced fractures with open reduction and internal fixation, which allows better control of displacement and immediate institution of hand therapy. This minimizes the risk of tendon adhesion, ligament shortening, and capsular contraction that can occur rather early with hand fractures treated with prolonged immobilization.

Fractures of the Bases of Metacarpals Two Through Five and/or Subluxation of Their Articulations with the Carpus

A direct blow can fracture the base of any metacarpal. A torquing dorsiflexion force to the hand and wrist can either fracture the bases of the fourth and fifth metacarpals or cause subluxation of their articulation with the capitate and hamate. These injuries occur frequently. Subluxation of the index and middle metacarpals at their articulation with the trapezoid and capitate, however, are relatively rare injuries. Unless a high index of suspicion is maintained, these injuries can be mistaken for carpal sprains and, if neglected, may result in chronic painful and stiff hand and wrist secondary to instability and posttraumatic arthritis.

Clinical Characteristics   The patient will present with tenderness localized to the base of the injured metacarpal. Often there is a bony prominence in the region of the base of the injured metacarpal. X-rays are obtained in the AP, lateral, and oblique planes. These will demonstrate the fracture of the involved metacarpal or subluxation at the carpometacarpal joint; if any doubt, lateral tomograms or computerized tomography can be used.

Treatment   The majority of these injuries can be treated in a closed fashion. When a reduction is necessary, adequate anesthesia can be obtained by using a hematoma block, a regional peripheral nerve block, or an IV regional anesthesia (Bier) block.

Nondisplaced fractures of the base of the metacarpals should be immobilized with a short-arm cast. Usually the digits do not need to be immobilized. Displaced fractures are reduced by traction with local pressure over the prominent proximal end of the distal metacarpal fracture. The injuries reduce easily but they can be unstable. If any instability is noted after reduction, these patients should be referred to an orthopaedic surgeon. Patients with these injuries should be followed-up closely, re-examined, and have repeat x-rays taken within 7 days. If there is subsequent redisplacement of the fracture fragments, the patient should be referred to an orthopaedic surgeon for consideration for open reduction and internal fixation.

Subluxations of the metacarpals with their carpal articulations generally occur dorsally and are easily reduced by pushing in a dorsal-to-palmar direction directly over the dorsum of the subluxed metacarpal while applying straight traction to the affected ray. After reduction, the wrist is placed in a short-arm cast with the wrist in slight dorsiflexion. It is essential that any recurrence of dorsal instability be detected with serial x-rays and close follow-up. If stability is maintained, these injuries should be immobilized for 4 to 6 weeks. Any resubluxation will require orthopaedic referral.

Fractures of the Thumb Metacarpal

Hyperabduction and hyperflexion of the thumb are the usual mechanisms for these injuries. Most common are the extra-articular transverse fracture of the thumb metacarpal and the Bennett and Rolando fractures, which are intra-articular fractures of the thumb metacarpal.

Clinical Characteristics Pain at the radial aspect of the wrist should alert the practitioner to suspect, in addition to these injuries, trauma to the trapezium, scaphoid, or radial styloid. Anteroposterior and lateral radiographs of the thumb are essential in making the correct diagnosis. The Robert's view, which is an AP view of the hyperpronated hand and wrist, will give an unobstructed view of the trapezium metacarpal joint and further aid in the accurate delineation of the fractures.

Treatment of Extra-Articular Fractures Extra-articular fractures of the thumb metacarpal are amenable to closed reduction and cast immobilization. Because of the wide arc of motion of the thumb, especially at the trapezial metacarpal joint, a less than anatomic alignment of the metacarpal fracture will not significantly alter the ultimate functional result. After adequate anesthesia either by hematoma block or IV regional anesthesia, gentle longitudinal traction on the thumb, either manually or by suspension in finger traps, and gentle manipulation of the fracture is followed by thumb spica cast. Angulation up to 15° can be tolerated with no loss of function. If an adequate reduction cannot be obtained or maintained, then referral to an orthopaedist is indicated.

Treatment of Intra-Articular Fractures Because they are intra-articular, Bennett fractures demand an accurate reduction (Fig. 4.39). The displacement of the fracture is actually the main metacarpal segment that is displaced in a dorsal and radial direction by the pull of the abductor pollicis longus. The small intra-articular fragment on the ulnar side of the metacarpal base is held in its anatomic position by the palmar oblique ligament, with reduction performed by realigning the thumb metacarpal to this small fragment. Because this fracture is frequently unstable after reduction and casting, it should be treated primarily with closed reduction and percutaneous pinning for stability, and thus should be primarily referred to an orthopaedist.

Dislocations of the Thumb Carpometacarpal Joint

Dislocations of the base of the thumb are relatively easy to reduce by gentle traction on the thumb and manipulation of the base of the

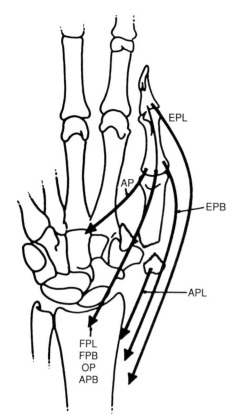

Figure 4.39. Bennett's fracture of thumb metacarpal and deforming forces. *EPL,* extensor pollicis longus; *EPB,* extensor pollicis brevis; *AP,* adductor pollicis; *APL,* abductor pollicis longus; *FPL,* flexor pollicis longus; *FPB,* flexor pollicis brevis; *OP,* opponens pollicis; *APB,* abductor pollicis brevis.

thumb metacarpal in a palmar-ulnar direction. These dislocations are unstable because of capsular incompetence and lax supporting ligamentous structures that are disrupted by definition; hence, these dislocations once reduced should be referred to an orthopaedist for percutaneous pinning.

Dislocations of the MCP, PIP, and DIP Joints

Although any MCP joint can be dislocated, the thumb appears to be the most vulnerable.

Clinical Characteristics

These dislocations are almost always dorsal, i.e., the phalanx is dorsal to the metacarpal. The mechanism of injury is a hyperextension force to the MCP joint. The articular surface of the proximal phalanx is displaced dorsally and proximally. A tear in the capsule allows dorsal migration of the proximal phalanx, or a tear through the volar plate of the MCP joint allows palmar migration of the metacarpal head.

Treatment

Fortunately, the thumb MCP joint dislocation is relatively easy to reduce. Gentle traction is used on the digit followed by applied pressure to the dorsum of the digit near the base of the proximal phalanx. This pressure is directed in a palmar and distal fashion. As the base of the proximal phalanx is brought just distal to the articular surface of the metacarpal, the digit will begin to relocate. It is imperative that collateral stability be assessed after reduction. Because of the frequency of associated collateral ligament injury, immobilization of the digit with the MCP joint flexed 50° is needed not only to prevent hyperextension of the digit but to allow collateral ligament healing. Immobilization can be with either a forearm-based thumb spica splint or cast. Protected motion can be started in therapy after 4 weeks of immobilization. If unable to reduce these dislocations closed, do not persist with more vigorous traction and reduction forces. Prompt referral to an orthopaedic surgeon is warranted for open reduction.

The mechanism of injury and reduction techniques for MCP dorsal dislocations of the index, middle, ring, and little fingers are the same as for the thumb. Treatment with forearm-based splint immobilization, maintaining the MCP joint in 50° of flexion, for 4 weeks will usually provide stability (Fig. 4.40). Not infrequently, these dislocations will be impossible to reduce closed because of soft tissue interposition and should be primarily referred to an orthopaedic surgeon for open reduction.

Fractures of the Metacarpal Shaft

Clinical Characteristics

These fractures may be transverse, oblique, or spiral. Transverse fractures usually result

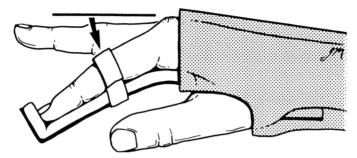

Figure 4.40. Outrigger splint.

from a direct blow to the dorsum of the hand. The oblique and spiral fractures usually result from a fall on the palmar or dorsal surface of the metacarpal heads or from an axial load such as punching with a closed fist. Displacement of metacarpal diaphyseal fractures is almost invariably an apex dorsal angulation, secondary to the force of the interosseous muscles. Oblique and spiral fractures tend to shorten and override more than transverse fractures. It is also important to recognize gross clinical rotational malalignment as the distal fracture fragment rotates relative to the proximal fragment. These deformities must be corrected when assessing the adequacy of the closed reduction.

Treatment

Many of these fractures can be treated non-surgically with an outrigger splint (shown in Figure 4.40), which should be worn for 4 weeks, followed by a removable splint in the same hand position with gentle active and active-assistive range of motion therapy to the wrist, MCP, and PIP joints. When treating this fracture conservatively, it is imperative to closely monitor the fracture alignment with serial radiographs to detect any displacement. The patient should be re-examined within 7 days after initial splinting to detect any changes in alignment. If the fracture displaces with more than 1 to 2 mm of shortening, 10° of dorsal angulation, or gross clinical malrotation or angulated fingers, the patient should be referred to an orthopaedist for consideration of open reduction and internal fixation.

Transverse fractures that are angulated and displaced should be reduced. Dorsal angulation can cause a cosmetic deformity as well as palmar hand pain secondary to a palmarly displaced metacarpal head, which can be uncomfortable for the patient when gripping objects tightly. Because of these problems, dorsally angulated fractures need to be reduced as anatomically as possible.

When treating these fractures, the physician should always examine closely for rotational malalignment. Although it is important to examine the digits from end on with the fingers extended for any gross evidence of malalignment, examination with the fingers flexed into the palm will make small malalignment more readily noticeable. The amount of angulation acceptable when treating these fractures conservatively depends on the particular metacarpal involved. A good rule for residual apex dorsal angulation of metacarpal shaft fractures is 10° for the index finger, 15° for the middle finger, and 20° for the ring and little fingers. The ring and little metacarpals are more mobile than the index and middle fingers because of their mobile carpometacarpal articulations, hence more angulation in the volar-dorsal plane is tolerated. Shortening greater than 1 mm or any rotatory malalignment should not be accepted, and a reduction should be attempted.

When the alignment does not fall within these limits, reduction under local or regional anesthesia should be performed, using straight traction on the involved digit with direct pressure in a dorsal-to-palmar direction over the apex of the fracture angulation. Once the fracture is reduced, a short-arm cast is applied with the wrist in neutral position or slightly dorsiflexed with an incorporated aluminum outrigger splint for 4 to 5 weeks. The fracture should be followed weekly with serial x-rays to rule out any displacement. Redisplacement after closed reduction or an inability to obtain initial fracture reduction within the limits outlined are indications for referral to an orthopaedist for surgical intervention.

Metacarpal fractures associated with significant soft tissue injury to skin, subcutaneous tissue, flexor and extensor tendons should be directly referred to an orthopaedist for possible operative intervention. Open reduction and rigid internal fixation of these fractures may ensure alignment and facilitate fracture healing and better treatment of the associated soft tissue injuries.

Spiral or oblique fractures tend to shorten and malrotate more frequently. These fractures, although they initially may be anatomically aligned, will frequently shorten and displace because of the force of the interosseous muscles. If these fractures are nondisplaced, they can be treated with simple immobilization with a forearm-based resting splint as previously described with the metacarpal fractures. Spiral or oblique fractures, however, do require close follow-up because of their propensity to displace. They should be x-rayed within 7 days for assessment of stability. If there is evidence of shortening of 1 mm or more, or evidence of digit malrotation on clinical examination, the patient should be referred to an orthopaedist for possible open reduction and internal fixation.

Fractures of the Metacarpal Neck

Clinical Characteristics

Fractures of the metacarpal neck result from punching with a closed fist in a manner that applies force to the dorsal aspect of the MCP joint. The MCP joint is displaced palmarly with the apex of angulation directed dorsally and usually impacted. Most commonly affected are the ring and little fingers.

Treatment

Because of the overall mobility of the ring and little finger metacarpal, these fractures tend to do well when treated nonoperatively with closed reduction because they can tolerate a less-than-anatomic union. Metacarpal neck fractures of the index and middle fingers should be addressed by an orthopaedic surgeon, because malalignment of the fracture is not well-tolerated by these digits. Nondisplaced metacarpal neck fractures of the index and middle fingers and those with angulation less than 10° can be treated with a simple forearm-based resting splint or cast with digital extension. Fracture angulation greater than 10° is an indication for referral to an orthopaedist. As with any hand trauma, AP and lateral radiographs are an essential component of the workup.

Fracture reduction requires either a hematoma block or IV regional anesthesia. When reducing fractures of the metacarpal neck, it is important to first disimpact the fragments. Disimpaction can be accomplished by flexing and distracting the MCP joint manually to 90° and gently manipulating the proximal phalanx in a radial-ulnar direction to disimpact the fracture fragments. Once the fracture has been disimpacted, the MCP joint can be extended and the fracture reduced by applying direct pressure with the thumb in a dorsal-to-palmar direction on the apex of the angulated fracture (Fig. 4.41). Fracture reduction with this maneuver will not succeed unless the fracture has been fully disimpacted.

Once reduced, the fracture should be immobilized in a forearm-based ulnar gutter splint that is well-molded over the area of the fracture. The MCP joint is kept in 70° of flexion and the PIP joint is extended. This will minimize joint stiffness during this period of immobilization lasting 4 weeks. As swelling subsides, the splint can loosen and the fracture may displace. Consequently, close follow-up is necessary (within the 1st week), and remanipulation or referral is indicated for any sub-

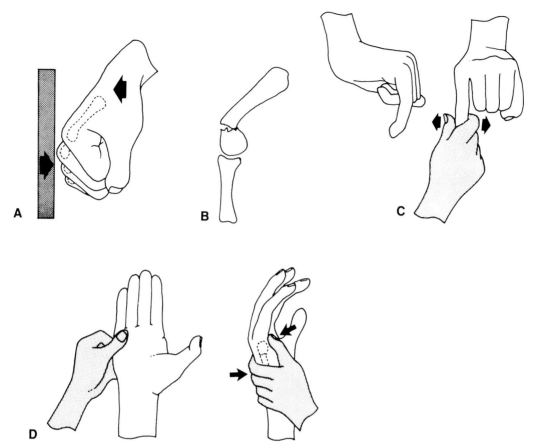

Figure 4.41. Boxer fracture of fifth metacarpal and reduction technique. *A*, mechanism of injury; *B*, dorsal angulation; *C*, disimpaction of fragments; *D*, reduction maneuver.

sequent displacement. After 4 weeks of immobilization, radiographs should be obtained out of plaster. If the fracture appears radiographically healed with no tenderness over the fracture site, then mobilization of the MCP and PIP joints can be commenced.

Phalangeal Fractures and Fracture-Dislocations of the PIP and IP Joints

Fractures of the phalanges are common injuries. Fractures of the proximal and middle phalanges are usually secondary to hyperextension or hyperabduction forces. They frequently involve the PIP and MCP joints. Phalangeal fractures that extend into the joint surface often indicate an actual fracture-dislocation. This must be kept in mind when evaluating these injuries, which will be discussed later in this chapter.

Distal Phalangeal and DIP Joint Injuries

Fractures of the distal phalanx are usually the result of a crushing-type injury. Often, these fractures have associated extensive soft tissue injuries to the tip or nail bed. These specific fingertip injuries have been discussed in an earlier section. Avulsion fractures of the terminal extensor tendon (mallet finger) have also been discussed. Fractures of the distal phalanx usually are slow to show radiographic evidence of healing.

Few fractures of the distal phalanx require more than symptomatic, protective splinting. The fracture should be treated and splinted until no further fracture tenderness is present. Isolated fractures of the distal phalanx can be treated with splints that immobilize the DIP joint and leave the PIP joint free, minimizing stiffness.

Middle Phalangeal and PIP Joint Injuries

Fractures of the middle phalanx can be treated using the same guidelines as for fractures of the metacarpal shaft. Fractures of the middle phalanx are often associated with a crush-type injury with significant soft tissue pathology. When there is accompanying soft tissue injury and dorsal extension apparatus involvement, it is imperative that the fracture alignment be anatomic and stable, allowing proper wound care and early motion. The threshold for referral to an orthopaedic surgeon should be low.

One particular fracture of the middle phalanx that needs to be highlighted is the commonly seen fracture of the palmar base (Fig. 4.42). This is an intra-articular fracture that is the result of a hyperextension or dorsal dislocation of the PIP joint, commonly seen in athletic activities. It is essentially an avulsion

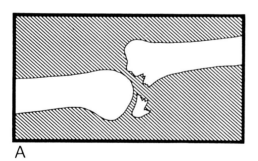

A

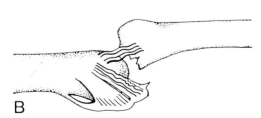

B

Figure 4.42. Volar plate avulsion of proximal interphalangeal joint. *A,* fracture of volar base middle phalanx with joint subluxation. *B,* volar plate attachment to fragment and tear of collateral ligament.

injury of the distal insertion of the volar plate. Often, this will lead to joint instability and dorsal subluxation, even after reduction of a dislocated joint. This injury should be recognized early and treated promptly, minimizing the chances of a chronically stiff or unstable PIP joint.

If the fracture fragment involves less than 40% of the articular surface seen on the lateral radiograph, the injury can frequently be treated nonoperatively. Treatment should allow protected early motion while maintaining a well-reduced joint. This can best be accomplished with dorsal extension block splinting, shown in Figure 4.43. Because of the initial dorsal joint subluxation, the reduced joint is more stable in flexion. Flexion of these PIP joints will also reapproximate the avulsed palmar plate. The initial position of the PIP joint should be the maximum extension that still maintains both a congruent PIP joint as well as apposition of the palmar fracture fragment. This should be documented with radiographs while in the splint. Once the dorsal extension block splint is applied and in place, active flexion of the PIP joint and extension of the joint within the confines of the extension block are encouraged. The follow-up includes serial x-rays. On a weekly basis, the splint is altered to allow 10° more extension. After a change in the splint allowing more extension, a congruent joint is documented with a lateral radiograph. If congruency is lost, the digits should be maintained in the previous degree of extension block. Once the PIP joint has been brought out to full extension over the course of 4 to 5 weeks, the splint can be discontinued and gentle strengthening exercises can be started.

The keys to proper treatment of this fracture are as follows: (*a*) closed treatment for injuries involving less than 40% of the articular surface; (*b*) dorsal extension block splinting, maintaining a congruent joint and apposition of the palmar plate or fracture fragment; (*c*) gradual extension of the splint, allowing more extension of the PIP joint on a graduated basis over 4 to 5 weeks; (*d*) when using the dorsal extension block splint, immobilization of the MCP joint to prevent

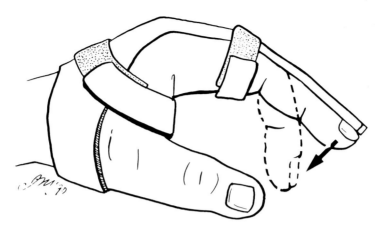

Figure 4.43. Dorsal extension block splint.

flexion, so that the forces can be directed at the PIP joint while in the splint; and (*e*) referral of injuries involving more than 40% of the articular surface or joint subluxation to an orthopaedist for possible surgical treatment.

Lesser injuries of the PIP joint are seen that do not begin with an obvious dislocation. Forces that laterally angulate, hyperextend, or hyperflex the joint may injure the capsule or its collateral ligaments. This is the classic "jammed" finger seen in sports. It is important to examine the collateral ligaments to assess any degree of instability. Because the PIP joint is essentially a hinge joint, laxity should be no more than 10° in either radial or ulnar directions with lateral stress. If there is tenderness about the joint with no gross instability, subluxation of the joint, or fracture on x-ray, this injury can be treated with buddy taping to an adjacent finger for stability for 2 to 3 weeks. Range of motion within the confines of the buddy taping is allowed. If gross instability or avulsion fracture of the collateral ligaments is seen on the AP radiograph with displacement greater than 1 mm, referral to an orthopaedic surgeon is indicated.

Proximal Phalangeal and MP Joint Injuries

As with metacarpal shaft fractures, fractures of the proximal phalanx can occur in a variety of configurations. Transverse, oblique, or spiral fractures often lead to angulation or shortening with a potential for rotational de-

formity. Proximal phalanx fractures tend to be palmarly angulated because of the pull of the intrinsic tendons. Similar fracture treatment guidelines are advised for the proximal phalanx fracture as for the metacarpal shaft fracture. Because of the close adherence of the dorsal extensor apparatus at the level of the proximal phalanx, proper treatment of these fractures is essential to minimize extensor adhesions and a subsequently stiff finger. Because of the functional benefits of early mobilization, many surgeons feel that surgical treatment of displaced fractures is indicated. Rigid stabilization with precise rotational control of the digit permits early mobilization. Unless the fracture is anatomically aligned by closed reduction or is a nondisplaced fracture, referral to an orthopaedic surgeon for possible open reduction and internal fixation may be indicated. If the fracture is anatomically aligned, continued nonoperative therapy is indicated. Immobilization should be with a forearm-based splint with the affected digit immobilized to the tip of the finger. The MCP joint should be in 70° of flexion and the IP joints extended. Immobilization should be for 4 to 5 weeks with supervised hand therapy instituted as soon as the fracture will allow, i.e., when there is no further fracture tenderness. Rigid internal fixation of these fractures allows virtually immediate postoperative mobilization.

Because many of these injuries are associated with a severe crushing force, many proximal phalanx fractures are comminuted and unstable. In such cases, they should be referred promptly to an orthopaedic surgeon for either internal or external fixation.

Suggested Readings

Bora FW Jr, ed. The Pediatric Upper Extremity. Philadelphia: WB Saunders Co., 1986.

Green D, ed. Operative Hand Surgery. New York: Churchill Livingstone, 1988.

Stern P, ed. Hand Clinics—Difficult Fractures of the Hand and Wrist. Philadelphia: WB Saunders Co., 1985.

Strickland J, ed. Hand Clinics—Flexor Tendon Surgery. Philadelphia: WB Saunders Co., 1985.

Taleisnik J, ed. The Wrist. New York: Churchill Livingstone, 1985.

Zook E, ed. Hand Clinics—The Perionychium. Philadelphia: WB Saunders Co., 1990.

Thoracic and Lumbar Spine

James C. Bayley, M.D.

Spinal disorders, especially low back pain, are endemic to modern industrialized society. Spine fractures can lead to significant morbidity and mortality. Tumors, both primary and metastatic to the spine, often contribute to the suffering and debilitation of patients with cancer. Metabolic and degenerative disorders cause problems in a large number of patients. After colds, low back pain is the next most frequent reason for patients to visit a primary care physician. Thus, familiarity with the evaluation, diagnosis, and initial management of problems in the thoracolumbar spine is crucial for those in the front lines of medical care.

This chapter includes a brief description of the anatomy and biomechanics of the spine. An algorithmic approach to the history taking, physical examination, and laboratory evaluation is included. Also included is a detailed summary of the presentation, diagnosis, and treatment of the more common back disorders with a discussion of conventional and alternative treatments of low back pain. Hopefully, the reader will be more comfortable when confronted with a Monday morning office full of patients with low back pain.

ANATOMY

The spine consists of a series of bones (the vertebrae) joined together by discs anteriorly and facet joints postero-laterally. These are held together by sets of ligaments and moved by muscles attached by tendons. The vertebral column protects and surrounds the spinal cord, which gives off segmental branches called nerve roots. These nerve roots then exit the spinal canal via neuroforamina to inner-vate the chest wall, abdominal cavity, extremities, and perineum. Two adjacent vertebrae with their surrounding structures and intervening disc are commonly referred to as the functional spinal unit.

The thoracic spine is curved in the sagittal plane with its apex posteriorly, forming a kyphosis. The thoracolumbar junction is ordinarily straight in both the anteroposterior (AP) and sagittal (lateral) planes, and the lumbar spine is normally curved with its apex anteriorly into lordosis. This combination of kyphosis and lordosis allows the center of gravity line to fall close to the spine, minimizing the energy expended in maintaining an upright position. These curves are not genetically programmed but are developmental because they are acquired during growth. Paralyzed infants who never sit do not develop a normal thoracic kyphosis or lumbar lordosis. Any curvature in the coronal plane is considered abnormal and is called scoliosis.

VERTEBRAL BODIES

Each spinal vertebra is morphologically similar to the one above and below, with subtle differences. They become progressively larger from the upper thoracic to the lower lumbar spine as well as broader and taller. Each vertebra is composed of the vertebral body anteriorly, which bears approximately 90% of the applied load. The vertebral bodies are convex anteriorly (Fig. 5.1) and concave posteriorly to allow room for the spinal cord and dura. The outer shell of the vertebra is thin cortical bone called endplates, which are at the superior and inferior sides in contact with the discs.

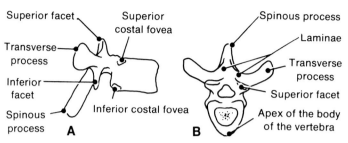

Figure 5.1. *A* and *B*, a thoracic vertebra. Lateral and superior views.

These endplates supply nutrition to the disc via diffusion, as the discs are avascular in adults. The inner part of the vertebra is filled with cancellous (trabecular) bone into which the bone marrow is packed. In adults, most hematopoietic marrow is located in the spine and pelvis. Thus, disorders of marrow cells, such as myeloma or lymphoma, will affect the vertebral bodies preferentially more than the appendicular skeleton.

The vertebral body is connected to the posterior elements by paired pedicles attached at its superior-posterior aspect. Each pedicle expands into four processes: the transverse process laterally for muscle attachments, the superior articular process for the facet joint with the next superior vertebra, the lamina for protection of the spinal cord, and the larger inferior articular process for the facet joint with the next inferior vertebra. The junction of the pedicle with the inferior articular process is also called the pars interarticularis and is the weakest part of the vertebra. The weakness of the pars becomes important in the conditions called spondylolysis and spondylolisthesis (discussed later in this chapter). Collectively, these bony elements from the pedicles on backwards are termed the posterior elements.

Thoracic vertebrae (T1-T12) differ from lumbar vertebrae in that they also serve as attachments for the ribs (Fig. 5.1). On the posterolateral corner of each thoracic vertebrae are joint surfaces called fovea. Each rib articulates with the superior fovea of one vertebra and the inferior fovea of the vertebra above. These paired costovertebral joints act as hinges for the ribs to move up and down during respiration.

The lumbar vertebrae (L1-L5) are larger than the thoracic vertebrae and more mobile because of the lack of support from the rib cage (Fig. 5.1). However, because L5 and, to a lesser extent, L4 sit down in and are attached to the pelvis by strong iliolumbar ligaments, they are relatively immobile. Maximal spinal motion occurs in the mid and upper lumbar spine (L1-L3) and especially at the thoracolumbar junction (T12-L1).

The sacrum (Fig. 5.2) consists of five fused vertebrae at the bottom of the spine. It acts as the keystone in the pelvis, transferring weight laterally from the spine through the immobile sacroiliac joints into the pelvis. At the inferior tip of the sacrum lies the coccyx, a vestigial tailbone. A true diarthrodial joint exists between the sacrum and coccyx that may be injured in falls on the buttocks or during childbirth. Painful disorders of the coccyx are referred to as coccydynia.

JOINTS

Each vertebra is connected to the next adjacent vertebra by three joints: two paired facet joints and one intervertebral disc. Each facet is composed of the inferior articular process from the upper vertebra joining with the superior articular process of the lower vertebra. These are true diarthrodial joints complete with facet capsules, synovial membrane, and fluid and articular hyaline cartilage. Ordinarily, the right and left facet joints are mirror images of each other. Because they are true joints, they may be affected by any disease process, either local or systemic, which affects articular cartilage. These joints are

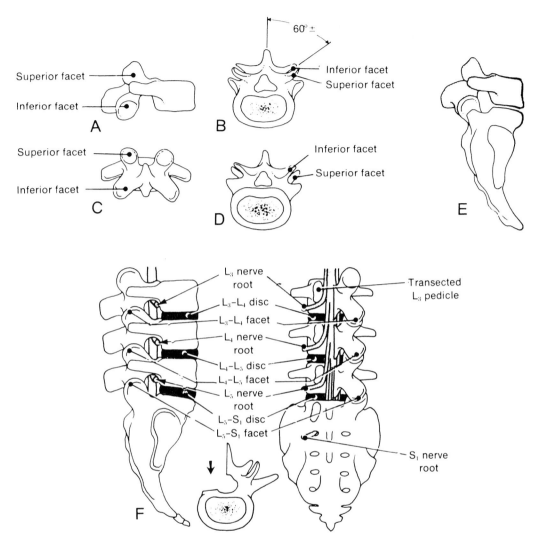

Figure 5.2. The lumbosacral spine. *A* and *B*, the 5th lumbar vertebra. Lateral and superior views. *C* and *D*, the 5th lumbar vertebra. Posterior and inferior views. *E*, the 5th lumbar vertebra, in articulation with the sacrum. *F*, the relationship of nerve roots to discs and the facet joints.

innervated by branches of the sinuvertebral nerve.

Thoracic facet joints are oriented in a sagittal direction so that flexion and extension as well as limited lateral bending are possible. The rib articulations provide some constraint to this motion so that the thoracic spine moves less and is more rigid than the cervical or lumbar spine.

Upper lumbar facet joints are similar to those in the thoracic spine. There is a gradual change from a sagittal orientation to a more coronal and transverse orientation through the lumbar spine so that lateral bending is increased as well as flexion and extension. Almost no rotation is possible, because the facet joints are mirror images of each other. The lumbosacral, or L5-S1 facet joint is a strong articulation, and because it is oriented at approximately 45° to the horizontal in both planes, it resists the large shear force generated by the lumbar lordosis.

INTERVERTEBRAL DISC

The third articulation between adjacent vertebrae is the intervertebral disc. This arises embryonically as the notochord around which the somites form; when persisting into adulthood, the intervertebral disc occasionally gives rise to midline tumors called chordomas. The disc is composed of an outer anulus fibrosus and an inner nucleus pulposus. The anulus consists primarily of type I collagen elaborated by fibroblasts and is structured as an interlocking series of circumferential layers that resist shear, distraction, and bursting forces generated in the nucleus. Only the outer third of the anulus is innervated. Unfortunately, the anulus weakens as it ages and is prone to tearing during twisting injuries.

The nucleus is composed primarily of type II collagen similar to articular cartilage, embedded in a matrix of proteoglycan and adsorbed water. Discs in children are approximately 80% water. This percentage decreases with age to approximately 30% in elderly patients. This age-related dehydration is commonly observed in MRI scans as a dark disc on T2 weighted images and is commonly labeled by the radiologist as disc degeneration, despite being a normal phenomenon of aging. The combination of collagen for strength and water and proteoglycan for cushioning gives the disc unique properties of limited compressibility, load bearing, and motion. The matrix is actively elaborated by embedded cartilage cells, which obtain nutrition by passive diffusion from the adjacent vertebral endplates but function anaerobically. There are no blood vessels, lymphatic channels, or nerve fibers in the nucleus.

LIGAMENTS

All bones are connected by ligaments that function to limit excursion of joints by becoming tight at the extremes of motion. The primary stabilizers of the thoracolumbar spine

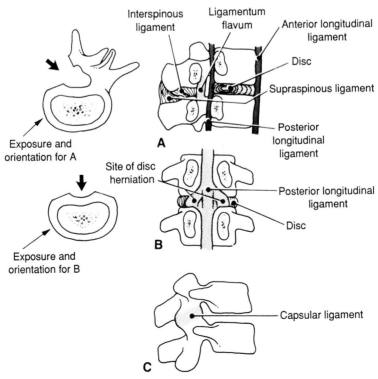

Figure 5.3. *A–C*, ligaments and discs of the dorsolumbar spine.

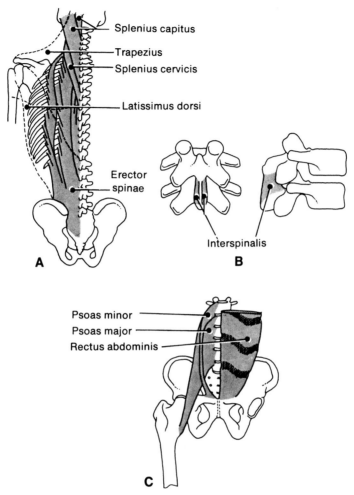

Figure 5.4. Musculature of the back. *A*, splenius and erector spinae muscle groups. *B*, interspinalis, posterior and lateral views. *C*, flexors of the lumbosacral spine.

are the anterior longitudinal ligament, which is anterior to the spine, the posterior longitudinal ligament posterior to the vertebral body, and the interspinous ligaments between the spinous processes and the facet capsules (Fig. 5.3). The posterior longitudinal ligament and interspinous ligament limit flexion (forward bending) of the spine while the anterior longitudinal ligament resists excessive extension (backwards bending). The facet capsules resist lateral bending. Also important is the ligamentum flavum that protects the spinal contents posteriorly and is the most elastic structure in the body. Overgrowth of this ligament results in spinal stenosis.

MUSCLES

Four basic sets of muscles are attached to the thoracolumbar spine (Fig. 5.4). Posteriorly, the most superficial layer includes the latissimus dorsi, trapezius, rhomboids, and levator scapulae, which function to move or stabilize the upper extremity. The intrinsic muscles of the spine are deep to this layer and are comprised of the erector spinae, interspinalis, and transversalis muscles. These are attached in various combinations from one of the posterior elements to another, and function to extend, rotate, and laterally bend the spine. Continuous and coordinated activity of these muscles balances the spine during sitting or standing. Spasms of these muscles can be painful and cause an involuntary list or bend of the spine in the direction of the spasm.

The third set of muscles, the psoas major and minor, attach to the anterior aspect of the lumbar vertebral bodies and function as hip flexors if the spine is stabilized, or as spine flexors if the hips are held immobile. Infection and tumors in the vertebral bodies may travel along the psoas muscles to the anterior thigh. The final set of muscles is the abdominal wall, composed of the rectus abdominis, the external oblique, internal oblique, and transversus abdominis. These counterbalance the extension force of the posterior intrinsic muscles but are often overlooked as part of the spine.

The different sets of muscles act in concert to balance the spine just as the guide wires of a tent support the central pole by pulling down. Thus, a muscle spasm will deviate the spine in the direction of pull of the particular muscle, whether lateral tilt, rotation, flexion or extension. Similarly, a significant difference in strength or flexibility of opposing muscle groups may result in abnormal posture or excessive muscle fatigue or weakness.

NERVOUS STRUCTURES

The spinal cord conducts nerve impulses from the periphery to the brain (sensory afferents) and from the brain to the periphery (motor efferents). This is a two synaptic relay system. Interruption of the relay between the primary (brain) and secondary (spinal cord) neurons results in loss of inhibition, leading to hyperexcitability, hyperreflexia, and clonus. Interruption of the secondary neurons (peripheral nerves) results in flaccid paralysis and areflexia.

The spinal cord gives off segmental nerves that form predictable patterns of innervation (peripheral nerves) in the appendicular skeleton, although there may be minor variations in individual patients. The thoracic nerve roots innervate the intercostal muscles after exiting the spinal canal under the pedicles. They are primarily sensory in a dermatomal pattern

with T4 at nipple level, T10 around the umbilicus, and L1 at the groin.

The lumbar nerve roots are involved in the innervation of the legs (Fig. 5.5). L2 through L4 combine in the midsubstance of the psoas muscles into the femoral plexus, which travels anteriorly into the pelvis to end as the femoral nerve. Portions of L4 as well as L5, S1, and S2 combine into the sciatic nerve anterior to the sacroiliac joint. The dermatomes in the legs wrap around laterally to medially so that L3 innervates the medial thigh, L4 the medial knee, L5 the anterior calf and dorsal foot, and S1 the posterior calf and sole of foot. Motor

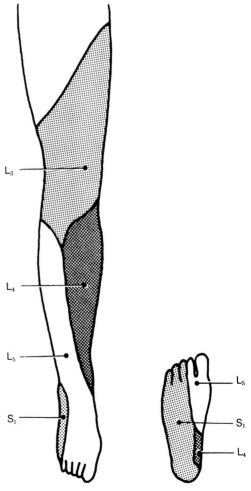

Figure 5.5. Sensory distribution of nerve roots, L-3 through S-1.

function is usually L3 and L4 to the hip flexors, L4 and L5 knee extensors, L5 foot dorsiflexors and S1 foot plantar flexors. The knee reflex is primarily L4, and the ankle reflex primarily S1. The remaining sacral nerve roots, S2 through S4, innervate the perineum, including perirectal and vaginal sensation, and control rectal and urethral sphincter tone.

The spinal cord ends at L1-L2 in 90% of people. Thus, lesions located in the spinal canal above L1 will affect the spinal cord, resulting in upper motor neuron lesions and hyperexcitability, whereas lesions below L1 will cause lower motor neuron symptoms such as paralysis and hyporeflexia.

The motor branch leaves the spinal cord as the ventral ramus, joins the dorsal ramus laterally in the spinal canal, and proceeds out the neural foramen as the peripheral nerve. The sensory ganglion where the sensory nerve cell nucleus lies is normally located in the neural foramen. After exiting the foramen, the nerve root gives off a sensory branch called the sinuvertebral nerve, which innervates the structures around the vertebral column: dura, facet joints, ligaments, and most importantly the outer third of the annulus of the disc. Because the sinuvertebral nerve innervates so many structures around the spine itself, pathologic lesions are often difficult to localize to any specific structure in the spine.

As the nerve root enters the foramen, it is bordered superiorly by the pedicle of the same number (i.e., L4 nerve root under L4 pedicle), posteriorly by the superior articular facet of the next lower vertebra, anteriorly by the posterior vertebral body, and inferiorly by an empty space. It reaches the level of the next lower disc far laterally, outside the foramen. Thus, the L4 nerve root will not be affected by an L4-L5 disc herniation unless in the far lateral position. Instead, a particular disc herniation will affect the next lower nerve root as it exits the spinal canal before the foramen.

VASCULAR SUPPLY

The arterial supply to the spine and associated structures comes as direct branches of the aorta and iliac arteries. In the thoracic spine, the segmental vessels from the aorta branch posteriorly at the level of the midvertebral body. Secondary branches then divide to supply the vertebral body, muscles, facet joints, and adjacent structures. A terminal branch joins the nerve root just lateral to the foramen and travels with this nerve root as the subcostal artery under the ribs. Unfortunately, the blood supply to the thoracic spinal cord is tenuous. Usually, only one or two of the segmental vessels send a significant branch to the spinal cord along the nerve root to anastomose with the anterior spinal artery that runs up and down along the entire length of the cord. This major blood supply to the cord enters between T4 and T10, usually on the right side as the artery of Adamkiewicz. This artery is neither large nor consistent in location. Thus, there is a significant risk of ischemic infarction of the cord during manipulation of or surgery on the thoracic spine.

In the lumbar spine, there is less need for vascular input to the cord as it ends at L1-L2, becoming the cauda equina. Because there are only peripheral nerves involved, the risk of vascular injury is much less. Aside from the branching of the aorta into iliac arteries at L4, the segmental supply to surrounding structures is the same as in the thoracic spine. The venous drainage of the spine is profuse. There is a large network of veins in the epidural space called Batson's plexus, which drains the vertebral bodies, dural space, muscles, facet joints, and segmental nerve roots. This receives tributaries from the pelvis and abdominal cavity in the lumbar spine and thoracic cavity in the thoracic spine. Significantly, these venous channels lack valves. Cancer cells may lodge in these valveless venous sinuses and, because flow is sluggish, become lodged as metastatic implants. Thus, tumors or infections in the genitourinary, gastrointestinal, or respiratory tracts can enter the spine hematogenously and produce foci of metastases or infection easily. This is why metastases to the spine are so common in patients dying of malignant tumors.

The lymphatic drainage is via the thoracic duct.

BIOMECHANICS

The spine has four purposes. Primarily, it supports body weight along with anything carried above the level involved. Evolutionary development of the backbone allowed vertebrates to resist gravity, ultimately culminating in the human's upright posture. To maintain this posture, the spine is balanced by a cervical lordosis for straight-ahead vision, a thoracic kyphosis for posture, and a lumbar lordosis for balance over the feet in bipedal locomotion. Although these curvatures are developmental, growth eventually imprints these curves into the bony anatomy of the spine, altering the shape of the vertebral bodies accordingly. Posture is maintained by the balance of the spinal muscles, primarily the abdominals for anterior support, and the long and short intrinsics muscles posteriorly. By maintaining a relatively constant tension, these muscles hold the spine upright. Excessive contraction of one set of muscles will pull the spine toward that side, as often occurs with muscle spasms after an injury. Similarly, chronic shortening or contraction of a muscle may cause an imbalance in posture.

The spinal curvature and the location of the center of gravity just anterior to the spine results in a compression side (the vertebral bodies anteriorly) and a tension side (the posterior ligament complex). Thus, 90% of weight is born by the vertebral bodies and discs anteriorly, while 10% is transmitted through the facet joints. Failure of either the compression side or the tension side may result in catastrophic spinal instability.

A second purpose of the spinal column is protection of the spinal cord and nerve roots. This is accomplished posteriorly by the strong lamina and spinous process and anteriorly by the large vertebral bodies that are resistant to compressive loading. However, this resistance decreases with metabolic, neoplastic, or infectious insults, which decrease bone mass and resistance to compression and thus may lead to spinal cord or nerve root compromise.

A third function of the spine is as an attachment point for muscles and ligaments responsible for moving the upper and lower extremities. Similarly, if the extremities remain fixed, these appendicular muscles help to move the spine.

The final function is as the primary site for hematopoietic marrow in the adult. In children, most of the skeleton as well as liver and spleen produce blood cells. In adults, these areas shrink to include only the pelvis and spine. Any process that produces diffuse involvement of the bone marrow in the spine (such as myeloma) may result in anemia, leukopenia, and thrombocytopenia, as well as problems in the vertebrae.

EVALUATION OF PATIENTS WITH BACK PAIN

When confronted with an office full of patients on a Monday morning and the first three chief complaints are low back pain, it is tempting to cut corners and proceed directly to an x-ray or MRI. Unfortunately, these and other tests do not always correlate with specific symptoms or disease processes. Thus, the history and physical examination are still crucial to developing the differential diagnosis. Laboratory tests may confirm a clinical suspicion but should never be relied on as the primary diagnostic modality.

HISTORY

The history begins with the chief complaint, usually back pain. Rarely, a deformity or neurologic symptoms may be the presenting complaint. The onset of pain is particularly important, especially whether it was traumatic and sudden or gradual and insidious. Frequently, patients associate the onset of pain with a particular event even though they may not be causally related. If there was trauma, the issue of compensation or litigation may arise (see below), explaining the need of some patients to blame their problems on a particular compensable event.

Since the onset of the pain, has the pain changed appreciably, and if so, how? Worsening pain should prompt the clinician to be more aggressive with the workup, whereas improving symptoms usually connote a benign or self-limited process. Is the pain continuous or episodic? Constant pain is worrisome. If the pain is changing, what makes it better and what makes it worse? Is the pain different at different times? Mechanical low back pain usually is better at night and while lying down, whereas malignancies, infection, or other serious disorders are often unaffected by posture and are usually worse at night. The pain of herniated discs is worse while sitting and better walking, whereas the symptoms of spinal stenosis are aggravated by being upright and walking and improved when sitting.

It is useful to categorize the pain into one of four types based on location: local (confined to the low back), referred (buttocks and posterior thigh), radicular (following the course of a nerve such as T10 towards the umbilicus or L5 to the big toe), and spasmodic (shooting up and down the spine, secondary to a local muscle spasm or cramp in the back). The character of the pain is often helpful. Sharp stabbing or knifelike pain is usually indicative of a muscle spasm, whereas burning or throbbing may be caused by nerve irritation or compression. Any associated numbness, tingling, paresthesias, loss of muscle control, or other neurologic symptoms should be ascertained. Prior treatments and their efficacy are important to determine, because pain that has not responded to two physical therapy courses carries a bad prognosis for recovery, regardless of the etiology. Does the pain change with Valsalva maneuvers such as coughing, sneezing, or straining? A positive response often indicates nerve root or spinal cord involvement, because Valsalva maneuvers increase the pressure on the nerves via the epidural venous plexus.

Finally, other complaints such as weight loss, fevers, chills, anorexia, nausea, vomiting, and other systemic symptoms should be elicited along with relevant medical and surgical histories, medications, and allergies. Positive response to these questions may indicate spinal involvement by more generalized diseases.

There are a series of positive responses, or red flags, in the history that should alert the clinician to the possibility of a serious condition. Night pain, especially that which forces the patient to arise or pace, is often a warning sign of infection or malignancy. Morning stiffness that improves with exercise often indicates a rheumatologic etiology such as ankylosing spondylitis, Reiter's syndrome, or Lyme disease. Obviously, weight loss or malaise may indicate malignancy, and spiking fevers can be associated with infection. Finally, neurologic symptoms such as sciatica (pain radiating down the back of the thigh to below the knee) are associated with nerve root involvement, whereas bilateral nerve symptoms or loss of sphincter control may indicate cauda equina or spinal cord involvement.

PAIN DIAGRAMS (FIG. 5.6)

Pain diagrams are extremely helpful in identifying patients with functional overlay or nonorganic complaints. While in the waiting area, patients are given a blank body diagram (Fig. 5.6) with instructions to mark all areas of pain, numbness, tingling, or other abnormal sensations on the figure. Patients with organic mechanical low back pain will mark their low back, buttocks, or upper thighs. Radicular pain will have marks following the course of the particular nerve root affected such as anterior thigh for L4 or posterior calf and foot for S1. Occasionally, the patient will draw a face or hair on the blank figure, which indicates a positive self image.

On the other hand, patients with functional overlay (formerly called malingering) or significant psychologic components to their back pain will often label areas outside their body as painful, which is clearly impossible. Occasionally, sharp objects are drawn impaling a part of the body, or blood dripping from an area without wounds. These and other bizarre images are nonorganic manifestations and

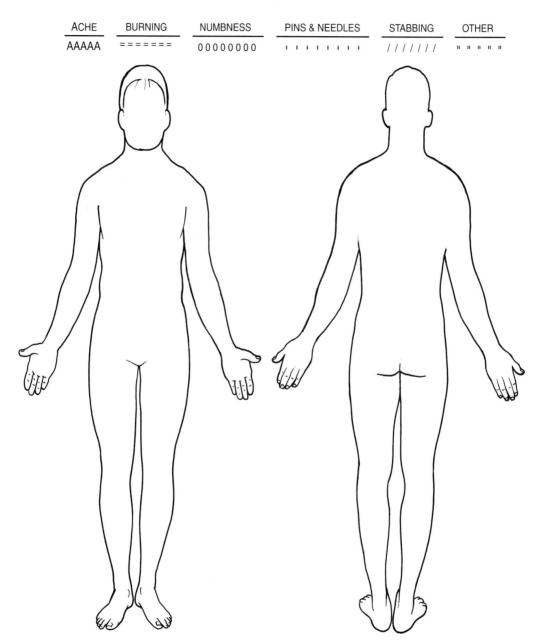

Figure 5.6. Pain drawing grid assessment.

point to an unhappy, poorly adjusted or hostile patient.

Other objective measures, such as the Oswestry pain score, the North American Spine Society (NASS) functional pain questionnaire, or the Minnesota Multiphasic Personality Inventory (MMPI), may give more objective detail about the patient's subjective complaints of pain but are beyond the scope of this chapter.

PHYSICAL EXAMINATION

The patient should be undressed and robed in a loose-fitting gown with the back open. Underwear may be left on, but shoes should be removed. During the history, the clinician observes the patient informally as to comfort level, ease of movement, and favored positioning. During the examination, the patient is asked to walk around the examination room to determine gait. A normal gait is called heel-to-toe, which is heel strike followed by stance phase (full foot contact) and then toe off in a coordinated fashion on both sides. An antalgic gait occurs when standing on one of the legs is painful, causing the patient to avoid weight-bearing on that side as much as possible. A foot-drop gait occurs with weakness of foot dorsiflexion (anterior tibialis and extensor hallucis muscles, innervated by L5) causing the foot to slap at heel strike. A Trendelenburg gait is caused by hip weakness or pain and causes the patient to waddle and drop the affected hip while weightbearing on that side. A broad-based gait with imbalance is frequently associated with spinal cord dysfunction. The patient is asked to walk on the heels first and then on the toes to test muscle function in foot dorsiflexors (L5) and ankle plantar flexors (S1).

Next, the back is inspected for scars, deformity (scoliosis, increased or decreased lordosis, or excessive thoracic kyphosis), skin lesions (heating pad burns or ecchymoses), hairy patches or dimples (indicative of spinal dysraphism), shoulder alignment, balance, and pelvic obliquity (indicating true or functional leg length inequality).

Palpation of the midline spinous processes may reveal a forward step-off as seen in spondylolisthesis. Paravertebral muscle spasm is felt as a tight or quivering muscle just lateral to the spinous processes. Masses, areas of fluctuation, and bony defects may be found by palpation. Tenderness to light touch is an important Waddell sign (see discussion on Waddell sign). Finally, palpation of the sciatic nerve just inferior to the ischial tuberosity may indicate a tender and inflamed nerve, and pressure over the greater trochanter may indicate trochanteric bursitis.

Percussion of the spine is rarely useful except in cases of spinal tumors or infection that may occasionally be painful to percussion. Pain on pressure over the kidneys at the costovertebral angle should point the way toward the urinary system as the source of the patient's back pain.

Range of motion of the spine and hips are evaluated next. The patient is asked to bend forward at the waist as far as pain free and then extend backwards in similar fashion. How the patient moves as well as how far he or she moves is observed. The angle of flexion and extension can be estimated as degrees from the vertical, or measured by a goniometer if accuracy is important. Alternately and more reproducibly, the part of the leg that the patient can easily touch can be listed as the point of maximal flexion such as knees, ankles, floor, etc.

During forward bending, the normal lumbar lordosis is reversed into a gentle kyphosis. Muscle spasm, ankylosis, or other abnormality may hinder this smooth transition and should be noted. Any forward slip may be exaggerated by forward flexion, and thoracolumbar scoliosis with a rib hump or lumbar prominence can be detected easily with the patient bent forward at the waist. Lateral bending is noted in degrees. Trunk rotation that is not an inherent motion of the lumbar spine but instead comes from the hips is evaluated as one of the Waddell signs. Range of motion of the hips and knees are best checked with the patient sitting or lying down. Many times the diagnosis of hip arthritis has been missed by skipping this important physical test.

The patient then sits on the examination table. A straight leg raising sign is elicited by asking but never forcing the patient to straighten the knee in front while sitting. The amount of hip flexion and knee extension obtained before pain in the leg occurs should be noted and compared with the supine straight leg raising test obtained with the patient lying down. A significant discrepancy between these values is a positive Waddell sign. To be truly positive, the straight leg raising (SLR) test must cause leg pain, not back pain alone. Occasionally, an SLR on one side will provoke leg pain on the opposite side, termed the crossed straight leg raising sign. This is 99% specific for a herniated disc on the painful side. The SLR tests for irritation of the sciatic nerve. To test for irritation of the femoral nerve, the patient is placed prone and the hip extended while the knee is flexed. If anterior thigh pain is elicited, this is a positive reversed SLR or flip test. Hip range of motion can be checked easily with the patient sitting on the examination table by stabilizing the knee with one hand and rotating the lower leg back and forth. A difference between sides or pain in the hip, buttock, or groin may indicate a painful hip condition such as osteoarthritis.

The knee reflex (L4) and ankle reflexes (S1) are elicited with the reflex hammer. If necessary, strength of the quadriceps (L4), extensor hallucis longus, and anterior tibialis muscles (L5) and gastro-soleus (S1) can be checked. Sensation or lack thereof can be checked with a paper clip or sterile pin; vibration sense for intact posterior columns is occasionally elicited by tuning fork as can be proprioception. Finally, the Babinski sign (up going is normal) and presence of clonus should be checked to evaluate for upper motor neuron disease. If long tract signs are present, the lesion must be higher than the lumbar spine since the spinal cord ends at approximately L1.

Finally, the patient is asked to lie down on the examining table. Again, the SLR test is elicited with the knee extended along with the hip range of motion test. A crossed leg test, or Faber (flexion-abduction-external rotation) test, is performed by placing the patient's ankle on the opposite knee with the hip flexed and externally rotated into a figure-four position. The knee is pushed downward, stressing the opposite sacroiliac joint. A positive pain provocation may indicate sacroiliitis caused by an infection in the sacroiliac joint or early ankylosing spondylitis. A reverse SLR test is performed by placing the patient prone and flexing the knee while extending the hip. This stretches the femoral nerve and is equivalent

to the SLR test for sciatica, but tests the L3 and L4 nerve roots that make up the femoral nerve.

WADDELL SIGNS

Originally described in 1980 by Gordon Waddell, this group of five signs is used extensively to identify patients with functional overlay. Functional overlay is the term currently used to denote patients formerly called malingerers—those with nonorganic signs who may be exaggerating or inventing symptoms, often for secondary gain.

The five signs are listed in Table 5.1. During the history and initial physical examination, the patient is observed for mannerisms and inconsistencies. Suspicion that the story given is untrue, exaggerated, or that the patient is out for secondary gain (money, disability, back massages, etc.) is counted as one positive Waddell sign. Simulation is performed by having the patient rotate his or her trunk back and forth in the standing position. Since the lumbar spine has no inherent rotation, this is accomplished by the hip joints and only simulates spine motion. If the patient complains of back pain during this maneuver, a positive Waddell sign is counted. Tenderness to light touch is documented by lightly pinching or rolling the skin of the back. Complaints of pain or the patient moving away from the examiner is a positive Waddell sign. Nonanatomic neurologic signs, such as numbness of the entire leg or global weakness in the

Table 5.1. Waddell Signs

1. General appearance: attitude and overreaction.
2. Tenderness:
   a. Superficial
   b. Nonanatomic
3. Simulation:
   a. Axial loading
   b. Trunk rotation
4. Distraction:
   a. Straight leg raising: sitting
   b. Straight leg raising: supine
5. Regional disturbances:
   a. Weakness
   b. Sensory

absence of central brain or cord involvement, is a fourth sign. Finally, a discrepancy in the SLR between lying and sitting can be identified by doing the SLR in both positions. Many patients with functional overlay will have no problem performing the SLR to 90° while sitting but will complain of severe pain in the back or leg at 20° while supine. This counts as the fifth Waddell sign.

In the original paper by Waddell, three or more positive signs correlated well with functional overlay or secondary gain. Many spine surgeons now use two or more as the threshold. Whichever is chosen, many papers have verified the use of Waddell signs to differentiate those who will do well with any particular treatment, whether it is therapy, surgery, or other, from those with functional overlay who will do poorly. Similarly, return to work within a reasonable time frame is inversely correlated with number of positive Waddell signs.

LABORATORY STUDIES

Laboratory studies should be used to confirm a clinically suspected diagnosis or to differentiate between two possibilities in the differential. Rarely will an x-ray or blood test be the primary indication of a particular disease, although there are exceptions such as an elevated erythrocyte sedimentation (SED) rate in infection, a characteristic MRI picture in metastatic cancer, or serum protein electrophoresis (SPEP) for myeloma. This is because many of the tests used in patients with low back pain are not specific, and have high rates of false-positive and false-negative predictive values. Additionally, many radiographic findings, including CT and MRI, are age related and do not necessarily reflect a pathologic disease state. However, laboratory studies remain a significant portion of the diagnostic triad.

X-rays

Plain x-rays give a two-dimensional picture of the three-dimensional spine. The routine series consists of AP (Fig. 5.7), lateral, and spot L5-S1. This last film, L5-S1, is done

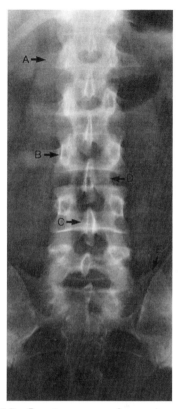

Figure 5.7. Roentgenogram of normal lumbosacral spine. *A,* transverse process. *B,* pedicle. *C,* posterior spinous process. *D,* lamina. *E,* sacrum.

because the pelvis often obscures the lower lumbar spine on the lateral x-ray. On the AP x-ray, the spine is checked for lateral deviation (scoliosis), rotation, missing parts such as an absent pedicle (often the first radiographic sign in metastatic cancer), fractures, and asymmetry. A standing AP can be used to check leg length inequality by determining abnormal pelvic tilt. The normal spine is straight and symmetrical on the AP film.

The lateral and spot films will show the normal lumbar lordosis (concave posteriorly). Abnormalities often noted include compression fractures, bone erosion, disc space narrowing (often part of the normal aging process), endplate erosion (seen in discitis), and facet osteoarthritis. Slippage of one vertebra on top of the one below may be visible and is always abnormal. Forward slippage is called as spondylolisthesis and backward slippage is called retrolisthesis.

Oblique x-rays are occasionally helpful to visualize the pars interarticularis (the junction of the five parts of the spine). This is the weakest part of the vertebra and may occasionally suffer a stress fracture (spondylolysis), the most common cause of back pain in the adolescent. The facet joints between adjacent vertebrae can also be seen more readily on the oblique films to check for osteoarthritis (spondylosis). Finally, the neuroforamina (exit points for the nerve roots) can be visualized on the obliques, although these are better evaluated by CT or MRI scan.

Dynamic lateral flexion/extension plain films are occasionally useful to document instability. These are best done standing, with the patient asked to bend forward and then backwards as far as possible without undue pain on each x-ray. Displacement forward or backward by more than 4 mm or angulation of more than 15° is considered potentially unstable. Lateral AP bending films to the left and right can be used to check the flexibility of the scoliotic curve, although in the primary care setting these rarely are used.

CT Scan

Initially used extensively to evaluate the soft tissues of the spine, disc, and spinal canal, the CT has largely been replaced by the MRI scan for soft tissue work. However, the CT scan is still useful to delineate the bony anatomy in cases where plain x-rays are unclear or ambiguous. CT gives direct transverse pictures of the three-dimensional spine, and a three-dimensional picture can be constructed with computerized reconstruction techniques. CT is useful to evaluate bony destruction, fractures, spinal canal dimensions, and facet joint abnormalities. Conditions in which this is particularly helpful include spondylolisthesis and spondylolysis, bone tumors, and facet asymmetry. If MRI is unavailable, CT is helpful for conditions such as herniated discs, spinal stenosis, and nerve root abnormalities. The benefit of CT is that it gives better bone detail than MRI, and is much cheaper. The

disadvantages are that soft tissues are all shown in various shades of gray and ionizing radiation is used. Also, any metallic artifacts will degrade or scatter the image.

Bone Scan

Technetium pyrophosphate radiolabeled bone scans provide a metabolic picture of the skeleton. Active osteoblasts pick up the radioactive tracer preferentially. Thus, any bone or part thereof that is actively incorporating phosphate into its matrix will be picked up as a hot spot on the bone scan. Conditions that stimulate the bone, such as osteoblastic tumors (both primary and metastatic), fractures (both stress and acute), disc or bone infections, osteoarthritis, and Paget's disease, will cause increased uptake and appear as dark spots on the bone scan. These various conditions can often be differentiated from each other by their characteristic patterns, especially with the use of single photon emission computed tomography (SPECT) bone scans, which give a CT type of image and are more sensitive than the plain bone scan.

Conversely, any process that causes bone to be less active will show up as a void on bone scan. These include large osteolytic tumors, some hemangiomas, and surgical bone resections. However, it is important to note that marrow diseases, such as lymphoma, leukemia, and myeloma, will be normal on the bone scan, because these conditions do not cause bony reaction.

MRI

Since its introduction in the 1980s in the United States, the MRI has become the gold standard test in many clinical situations. MRI shows primarily soft tissues, and in the spine, this refers primarily to the discs, spinal cord and nerve roots, blood vessels, and muscles. To a lesser extent, bones, tendons, and ligaments can be visualized. This is primarily because MR images hydrogen nuclei best, and the well visualized structures contain water, whereas the less well visualized structures are dry. In addition, MRI is useful in differentiating tumors from normal tissue and in identifying infections. Also, unlike CT scanning, MRI can give true pictures in any plane desired, whether sagittal, coronal, or transverse.

The major drawbacks to using MRI are expense (sometimes amounting to more than $1,000 per examination), degradation of the image by the presence of ferromagnetic implants, claustrophobia on the part of some patients, and the loss of clairvoyance in one case.

In the evaluation of back problems, MRI is primarily used to visualize the spinal cord, vertebral column, and enclosed structures. MRI is the test of choice in identifying infections around the spine such as tuberculosis and discitis, herniated discs, spinal stenosis, and other causes of radiculopathy. Spinal tumors, including metastases to bone and intradural and extradural extensions, are well visualized. By injecting Gadolinium intravenously, scar tissue from prior surgery can be differentiated from otherwise normal or pathologic structures such as recurrent disc herniations. To a large extent, MRI has supplanted myelography as the best test for spinal canal problems, because the latter is invasive and entails the risk of infection and spinal headaches.

Clinical problems where MRI is not useful include the evaluation of fractures in which x-rays and CT scans are more helpful, and in active spondylolysis where bone scanning is better.

Unfortunately, like other tests MRI is rarely diagnostic. Several authors have found a high false-positive rate of up to 30% in normal healthy asymptomatic volunteers. This error rate approaches 65% in older patients. Thus, any abnormality seen on an MRI scan must be correlated with the patient's history and physical examination to arrive at a clinical diagnosis. MRI should be used to confirm or localize a clinically suspected diagnosis, not as a fishing expedition for possible spinal pathology.

Blood Tests

As with the MRI, blood tests will most commonly support or clinch but rarely provide a clinical diagnosis. A complete blood count (CBC) is rarely useful, except as a marker for anemia in marrow-occupying lesions or occasionally in infections. The erythrocyte sedimentation rate (ESR) is one blood test that should be used more frequently. An uncommon but potentially serious cause of back pain is bacterial infection, either in the disc (discitis), vertebra (osteomyelitis), or epidural space (epidural abscess). In all three, the ESR as well as the C-reactive protein (CRP) are significantly elevated early in the disease process when the infection is contained in the affected structure and before systemic spread resulting in sepsis. These are often the only blood tests that are abnormal, because frequently the white blood cell count (WBC) is normal before systemic spread. Thus, if there is any question of a spinal infection, an ESR should be ordered and may occasionally save the patient and clinician from a potentially disastrous delayed diagnosis or misdiagnosis.

Metabolic problems such as hyperparathyroidism, tumor induced hypercalcemia, renal abnormalities, hypothyroidism, etc., that affect the skeletal system can be picked up by blood tests, but usually these diagnoses are suspected on other grounds rather than initially presenting in the spine. In general, the following tests will cover most spinal abnormalities: CBC, ESR, Ca, Phos, BUN, Creat, Glucose, thyroid levels, and alkaline phosphatase. The alkaline phosphatase may be elevated in any abnormality involving bone destruction or excess activity and thus is nonspecific.

Finally, rheumatologic tests should be considered with any possibility of inflammatory arthritis, such as lupus (ANA), rheumatoid arthritis (Rheumatoid factor), ankylosing spondylitis (HLA B-27), and Lyme disease (Lyme titer). Except for ankylosing spondylitis, these inflammatory spondyloarthropathies almost always affect the spine late in the disease course. However, because ankylosing spondylitis usually begins in the axial skeleton (often in the sacroiliac joints), back pain is frequently the primary initial complaint (see "Spondylolysis and Spondylolisthesis"). Thus, in any otherwise healthy young patient with back pain, the diagnosis of ankylosing spondylitis must be considered, and an HLA B-27 positive test may point the way to this diagnosis.

COMMON SPINAL CONDITIONS

The aim of the workup is to obtain a diagnosis so that treatment can be initiated. It has been estimated that an exact pathologic diagnosis will be discovered in less than 50% of patients with low back pain. However, because so many of the identifiable causes of low back pain are serious with such capacity for spinal destruction and instability, the diagnostic algorithm discussed above should be followed. This section describes many common etiologies of back pain as well as early management strategies.

SPONDYLOLYSIS AND SPONDYLOLISTHESIS

There is generally much confusion about these terms. *Spondylos-* denotes spine, *-lysis* derives from broken, and *-listhesis* denotes slipped. Thus, a spondylolysis by common usage refers to a stress fracture of the pars interarticularis, whereas a spondylolisthesis refers to one vertebra slipping forward relative to the one below. The term anterolisthesis is equivalent to although less common than spondylolisthesis, while the term retrolisthesis denotes slipping backwards. Spondylosis, however, has come to mean abnormal spinal degenerative disease, or osteoarthritis of the spine, and is discussed separately.

Spondylolysis (Fig. 5.8) is a fracture through the pars interarticularis of a vertebra. It is most common at L5 but may occur in any vertebra. Usually, this is a stress fracture where this weakest part of the vertebra is consistently overloaded and finally snaps. Spondylolysis commonly occurs in adolescents, with an increased prevalence in football linemen, ballet dancers, gymnasts, and rowers. Common to all these activities is prolonged or repetitive extension of the lumbar spine. One population-based series found a prevalence of 4% in healthy first graders, increasing to 5.8% in the same adolescents 10 years later. This study was based on a radiographic survey of all children in a town in northern Pennsylvania, so it probably represents a true prevalence rate. Some, but not all of the children were asymptomatic, and many had

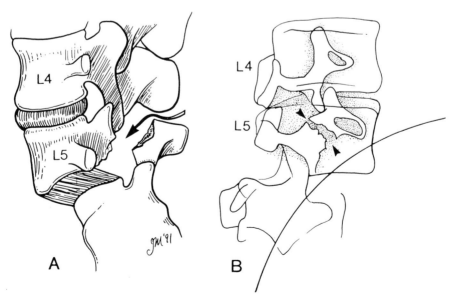

Figure 5.8.   *A,* lateral view of spondylolytic spondylolisthesis. *B,* spondylolysis. 45° oblique view of the lumbar space will show a defect in the pars interarticularis.

no recollection of any spinal trauma. Significantly, no cases of spondylolysis have been found in an autopsy series of 500 stillborn infants. Therefore, spondylolysis is not a congenital defect. A group of Eskimos that were studied in Alaska have a higher than 50% prevalence rate of spondylolysis, indicating that both genetic and traumatic factors are involved in the etiology of this condition.

The usual, but by no means only, presentation of spondylolysis is the teenage athlete with sudden or gradual onset of low back pain. In fact, spondylolysis is the most common cause of back pain in the adolescent. The pain is usually localized to the lower back and is aggravated by extension, relieved by bending forward or resting, and may radiate to the buttocks and posterior thighs. Morning stiffness is common and the causative activity is usually too painful to be continued. Night pain is extremely rare.

On examination, there may be tenderness in the lumbar spine with muscle spasms. Neurologic examination is usually normal, and frequently the hamstrings are abnormally tight. Active extension is painful, and the patient will usually avoid this activity.

Laboratory tests are normal with the exception of the x-ray. Because the pars interarticularis is oblique to the coronal and sagittal planes, routine AP and lateral films will frequently fail to visualize the fracture. Thus, oblique x-rays are indicated that will profile the pars. Occasionally, even oblique films miss the fracture, so a CT scan can be used in cases with negative plain films and a high index of suspicion.

The same set of symptoms can occur in an incipient but incomplete stress fracture, which will not be seen on x-ray or CT scan. Thus, a bone scan or, if available, a SPECT scan is often useful to detect the increased bone activity around an incipient stress fracture.

Once the diagnosis has been made, treatment is initially symptomatic. Avoidance of the offending activity is mandatory until symptoms disappear. Nonsteroidal anti-inflammatory drugs (NSAIDs) can be used but will not speed healing. Physical therapy to stretch the tight hamstrings and improve lumbar strength and flexibility is helpful. Promotion of antilordotic posture may ease the pain.

If these conservative treatments fail, a trial of immobilization in the Boston brace should be considered. This orthosis is a plastic lumbosacral orthosis that is fitted in an antilordotic position. This positioning promotes contact of the two sides of the fracture and has been found to heal the defect in 54% of patients at follow-up x-ray. More importantly, it alleviates pain in a significant majority of adolescents and allows gradual resumption of full activities after cessation of symptoms. The brace is ordinarily worn for at least 3 months and then a weaning process is begun; after 9–12 months, the brace can be discarded.

If all conservative treatment fails, surgery may be the only option. Traditionally, a posterolateral fusion of the slipped vertebra to the one below is the standard technique, since initial attempts to heal the lytic defect by bone grafting resulted in a high failure rate. Wiltse has reported a better than 90% success rate with simple posterolateral fusion without instrumentation in alleviating back pain, radicular symptoms, and the hamstring tightness. Most patients were able to resume full activities without restriction after 6 months.

If the spondylolysis is present at L4 or above, direct repair of the fracture with bone grafting and circular wiring or screw insertion can be done. This avoids the necessity of fusing two vertebrae together and thus may retain more lumbar spine motion; however, in most series, this procedure has a higher failure rate and is technically more difficult. Thus, the Wiltse posterolateral fusion remains the gold standard for surgical treatment of spondylolysis.

Spondylolisthesis is the slipping of one vertebra forward on top of another. It is generally secondary to a spondylolysis, but occasionally may result from abnormal facet joints, pathologic bone (as in Paget's disease), or surgical removal of enough bone to allow instability. On x-ray, spondylolisthesis is measured as the amount of forward slip on the standing lateral x-ray compared with the AP length of the lower vertebral body. This can be denoted as a percentage, e.g., 40% slip, or as a grade, where grade 1 denotes a slip of from 1% to 25%, grade 2 as 25% to 50%, grade 3 as 50% to 75%, and grade 4 as more than 75% forward slip. Currently, many authors group grade 1 and 2 into low-grade slips and grade 3 or 4 as high-grade slips, because recommended treatment differs for the two categories.

Low-grade slips can be treated in the same fashion as simple spondylolysis, with conservative treatment having a high rate of success. However, high-grade slips are treated surgically with fusion as soon as discovered, because these tend to progress to higher degrees of slips, are refractory to conservative treatment, and are usually symptomatic. Once again, posterolateral fusion is the gold standard, although many surgeons also will perform a decompression of the loose posterior elements at the same time, and frequently surgical instrumentation (screws, rods, or plates) is added to improve fusion rates and clinical success.

The preceding discussion applies primarily to spondylolysis and spondylolisthesis discovered and treated in the adolescent. A frequent clinical problem encountered is the adult with sudden or gradual onset of back pain who is found to have spondylolysis or a low-grade spondylolisthesis on lateral x-ray. Usually, these patients have no history of back problems, even during adolescence, and frequently the onset of back pain comes after a work-related injury. It is simplistic to ascribe the patient's current back pain to spondylolysis, because these are not commonly new fractures, evidenced by the usually negative bone scan. At times, another condition may cause the back pain such as a herniated disc, muscular strain, or compensation related back pain. Thus, the patient should still be worked up for other causes of back pain before the current episode is ascribed to spondylolysis. However, if nothing else is found, spondylolysis can present suddenly in middle age. Current thinking is that a disc injury or degeneration will allow a sudden increase in slip leading

to the episode of back pain in a previously asymptomatic individual. These patients will present just as in adolescents, with primary back pain plus or minus leg pain and tight hamstrings. Radicular pain is more common in the adult, probably from foraminal narrowing above the slip, and athletics are not usually involved. Extension of the lumbar spine is more painful than flexion, and the neurologic examination is often positive for mild L5 nerve deficits (weak ankle and great toe dorsiflexion, numbness of the big toe and top of foot). The radiographic workup is the same as previously described, except that the bone scan is almost always negative, indicative of a chronic or longstanding lysis.

Treatment in the adult is directed more at functional improvement rather than healing the fracture. Thus, physical therapy is more important, with postural exercises and lumbar muscle and abdominal strengthening. Reliance on modalities such as heat, ultrasound, and other passive modalities should be avoided. Braces are usually ineffective and many adults will not wear them, although a simple corset for support is often helpful. Injection of corticosteroids with Xylocaine into the spondylolysis is often used both diagnostically and therapeutically. If successive injections into the pars defect relieve the pain temporarily but the pain returns, surgical treatment is usually effective, because the injections help confirm that the pars fracture is truly the cause of the patient's symptoms. If no relief is obtained from the injections even temporarily, a more thorough search for the cause of the patient's pain must be undertaken.

If surgery is ultimately undertaken, the same protocol is followed as with adolescents, except that instrumentation is more often used to assure a higher fusion rate. Reduction of the slip by instrumentation can lead to unintended L5 nerve stretch, causing chronic and unrelieved radicular pain, and should be avoided if possible. Treatment for high-grade spondylolistheses is difficult and has a high complication rate, and fortunately, this condition is extremely rare in adults.

Finally, pseudospondylolisthesis, or degenerative spondylolisthesis, occurs in older patients caused by extensive osteoarthritis of the lumbar facet joints. This most commonly occurs in women at L4-L5 and when the pars is intact. Because the presentation is usually as spinal stenosis, this will be discussed in that section.

SPINAL INFECTIONS

Although rare, spinal infections are potentially more dangerous than any other spinal problem. Before the advent of effective antibiotic therapy, tuberculosis of the spine was extremely common. In fact, surgical treatment of this problem led to the development of many surgical techniques still used today for other maladies (anterior debridement, posterior fusions). Now that tuberculosis has receded from the clinical experience of many physicians, spinal infections are not often part of the common differential diagnosis. A high index of suspicion is necessary to avoid missing one of these potentially lethal infections.

Infection in the spine commonly occurs in two age groups: children and debilitated older adults. In children, the edges of the vertebral endplate and outer disc are vascularized. Because most infections enter the spine hematogenously, bacteria may circulate to these vascular areas of the disc, lodge in the vascular sinusoids present there, and set up a nidus of infection. The bacteria then invade the nonvascularized disc where host defense mechanisms will not reach and gradually develop an abscess cavity or infiltrative infection. In children, the most frequent organism is Staphylococcus aureus, although streptococcus can occur in neonates and other bacteria in immunocompromised individuals. Only rarely can a prior source of infection be identified in children.

In adults, there is usually a preceding source of infection elsewhere in the patient, such as endocarditis, skin ulcer, urinary tract infection, or pneumonia. The bacteria then spread hematogenously and lodge in the venous channels next to a degenerated disc or bone, setting up an infection. These patients are usually debilitated with pre-existing risk factors such as diabetes, alcoholism, chronic urinary catheterization, etc., which predispose them to frequent bacteremia. The organism is often staphylococcus, but almost any bacteria or fungus may be involved.

Regardless of age, the common presenting symptom is unremitting back pain. This pain usually is present both day and night, often is worse at night, and is not posture dependent (unlike mechanical back pain). Many times the patient will be awakened from sleep and will pace the hall, a red flag in the history. Characteristically, the pain worsens gradually and the patients may return many times to the practitioner complaining of worsening back pain. This clinical picture should alert one to possible spinal infection and the workup should be aggressive. Radicular or myelopathic symptoms (gait abnormalities, saddle anesthesia, or urinary incontinence) present late in the course and indicate a serious prognosis. The pain is usually deep and difficult to localize, although it will generally be around the area of the infection. In normal children, back pain is a rare complaint, even when an important test at school is scheduled. Thus, any child complaining of back pain should be investigated early and aggressively, because discitis is one of the common causes of back pain in children.

The physical examination is usually noncontributory except that occasionally tenderness to percussion is found. Outward sign of infection is almost never present around the spine such as erythema, drainage, or lymphangitis, because the infection remains deep in the spine.

Infection is one case in which laboratory tests are diagnostic. Usually the WBC is normal. However, the ESR is sensitive and will be elevated early, often near 100 mm/hour. Thus, if there is any suspicion of infection, the ESR should be obtained. Once the probability of infection is considered, the MRI is an excellent study to locate the infection and ascertain the extent of spread. Characteristically, pus can be visualized as a cavity in the disc or bone with high intensity on T2 weighted images. Because most infections begin in the disc, any disc abnormality affecting the bone on both sides on the lateral x-ray should be suspected as being discitis. This is especially true in children in which frequently the only early radiologic sign is endplate erosions or indistinctness on both sides of the disc.

Treatment depends on obtaining the organism and prescribing the appropriate antibiotic. In children, the most common organism is Staphylococcus aureus; therefore, a presumptive diagnosis can be made and IV anti-staphylococcus antibiotics given. If the clinical course does not improve rapidly, then biopsy or aspiration should be performed to identify the organism. In adults, however, any organism is possible, thus direct isolation of the organism is mandatory. Often, the bacteria can be identified from blood cultures or culturing the primary site of infection. However, cases of simultaneous infection with two or more organisms have been reported, especially in the compromised host, thus direct aspiration or biopsy of the spine is frequently necessary in adults. This can be performed radiographically with CT guided fine needle aspiration under local anesthesia.

Ordinarily, 6 weeks of intravenous antibiotics will be necessary, with consultation of infectious disease specialists to monitor antibiotic levels and efficacy. Occasionally, 2 weeks of IV antibiotics followed by 4 weeks of effective oral antibiotics can be given in children, although effective bactericidal levels must be assured. In children, a rigid brace is recommended to rest the infected spinal segment and prevent bone collapse. In adults, a brace is helpful to lessen pain but will not usually prevent collapse into kyphosis or scoliosis.

If the infection is left untreated or ignored, consequences may be severe. The bacteria gradually form an abscess that will eventually break out of the disc or bone. If breakout occurs anteriorly, a retroperitoneal or intrapleural abscess will occur. If the psoas muscle is involved anterolaterally, the abscess may track into the medial thigh. Most severe is posterior extension into the spinal canal. This will lead to an epidural abscess with compromise of the spinal cord or nerve roots. Often, this catastrophic event (paraplegia) is the first presentation of a previously ignored or downplayed episode of discitis. Once the neurologic structures are involved, surgical debridement as soon as possible is mandatory.

If an abscess is present on MRI or if neurologic compromise is evident, surgical debridement is recommended. This can be performed posteriorly via a laminectomy, although most surgeons will approach the problem anteriorly via a thoracic or retroperitoneal approach. Effective drainage of the abscess, debridement of the necrotic bone and soft tissue, and adequate stabilization with bone graft or instrumentation can be performed usually with good results.

To summarize, spinal infections are dangerous and must be diagnosed and treated aggressively to avoid catastrophe.

SPINAL TUMORS

Primary spinal tumors are extremely rare. Benign tumors include osteoid osteoma, osteoblastoma, eosinophilic granuloma, and chondroblastoma. Aggressive but theoretically benign spinal tumors include giant cell tumors and chordomas. Malignant primary tumors include osteosarcomas, chondrosarcomas, malignant fibrous histiocytomas, and fibrosarcomas. All are extremely rare in the spine. Included in the list of primary spinal malignant tumors is multiple myeloma and lymphoma, which, because they actually arise from marrow elements, will be discussed separately.

Primary bone tumors usually present with pain, localized to the particular area of the spine. Occasionally, a mass will be the chief complaint if the tumor occurs in the posterior part of the spine. Characteristically, the pain from osteoid osteomas, most common in young patients, will be intense at night and relieved almost completely by aspirin. In children, scoliosis caused by muscle spasm will often be found, but the neurologic examination will be normal. X-rays will suggest the presence of an abnormality; therefore, the workup should include MRI, CT scan, or bone scan, depending on tumor type. Blood tests are normal. Treatment depends on tumor type and aggressiveness. Primary bone tumors should be referred to a specialist in this type of pathology.

Malignant bone tumors are almost always metastatic. The five most common tumors that metastasize to bone are breast, prostate, lung, renal, and thyroid, accounting for 80% of primary sites. Metastases to the spine are found at autopsy in 75% of patients who have died of cancer. Most commonly, the primary site will be known before discovery of the spine lesion, although occasionally a clinician is faced with a patient with back pain of unknown etiology, which turns out to be secondary to a metastasis.

These patients usually present with back pain, again of an unremitting nature and gradually worsening. Night pain is common along with weight loss, cachexia, and other systemic signs of cancer. Frequently, radicular or spinal cord symptoms are present, as the tumors invade the epidural space causing cord or root compression. This neurologic pain is often severe and unremitting, described as agonizing and sharp while the back pain is deep and aching. Occasionally, a catastrophic collapse of a pathologic fracture will cause sudden paraplegia that is usually irreversible.

The physical examination of the spine may reveal deformity following pathologic fracture, overlying masses, and tenderness to percussion. The neurologic examination will often be positive for radicular or myelopathic signs. Obviously, other nonspine physical findings will depend on the spread of the tumor to other organ systems such as the lung, brain, etc.

Radiographic evaluation begins with plain x-rays of the affected area. This will indicate any pre-existent bony collapse or pathologic fractures. Impending collapse can often be predicted on plain x-ray, although it has been estimated that at least 60% of the vertebral body must be destroyed before plain x-rays are positive. Often, the first radiographic sign is the loss of a pedicle on AP x-ray (denoted as the winking owl sign) as the tumor that begins in the vertebral body grows down along the pedicle destroying it from inside out.

MRI is by far the best test to detect occult or overt malignancies in the spine. Tumors have a characteristic MRI appearance and almost always spare the disc space, differentiating tumors from bone destroying infections (see "Spinal Infections"). In addition to the suspected site, MRI of the entire spine can be done to search for other metastatic sites that might prove more dangerous in the long run and also require treatment.

Treatment depends on several variables. Paramount is the length of expected survival. A patient with only a few weeks or months to live should not be subjected to a lengthy surgical procedure just to restore spinal stability when a simple brace might suffice. In general, most surgeons will use 6 months of expected survival as a cutoff for surgical stabilization. Of secondary importance is the tumor type. For instance, osteoblastic prostate carcinoma may be slow growing and rarely cause vertebral collapse. Others such as squamous cell carcinoma of the lung or renal cell carcinoma are aggressive and result in significant spinal collapse. Whether the tumor is radiosensitive or chemosensitive will determine treatment options. Finally, the degree of actual or predicted vertebral collapse and instability will indicate whether a brace, surgery, or no stabilization is required. Harrington has reported that any tumor with major involvement of the vertebral body or collapse, or one that involves neurologic compromise and bony involvement should be surgically stabilized, if life expectancy is appropriate. Malignancies involving the spine should be referred to an orthopaedist or other specialist as soon as possible so that adequate stabilization, biopsy, or decompression can be performed as required.

Finally, multiple myeloma and lymphoma technically are classified as spinal tumors. In fact, myeloma is the most common malignant primary spine tumor. These tumors usually present with systemic signs such as anemia, fevers, infections, or bleeding consistent with the systemic nature of these diseases. When present in the vertebrae, often the first sign is a compression fracture and subsequent back pain. The plasma cells or malignant lymphocytes infiltrate the bone marrow spaces causing destruction of the cancellous (marrow) bone but not the cortical bone. Thus, the vertebra is hollowed out and collapses as a compression fracture. The radiographic picture appears identical to a benign osteoporotic compression fracture; therefore, a high index of suspicion for myeloma must be weighed when evaluating patients with otherwise routine compression fractures (see below). MRI is rarely helpful in myeloma and lymphoma, because the marrow signals may be similar to normal bone marrow. Bone scan is almost always negative.

Blood tests including the ESR almost always will be abnormal. The SPEP will reveal a monoclonal spike, and the patients will usually be anemic and leukopenic secondary to marrow replacement by malignant cells. The SPEP may be normal in light chain disease. In this situation, the urine protein electrophoresis will be diagnostic.

Treatment of myeloma is rarely surgical, although occasionally a biopsy of a spinal lesion is required. Once the diagnosis is made, a brace can be prescribed for comfort of any pathologic compression fractures. Chemotherapy is the treatment of choice, although expected survival from myeloma is not good.

HERNIATED DISCS

Low back pain is common. Approximately 80% of the general population will suffer at least 2 weeks of back pain at some time during their lives. Of these, approximately 10% are related to disc herniations. Before 1934, cartilage-containing masses that were compressing nerves in the lumbar spine were thought to be tumors arising de novo from the disc. In that year, Mixter and Barr published a landmark paper explaining that these cartilage masses were in fact protrusions of normal disc

tissue into the spinal canal, which caused back and radicular pain. This ushered in the era of the disc.

The normal disc is composed of two parts: the inner nucleus pulposus and the outer annulus fibrosis. The nucleus begins during childhood as a well-hydrated compressible gel, gradually changing through life into a more fibrous, dehydrated, degenerated lump of cartilage as one ages. The disc is responsible for cushioning and supporting the loads on the spine as well as functioning as the joint between vertebrae. The nucleus is contained by the outer annulus, which is composed of tough type I cartilage in a circular orientation around the nucleus that resists shear and tensile forces. The outer third of the annulus is innervated, but not the inner two-thirds or the nucleus. Unfortunately, both age-related and trauma-related changes can occur in the annulus, predisposing it to tearing or other injury, usually during twisting activities. If an annular tear is incomplete but involves the outer innervated portion, back pain can result as so-called discogenic back pain (see "Miscellaneous Causes of Low Back Pain"). If the tear is complete, the nucleus may protrude or herniate outward. Because the weakest part of the annulus is at the posterior-lateral corners, most disc protrusions occur in these spots where the nerve roots are located. Thus, a herniated disc may cause back pain or radicular pain, depending on the size, extent, and location of the protrusion.

In the past, when myelography was the test of choice for diagnosis of disc herniations, it was assumed that the size of the herniation determined the degree of pain and dysfunction, because the myelogram is usually read as showing either nerve root compression or normal findings (no gradations). With the advent of CT scanning and subsequently MRI, which is able to measure the size of a disc herniation, it has been discovered that there is often a poor correlation between the size of a disc herniation and the degree of pain. In fact, Boden has shown that there may be a 10% rate of asymptomatic disc herniation in normal healthy volunteers. This has led to the conclusion that it is the disc material itself, not the mechanical pressure, that causes radiculopathy. In fact, several studies have shown that disc material induces changes in the nerve roots in contact with the disc material, including elevated substance P levels and various inflammatory products. This may be why NSAIDs and epidural steroids are often effective in treating radiculopathy from herniated discs.

Patients with a herniated disc usually present with a history of back pain that subsequently evolves into leg pain, usually unilateral because of the relative strength of the annulus in the midline forcing the disc rupture postero-laterally. There is often a history of trauma or lifting, especially when compensation issues are involved, although only approximately 40% of patients can remember the exact incident that initiated the pain. Certain occupations are involved at a higher rate than the general population, such as nurses, heavy laborers, and truck drivers. The average age of these patients is 37; this condition is rare in teenagers and the elderly. Smokers have a higher rate of disc protrusion than nonsmokers, and there is often a family history of disc problems. Interestingly, no animals are known to rupture discs, although many dogs suffer from other spinal problems seen in humans, such as spinal stenosis. Thus, disc herniation in humans is a common problem in industrialized society of multifactorial origin.

The most common location of the herniated disc is at L4-L5, followed closely by L5-S1, and then much less often at upper lumbar discs. If at L4-L5, the L5 nerve root is usually affected, resulting in pain down the back of the thigh to the lateral calf and anterior foot. If at L5-S1, the S1 nerve root is affected, with pain in the posterior calf and sole of the foot. The pain is usually worse with Valsalva maneuvers such as coughing, sneezing, or straining. Sitting is usually more uncomfortable than standing, although if the disc fragment has become dislodged from the main part of the disc, occasionally sitting is better. Lying down is commonly best, and night pain is not usually significant. Numbness, tingling,

paresthesias, or other neurologic symptoms may accompany the pain. The patient often perceives the affected leg to be weaker than the other leg. Bowel and bladder disturbances are rare and should raise the possibility of a cauda equina syndrome.

If a higher lumbar disc is involved, the pain will radiate into the anterior or medial thigh, and more proximal muscles will be involved, such as the quadriceps in an L3-L4 herniation. Pain down the back of the thigh that stops above the knee should not be considered as sciatica, since it is usually referred pain from the annulus or other spinal problems.

On examination, the patient may limp on the affected side. Commonly, a list or bend to the opposite side is seen, as if the patient does not want to press on the affected nerve by leaning toward it. Depending on the nerve root involved, various combinations of weakness may be encountered, such as inability to walk on the toes for an L5-S1 herniation or on the heels for an L4-L5 protrusion. Reflex changes may be present, such as loss of the ankle reflex at S1. Muscle spasm may be present in the lumbar spine. The straight leg raising test (SLR) is usually positive for lower lumbar herniations, because the nerve root is stretched over the irritating cartilage lump with this maneuver. However, this test becomes less reliable in patients over the age of 40. For upper lumbar herniations, the reverse SLR (stretch of the femoral nerve) may be positive. A positive bowstring sign (tenderness of the sciatic nerve or branch behind the knee) with SLR is often present, especially in young patients. Finally, a crossed SLR, in which straightening one leg causes radicular pain in the opposite affected leg, is 99% specific for a herniated disc.

Laboratory workup of a suspected herniated disc is relatively straightforward. Plain x-rays are rarely useful because discs are invisible to plain x-rays. The MRI has become the gold standard in visualizing the cord, dura, nerve roots, and discs, but because of the relatively high false-positive rate, any findings must be correlated with the history and examination. CT scans are useful but not as distinct as the MRI. Bone scans and blood tests are not helpful, except to rule out other diagnoses such as spondylolysis or spinal infections.

Once the diagnosis of an acute herniated disc has been made, treatment is initially conservative. Approximately 80% of patients will be successfully treated with conservative (nonoperative) methods of which there are innumerable types. Rest is advised for the acute episode, with analgesics, NSAIDs, and muscle relaxants provided short-term. One study showed that 2 days of bedrest were as effective as 2 weeks, so prolonged bedrest should be discouraged. Activity should be at whatever level the patient can withstand without undue pain. Physical therapy may help regain spinal motion and muscle strength but has not been shown to heal the disc more quickly. Currently in vogue is the McKenzie approach with enforced extension of the spine. Modalities such as heat, ultrasound, massage, transcutaneous electrical nerve stimulator (TENS) units, and electrical stimulation may make the patient feel better but have not been subjected to prospective trials. In fact, a recent Health Care Financing Administration (HCFA) report states that these methods should be discouraged because they do not work.

One study has shown that short-term chiropractic manipulation may have a role in the treatment of acute back pain with or without sciatica. Rolfing, acupuncture, herbal therapy, moxibustion (heated glass globes applied to the skin), and other nontraditional therapies have many adherents and may be tried at the clinician's discretion but have not been rigorously tested.

If an adequate trial of effective conservative treatment has failed, if the patient is getting rapidly worse, or if the clinician deems it beneficial, epidural steroids may be effective. As noted above, disc tissue is inflammatory to nerve tissue, so washing out or suppressing the inflammatory products around the herniation may have a role in reducing nerve pain. Steroids can be given orally but may have complications in the gastrointestinal tract or endocrine system. Classically used are epidural steroids in which a large volume of steroid solution is infiltrated into the epidural space, but because of the location of most herniations, these injections may not reach the site of nerve root irritation. The most efficient method for delivery of steroids to the nerve root is via selective extraforaminal nerve block, after the offending disc and nerve root have been located by scanning. This requires fluoroscopy and technically is more difficult than epidural steroids but is more effective. Ordinarily, injected steroids are used for an acute attack of radiculopathy caused by a herniated disc, but it should be noted that a prospective randomized trial failed to find any significant difference between steroids and placebo.

If the aforementioned treatments fail, surgical disc removal is an excellent option. Standard discectomy formerly consisted of a large laminectomy, big incisions, and muscle trauma. Currently, microdiscectomy with loupe or microscopic magnification has become standard, with incisions less than 5 cm long, unilateral exposure, and 1-day hospitalizations. In this operation, only the disc fragment that is in direct contact with the nerve root is removed, and fusions are not indicated. Results in most series have been 85 to 95% good to excellent with early return to work. Leg pain, not back pain, is the symptom best relieved by this procedure. Muscle strength often improves, but numbness and reflex loss may persist no matter what the treatment. A few complications can occur with this operation. General anesthesia is usually required, although a few surgeons operate under local anesthesia. Nerve injury can occur with a rate of less than 2%, and infection can happen with any open procedure. The smaller incisions carry an increased risk that a significant piece of disc will be missed, resulting in failure to relieve pain and a subsequent need for reoperation. Endoscopic discectomy is still investigational at this point but may soon be perfected. Chymopapain, popular in the 1980s, has been withdrawn secondary to anaphylactic reactions to the enzyme. Recent enthusiasm for laser discectomy, in which the center of the disc is dissolved by laser light, has waned with the relatively high complication rate of nerve injury. Thus, the excellent results make microdiscectomy the procedure by which all others will be measured.

Finally, the rare but significant clinical problem of cauda equina syndrome must be noted. If a disc herniation occurs in the midline, compression of the thecal sac and central (sacral) nerve roots will occur. If the disc herniation is large enough, the sacral nerve roots will cease to function, leading to loss of bowel and bladder control, and saddle (down the back of both legs) anesthesia. This is a true surgical emergency, because the longer the nerve roots are compressed, the slower is the recovery. Thus, any patient who presents with bilateral leg pain or neurologic dysfunction and sphincter control difficulties requires an immediate MRI scan and surgical decompression.

INFLAMMATORY BACK PAIN

The most common systemic inflammatory disorder to involve the lumbar spine is ankylosing spondylitis. This disorder characteristically starts in the sacroiliac joints, most commonly and severely in young males. The lumbar facet joints can be the first involved, and peripheral joints are only involved later in an outward radiating (hips, knees, ankles) fashion. Thus, the initial symptom reported most often is low back or buttock pain. Rarely is there any radicular component, because the nerves are not involved. Morning stiffness is extremely common, and improvement with activity or exercise should make the clinician suspect this diagnosis.

On examination, patients with ankylosing spondylitis are stiff; thus, the original common name was "stiff man" syndrome. Forced motion in the sacroiliac joints (Faber test) will usually be painful, and the range of motion of the lumbar spine and the hip joints are usually less than predicted. The neurologic examination is normal, as are all blood tests except for HLA B-27. This marker occurs in approximately 20% of the normal population but occurs in 99% of patients with ankylosing spondylitis.

X-ray evaluation of the lumbar spine and pelvis will often show sclerosis of the sacroiliac joints. Later in the disease process, the lumbar vertebrae show a characteristic squaring off of the normally rounded upper and lower vertebral endplates. As the disease progresses, the discs in the spine, both lumbar and eventually thoracic and cervical, become ossified, limiting spinal motion and functionality and turning the spine into one long bone. Occasionally, a bone scan is required initially that will show significantly increased uptake in the pelvis and sacrum around the sacroiliac joints.

Treatment initially is with NSAIDs. Response to indomethacin is often dramatic, and occasionally a patient will require up to 150 mg/day to alleviate stiffness and pain. Physical therapy should be advised to teach flexibility and postural exercises, but will not stop the disease process. In fact, nothing currently available stops the inexorable ossification of the lumbar discs. Thus, the patient should be encouraged to remain as active as possible and, most importantly, to maintain an upright posture, because the spine will eventually ankylose in whatever position is typically assumed. Braces may help enforce a good posture but should not be worn all the time, because this fosters dependence on the external support and weakens muscles.

Surgical treatment of the spine is hazardous at best. Ordinarily, this is reserved for patients with extreme kyphosis in the neck or lower back who cannot look ahead or keep their balance. The procedures involve osteotomies (breaking the spine under anesthesia) followed by realignment and fusion with instrumentation. This is risky in terms of blood loss and infection and, most significantly, to the spinal cord in which many cases of iatrogenic quadriplegia have been reported.

Because the spine eventually becomes one long bone, fractures with even trivial trauma can have catastrophic results. When the spine is fractured, the two ends form large levers, and any movement can make the broken ends move, damaging the spinal cord. Thus, any patient with ankylosing spondylitis involved in trauma, even a minor fall, who complains of increased spine pain should be assumed to have a fracture until ruled out. This may require sophisticated x-rays, CT scan, or even a bone scan to delineate the anatomy; therefore, the evaluation is best performed by a center with experience in trauma.

Other inflammatory diseases such as Reiter's syndrome, rheumatoid arthritis, Lyme disease, and polymyalgia rheumatica can rarely involve the spine. Rheumatoid arthritis in the spine is almost always confined to the cervical spine. The diagnosis of these other conditions will usually be suspected before thoracolumbar spine involvement. Treatment is that which is appropriate for the generalized disease process, i.e., antibiotics for Lyme arthritis, medications for rheumatoid arthritis, etc.

SPONDYLOSIS (OSTEOARTHRITIS OF THE SPINE)

Many anatomic, physiologic, and radiographic changes occur in the normal spine as it ages. Thus, separating out what is part of the normal aging process from what may be clinically significant in any individual patient is often problematic. Almost everyone over the age of 50 will have radiographic evidence of degeneration either in the disc, facet joints, or bones. Yet, the prevalence of low back pain is actually lower in patients over the age of 50 than in people from 30 to 50 years old.

However, a small number of patients will suffer from what is eventually diagnosed as spondylosis (not spondylolysis). These patients are usually over the age of 50, and the pattern of pain is akin to the complaints seen in any other arthritic joint. Commonly, these patients present with low back pain referred to the buttocks and posterior thighs. Any radiation below the knees should raise the suspicion of spinal stenosis (see below). Morning stiffness is extremely common, and the pain is usually aggravated by extension of the spine as more pressure is transferred to the facet joints during extension than flexion. The pain is not aggravated by Valsalva maneuvers, and aerobic exercise such as walking usually improves the pain. It is also important to inquire about night pain, worsening pain, and systemic factors so as not to miss one of these red flags that might indicate a more serious disorder.

On examination, range of motion of the spine is usually restricted. It is vital to check the range of motion of the hips when evaluating these patients, because concomitant osteoarthritis of the hips may turn out to be the true cause of the buttock and thigh pain, and can be markedly helped by hip replacement. The neurologic examination is usually normal. Radiographs of the lumbar spine characteristically show severe degeneration of the facet joints and discs. Decreased lordosis on the lateral x-ray and degenerative scoliosis on AP x-rays are common. Unless there are associated neurologic findings or symptoms, MRI is not indicated. CT scans can be helpful in preoperative planning, although routine use in the evaluation is not indicated. Most importantly, a thorough search must be made for more serious spinal or extraspinal causes before ascribing the patient's symptoms to osteoarthritis of the spine.

Treatment is analogous to the treatment of any arthritic joint. NSAIDs are often beneficial but must be taken at an adequate dosage, and the type of NSAID must be chosen that does not cause side effects such as gastrointestinal irritation or fluid retention. A once-a-day NSAID is best so that the patient does not become confused. Additionally, the patient must be instructed that the NSAID is a true medication to be taken on schedule, not just p.r.n. (when necessary) as often occurs. Lumbar supports, such as a corset or occasionally more rigid lumbosacral plastic orthosis, may help in alleviating symptoms, especially when the patient does not want to give up a painful activity such as gardening, etc. The support must not be worn all the time. Bedrest is absolutely contraindicated.

Exercises, whether supervised by a therapist or on their own, are helpful. Pool therapy is beneficial because it improves aerobic fitness, range of motion, and general health. Logistically, it may be difficult. Once serious spine pathology has been ruled out, the patient should be encouraged that this is not a serious life-threatening condition, and that whatever activities the patient likes to do that do not cause significant pain are appropriate. In general, most patients are able to accommodate their lifestyle so that they can live with any restrictions.

Surgery is rarely helpful, except in cases of extreme deformity such as rapidly collapsing degenerative scoliosis, or in the case of concomitant spinal stenosis.

SPINAL STENOSIS

Spinal stenosis is closely associated with spondylosis. Technically, this term indicates any condition that causes decreased caliber (diameter) of the lumbar spine whether caused by tumor, fracture, or osteoarthritis, etc. By common use, it has come to mean the clinical syndrome of decreased lumbar spinal canal size caused by disc and facet degeneration or, occasionally, by a disc herniation in an older patient.

As noted above, as the spine ages, degeneration occurs in the facet joints and discs. This degeneration causes infolding of the ligaments and other soft tissues around the spinal canal, as well as hypertrophy of the facet capsules and bony osteophytes in the facet joints. When the spinal canal diameter is narrowed below 100 mm^2, the clinical picture of spinal stenosis usually occurs (Fig. 5.9).

Patients with spinal stenosis present with low back or leg pain in the upright position. Characteristically, they can walk upright only for a limited distance and then must either sit or otherwise bend at the waist to alleviate pain. This is because the upright position narrows the spinal canal slightly in everyone; a patient with a restricted spinal diameter caused by spinal stenosis then effectively shuts off the blood flow to the spinal nerve roots and dorsal root ganglia, which become ischemic. This results in pain in the back and legs that is relieved only by re-establishing blood flow to the nerve roots by flexion of the spine.

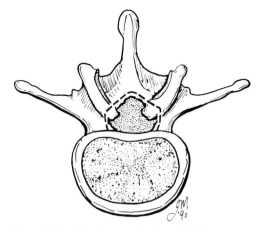

Figure 5.9.   Spinal stenosis. Facet joint hypertrophy with thickening of the capsule and ligamentum flavum diminishes available space of the cauda equina. The dotted line marks the normal shape of the canal.

These patients can walk a reproducibly specific distance before stopping. They often lean on the cart in the grocery store and avoid prolonged shopping or standing because of the pain. Loss of bowel or bladder control is not associated with this condition, because the dorsal root ganglia for the sacral nerve roots are never involved. Valsalva maneuvers are not usually provocative of the pain. There may be a history of relative waxing and waning of the symptoms, but usually the distance walked has been gradually decreasing for months or years. Physical examination is usually not particularly helpful. The neurologic examination is usually negative, except that prolonged extension may cause symptoms. Range of motion of the hips should be checked to rule out painful osteoarthritis of these joints. It is important to check the pedal pulses, because vascular claudication can cause the same symptoms. In fact, the leg pain of spinal stenosis is commonly called pseudoclaudication. To differentiate these two, the provocative maneuver should be determined. In spinal stenosis, the patient bends forward to relieve the pain, whereas in vascular claudication, the patient simply stops to rest the legs without having to bend forward. If there is any doubt, noninvasive vascular studies can be checked to determine arterial insufficiency. Significantly, patients with spinal stenosis cannot walk far upright but can often bicycle for long distances, since the spine becomes flexed in bicycling.

Radiographs are not helpful except in the case of degenerative spondylolisthesis. This condition usually occurs in older women and results from degeneration of the facet joints, most often at L4-L5. The forward slippage of L4 on L5 can result in pinching of the spinal canal and symptoms of spinal stenosis. The imaging study of choice is the MRI because it will show the spinal canal, nerve roots, discs, and joints. The true diameter of the canal can be determined, because cross-sectional areas below 100 mm^2 are highly correlated with the clinical symptoms of stenosis. The CT scan is a good alternative, especially when the bony anatomy is to be evaluated. Blood tests are normal, except in the case of other spinal or systemic pathology. Spinal stenosis is one disease in which EMGs are important to rule out peripheral neuropathy from diabetes or other neurologic disorders. Surgical treatment will not be helpful if the problem is caused by an intrinsic neurologic disease with coexistent spinal stenosis.

Treatment falls into one of three categories. Conservative treatment includes NSAIDs and a graded exercise program. Education is paramount. Often, the patient is relieved to hear that they do not have a serious spinal disorder such as cancer and are relatively happy adjusting their lifestyle to accommodate their walking restrictions. Lumbar corsets usually are not helpful and in many cases will make the symptoms worse by forcing the spine into an extended position. Physical therapy is rarely helpful except as an encouragement to exercise. Many patients cannot walk long distances but can bicycle or swim for extended times because these activities do not extend the spine. Thus, this type of exercise should be encouraged. Basically, the patient is instructed to listen to their back but to remain active. There is no need to restrict activities beyond those that are significantly painful. Spinal stenosis can be accommodated for many years without any drastic treatment necessary if the patient is happy with this situation or if there are major risk factors to more invasive treatment.

A second line of treatment is epidural steroids. Because part of the pathologic condition is inflammation or swelling of the facet joints, discs, and nerve roots, reduction of this inflammation may have a salutary effect in spinal stenosis. Commonly, epidural steroids are given as a series of one to three injections in the midline over a 6-week period. Results can be up to 60% long-term relief, although the injections may have to be repeated 6 to 12 months later. Many patients are happy receiving an occasional series of epidural steroids for the bad times and accommodating to the other less severe periods.

If all methods of treatment fail, surgery is an appropriate last resort. Decompression combined in some cases with fusion has an 80 to 90% success rate initially, although in one series these results deteriorated with time. The aim of surgery is to increase the distance the patient can walk without symptoms so that activities such as shopping, golf, walking, or hiking can be resumed. Often, a gratifying improvement in the patient's outlook, activities, and enjoyment of life can be achieved with this relatively safe surgical decompression. The risks of surgery are primarily those associated with general anesthesia and blood loss, and neurologic complications are rare. The major deficiency is that surgery does not cure concomitant neurologic disorders such as diabetic neuropathy, occasionally responsible for a poor surgical outcome.

OSTEOPOROTIC COMPRESSION FRACTURES

Compression fractures are a significant problem in elderly patients, second only to fractures of the hip as a source of morbidity in this group. Significant loss of trunk height is extremely common as people age, due to multi-level disc degeneration and to symptomatic or asymptomatic thoracolumbar compression fractures. Unfortunately, little can be done to prevent these from occurring other than to treat osteoporosis as a systemic disorder. This treatment classically involves weightbearing exercise, effective hormonal replacement in the appropriate patient, calcium supplementation throughout life (especially important in younger women), and treatment of other conditions that cause osteoporosis such as hyperthyroidism and hypothyroidism, prolonged steroid use, hyperparathyroidism, calcium and vitamin D deficiency, etc.

Compression fractures remain a significant problem in today's elderly. The patient usually presents with the acute onset of upper or lower back pain, often following a trivial injury. Neurologic complaints or symptoms are rare except in longstanding severe kyphosis. Many times, the patients present only with a slowly developing loss of truncal height or are brought in by family members because they are "shorter than they used to be." At this point, x-rays will show the compression fractures; however, the age of the fracture cannot be predicted from an x-ray. In general, if there is an acute event, it must be presumed that the fracture is new. The most important part of the evaluation is to workup the patient for treatable causes of osteoporotic fractures such as multiple myeloma or other etiologies. One cannot simply assume that a compression fracture is due to postmenopausal osteoporosis until other causes have been eliminated.

Treatment of the acute fracture remains supportive. A brace can be comfortable, provided it does not aggravate any symptoms of spinal stenosis, and it is eventually weaned off. Pain medications should be prescribed, but avoiding dependency may be difficult. Gradual resumption of full activities should be encouraged. Swimming or pool therapy may help the patient increase aerobic fitness most rapidly. Bedrest is absolutely contraindicated because bedrest will result in a patient never regaining functional activities. Obviously, any treatable symptoms should be treated aggressively. With the recent introduction of effective medical treatments for osteoporosis, such as hormonal therapy and alendronate, osteo-porotic compression fractures may be less of a clinical problem in the future.

MISCELLANEOUS CAUSES OF LOW BACK PAIN

There are innumerable other causes of low back pain. A partial list includes intrinsic spinal problems such as acute fractures, scoliosis, and muscle strains. Extrinsic causes include gynecologic problems, renal abnormalities (infections, tumors, kidney stones), retroperitoneal tumors (pancreatic cancer), aortic aneurysms, and occasionally cardiac etiologies. Most of these will be obvious based on the other systemic signs present.

After the full workup is pursued, and no specific diagnosis can be made, the clinician is left with the dilemma of what is the cause of the low back pain. It has been estimated that the full workup detailed in the preceding text will yield a specific diagnosis in less than 50% of cases. Without a specific diagnosis, nonspecific treatment occurs.

Many theories exist as to the true etiology of nonspecific low back pain. In the acute situation, it is commonly labeled low back strain or sprain, implying injury to the muscles or ligaments, respectively. As anyone who participates in athletics knows, muscular strains or sprains rarely last longer than a few days, or at most, a few weeks. Thus, calling acute low back pain that is caused by a specific injury a sprain or strain is adequate for the first few weeks, but thereafter it must be caused by another factor.

Currently, the favored causative structure is the disc. Because the outer third of the annulus is innervated, tears or irritation of the outer annular fibers can be felt as low back pain. Thus, a commonly used synonym for low back strain is discogenic low back pain, similar to the pain encountered in an acute disc herniation but without the radicular component. Characteristically, the pain presents with the acute onset of back or buttock pain after a twisting, bending, or lifting injury. This is especially true for compensable situations such as at work or after a motor vehicle accident. Low back pain is most common in ages 30–50, with a bell-shaped curve on either side of the age distribution. Usually, a severe initial episode occurs followed by the development of a chronic ache or pain in the low back, buttocks, or posterior thighs. The pain is normally aggravated by maneuvers that increase pressure on the disc, such as carrying, lifting, or twisting. Bending forward and sitting, which doubles the pressure in the disc, are especially painful, whereas extension and lying down usually relieve the pain. Often, the patient is stiff in the morning, after which the pain is tolerable until later in the day when, as the disc is compressed with upright activities during the day, the pain worsens again. The patient may have had prior episodes of back pain, and the family history is often positive for relatives with similar problems. Again, during the history phase of the workup, the presence of red-flag symptoms must be sought to direct the workup towards more serious pathologic etiologies.

On examination, the patient is usually uncomfortable. Muscle spasm may be present in the more acute situation, but no masses should be palpable. There may be a list or involuntary bend away from the affected side, if there is one. The neurologic examination is usually normal or noncontributory, and straight leg raising will cause low back pain, not sciatica. Physical signs for other etiologies must be sought. Waddell signs are especially important to detect the presence of malingering or functional overlay, which will decrease effectiveness of treatment and herald a poor prognosis for recovery.

Laboratory tests are almost always normal, with the exception of the x-ray and MRI, which will show nonspecific age-related changes. Most importantly, any suspicion of a more dangerous etiology such as infection, tumor, etc., should prompt laboratory investigations in that particular direction.

To confirm the diagnosis of discogenic low back pain, an old test called discography has once again become popular. Originally used in the 1960s to confirm disc ruptures before the advent of axial imaging (CT scanning),

discography fell into disrepute when Holt found a high false-positive rate in asymptomatic convicts. As currently performed, discography involves placement of a needle under sterile conditions into the lumbar discs, usually L3-L4, L4-L5, and L5-S1. Hypertonic dye is then injected under fluoroscopic control, and the morphologic appearance of the inner nucleus is visualized radiographically. Any leakage of dye from the nucleus into or through the annulus can be seen, indicating a tear in the annular fibers. Most importantly, the patient is questioned blindly as to whether each injection reproduces their low back pain, which is then graded as concordant (for the exact pain), similar, dissimilar, or none. Reproduction of the patient's typical pain (concordant) confirms the diagnosis of that disc as the source of the problem. Discography is thus a useful test to indicate the diagnosis. Complications include infection (less than 1%), nerve injury, and inadvertent cerebrospinal fluid leakage if needle placement is incorrect. This procedure is also intensely painful because it aims to reproduce the patient's pain.

Anecdotal evidence recently has shown that steroid injection into the painful disc at the time of discography may help a significant percentage of patients, some for prolonged intervals. However, no prospective trials of intradiscal steroids have been published. The problem with discography arises from the dilemma of what treatment to follow after delineation of the painful lesion.

Because back pain is so common, treatment of low back pain has been extremely varied. Standard medical treatment includes brief periods of bedrest in the acute situation with NSAIDs, muscle relaxants, or narcotic analgesics prescribed depending on the severity. Hospitalization should be avoided because it may foster the unfortunate idea that this is a serious medical condition. Prolonged bedrest is also contraindicated. Physical therapy is often helpful, both to improve lumbar range of motion as well as to show the patient that gradual resumption of exercise is beneficial. Modalities such as heat, ultrasound, and TENS units have never been proven effective in prospective trials, although they may make the patient temporarily feel well. Swimming or pool therapy is also beneficial, because the disc is weightless in water and may have time to recover. In well-run prospective trials, no specific conservative treatment has been shown to affect the course of discogenic low back pain, which is usually one of gradual recovery over 6 weeks in 80% of patients. Once the workup has eliminated the possibility of a serious underlying medical cause, the clinician should reassure the patient that the problem will gradually improve and that expensive or dangerous tests and invasive therapies are not indicated.

Failure of standard medical treatment has opened the door to all kinds of nontraditional "cures." Chiropractic treatment of low back pain has evolved considerably since its introduction by Palmer in the 1890s. Many patients report significant relief, sometimes long-lasting with a few simple manipulations. A recent prospective trial has shown higher success rates with a short course (not more than 6 weeks) of chiropractic care. Why this works has never been successfully explained, although manipulative therapy does alter positions and forces in the facet joints and discs. Other therapies include acupuncture, Rolfing, herbal therapy, moxibustion, fire walking, gravity boots, etc. None of these are proven, although if the patient experiences relief with any treatment that is nontoxic and not too prolonged or expensive, such treatment should be allowed. Insurance payment for these, however, may not be forthcoming. No treatment should delay the search for a more dangerous medically treatable disorder.

Aside from anecdotal reports of intradiscal steroids helping low back pain, spinal injections are rarely helpful for discogenic low back pain. If there is suspicion of spondylosis as the cause, facet injections may be diagnostically and sometimes therapeutically effective. Trigger point injections are invasive, costly, and do not help. Epidural steroid injections similarly are not indicated because of the risk of inadvertent dural penetration and unproven effectiveness.

Surgery has been uniformly ineffective to date. One study, a meta-analysis of all papers on spinal fusion for low back pain, documented a 54% rate of failure for posterior fusion, with a high reoperation rate. Additionally, posterior fusion, especially that involving the use of spinal instrumentation (screws and rods), is expensive. Radiographic fusion, which many surgeons use as the measure for success, can be technically achieved, but relief of symptoms often does not correlate with this achievement.

Recently, intradiscal fusion using threaded cages or screws has been advocated, performed either anteriorly, posteriorly, or laparoscopically through the abdomen. Preliminary studies are promising, but no long-term results are available, and only time will tell if these invasive therapies are successful. Disc replacement is on the horizon, but none have been successfully implanted in humans to date.

A brief word should be made about compensation-induced low back pain. In our litigious industrial society, low back pain is the most frequent cause of disability, costing up to $40 billion per year in direct and indirect costs. Clearly, there are some back injuries that are work related and should be covered. However, the majority of low back disabilities are prolonged by overreliance on expensive and dangerous therapies, and their duration is excessively lengthened by the adversarial nature of the legal process. Ideally, early institution of effective treatment and job modification or retraining should get the patient back to gainful employment as soon as possible with a minimum of cost to society. This is currently not the case, because the legal process drags the proceedings out for the benefit of the lawyers, clinicians, and therapists and to the detriment of the patient. Effective resolution of the problem is a societal and not a medical endeavor.

SUMMARY

This chapter hopefully will have given the clinician a useful algorithmic approach to the investigation and treatment of thoracolumbar spinal disorders. Included in the suggested readings list are papers and books that the author has found helpful, should the reader desire more detailed or alternate sources of information.

SUGGESTED READINGS

Anon. Acute low back pain problems in adults: Assessment and treatment. Agency for Health Care Policy and Research Clinical Practice Guidelines—Quick Reference Guide for Clinicians 1994;14:1–25.

Bradford DS, Lonstein LE, Moe JH, et al. Moe's Textbook of Scoliosis and Other Spinal Deformities. 2nd ed. Philadelphia: WB Saunders Co, 1987.

Errico GJ, Bauer RD, Waugh T. Spinal Trauma. Philadelphia: JB Lippincott Co, 1990.

Floman Y, ed. Disorders of the Lumbar Spine. Rockville, MD: Aspen Publishers, 1990.

Frymoyer JW. Medical Progress: Back pain and sciatica. N Engl J Med 1988;318:291–300.

Frymoyer JW, Newberg A, Pope MH, et al. Spine radiographs in patients with low back pain. J Bone Joint Surg 1984;6A:1048–1055.

Fredrickson BE, Baker D, McHolick WJ. The natural history of spondylolysis and spondylolisthesis. J Bone Joint Surg 1984;66A:699–707.

Harrington KD. Metastatic tumors of the spine: diagnosis and treatment. J Am Acad Orthop Surg 1993;1:76–86.

Hensinger RN. Current Concepts Review: spondylolysis and spondylolisthesis in children and adolescents. J Bone Joint Surg 1989;71A:1098–1107.

Turner JA, Ersatz M, Herron L, et al. Patient outcomes after lumbar spinal fusions. JAMA 1992;268:907–911.

White AA, Panjabi MM. Clinical Biomechanics of the Spine. 2nd ed. Philadelphia: JB Lippincott, 1990.

Hip and Pelvis

Gerald G. Steinberg, M.D., and Eric A. Seybold, M.D.

ESSENTIAL ANATOMY

Like the shoulder, the hip is a ball-and-socket joint that attaches to the body axis through a bony girdle. However, there are major differences that are important for understanding the normal function of the pelvis and hip, as well as the manifestations of disease.

In contrast to the shoulder girdle, the pelvic girdle is relatively fixed to the body axis. The pelvic girdle is capable of significant movement with the body axis only through its joint at the lumbosacral junction. The pelvis is attached to the body axis by the abdominal and spinal muscles and by the stout ligaments of the relatively immobile sacroiliac joints. Because of this immobility, a primary abnormality of the hip or pelvis may create a secondary abnormality in the lumbar spine or at the knee. For example, a patient with a severe flexion contracture of the hip will not ambulate bent forward. The patient will develop a compensatory increase in lumbar lordosis and/or flexed posture at the knee. Also, a primary abnormality in the lumbar spine or knee may create a secondary abnormality in the hip. These abnormalities must be distinguished when examining a patient with an apparent hip problem.

The shoulder and hip joints are ball-and-socket types, whereas the shoulder socket is small and flat, providing little inherent stability to the joint. The articular surface of the acetabulum, however, is large and deep, providing substantial mechanical stability. Therefore, the muscles about the hip are responsible more for postural than for articular stability.

The ligaments of the joint are responsible for limiting motion of the hip at the extremes.

Unlike the shoulder, the articular surface of each hip is a weightbearing surface constantly subjected to high loads. This makes the hip more vulnerable to developing clinical symptoms. Several areas of functional and anatomic detail are important for evaluating and treating disorders of the hip. These areas include the following: (a) x-ray anatomy, (b) bony and ligamentous structure of the pelvis and hip, (c) muscular control of the hip joint, (d) innervation and blood supply, and (e) relationship of the hip to major nerves and vessels of the extremity.

X-RAY ANATOMY

Figure 6.1 shows an anteroposterior (AP) projection of the pelvis and hips with important elements labeled.

BONE AND LIGAMENT STRUCTURE OF THE PELVIS AND HIP

Each hemipelvis is formed by the fusion of the pubis, ischium, and ilium. These bones emerge from separate centers of ossification and fuse into a single bone by early adolescence. Before maturity, x-rays show a normal lucency traversing the acetabulum. This is the triradiate cartilage, which is the site of fusion of the three bones of the hemipelvis. Several cartilaginous (epiphyses or) apophyses are clinically important in the immature individual: the iliac crest, anterior superior and anterior inferior iliac spines, and ischial tuberosity (Fig. 6.2). These begin to ossify by midadolescence but do not fuse to the underlying bone

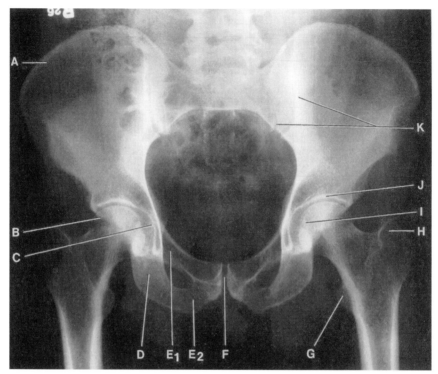

Figure 6.1. AP x-ray of the pelvis and hips. Important points of bony anatomy are noted: *A,* iliac crest. *B,* posterior acetabular margin. *C,* medial acetabular wall. *D,* ischium. *E,* pubis. *E1,* superior ramus. *E2,* inferior ramus. *F,* symphysis pubis. *G,* lesser trochanter. *H,* greater trochanter. *I,* fovea of femoral head. *J,* acetabular dome. *K,* sacroiliac crest.

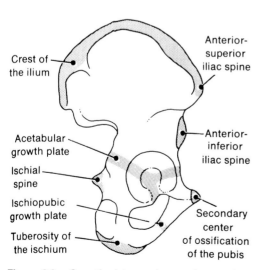

Figure 6.2. Growth plates and secondary centers of ossification of the hip.

until the mid-to-late twenties. Recognition of these apophyses is important in evaluating certain traction injuries about the pelvis and in evaluating x-rays of individuals before full ossification.

The pelvic ring is formed by the junction of each ilium at the sacrum posteriorly and the junction of each pubis at the symphysis pubis anteriorly. The pelvic ring is stable because of the tremendously strong ligaments of the sacroiliac joints and the symphysis pubis and the locking orientation of the sacroiliac joint facets. Many ligaments stabilize each sacroiliac joint. The most important are the short interosseous sacroiliac ligaments and dorsal sacroiliac ligaments (Fig. 6.3). The short interosseous ligament is a strong structure that forms the fibrous portion of the sacroiliac joint. Only the inferior portion of the sacroiliac joint is a true synovial joint. Above this region is a fibrous ankylosis, and the short

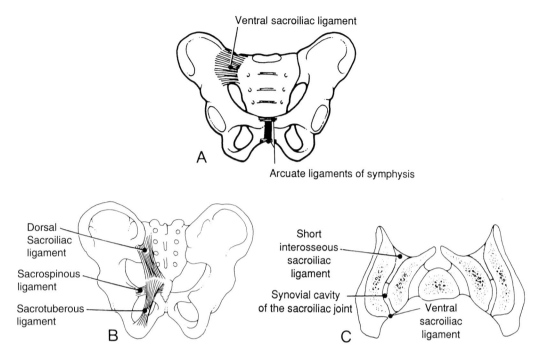

Figure 6.3.   The stabilizing ligaments of the sacroiliac joint and symphysis pubis. *A,* anterior view of the stabilizing ligaments. *B,* posterior view of the stabilizing ligaments. *C,* coronal section of the sacroiliac joint.

interosseous ligament forms the fibrous structure. The dorsal sacroiliac ligament passes from the lower third of the sacrum vertically and obliquely upward across the joint to the ilium (Fig. 6.3B).

Anteriorly, the pelvic ring is closed by the joint at the pubic symphysis, which is stabilized by a fibrocartilaginous disc and by two ligaments that merge into the disc (Fig. 6.3A). Whereas the ligaments of the symphysis are strong, the stability of the joint is helped by the structure of the pelvis, which is designed to transmit compressive force across this joint. This reduces the tendency for any distraction or displacement of the joint and helps maintain pelvic stability.

By virtue of its stability, the pelvic ring can withstand the routine forces of bearing weight, effectively transferring body weight across the hip joints to the lower extremities. Because of such inherent stability, an injury of tremendous force is required to produce a dislocation or displaced fracture of the pelvis.

A lesser force can cause injury in the pregnant patient because changes in hormonal balance impart increased elasticity to the pelvic ligaments. This increased elasticity accommodates the process of childbirth but weakens the ligaments and makes them more vulnerable to sprain.

Hip Joint

Each part of the hemipelvis participates in the formation of the acetabulum (Fig. 6.4). The superior ramus of the pubis and the body of the ischium form its anterior and posterior walls, respectively. The body of the ilium forms the superior acetabular wall. The posterior ilioischial column connects with the anterior iliopubic column to form the strong arch of bone making up the superior acetabulum. The anterior columns form a bridge between the two posterior columns and function as a compression-resisting strut for the medially directed forces generated at the hips. As the anterior and posterior acetabular walls

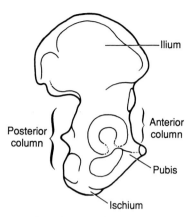

Figure 6.4. The right hemipelvis showing the convergence of the ilium, ischium, and pubis in the formation of the acetabulum. The posterior and anterior columns are marked.

converge inferiorly, an inferior medial deficiency forms the acetabular notch (Fig. 6.5).

The surface of the acetabulum is composed of an incomplete ring of hyaline cartilage that surrounds the central acetabular fossa, which in turn merges with the acetabular notch inferiorly. The fossa contains the ligamentum teres and does not have a hyaline cartilage covering. The walls of the acetabulum are expanded by a fibrocartilaginous extension called the acetabular labrum. Inferiorly, the labrum continues across the acetabular notch as the transverse acetabular ligament (Fig. 6.5). The labrum and transverse acetabular ligament extend beyond the hemisphere of the femoral head, deepening the acetabulum and increasing its coverage to approximately two-thirds of the head.

The capsule of the hip joint extends from the femur to the acetabulum, overlying the acetabular labrum proximally. The capsule inserts on the femur along the intertrochanteric line anteriorly and on the distal aspect of the femoral neck posteriorly. The capsule is composed of four recognizable ligaments. The strongest ligament is the iliofemoral ligament (Fig. 6.6), which is the main capsular restraint to extension and internal rotation.

The synovial membrane of the capsule completely lines its surface and reflects back along the neck of the femur where the capsule

makes its femoral attachment. Completely covering the femoral neck is the synovium, ending at the peripheral border of the cartilage of the head of the femur. The entire femoral head and most of the neck are intrasynovial (Fig. 6.7). This anatomic circumstance allows a septic arthritis to develop from a focus of metaphyseal osteomyelitis of the femoral neck.

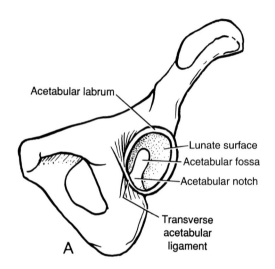

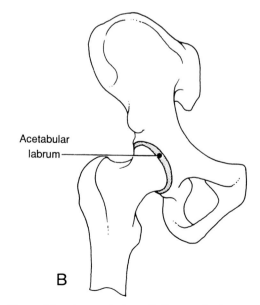

Figure 6.5. *A,* acetabulum. *B,* fibrocartilaginous acetabular labrum containing the femoral head.

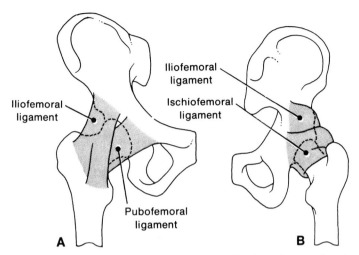

Figure 6.6.   Ligaments of the hip joint. *A,* anterior view. *B,* posterior view.

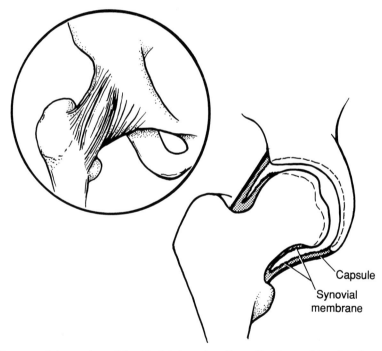

Figure 6.7.   The synovial covering of the hip joint renders the entire femoral head and most of the femoral neck intrasynovial.

Proximal Femur

The neck of the femur forms an angle of approximately 135° with the femoral shaft in the coronal plane (Fig. 6.8). In the sagittal plane, the average angle of anteversion (apex posterior) is approximately 15° in the adult. The angulation of the proximal femur provides improved range of motion as it brings the femur away from the acetabulum, providing better clearance. This angulation, how-

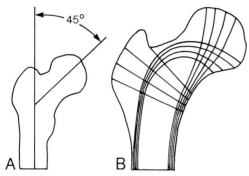

Figure 6.8. Architecture of the upper end of the femur. *A,* neck of the femur angulates medial to the axis of the femoral shaft. *B,* trabecular architecture parallels the lines of tension and compression within the bone.

ever, causes weightbearing forces to generate substantial bending moments in the proximal femur that dictate the pattern of bony architecture. The trabecular architecture of the upper end of the femur is oriented to bear these forces of tension and compression most efficiently (Fig. 6.8). This is a demonstration of Wolff's fundamental law of bony architecture, in which bony form accommodates function and applied force.

The lateral placement of the hip joints provides increased stability when an individual stands stationary in double-limb stance. However, during single-limb stance while walking or running, the lateral placement of the hip joints necessitates strong abductor muscle force to maintain stable, erect posture. Figure 6.9 shows the abductor muscle group mechanics across the hip. Assuming an equilibrium, that is, someone standing on one leg maintaining an erect posture, the forces of the abductor muscles exerted on the greater trochanter must balance the forces of body weight exerted on the pelvis. To maintain a stable, erect posture, abductor muscle forces are high and are the dominant force across the hip joint. Abductor muscles are consequently subject to considerable wear and tear. Deficiencies in these muscles lead to abnormalities of hip function during many activities of daily living, such as walking, running, and stair

climbing. This will be addressed in more detail later in this chapter.

The abductor muscles have a broad attachment to the proximal femur at the greater trochanter, which forms the upper pole of the body of the femur. The greater trochanter also provides the site of attachment for the external rotators. The lesser trochanter arises posteromedially at the junction of the neck and shaft of the femur, providing attachment for the major hip flexor, the iliopsoas. The bony ridge on the posterior surface of the proximal femur, just distal to the greater trochanter, is the site of attachment of the direct tendon of the gluteus maximus, which is the major hip extensor (Fig. 6.10). The head and trochanters of the femur develop as epiphyses that begin to ossify in childhood; the capital femoral epiphysis begins to ossify during the first year of life, the greater trochanter at 5

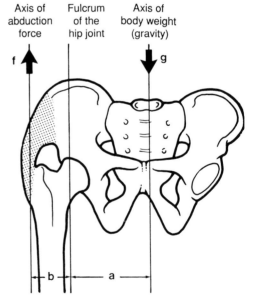

Figure 6.9. Mechanics of the abductors: a = the distance or moment arm along which gravity or body weight acts with one extremity weightbearing; b = the abductor moment arm; *g* = the force of gravity or body weight; f = the abductor force. At equilibrium (when an individual stands stationary on one leg) f × b = *g* × a. Consequently, f = *g* × a/b. In this individual, the ratio of a to b is approximately 3. Consequently, f = 3*g*. (When *g* = 70 kg, f = 210 kg.)

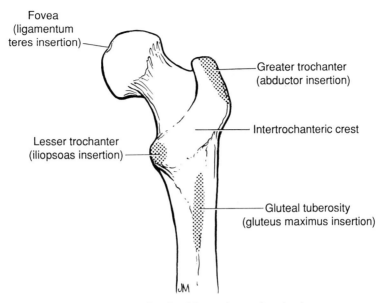

Fovea
(ligamentum
teres insertion)

Greater trochanter
(abductor insertion)

Intertrochanteric crest

Lesser trochanter
(iliopsoas insertion)

Gluteal tuberosity
(gluteus maximus insertion)

Figure 6.10. Proximal femur (posterior view).

years, and the lesser trochanter at 9 years. These all fuse with the metaphysis in adolescence, with the capital epiphysis fusing last. Like all epiphyses, they are vulnerable to traumatic separation, but the capital femoral epiphysis is most vulnerable to slippage.

The femoral head is approximately two-thirds of a sphere and is covered by articular cartilage, except at the insertion of the ligamentum teres. The femoral neck is smaller than the femoral head, providing improved range of motion so that the neck does not impinge on the margins of the acetabulum.

MUSCLES CONTROLLING THE HIP JOINT

Numerous short and long muscles control the hip joint. The main function of the musculature is to meet the requirements of efficient walking—to maintain stability of the weight-bearing leg despite continued change in limb and body position, and to move the body forward. Stability is gained by muscle action to resist the force of gravity that acts to pull the body downward. Because the human frame is top-heavy with much of its mass above the pelvis, large muscular forces are required to maintain stability. Also, because the center of

gravity must move from behind the supporting stance phase foot to ahead of the stance phase foot to move the body forward, the demands on the muscles are constantly changing. The force to propel the body forward is derived from accelerating the swing phase limb during the gait cycle and positioning the stance phase limb to allow the body to fall forward. Hip muscles participate in both these functions. The gait cycle presents complex and progressively changing demands on the hip musculature. Abnormalities of these muscles, which cause weakness or pain, distort the gait cycle, producing a limp. It is convenient to think of the muscles in functional groups when describing muscular control; however, an individual muscle may contribute to more than one functional movement. These groups are described as the abductors, flexors, adductors, extensors, and rotators. The innervation of these muscles will be noted so that the physician can interpret the effect of neurologic disorder on hip function.

Abductor Group

The origins and insertions of the gluteus medius, gluteus minimus, and tensor fascia

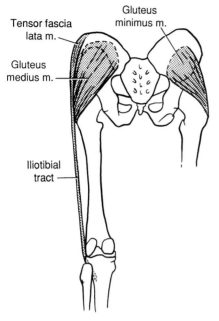

Figure 6.11. Abductors of the hip.

lata are demonstrated in Figure 6.11. The tensor fascia lata extends its tendinous fibers with the fibers of gluteus maximus to form the iliotibial tract on the lateral aspect of the thigh. Muscles of this group are innervated by the superior gluteal nerve, which is composed mainly of fibers from the fourth and fifth lumbar nerve roots. The muscles of this group are required to maintain pelvic stability during the stance phase of gait. During stance phase, body weight forces the bearing hip into adduction. Unless the abductors contract with normal strength, there is an excessive pelvic tilt. With deficient abductor function, the individual will compensate by leaning the trunk over the stance phase limb. This compensatory gait pattern is called an abductor lurch (Figs. 6.12 and 6.13) and reduces forces across the hip.

Hip Flexors

The primary flexors of the hip are the iliopsoas, rectus femoris, and sartorius. The pectineus and tensor fascia lata also function as flexors. The strongest flexor is the double-bellied iliopsoas muscle (Fig. 6.14). The iliopsoas is innervated by the femoral nerve, which is composed of fibers originating from the second through fourth lumbar segments. The sartorius and rectus femoris muscles are less powerful flexors and are innervated by the femoral nerve. During gait, hip flexors are important as swing phase is initiated. These muscles contract to accelerate the leg forward. A patient with weak hip flexors circumducts the leg and compensates further by pivoting the body about the opposite stance phase foot, giving the characteristic circumduction limp. The hip flexors are also important in elevating the limb during stair climbing and in such activities as kicking. With kicking, the rectus femoris contracts strongly and its origin through an apophysis at the anterior inferior iliac spine may be avulsed in adolescence.

Adductor Group

The adductor group is comprised of five muscles: the adductors longus, brevis, and

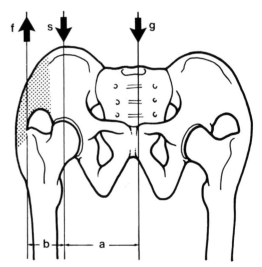

Figure 6.12. Calculation of force (s) acting on the hip joint during normal gait; a = gravity or body weight moment arm with right extremity weightbearing; b = abductor moment arm; g = the force of gravity (body weight); f = abductor force. At equilibrium $f \times b = g \times a$, $f = g \times a/b$. If $a/b = 3/1$, then $f = g \times 3$. When $g = 70$ kg, $f = 210$ kg. The force across the hip is $s = g + f = 70 + 210 = 280$ kg.

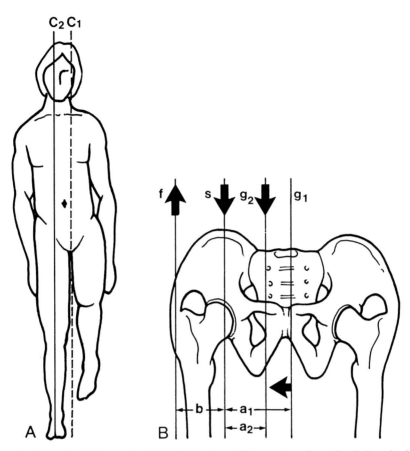

Figure 6.13. Leaning gait (abductor lurch). *A,* illustrates shift in center of gravity during single limb stance with individual leaning forward the stance phase side; c_1, normal axis; c_2, axis with leaning. *B,* calculation of hip joint force; a_1, gravity moment arm in normal gait; a_2, gravity moment arm during leaning gait. $f \times b = g_2 \times a_2$. If $a_2/b = 2$, then $f = 2g_2$. When $g_2 = 70$ kg, $f = 140$ kg. $s = f + g_2 = 210$ kg.

magnus; the gracilis (Fig. 6.14); and the pectineus (Fig. 6.15). The adductors longus and brevis, the gracilis, and much of the adductor magnus are innervated by the obturator nerve. The posterior portion of the adductor magnus, which is predominantly an extensor of the hip, is innervated by the sciatic nerve, whereas the pectineus is innervated mainly by the femoral nerve. Like the hip flexors, these muscles are largely controlled by the second through fourth lumbar segments.

The adductor group has a varied role during gait. At the beginning of stance phase, the adductor magnus is important in assisting the hip extensors to resist flexion of the hip. The adductor longus acts as a hip flexor at the end of the stance phase and as an extensor at the end of the swing phase.

Extensor Group

The extensors consist of the gluteus maximus and hamstring muscles, including the long head of the biceps femoris, the semitendinosus, and the semimembranosus. Also an extensor, is the posterior portion of the adductor magnus (Fig. 6.16). The gluteus maximus is innervated by the inferior gluteal nerve, which is predominantly composed of fibers from the fifth lumbar and first sacral segments. The hamstrings are all innervated by

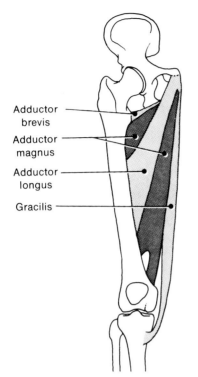

Adductor brevis
Adductor magnus
Adductor longus
Gracilis

Figure 6.14.   Adductor of the hip (anterior view).

the sciatic nerve, with fibers originating from the fifth lumbar through second sacral segments.

Primarily, the hip extensors are responsible for preventing hip and trunk flexion during gait, especially during the early stance phase of gait. The extensors are also responsible for slowing down the accelerating swing phase leg at the end of swing phase. If these muscles fail to function properly, gait becomes unsteady. The gluteus maximus, along with the adductor magnus, is also responsible for climbing and rising from a sitting posture.

External Rotators

Extending across the posterior aspect of the hip are the short external rotators, including the piriformis, superior and inferior gemelli, obturator externus and internus, and the quadratus femoris (Fig. 6.17). Except for the obturator externus, which is innervated

by the obturator nerve, the short rotators are innervated by a branch of the sacral plexus.

Internal Rotators

There are no pure internal rotators of the hip. A number of muscles provide internal rotation as well as other functions. For example, the anterior fibers of the gluteus minimus may internally rotate the hip.

INNERVATION AND BLOOD SUPPLY

Innervation

Branches of the lumbar and sacral plexus innervate the hip joint. These nerves derive from the second through fifth lumbar segments. Several of the branches originate from the obturator nerve. The other branches of the obturator nerve innervate the anterior portion of the knee joint, which helps explain why patients with hip disorders may have anterior knee pain in the absence of significant pain about the hip. Occasionally, knee pain may be referred to the hip.

Blood Supply

Blood supply to the hip in general is profuse, but blood supply to the femoral head is tenuous. The femoral head blood supply is carried by a retinacular arterial system that runs along the neck of the femur. There are two major retinacular systems: the posterior superior and the posterior inferior. These vessels are supplied by perforating capsular branches that derive from an extracapsular arterial ring, formed predominantly by the medial femoral circumflex artery with contributions from the lateral circumflex vessel. When the epiphyseal growth plate is well formed, no metaphyseal vessels traverse the plate to help supply the femoral head. This renders the head particularly susceptible to vascular interruptions. Consequently, avascular necrosis is commonly seen in a child with a femoral neck fracture. This circumstance may also explain the development of avascular necrosis in the pediatric patient after pyogenic arthritis. The increased pressure in the joint may

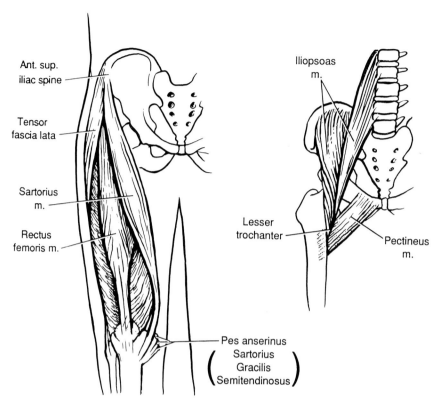

Ant. sup.
iliac spine

Tensor
fascia lata

Sartorius
m.

Rectus
femoris m.

Iliopsoas
m.

Lesser
trochanter

Pectineus
m.

Pes anserinus
(Sartorius
Gracilis
Semitendinosus)

Figure 6.15.   Flexors of the hip. The primary flexors are the iliopsoas (most powerful), and the rectus femoris and sartorius (less powerful).

occlude the retinacular vessels, and the epiphyseal plate may block any communication between the femoral neck metaphyseal vessels and the femoral head epiphyseal vessels.

In the adult, after closure of the epiphyseal plate, anastomosis occurs between the metaphyseal and the epiphyseal vascular systems. Therefore, the femoral head is at reduced risk, but the blood supply still remains tenuous. For example, in the adult with a displaced intracapsular fracture of the neck, the metaphyseal vessels traveling into the head and the subsynovial retinacular vessels may be disrupted. This can result in aseptic necrosis of the head of the femur. In most individuals, the artery carried in the ligamentum teres does not supply adequate circulation to prevent avascular necrosis. Avascular necrosis can also be seen in patients who have sustained a dislo-

cation of the hip, tearing and stretching the arterial system. Because of this potential for avascular necrosis, a dislocation of the hip must be treated as an orthopaedic emergency.

RELATIONSHIP OF THE HIP JOINT TO THE GREAT VESSELS AND NERVES

The sciatic nerve emerges from the sacral plexus through the greater sciatic notch between the piriformis and the obturator internus (Fig. 6.18). In the sciatic notch, the sciatic nerve is vulnerable to injury from pelvic fractures and, distal to the notch, vulnerable to injury from posterior dislocation of the femoral head. The femoral artery, vein, and nerve enter the thigh lying on the iliopsoas and pectineus muscle. They are cushioned by these muscles and are not likely to

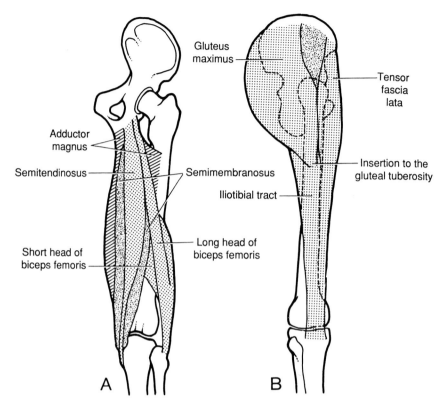

Figure 6.16. Extensors of the hip. *A,* posterior view of the hamstring muscles. *B,* lateral view of the gluteus maximus and its relationship to the tensor fascia lata and the iliotibial tract.

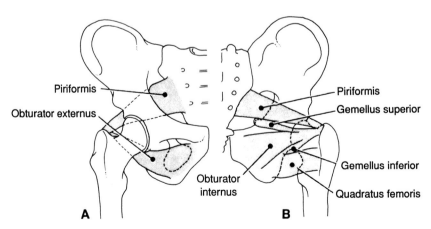

Figure 6.17. Pure external rotators. *A,* anterior view. *B,* posterior view.

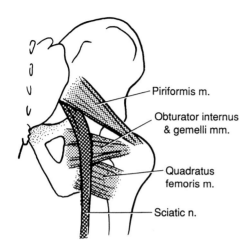

Figure 6.18. Relationship of the sciatic nerve to the posterior aspect of the hip joint and the external rotators.

be injured by hip dislocation or pelvic fractures.

EVALUATION OF THE PATIENT WITH HIP SYMPTOMS

HISTORY

Pain is usually the chief complaint of patients with hip problems. These patients may present with pain over the anterior or lateral aspect of the hip, in the groin, or more medially in the region of the adductors (corresponding to the obturator nerve distribution). Pain may radiate distally to the knee. Pain referred to the hip may be secondary to spinal problems, which must be considered in the differential diagnosis of patients with "hip" pain.

Most patients with hip pain have increased pain with activity. Measurements of joint forces reveal that peak forces at the hip can exceed four times body weight when going from a slow to fast walking speed. Jogging can increase this force up to six times body weight. This increased force is generated primarily by the muscles about the hip. Those who complain of pain at rest usually have some inflammatory component to the disease they have. An infectious or neoplastic process may

be present. Many patients will report increased pain as they begin activity. Pain is increased when the patient loads a joint that has been at rest. As the joint accommodates the new level of activity, pain subsides.

Patients with chronic progressive disease, such as osteoarthritis, report progressively severe pain. They often report prior problems, e.g., injury or childhood disease including developmental dysplasia, avascular necrosis, or slipped capital femoral epiphysis. Adults with avascular necrosis may describe the onset of pain months or years after cortisone use. Excessive alcohol ingestion may be a contributing cause of avascular necrosis.

Patients will complain of stiffness, which may be worst in the morning or may be a more constant problem affecting many activities of daily living. To obtain an accurate analysis, patients should be questioned to determine their impairment in the activities of walking, dressing, stair climbing, and foot hygiene.

PHYSICAL EXAMINATION

The patient must be adequately undressed for proper examination. Inspection normally reveals a level pelvis. Pelvic obliquity suggests leg-length discrepancy or scoliosis, which may or may not be associated with hip disease. Range of motion of the spine will help demonstrate any true spinal abnormality. Contracture of the hip may cause a compensatory obliquity of the pelvis. If inspection of the pelvis is difficult because of the patient's size, palpation should be performed at the bony prominences to determine position and symmetry.

Observe the resting posture of the hip. The ligaments of the hip are so oriented that pressure in the joint space is least when the hip is slightly flexed, abducted, and externally rotated. Therefore, patients with an acute synovitis or effusion tend to maintain the hip in this position.

The Trendelenburg's test is performed following inspection. The patient is asked to stand on one leg and lift the other leg with the hip and knee flexed. Normal patients will lift the pelvis contralateral to the stance limb. Patients with deficient abductor muscles or a hip disorder that causes pain on contraction of the muscles have an impairment of this normal mechanism. Consequently, these patients will allow the pelvis to drop contralateral to the stance phase side or may shift the upper body over the stance phase leg to reduce muscular demand (Fig. 6.13).

The patient's gait should be observed. Many limps are secondary to abnormality of the hip. The antalgic limp results from decreased time in the stance phase on the painful side, producing an abnormality in the normal rhythm. The short-leg limp is secondary to leg-length inequality, which may be associated with hip disease. There is an obvious increase in the up and down movement of the head and shoulders. This occurs when the body falls onto the shortened stance phase leg and then rises up on the long contralateral leg when stance phase begins on that side. The abductor sway is characterized by increased sway of the head and upper body over the stance phase limb. As noted above, this may be associated with a painful hip or with chronic weakness of the hip abductor muscles.

After observation of gait, the hip is palpated to elicit areas of tenderness. Tenderness may be present over the greater trochanteric bursa or ischial bursa. Palpation over the posterior superior iliac spine often reveals tenderness that may be a trigger zone for spinal pain, or there may be pain in this area from sacroiliac disease. Tenderness can be present in various muscles, such as the tensor fascia lata or gluteus maximus.

Leg lengths are measured after palpation. Reliable measurement of true leg length can be obtained by noting the distance from the anterior superior iliac spine to the medial malleolus. Range of motion should be determined. Flexion contracture of the hip is often noted with serious hip disease. This is detected with the patient supine, as demonstrated in Figure 6.19. When checking abduction and adduction of the hip, it is also important to isolate hip motion from pelvic motion on the lumbosacral spine. Following range of mo-

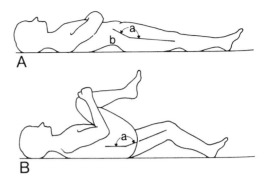

Figure 6.19. Demonstrating flexion contracture of the hip. *A,* with the patient lying supine and both hips extended, there is an increased lumbar lordosis (*b*) compensating for the true flexion contracture (*a*) of the hip. *B,* with the right hip flexed to flatten the lordosis, the true flexion contracture of the left hip becomes apparent.

tion, strength of muscle groups can be determined.

NONTRAUMATIC CONDITIONS IN ADULTHOOD

DEGENERATIVE ARTHRITIS OF THE HIP

Osteoarthritis is one of the most common diseases affecting the adult hip. This condition is often secondary to an underlying abnormality of the hip, such as developmental dysplasia, Legg-Calvé-Perthes disease, or slipped capital femoral epiphysis. In some cases, however, there is no identifiable cause, and in those situations the osteoarthritis is considered primary or idiopathic. The pathophysiology of osteoarthritis is reviewed in Chapter 12. As a result of these changes, motion in the hip becomes progressively restricted, first by painful synovitis and muscle spasm, then by secondary soft tissue contracture. In more advanced stages of the disease, there is loss of joint congruity, osteophyte formation, and mechanical block to motion superimposed on the soft tissue contracture.

Pain in osteoarthritis can be caused by this synovitis or by muscle spasm, capsular contracture, and pain fibers in bone and reparative granulation tissue.

Clinical Characteristics

The patient presents with pain, which may be felt in the groin, buttock, anterior thigh, or knee. Pain is usually worse with weight-bearing, although there may be pain at rest. Initially, the pain may be intermittent, but with time it becomes more frequent, lasts longer, and becomes progressively severe. The patient may limp, which may be an antalgic limp or an "abductor sway" (Fig. 6.13).

Motion is restricted and may be demonstrable as a flexion contracture. Abduction and internal rotation are usually more restricted than adduction and external rotation. The leg shortens with advanced disease. X-ray of the hip demonstrates varying changes, including narrowing of the joint space, subchondral bone irregularity with cyst and osteophyte formation, sclerosis of the subchondral and trabecular bone, and lateral or superolateral subluxation of the femoral head.

Conservative Treatment

Conservative measures can be helpful in reducing the symptoms and associated disability of degenerative arthritis of the hip. One of the most important measures of conservative treatment is reducing the stress across the joint. The patient should walk less and avoid running, jumping, climbing stairs, and other impact-type activities. An overweight patient can reduce the stress on the hip by losing weight. In Figure 6.12, if body weight was 90 kg instead of 70 kg, the force across the hip joint would be 360 kg, not 280 kg. This is nearly a 25% difference. A cane is another effective means of reducing stress across the hip. A cane used on the side opposite the affected hip can reduce hip joint force by as much as 30%. The cane should be approximately 1 to 2 inches longer than would be necessary to reach the ground when held in a weightbearing grip with the elbow fully extended.

Although rest reduces symptoms, it also produces atrophic muscular weakness. Consequently, a patient should maintain muscular strength by performing daily exercises that are of low stress. Range of motion exercise will help to preserve motion. Muscle strengthening and range of motion exercises as outlined in Figure 6.20 are recommended if well tolerated. The patient should omit any exercise that produces pain. If these strengthening exercises are painful, the patient may perform isometric exercises. In addition to these exercises, a regular swimming or stationary bicycle program is beneficial. These are excellent general conditioning activities and will not lead to the type of joint stress and increased wear that impact activity would. It is difficult for a patient to maintain optimum weight without an exercise program.

The use of heat or cold may reduce the symptoms of osteoarthritis of the hip. Anti-inflammatory medication (aspirin, nonsteroidals, and corticosteroids) may provide relief from pain of synovitis associated with osteoarthritis. Systemic corticosteroids have serious side effects and should be avoided in routine treatment of osteoarthritis. Intra-articular steroid injection may be beneficial and can be employed on a limited nonrepetitive basis. Although nonsteroidal anti-inflammatory drugs can be beneficial, evidence suggests that prolonged use of these medications may impair the reparative processes about the diseased hip, and bones may deteriorate more rapidly.

Surgical Treatment

When conservative treatment is unsuccessful, surgical treatment is considered and orthopaedic referral is necessary. Three forms of surgical treatment are commonly considered.

Arthrodesis of the hip provides pain relief by surgical ankylosis of the joint. The patient trades movement for a stable, painless hip. It is usually indicated in severe posttraumatic and postinfectious unilateral arthritis in young otherwise healthy patients. Generally, normal low back, ipsilateral knee, and contralateral hip function are prerequisites for a hip fusion. If arthrodesis is successful, more than 20 years of good function can be anticipated.

Osteotomy of the femur or pelvis attempts to improve the weightbearing condition of the hip by changing the weightbearing relationship of the femoral head and acetabulum.

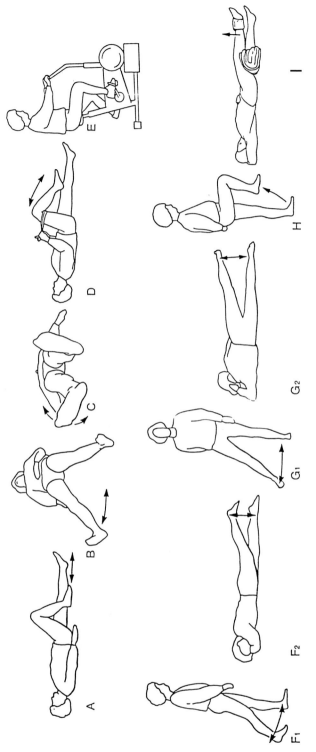

Figure 6.20. Exercises for the hip. A through E, range of motion exercises. A, sliding flexion while supine. B, sliding abduction/adduction while supine. C, internal and external rotation while supine (this can be repeated with the hip flexed). D, active and self-assisted further flexion using hands or exercise strap. E, stationary bicycle with low resistance on pedal. F through I, strengthening exercises. F, hip extensor strengthening, erect (F_1) and prone (F_2) (more advanced). G, hip abductor strengthening, erect (G_1) and side-lying (G_2) (more advanced). H, hip flexor strengthening, supine (see Fig. 6.23A) and erect (more advanced). I, quadriceps strengthening.

An attempt is made to increase the weight-bearing area of the hip to decrease the relative force per unit area and to bring the femoral head into a more "congruous" relationship with the acetabulum. This procedure should be done relatively early in the arthritic process while the patient still has a good range of motion. Therefore, early orthopaedic referral is important, particularly for younger patients. Recent data indicate that approximately 20% of patients require some form of major surgical reconstruction within 5 years of the index osteotomy. The subsequent reconstruction rate corresponds directly to the amount of arthritis present at time of initial osteotomy.

The most common therapy for osteoarthritis of the hip is total hip arthroplasty. Over 125,000 total hip arthroplasties are performed annually in the United States with two-thirds performed in patients over 65 years old. Recent prospective studies indicate dramatic improvement in quality of life, physical function, social interaction, and overall health. These improvements are realized as early as 12 weeks after surgery. Most patients are kept on protected weightbearing on the operated hip for 6 to 12 weeks and will require inpatient or outpatient physical therapy for gait training and strengthening. Full weightbearing is typically allowed after the second or third postoperative month.

The technique of this procedure, as well as the design of the prosthesis used, has improved substantially over the last 30 years. Methylmethacrylate cement continues to be the most common means of fixation of the prosthetic component to the bone. There have been significant advances in cement preparation and application that improve the bonding of cement to bone and strengthen the bone cement. Over the last decade, a prosthesis with porous-coated surfaces has been developed. This type of prosthesis eliminates the need for cement because bone ingrowth occurs to the microporous coating, and the bone ingrowth provides long-term fixation. More recently, prostheses with hydroxyapatite coating have been developed. This coating encourages the bone to grow onto the surface of the prosthesis and also provide long-term fixation. At this point, comparative follow-up studies show a decreased rate of loosening of porous ingrowth acetabular components in comparison to cemented acetabular components. Uncemented femoral components, however, have not shown a decreased loosening rate in comparison to a cemented component. Currently, most total hip replacements are performed using cement fixation for the femoral component and bony porous ingrowth for fixation of the acetabular component (Fig. 6.21). In younger patients, uncemented components are used increasingly on the femoral side as well. This practice is based on the expectation that the uncemented components that have been designed most recently will provide a more durable and more physiologic prosthetic replacement of the femur.

Operative time is approximately 3 hours with blood loss typically between 1 to 2 units

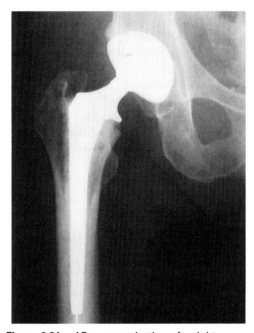

Figure 6.21. AP x-ray projection of a right "hybrid" total hip replacement with cemented femoral component and uncemented acetabular component. Note the loss of the endosteal outline of the femur adjacent to the distal half of the prosthesis because of excellent intrusion of bone cement obliterating the normal cortical margin.

during surgery. Most patients elect to donate their own blood for subsequent autologous transfusion. Survivorship studies on total hip arthroplasties have revealed a 10 to 40% incidence of radiographic loosening at 10 years, although the revision rate is significantly lower because many of these hips continue to function well despite the radiographic findings. Early loosening (first 5 years) is more commonly seen about the femoral component at the prosthesis cement interface. Late loosening is more associated with the acetabular component. The need for revision surgery at 20 years correlates inversely with age at time of primary hip replacement. One of the major clinical problems that develops in the intermediate to long-term period following hip arthroplasty is osteolysis. This condition may present in a patient who has a painless, well-functioning implant. Radiographically, it presents as areas of lucency within bone adjacent to the prosthesis. The localized osteopenia or rarefaction may extend into the cortical bone. Osteolysis is a result of inflammation caused by microparticulate wear debris generated from the polyethylene acetabular surface. This wear debris can be "pumped" into the interface between prosthesis and bone, or cement and bone. These micron and submicron particles can generate an intense inflammatory reaction leading to areas of aggressive bone loss. Many improvements in component design and fixation techniques have been implemented to address this problem, which now seems to be on the decline.

Several acute complications can occur after hip arthroplasty that are significant, and standard prophylactic measures are usually employed to avoid them. Deep venous thrombosis and thromboembolic disease are common after total hip replacement. Typically, either warfarin or a low molecular weight heparin is used as a prophylactic agent. Immediate postoperative infection has been successfully prevented by the standard use of perioperative antibiotics given preoperatively and for a period of 24 hours postoperatively. The most common antibiotic agent is a first generation cephalosporin. The overall risk of infection is 1% over the lifetime of the prosthesis. Other complications that occur include heterotopic ossification, thigh pain, periprosthetic fracture and dislocation of the prosthetic hip, particularly within the first 3 months. Despite these potential complications, primary total hip arthroplasty remains a highly successful procedure with many studies documenting that over 90% of patients achieve a good to excellent result. The surgery provides the great majority of patients with a durable, long-term, pain-free functioning hip.

INFLAMMATORY ARTHRITIS OF THE HIP

Chapter 12 describes the various arthritides. Arthritis can affect the hip or any other synovial joint. Any patient who appears to have synovitis of the hip that is refractory to treatment should be referred for orthopaedic or rheumatologic evaluation. A variety of conditions must be considered, including rheumatoid arthritis, spondyloarthropathies, collagen vascular disease, crystalline arthritis, primary and metastatic malignancy, pigmented villonodular synovitis, avascular necrosis (see below), and infection (see below).

INFECTIONS OF THE HIP

Adult patients rarely develop septic arthritis of the hip. Those patients who develop septic arthritis are frequently immunocompromised, e.g., patients with diabetes or renal failure, or those taking corticosteroids or chemotherapeutic agents. The intravenous drug abuser is also at increased risk. A healthy patient who develops septic arthritis presents acutely ill with high fever, exquisite pain, and decreased motion. An immunocompromised patient may present without high fever and may not appear acutely ill. Range of motion may not be as painful.

Tuberculosis can occur in the hip joint as in any other synovial tissue. Pain, limited motion, subcutaneous abscess, or draining sinus may be part of the presentation. In the advanced stages of this disease, x-ray changes are significant and demonstrate bone and joint destruction.

A patient suspected of having infectious arthritis of the hip must undergo joint aspiration and should be referred immediately to the orthopaedist.

AVASCULAR (ASEPTIC) NECROSIS OF THE ADULT HIP

Avascular necrosis of the femoral head is well recognized in association with fractures of the femoral neck and dislocations of the femoral head in both adults and children. Fracture of the femoral neck is associated with a 15 to 30% risk of avascular necrosis. Dislocation of the hip is associated with a 10 to 15% risk of avascular necrosis. The cause of avascular necrosis of the femoral head after direct hip trauma is primarily the result of an interruption of the arterial supply to the femoral head secondary to the injury. Evidence suggests that avascular necrosis also may be the result of a short duration shower of fat emboli that can occur after significant trauma. Avascular necrosis of the femoral head without recognizable injury is not well understood and may be multifactorial. In patients with sickle cell disease, avascular necrosis is thought to be associated with vascular thrombosis. Avascular necrosis commonly has been associated with alcoholism and long-term steroid use. The risk of developing avascular necrosis after brief exposure to corticosteroids occurs uncommonly and is not well understood, but the potential risk is certainly great enough to justify caution when prescribing systemic corticosteroids for prolonged periods. There is no known risk of avascular necrosis after single or repeated trigger-point or intra-articular injections. Avascular necrosis has also been noted in gout, Gaucher's disease, caisson disease, and in patients with altered hemostasis. In several large series of patients with avascular necrosis, the idiopathic category remains the largest group followed by alcohol-related or corticosteroid-induced. Venous compression has been implicated as a cause for avascular necrosis, especially in decompression sickness, pregnancy, or thrombophlebitis. Embolic causes typically are centered on fat emboli as the inciting event. Intraosseous fat embolism not only directly obstructs blood flow but is also hypothesized to mediate vascular occlusion through an intermediary pathway of localized intravascular coagulation.

The pathologic change associated with the early phase of this disease is a segmental necrosis of the femoral head. The overlying articular cartilage is unaffected. With time, there is reparative tissue ingrowth with resorption of necrotic bone accompanied by formation of new bone on necrotic trabeculae. With resorption, the area of segmental necrosis weakens, and a subchondral fracture can occur. Patients often have a marked increase in pain when the fracture occurs.

Avascular necrosis is clinically categorized in stages based on the x-ray appearance of the hip. The condition is frequently bilateral in nontraumatic cases.

Clinical Characteristics

Patients with avascular necrosis may be asymptomatic in the earliest stages. In the early stages, plain radiographs are often normal. MRI is the best single imaging study to establish the diagnosis with a specificity of 98%. However, it is not uncommon for patients who present with pain in one hip to already have subtle x-ray or MRI changes on the asymptomatic opposite side. Patients who are symptomatic present with pain in the groin and anterolateral hip. Pain may be in the thigh or radiate to the knee. In some patients, an episode of severe pain develops after a period of milder pain; this is frequently at the time of subchondral fracture. The patient may have an antalgic limp or an abductor sway. Motion is restricted by pain in the early stages of the disease and by mechanical obstruction in the later stages when secondary degenerative arthritis develops.

Treatment

Treatment of this condition is surgical, and orthopaedic referral is necessary. In the early stages before collapse, a "core decompression" of the avascular segment can be performed by drilling into the head from the lateral femoral cortex. This decompression may be followed by healing. Once any collapse occurs, this form of treatment is not predictable, and other procedures, including osteotomy, debridement, grafting, and hip arthroplasty, must be considered. Early referral of the patient is important to salvage the femoral head.

BURSITIS

Bursitis about the hip is a common condition secondary to inflammation of one of the three major bursae about the hip: the trochanteric bursa, the iliopsoas bursa, and the ischiogluteal bursa. These bursae facilitate the gliding of musculotendinous or ligamentous structures. Bursitis may be secondary to direct injury or overuse of the adjacent musculotendinous structures or degenerative changes in these structures. Because bursae are lined by true synovial tissue, bursitis also can occur with systemic disease, causing synovitis.

Trochanteric Bursitis

The trochanteric bursa is a large bursa that lies between the greater trochanter and the overlying junction of the gluteus maximus and tensor fascia lata, as these merge to form the fascia lata and iliotibial tract (Fig. 6.22).

Clinical Characteristics

Patients complain of pain over the lateral aspect of the hip; frequently radiation occurs into the lateral thigh and posterolaterally toward the posterior aspect of the trochanter and into the buttock. Patients complain of pain when they turn onto the affected hip or with hip movement, particularly rotation. The pain may develop abruptly or insidiously and may be mild or severe. Tenderness is present over the trochanter laterally and posterolaterally, but swelling or redness rarely is present. Rotation of the hip may increase pain, especially if this is combined with compression over the trochanter. X-rays are usually noncontributory, but they should be obtained to rule out other conditions. Signs of soft tissue swelling or calcification may be present in the adjacent tendinous structures. Fracture of the greater trochanter in the elderly patient with osteoporosis can mimic trochanteric bursitis.

Treatment

Treatment consists of rest, heat or ice, and the use of nonsteroidal anti-inflammatory medication. Local steroid injection also can be helpful, but one must be careful to inject this in the bursa and avoid intratendinous injection.

Ischiogluteal Bursitis

This is inflammation of the bursa between the ischial tuberosity and the overlying gluteus maximus. Ischiogluteal bursitis usually is associated with injury or with occupations requiring long periods of sitting.

Clinical Characteristics

The patient complains of pain over the ischial tuberosity that is aggravated by sitting, and the pain may radiate into the posterior thigh. Tenderness is present overlying the ischial bursa, but swelling is rarely noted. X-rays are usually noncontributory.

Treatment

Treatment is the same as for trochanteric bursitis. Resolution usually occurs in 1 to 2 weeks.

Iliopsoas Bursitis

This is inflammation of the iliopsoas bursa, located between the iliopsoas muscle and the

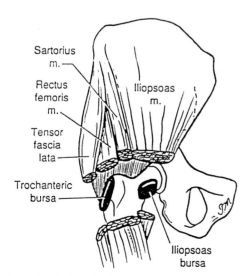

Figure 6.22. Trochanteric and iliopsoas bursae of the hip joint, anterior view.

pelvis proximally and the hip capsule and psoas tendon distally (Fig. 6.22). Communication between the hip joint and psoas bursa is common.

Clinical Characteristics

Pain is felt in the groin and may radiate into the anterior aspect of the thigh. The pattern of pain is difficult to distinguish from true hip arthritis. The patient may complain of pain on walking. Local tenderness is difficult to elicit because the structures are deep. Pain may occur with deep palpation over the anterior aspect of the hip. Pain is increased with flexion of the hip against resistance or with hyperextension of the hip. X-rays are noncontributory.

Treatment

Treatment consists of rest, heat, ice, and nonsteroidal anti-inflammatory medication. When treating bursitis in any location, a gentle program of stretching exercise within the limits of pain and active exercise of the involved muscles should be instituted once pain has subsided. Brief, frequent periods of exercise are recommended, as opposed to one long period of exercise that tends to produce fatigue and may cause reinjury. If symptoms persist after 2 weeks of treatment, orthopaedic referral is indicated.

THE SNAPPING HIP: COXA SALTANS

Coxa saltans, or snapping hip, is characterized by an audible snapping or popping that occurs with flexion and extension of the hip with normal activity. Coxa saltans often is associated with pain and can have several causes. This condition can result from the gluteus maximus or the iliotibial band sliding over the greater trochanter (external type) or the musculotendinous iliopsoas snapping directly over the femoral head, iliopectineal eminence, or iliopsoas bursa (internal type). Intra-articular pathology, such as synovial chondromatosis, loose bodies, fracture fragments, and capsular or labral tears (posterior-superior portion), also can be a source for a painful clicking sensation in the hip.

Clinical Characteristics

Patients with external type snapping (most common) typically present with a gradual history of snapping in the region over the greater trochanter, which may be painful. When the external type of coxa saltans is suspected, the patient is placed on the unaffected side. The hip is then flexed actively by the patient with the examiner palpating the snap over the greater trochanter. The snapping can be blocked with finger pressure on the greater trochanter.

When internal coxa saltans is suspected, the patient is placed supine with the hip brought from a flexed and abducted position to an extended and adducted posture. This maneuver will often elicit a painful snapping or clicking sensation. Applying finger pressure over the iliopsoas tendon at the level of the femoral head can block the snapping and help corroborate the diagnosis of internal psoas snapping. Those with intra-articular disorders complain more of clicking than snapping. Labral tears or small fracture fragments are often associated with an acute traumatic episode.

There is uncertainty as to the best method to radiographically investigate coxa saltans. Iliopsoas bursography is the definitive and single most useful procedure. MRI is indicated only when plain films are negative and labral tears or intra-articular disorders are strongly suspected.

Treatment

Many people experience benign painless snapping in which no treatment is required. If snapping is of recent onset (less than 6 months), intermittent, conservative therapy consisting of rest and anti-inflammatory medication followed by a stretching program under the guidance of a physical therapist will usually be adequate. Surgical treatment is reserved for those who do not benefit from at least 12 months of therapy. External snapping is treated with removal of the trochanteric bursa and often lengthening of the iliotibial band. Internal snapping that fails conservative therapy can be treated in a similar fashion with lengthening of the iliopsoas tendon.

Intraarticular snapping, whether caused by bony or soft tissue disorders, can often be addressed arthroscopically. The last decade has seen significant advancement in the surgical technique, patient application, and clinical efficacy of hip arthroscopy over conventional open arthrotomy for retrieval of loose bodies, debridement of symptomatic labral tears, or synovectomy.

PERIARTICULAR MYOFASCIAL PAIN SYNDROMES

Many varieties of myofascial pain syndromes occur about the hip joint. These syndromes usually occur in middle-aged or older patients. The pain site varies in location according to the specific muscular unit that is involved. The pathophysiology is not clear, and some authors argue the existence of these syndromes. Nevertheless, many patients present with localized muscular pain and consistent areas of tenderness (trigger points). These areas of tenderness may be somewhat firm, or the muscle may have a cordlike thickening. The distinction of these syndromes depends on the location of pain and tenderness and a fairly characteristic pattern of referred pain (as noted below).

Gluteus Medius Syndrome

Pain is felt over the upper and midportion of the gluteus medius. Referred pain may be felt in the posterior or lateral thigh (Fig. 6.23). Passive stretch or contraction against resistance may aggravate the pain.

Gluteus Maximus Syndrome

Pain is felt more centrally in the buttock. Referred pain may be felt in the posterior thigh (Fig. 6.23).

Tensor Fascia Lata Syndrome

Pain is felt more anteriorly over the tensor fascia lata muscle with referred pain to the lateral and anterolateral thigh. Pain may go below the knee (Fig. 6.23).

Hamstring Syndrome

Pain is felt over the ischium or proximal thigh posteriorly and is associated with tenderness in the region of the hamstring origin and muscles.

Piriformis Syndrome

Pain is felt in the region of the sciatic notch (Fig. 6.23). Referred pain may be felt more generally in the buttock, posterior thigh, or lower leg. Because of the proximity of the adjacent sciatic nerve, a patient with "sciatica-type" pain may present with inflammation of the piriformis. Local tenderness is present over the piriformis. Pain may be increased with passive forced internal rotation or resisted external rotation. Patients may complain of pain in the rectal or vaginal area, which can be reproduced on rectal or vaginal examination by fingertip pressure just at and medial to the ischial spine.

Treatment

In all of the myofascial pain syndromes, rest, heat or ice, and oral anti-inflammatory medication may be helpful. Injection with a local anesthetic with or without depository steroid may be helpful, but intratendinous injection must be avoided. Success has also been reported with "cold spraying" of the affected muscle using a fluoromethane spray followed by manual stretching.

SACROILIAC SYNDROME

Inflammation of the sacroiliac joint can occur with a variety of the spondyloarthropathies. Reiter's syndrome, psoriatic arthritis, ankylosing spondylitis, and inflammatory bowel disease commonly occur with sacroiliitis. In other patients, there may be sacroiliac pain without other signs of spondyloarthropathy. Pain may be from true synovitis of this joint, or from inflammation of the overlying muscles or ligaments.

Clinical Characteristics

Pain occurs over the sacroiliac joint region with referred pain into the lower buttock and

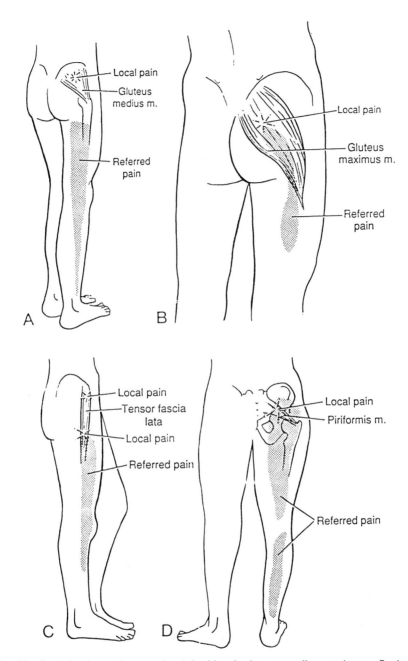

Figure 6.23. Myofascial pain syndromes about the hip. *A,* gluteus medius syndrome. *B,* gluteus maximus syndrome. *C,* tensor fascia lata syndrome. *D,* piriformis syndrome.

thigh. Pain over the greater trochanter and groin pain may also be present. Tenderness is present over the sacroiliac joint and in the region of the posterior superior iliac spine. The Patrick's test may elicit pain in the in-

volved joint. With the patient side-lying, strong compression of the pelvis may cause pain. Hyperextension of the hip may also produce pain. X-rays frequently show no significant change. In the case of spondyloarthropathy, however, there may be irregularity or osteopenia of the subchondral bone leading to "blurring" of the joint space. These changes are most commonly seen in the lower (synovial) part of the joint. Patchy areas of lucency and sclerosis may develop. With further progression, marked narrowing of the joint space occurs, and ankylosis can be present.

Treatment

When sacroiliitis is a manifestation of an underlying spondyloarthropathy, treatment is dictated by the underlying inflammatory disease. In isolated cases of sacroiliac syndrome, symptomatic relief can be achieved by rest, application of local heat or ice, and use of nonsteroidal anti-inflammatory medication. A sacroiliac belt may also be helpful.

TRAUMATIC DISORDERS OF THE PELVIS AND HIP

PELVIC SPRAINS

Because of their strength, disruption of the sacroiliac joints and pubic symphysis only occur as a result of severe injury. Because the pelvis is a stable bony ring (see "Essential Anatomy"), injuries that involve actual displacement of one of the pelvic joints usually occur in conjunction with a secondary site of injury elsewhere in the bony ring. For example, a disruption of the symphysis may occur in conjunction with a sacroiliac dislocation, sacral fracture, or iliac fracture.

Women in the later stages of pregnancy are more subject to sprains of the pelvic ligaments with lesser degrees of injury. Also, isolated pubic symphysis sprains can occur as a result of a fall directly onto the symphysis or perineum, such as when an individual slips off a bicycle seat onto the frame.

Clinical Characteristics

Sprain of the sacroiliac joint is associated with pain over the region of the joint and posterior superior iliac spine with referral into the buttock and thigh. Sprains of the pubic symphysis are associated with pain in that region. Pain is referred into the groin and inner thigh and may be bilateral. Localized tenderness is present in the region of the joints. Weightbearing can increase pain, and transfer of weight from one extremity to another may aggravate symptoms. In pregnancy, pain may persist until delivery. X-rays are usually noncontributory, except if there has been actual displacement of the joint. Cases with displacement are usually the result of violent trauma, and sacroiliac or symphyseal dislocation is often associated with a fracture of the pelvic ring.

Treatment

In the case of obvious displacement of the sacroiliac joint or pubic symphysis, orthopaedic consultation should be obtained immediately for further evaluation and treatment. Even if no obvious abnormality is found on x-ray, orthopaedic consultation should be obtained when there is a history of violent injury and when significant pubic symphysis or sacroiliac injury is suspected.

In other circumstances, treatment is rest, heat or ice, and nonsteroidal anti-inflammatory medication. During pregnancy, medication is usually avoided. After a brief period of rest, activity can be increased progressively within the limits of pain as tolerated. Some patients benefit from a sacroiliac belt.

MUSCULAR STRAINS AND AVULSION INJURIES

Muscular strains are distinguished from the myofascial pain syndromes by the recognition of their immediate onset after an injury. These injuries are secondary to violent stretch or contraction of the muscle against resistance, or less often as a result of blunt impact. Contusion of the muscle can occur anywhere in its substance and can disrupt the fascial muscular envelope as well as the actual muscle fibers. Bleeding occurs with associated swelling and ecchymosis. Local tenderness is present and pain occurs with passive stretch or active contraction of the muscle. The area of hematoma may become the site of abnormal bone formation, which can prolong pain and swelling and cause limited motion secondary to muscular contracture; this is known as myositis ossificans.

Any of the major muscle groups about the hip can be injured. A common injury is the "groin pull." This is an injury of the adductors. It is often secondary to forced abduction of the hip in a fall, twisting injury, or collision. Pain is felt at the adductor tubercle, about the inferior pubic ramus, or within the adductor tendon region.

An abrupt, strongly resisted, sudden hip flexion, which might occur in a kicking injury, produces a strain of the iliopsoas or rectus femoris muscles. Pain is felt over the anterior iliac spine or anterior aspect of the hip. Tenderness is present in these regions and pain occurs with passive extension or active flexion.

In adolescence, passive stretch or strong contraction against fixed resistance may produce avulsion injuries of a musculotendinous unit. This occurs because these muscles join the bone at the apophyses that are still unfused during adolescence. An abruptly resisted hip flexion, which might occur when a kick is blocked, may cause avulsion of the rectus femoris at the anterior inferior iliac spine, avulsion of the sartorius at the anterior superior iliac spine, or avulsion of the lesser femoral trochanter by the iliopsoas. Severe stretch of the hamstrings, which can occur doing the splits, may cause avulsion of the hamstrings from the ischial tuberosity. Abruptly opposed hip adduction or hip extension, which may occur during a fall or the splits, can avulse the origins of the adductor group from the inferior pubic ramus and ischial tuberosity.

Clinical Characteristics

Pain and tenderness are localized to the injured muscle or its site of origin or attachment. There may be associated swelling and ecchymosis. Passive stretch or voluntary contraction is painful and may be inhibited.

X-rays may show avulsion injuries at the bony apophyses.

Treatment

If gross disruption of the musculotendinous unit is suspected or there is an avulsion injury on x-ray, orthopaedic referral should be obtained. The orthopaedist must then decide whether immobilization is indicated or whether actual repair of the injury should be considered. These injuries rarely require operative repair.

For the majority of these injuries, the goal of treatment is reduction of symptoms, allowing a comfortable period of rest and restricted activity for healing to occur. The duration of restriction and symptomatic treatment depends on the severity of injury.

Initially, rest, use of crutches, and application of ice are helpful. When there is injury to a muscle belly, it is helpful to provide support to reduce symptoms and further minimize intramuscular bleeding and swelling. For injuries about the hip, a pelvic elastic bandage spica is effective. Another helpful device is elasticized shorts that provide good muscular support.

If the injury is minor with little swelling, mild tenderness, and no pain with weightbearing, it usually resolves over several days. Stretching and active exercise may progress as soon as symptoms allow. Ice is applied initially, and after the first 24 to 48 hours, applications of heat may be helpful.

When a patient has severe injuries with marked swelling and tenderness several hours after injury and significant pain with weightbearing, a more major disruption of the muscle tissue is presumed. Treatment is initiated with rest and ice, and the patient is instructed in crutch use. This treatment must continue for several weeks and then, as pain recedes, stretching and active exercise and increased weightbearing may begin. Pain is used as a guide to initiation and progression of activity. Return to sporting activity is allowed when the patient feels pain-free during activities of daily living and has regained nearly full motion and strength. With a severe hamstring pull, it is not uncommon to have patients restricted for 2 months.

SPRAINS AND DISLOCATIONS OF THE HIP JOINT

Sprains

Sprains of the hip joint are secondary to the same kinds of forces that cause dislocations but are of a lesser magnitude. Also, it must be remembered that the hip joint is intrinsically stable and, except with violent force, is not subject to sprain or dislocation. Therefore, sprains of the hip are much less common than those of the knee or ankle. When this injury occurs, synovitis may be associated with the stretch or partial tear of the hip capsule and ligaments.

Clinical Characteristics

Sprain of the hip joint is characterized by pain and limited motion in the hip after acute injury.

Treatment

Treatment includes rest and ice. For minor sprains, as comfort returns within 24 to 48 hours, weightbearing may be resumed, and range of motion and strengthening exercises begun. With more severe injuries, a more prolonged period of rest and restricted weightbearing is recommended.

Dislocations of the Hip Joint

Hip dislocations are most prevalent among young patients whose bones are strong and whose activities carry the risk of violent injury. Elderly patients with more fragile bones are more likely to suffer a fracture of the hip.

The hip can dislocate in three directions: posterior, anterior, and central. The posterior dislocation is the most common. An acetabular fracture often occurs with dislocation of the hip, and the exact nature of the injury depends on the magnitude and precise direction of the forces applied.

Posterior Dislocation

Posterior dislocations are produced by forces that act along the axis of the femur, driving the femoral head posteriorly into the posterior acetabular wall. The most common mechanism of posterior dislocation is a motor vehicle accident in which the knee of the victim riding in the front seat strikes the dashboard. With the hip flexed and adducted, the head of the femur is driven over the posterior rim of the acetabulum (Fig. 6.24) as it bursts

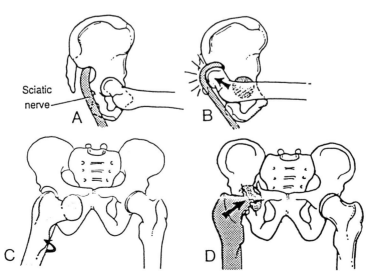

Figure 6.24. Dislocation of the hip. *A,* normal articulation. *B,* posterior dislocation with sciatic nerve on stretch. *C,* anterior dislocation. *D,* central dislocation.

through the posterior capsule and ligament. When the hip is flexed but in less adduction, a fracture through the posterior wall of the acetabulum may occur. Approximately 10% of posterior dislocations have associated fractures of the femoral head or neck. These fractures are at highest risk for developing osteonecrosis and posttraumatic degenerative arthritis.

Clinical Characteristics The patient presents with complaints of hip pain. The hip is usually adducted and internally rotated and shortened (Fig. 6.25). Evidence of sciatic dysfunction may be present with numbness, tingling, and muscular weakness or absence of muscular function in the sciatic distribution. X-ray will demonstrate the dislocation. A true lateral film of the hip is often necessary to confirm the direction of dislocation.

Anterior Dislocation

The anterior dislocation is rare (10% of all dislocations) and is produced by a violent force that externally rotates the extended hip. The head of the femur disrupts the anterior infe-

rior capsule and may come to rest over the pubis or may lodge in the obturator foramen (Fig. 6.24).

Clinical Characteristics Pain is felt in the hip and anterior and medial thigh. The hip is usually held in slight abduction, in relative extension, and in external rotation (Fig. 6.25). X-rays demonstrate the dislocation.

Central Dislocation

Central dislocations are produced by violent forces that drive the head of the femur through the medial wall of the acetabulum (Fig. 6.24). This injury can be produced by a variety of combined forces.

Clinical Characteristics The patient presents with severe pain in the hip, groin, and anterior and medial thigh. The hip may be externally rotated or shortened slightly. X-rays demonstrate the dislocation with medial wall fracture.

Complications of Dislocation

The immediate complication of posterior dislocation of the hip is injury to the sciatic nerve (Fig. 6.24), which may affect its peroneal or tibial branches. Sciatic nerve injuries occur in approximately 10% of posterior hip dislocations. Peroneal injury is more common and manifests as decreased sensation of the anterolateral leg and dorsum of the foot with weakness or inability to dorsiflex the ankle and toes. Posterior tibial nerve dysfunction manifests as decreased sensation on the posterior aspect of the lower leg, and plantar aspect of the foot and heel with weakness or inability to plantar flex the ankle or toes.

The other complication of dislocation of the femoral head is interruption of the blood supply to the head, leading to avascular necrosis. The risk of osteonecrosis increases with time delay of more than 6 to 12 hours between injury and time of reduction. This can be associated with actual tearing of the vessels, or there may be interruption secondary to stretch of these vessels. The effects of this vascular

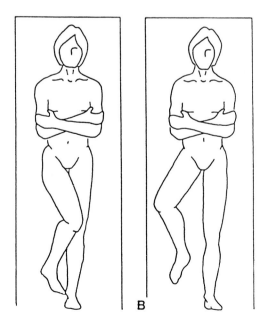

Figure 6.25. Postures of hip dislocation. *A,* posterior dislocation. *B,* anterior dislocation.

interruption may not be noted for months or years following the initial injury.

Given the potential for sciatic nerve injury and interruption of the blood supply, dislocations of the hip must be reduced as rapidly as possible. The sciatic nerve is put on stretch by the protruding femoral head, and removal of this deforming force is important to reduce the potential for increasing nerve injury. Also, stretching of the vessels supplying the femoral head may cause ischemia, and with reduction those blood vessels that are not actually disrupted can resume circulation and minimize the subsequent development of avascular necrosis. Finally, dislocation of the hip often causes injury to the articular cartilage, and it is not uncommon for these patients to develop some degree of posttraumatic arthritis.

Treatment

Dislocations of the hip are often associated with other injuries secondary to violent force. Consequently, comprehensive evaluation and support of the patient are necessary before treatment of the hip dislocation. It is especially important to check for ipsilateral knee injury. Reduction of the dislocated hip is an orthopaedic emergency, thus orthopaedic referral should be made immediately. In circumstances in which orthopaedic referral is not possible or may be delayed for several hours, the primary care physician should proceed with reduction of the hip. Such reduction should only be performed with good pain control and muscle relaxation. This can often be achieved in the emergency department in an otherwise stable patient, taking care that full resuscitative facilities are available.

For posterior dislocation, the hip can be reduced with the patient either supine or prone. The more common method is with the patient supine (Fig. 6.26). The hip is flexed. An assistant stabilizes the pelvis, and the operator applies traction to the leg from behind the flexed knee. The hip is often in adduction initially, and the operator should not attempt to correct this position initially. Traction should be applied along the line of the limb and maintained as the hip is brought gently

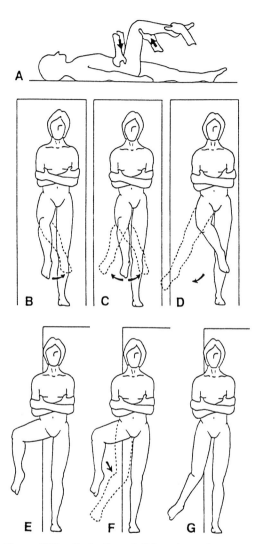

Figure 6.26. Reduction of dislocations. *A* through *D,* posterior dislocation. *A,* upward traction with hip flexed progressively to 90°. *B,* external rotation while continuing traction. *C,* alternate external and internal rotation while continuing traction. *D,* extension and abduction while maintaining traction and external rotation. *E* through *G,* anterior dislocation. (Note the position of the patient at the edge of the examining table.) Maneuver begins with strong traction to the hip through the flexed knee. *E,* hip abducted while maintaining flexion. *F* and *G,* reduction accomplished with continued traction and usually some internal rotation; adduction and extension complete the maneuver.

into flexion to a position of approximately 90°. With continued traction, the hip can be gently rotated using the lower leg as a lever. Reduction usually occurs with external rotation, but it may be necessary to alternate gentle internal and external rotation.

With reduction of the hip, there is usually a palpable and at times audible click. This is less apparent with posterior rim fractures. Also, certain dislocations are unstable, and redislocation will occur if traction is released and the hip allowed to internally rotate in flexion.

An x-ray is obtained after reduction and is inspected to confirm a congruous reduction of the hip to evaluate the presence of any acetabular or femoral head fractures or intraarticular fragments. Only after reduction is thin section CT scan imaging useful for delineating the bony detail of the injury. A CT scan of the hip should not be performed before reduction because it consumes precious time and provides only marginal additional information with the hip in the dislocated position.

If this supine method is not successful, the patient is placed prone with the hip flexed over the end of the table. In this position, gravity works with the operator to facilitate reduction. Access to the patient is limited, however, so the patient must be breathing in a normal spontaneous way and must be cooperative to do this safely. While considerable traction is necessary, excessively rough or ballistic-type movements should be avoided. If reduction is not possible, the patient must be prepared for general or spinal anesthesia and possible open reduction, which are preferable to traumatic manipulation. In this situation, orthopaedic referral becomes mandatory.

For anterior dislocation, the technique of reduction is strong, continuous traction along the line of the femur with the patient supine (Fig. 6.26). The hip is usually externally rotated and abducted, and traction should be applied to the femur in this position. Traction is continued with progressive flexion of the hip. Usually, internal rotation and then extension with adduction will complete the reduction. As with posterior dislocation, repetitive traumatic attempts at reduction should be avoided. If these measures are not successful, the patient must be prepared for general anesthesia and possible open reduction. In this situation, orthopaedic referral becomes mandatory, even if delay is necessary.

After reduction of the hip, an x-ray is obtained to confirm congruous reduction and to rule out fractures of the acetabulum or femoral head.

The central dislocation of the hip is actually a combination of fracture of the medial and superomedial acetabular dome and medial displacement of the femoral head. Prolonged longitudinal traction is usually necessary to effect reduction. This fracture dislocation may be unstable, and operative methods may be necessary. Definitive treatment of this injury requires orthopaedic referral.

Postreduction Care and Rehabilitation

If the hip is stable after reduction of a simple dislocation, patients are maintained in skin traction for 1 to 2 weeks. When patients are comfortable and have regained good leg control, they may get up with light partial weightbearing using crutches. Limited range of motion exercise can begin. In the case of posterior dislocation, patients are instructed to avoid flexion beyond 90° and combinations of flexion with internal rotation or adduction. Weightbearing may be slowly progressed using the rule of no pain/no limp. Full weightbearing is allowed when patients can ambulate without pain or limp and have regained good strength. This is usually possible by 6 weeks. Follow-up x-rays are obtained at this point. If the patient has been nonweightbearing, disuse osteopenia of the hip may be present. This is a good sign, indicating that the femoral head blood supply is intact. The femoral head of a patient with avascular necrosis may not show this disuse osteoporosis because the bone resorption that is the basis of disuse osteoporosis requires intact circulation.

FRACTURES OF THE HIP

Fractures of the hip are most prevalent among elderly women in whom osteoporosis is common. In this group of patients, the forces that produce these fractures are often surprisingly mild. A fall from which a younger person may get up with a sore hip and limp can cause a fracture in the elderly patient. Most commonly, fractures occur from a fall directly onto the hip. In some circumstances, a twist of the weightbearing extremity when a patient is trying to avert a fall may result in fracture. The architecture of the upper end of the femur is well suited to resist the forces of weightbearing. In the elderly osteoporotic patient, however, the upper end of the femur is not as well suited to resist twisting and shearing forces, and it is often these forces that result in hip fracture.

Hip fractures may be classified into two large groups: fractures of the femoral neck (subcapital or transcervical) and fractures of the intertrochanteric region (Fig. 6.27). The femoral neck fractures are usually intracapsular, and the intertrochanteric fractures are extracapsular. The importance of this distinction derives from the vascular anatomy of the head and neck of the femur (as summarized in the section "Blood Supply"). Intracapsular femoral neck fractures may disrupt the blood supply to the femoral head, resulting in avascular necrosis. Because the younger patient with a hip fracture has usually been subject to greater violence than the elderly patient, there is often more tissue injury, and as a consequence, there is a higher rate of avascular necrosis in the young patient. Most fractures of this type, whether intracapsular or extracapsular, are unstable and displaced. A minority of these injuries are firmly impacted and may withstand substantial weightbearing forces. These patients may be able to ambulate on the fracture with only mild or moderate pain.

Clinical Characteristics

The elderly patient has fallen or twisted a hip, whereas a younger patient has been subject to much more substantial injury. The patient complains of pain in the hip, groin, or thigh and is unable to bear weight or move the extremity. The uncommon exception is the patient with an impacted femoral neck fracture in which there is moderate stability and only mild pain. The injured extremity is usually shortened and externally rotated, although minimally displaced and impacted fractures may not show this deformity. Motion is painful and limited. X-rays of the hip and pelvis demonstrate the fracture. In minimally displaced, impacted fractures of the femoral head, the fracture line may be difficult to see.

Treatment

Most of these injuries are treated surgically with reduction and internal fixation using bone screws or screw/plate devices (Fig. 6.28). In displaced femoral neck fractures in elderly patients, prosthetic replacement of the femoral head is commonly performed. This is true when displacement is severe, osteoporosis is significant, and definitive treatment is delayed. All of these factors increase the chances of

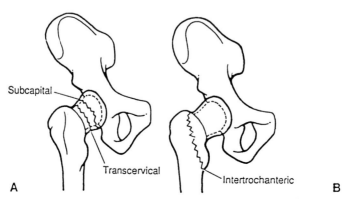

Figure 6.27. Fractures of the hip. *A*, intracapsular. *B*, extracapsular (intertrochanteric).

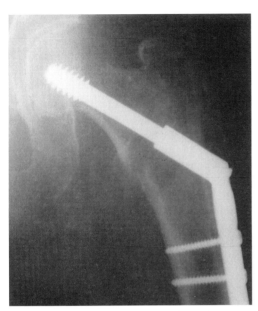

Figure 6.28. A/P x-ray of intertrochanteric fracture of the left hip fixed with a compression screw plate. This fracture has healed so that it is difficult to visualize the fracture line.

avascular necrosis and problems with healing, even with fixation.

In the elderly patient with a fractured hip, the primary practitioner must first identify the presence and nature of the fracture. Once this is done, orthopaedic referral should be made promptly. It is important to proceed with comprehensive evaluation of the patient's medical status, because these patients require surgical treatment. The primary care practitioner should coordinate the timing of surgery with the treating orthopaedist based on the patient's medical status. It is important to optimize the patient's condition before surgery, and this can usually be done within the first 24 to 48 hours.

FRACTURES AND DISLOCATIONS OF THE PELVIS

Because of the stability of the pelvic ring, fractures of the pelvis, unless they involve the osteoporotic bone of the elderly, are usually caused by violent forces. These injuries are commonly the result of a fall from a height or impact during a motor vehicle accident.

Fractures and dislocations of the pelvis can be associated with massive hemorrhage, and severe genitourinary and rectal injury. Therefore, evaluation of patients with pelvic fractures must include assessment of hemorrhage and hypotension and evaluation of the genitourinary and lower gastrointestinal systems. The pelvis is commonly thought of as a rigid ring. Therefore, for the shape of the pelvic ring to be distorted, it must be disrupted at two points. The example of a "pretzel ring" is helpful. One cannot imagine breaking a crisp pretzel ring in only one location by applying a compressive or shearing force; it will break in two locations. Of course, the pelvis is not a truly rigid ring. There are two rigid half-rings that are connected at the symphysis and sacroiliac joints, and these joints provide yield points during applied stress. These yield points allow isolated fractures of the pelvic ring to occur and to present with a nondisplaced or minimally displaced appearance. When a fracture occurs, the pelvis yields at the sacroiliac joints or symphysis, or there may be some deformation in the bony ring. If the deformation of the symphysis or sacroiliac joint is slight, it may not be readily apparent on x-ray. When there is displacement at one site in the bony pelvic ring, one must anticipate and search for the second site of ring disruption. For example, a widely displaced dislocation of the symphysis pubis anteriorly will be associated with a posterior iliac fracture, sacral fracture, or sacroiliac dislocation posteriorly (Fig. 6.29).

Pelvic injuries can be classified as "closed ring" or "open ring" fractures (Fig. 6.29). The closed ring injuries include the nondisplaced and minimally displaced single rami or two ipsilateral rami fractures and fracture near or subluxation of the symphysis pubis or sacroiliac joint without significant dislocation. These injuries are stable and usually can be treated symptomatically with rest and then progressive mobilization. Open ring injuries involve double breaks in the pelvic ring and are more commonly unstable to either vertical or lateral plane forces. These injuries require more aggressive treatment, including skeletal traction and internal or external fixation. Fractures of

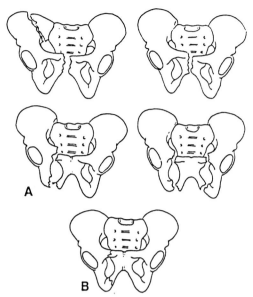

Figure 6.29. Fractures of the pelvis. *A,* four examples of open ring fractures. *B,* closed ring fracture.

the acetabulum must be considered as a separate category. These are evaluated based on the relative stability of the hip and disruption of the articular surface. They may occur with closed or open ring fractures of the pelvis.

Open ring fractures of the pelvis are more likely to be associated with injury to the genitourinary system or rectum. It is important to recognize this during the evaluation and initial treatment of patients with pelvic injuries.

Clinical Characteristics

The patient has been involved in a violent accident and, if conscious, will complain of pain that often girdles the hips or localizes unilaterally in the buttock or groin. Attempts to actively or passively move the lower extremities increase the pain. There may be obvious ecchymosis or swelling about the pelvis, groin, scrotum, or perineum.

Manipulation of the pelvis increases the pain. Downward pressure on the anterior superior iliac spine may be associated with posterior displacement or external rotation of the ilium if there has been disruption of the symphysis anteriorly or injury of the sacroiliac joint posteriorly. Downward pressure on the pubic symphysis may cause pain if there is injury at this location. Central compression over both trochanters or iliac crests may demonstrate medial-lateral instability of one or the other hemipelvis. Vertically directed force applied to the hemipelvis through the femur may demonstrate vertical displacement of the hemipelvis. These maneuvers help to demonstrate the location of the fracture and degree of stability.

Hematuria or urinary retention may be present. There may be blood in the urethral meatus, rectum, or vagina indicating injury in these locations. X-rays of the pelvis reveal the fracture.

Treatment

The role of the primary care practitioner is in the initial assessment and stabilization of the patient with a pelvic injury. Once the patient is stabilized, physical examination, including genitourinary and rectal examination, should be accomplished. With suspected genitourinary injury, urethrogram and cystogram are considered first, then intravenous pyelogram. Prompt orthopaedic referral is indicated.

Nondisplaced and minimally displaced closed ring fractures are usually stable and can be treated symptomatically with bed rest and progressive mobilization as symptoms allow. Usually, bed-to-chair activity and partial weightbearing are possible within 1 to 2 weeks. After the initial consultation, these patients can be followed by the primary practitioner. The treatment of open ring fracture of the pelvis must be deferred to the orthopaedic surgeon. Skeletal traction or internal or external fixation may be used based on the degree of instability and other characteristics of the fracture.

SUGGESTED READINGS

Allen WC, Cope R. Coxa saltans: the snapping hip revisited. J Am Acad Orthop Surg, 1995;3:303–308.

DeLee JC. Fractures and Dislocations of the Hip. In: Rockwood CA Jr, Greene DP, eds. Fractures in Adults. Philadelphia: JB Lippincott Co, 1984:1211–1356.

Fernbach SK. Avulsion injuries of the pelvis and proximal femur. Am J Roentgenol 1981;137:581–584.

Hely DP, Salvati EA, Pellicci PM. The Hip. In: Cruess RL, Rennie WR, eds. Adult Orthopaedics. New York: Churchill Livingstone, 1984:1209–1274.

Kane WJ. Fractures of the Pelvis. In: Rockwood CA Jr, Greene DP, eds. Fractures in Adults. Philadelphia: JB Lippincott Co, 1984:1093–1210.

Kasser JR. Orthopedic Knowledge Update 5. American Academy of Orthopaedic Surgeons, 1996.

Koval K, Zuckerman JD. Hip fractures I. Overview and evaluation and treatment of femoral neck fractures. J Am Acad of Orthop Surg 1994;2(3):141–149.

Koval K, Zuckerman JD. Hip fractures II. Overview and evaluation and treatment of femoral neck fractures. J Am Acad of Orthop Surg 1994;2(3):150–156.

Tometta P, Mostafavi HR. Hip dislocations: current treatment regimen. J Am Acad Orthop Surg 1997;5(1):27–36.

Knee

Dudley A. Ferrari, M.D.

Essential Anatomy

The knee is a weightbearing, modified-hinge joint. Its motion is controlled and stabilized by muscles and ligaments, as well as the shape of the opposing bone surfaces and their associated meniscal cartilages. The knee is a highly efficient structure that can provide support for the body and meet the changing demands of multiple locomotor tasks. Because it is subject to high forces exerted along lengthy lever arms (tibia and femur), the knee is vulnerable to injury during the course of normal daily activities and during sports.

Knee motion is a complex function. Flexion and extension of the knee require rotation and some degree of abduction and adduction. The rotation effect can be demonstrated by placing the fingers over the tibial tubercle and noting that the tibia internally rotates as the leg goes into flexion and externally rotates as it goes into extension. This rotation depends on the relative size of the medial and lateral femoral condyles, the shape of the tibial condyles, and the effects of the controlling ligaments (Fig. 7.1). As the femoral condyles move through their rotational arc, they both roll and slide on the tibial condyles (Fig. 7.2). If the femoral condyles did not slide, the femur would simply roll off the tibia posteriorly at the extremes of flexion. In fact, the rolling motion is combined with a sliding motion, and it is this combination that allows for the full arc of stable flexion of the knee. Rolling and sliding varies between the medial and lateral sides of the knee. The lateral condyle rolls more and the medial condyle slides more, producing external rotation as the knee goes into full extension. The rolling and sliding mechanism is passively con-trolled by the anterior cruciate ligament as the knee flexes and by the posterior cruciate ligament as the knee extends.

X-RAY ANATOMY

Figure 7.3 shows radiographs of the knee with important elements labeled.

Skeletal and Articular Structure of the Knee

Femur (Fig. 7.4)

The shaft of the femur extends from the trochanters to the condyles and is triangular in cross section with its apex. The apex posterior with its ridges is called the linea aspera. The shaft is slightly bowed with anterior convexity and inclines from the trochanters to the condyles in slight adduction. Posteriorly, the linea aspera provides insertion for the adductors and extensors of the thigh, whereas the anterior surface of the midshaft and the trochanteric area provide origin for the extensors of the knee. As the shaft approaches the condyles, it broadens laterally and medially, and the ridges of the linea aspera merge with the supracondylar ridges. These ridges outline a triangle, called the popliteal surface, to which no muscles are attached.

The femoral condyles are the rounded ends of the femurs that articulate with the tibia. Anteriorly, the condyles merge to form the patella articular surface. The medial condyle is larger in surface area than the lateral condyle, which diverges from the medial. Although the lateral condyle is smaller in total area, it is longer in length than the medial (Fig. 7.4). The condyles of the tibia are the widened platforms that articulate with the condyles of the femur (Fig. 7.5). The medial side is concave and the lateral side convex from front-to-back. The medial and lateral tibial condyles are separated by the intercondylar eminence, whose medial and lateral spines articulate with the femur. The cruciate ligaments maintain contact between the spines and the femur. The actual center of rotation may vary but in static systems is considered to be near the medial spine.

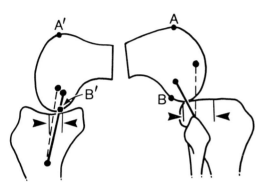

Figure 7.1. Unequal motion of the condyles is caused by the following: (1) The unequal length of the condyles. A to B is greater than A′ to B′ on the medial condyle. (2) The shape of the condyles. The medial tibial condyle is concave and the lateral is convex, allowing more posterior rolling. (3) The direction of the collateral ligament. The medial collateral is stretched faster and the lateral is more posterior, allowing the condyle to move farther back. (Adapted from Kapandji IA. The Physiology of the Joints. Edinburgh and London: E and S Livingstone, 1970:195,196.)

Anatomy of the lower extremities is such that the hips are wider apart than the ankles. Consequently, a physiologic valgus alignment is produced at the knee in order for the joint to remain parallel to the ground, biomechanically the most efficient orientation (Fig. 7.6).

Ossification Centers About the Knee

Three ossification centers are about the knee. The femoral condylar epiphysis is evident at birth and completes ossification by age 20. Ossification of the distal aspect of the femoral condyles can sometimes proceed in an irregular pattern, which must not be confused with osteochondritis (see "Nontraumatic Conditions of Childhood"). The tibial condylar epiphysis is usually evident at birth and completes ossification by age 20. This epiphysis includes the tibial tubercle as well as the tibial condyles. The patella ossifies from a single center that becomes radiologically evident by age 6. Ossification is completed during puberty.

Synovium of the Tibiofemoral Articulation

Figure 7.7 illustrates the three-dimensional form of the synovial space and the lines of attachment of the synovium to the articular borders of the femur and tibia. The menisci are included within the synovial space but the cruciate ligaments are excluded.

Within the synovium there can be shelves

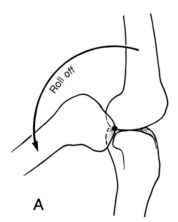

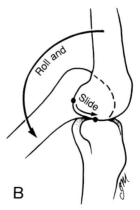

Figure 7.2. *A,* position of femur if only rolling occurred. *B,* normal rolling and sliding motion of the femoral condyles. Initial rolling is followed by sliding to maintain position on the tibial condyle.

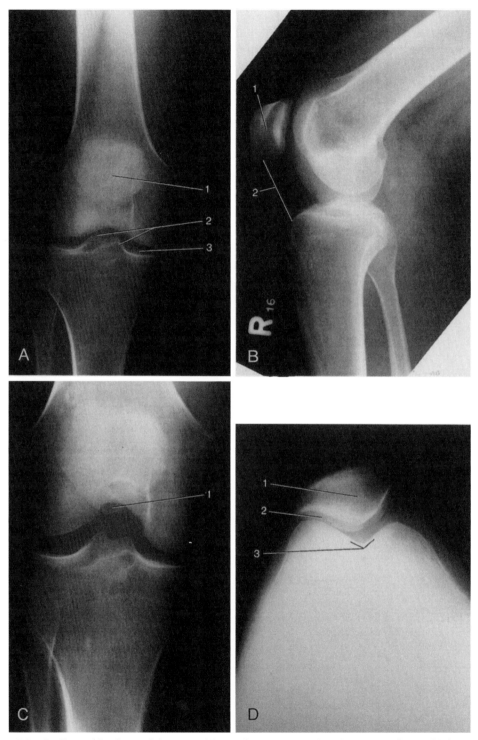

Figure 7.3.   Radiographic views of the normal knee. *A*, anteroposterior view; *1*, patella; *2*, tibial spines; *3*, medial joint space. *B*, lateral view; *1*, patella; *2*, patellar ligament. *C*, tunnel view; *1*, intercondylar notch. *D*, tangential view; *1*, patella; *2*, lateral patellar facet; *3*, trochlear groove.

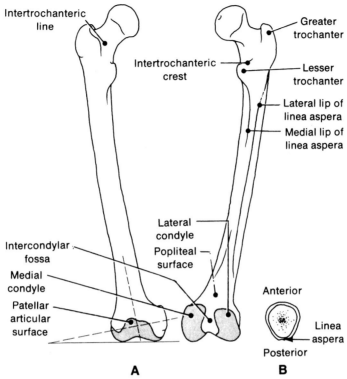

Intertrochanteric line

Greater trochanter

Intertrochanteric crest

Lesser trochanter

Lateral lip of linea aspera

Medial lip of linea aspera

Intercondylar fossa

Medial condyle

Patellar articular surface

Lateral condyle

Popliteal surface

Anterior

Linea aspera

Posterior

A

B

Figure 7.4. The femur. *A*, anterior and posterior views. *B*, cross section, midfemur.

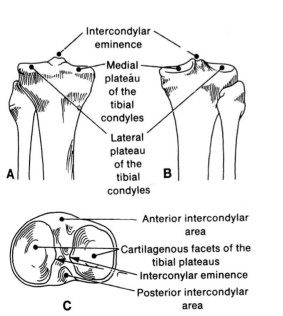

Intercondylar eminence

Medial plateâu of the tibial condyles

Lateral plateau of the tibial condyles

A

B

Anterior intercondylar area

Cartilagenous facets of the tibial plateaus

Interconylar eminence

Posterior intercondylar area

C

Figure 7.5. The proximal condyles of the tibia. *A*, anterior view. *B*, posterior view. *C*, superior view.

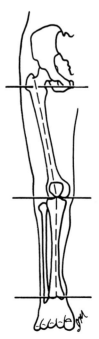

Figure 7.6. To keep the knee, pelvis, and ankle parallel to the ground, an angle is created by the wider pelvis and the knee.

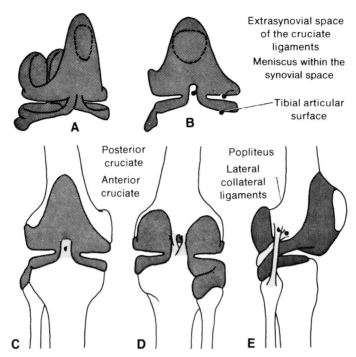

Figure 7.7. Synovial space of the knee. Diagrammatic cast of the synovial space. *A,* three-quarter anterior view. *B,* full-face anterior view. *C* through *E,* the cast of synovial space applied to the femur, patella, tibia, and fibula to indicate the margins of attachment of the synovial membrane to those bones.

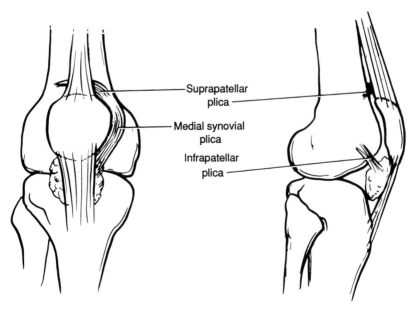

Figure 7.8. Suprapatellar plica divides the suprapatellar pouch and knee. Infrapatellar plica extends from the infrapatellar fat pad to the intercondylar notch. Medial plica extends from the fat pad to the suprapatellar plica.

or bands called plicae, which are the remnants of membranes that separated the compartments of the knee during embryonic development. There are three types of plicae, which vary in size (Fig. 7.8). The suprapatellar plica divides the suprapatellar pouch from the rest of the knee. The infrapatellar plica separates the medial and lateral compartments anterior to the cruciate ligaments. The medial plica originates from the medial synovium near the suprapatellar plica and extends to the infrapatellar fat pad. Also, the medial plica is the one band that often becomes symptomatic by being caught between the patella and medial femoral condyle or against the medial condyle alone, producing medial patellar pain. This will be discussed further in the section "Injury of the Patellofemoral Articulation."

Menisci

The two menisci are semilunar fibrocartilaginous wedges that rim and cushion each tibiofemoral articulation. The radius and circumference of the medial meniscus are larger than those of the lateral meniscus. Ends of the lateral meniscus attach to the intercondylar eminence, and ends of the medial meniscus attach to the intercondylar areas. Outer rims attach to the synovial membrane of the articular capsule (Fig. 7.9). The menisci sit on the tibial surfaces and assist in weight distribution through the knee. The medial meniscus shares half the load with the exposed weightbearing area of the tibial condyle. The lateral meniscus shares more of the weightbearing load than the exposed area of the lateral tibial condyle.

This weight distribution varies with activities (Fig. 7.10). The weightbearing area of the tibial condyle is posterior in flexion. The menisci become wedges that act as stabilizers in addition to accepting weight. In flexion the menisci are pushed back, and in extension they are pushed forward. In addition to these passive motions, the ligaments also affect the movement of the menisci. For example, the medial collateral ligament pulls the medial meniscus posteriorly during flexion and internal rotation of the tibia, and anteriorly during extension and external rotation of the tibia.

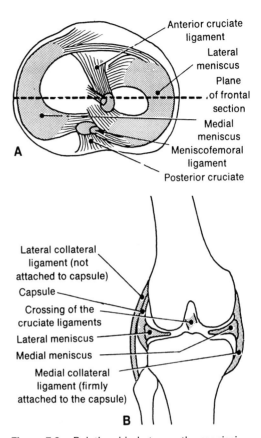

Figure 7.9. Relationship between the menisci, the capsule, and the ligaments of the knee. *A*, superior view of the menisci and cruciate ligaments. *B*, posterior view of a frontal section of the knee through the middle third.

On the lateral side, the popliteus muscle pulls the lateral meniscus posteriorly during flexion or during external rotation of the femur. The movement of the menisci is synchronous and obligatory. Consequently, abnormal stresses to the knee often produce meniscal tear. Because the lateral meniscus is less firmly attached to the capsule and more free to move about, it is injured less frequently than the medial meniscus.

Ligaments (Fig. 7.11)

The ligaments of the knee guide and check the movements of the articular surfaces. The lateral and medial patellar retinacula are continuations of the fascia lata and quadriceps tendon on their respective sides of the patella.

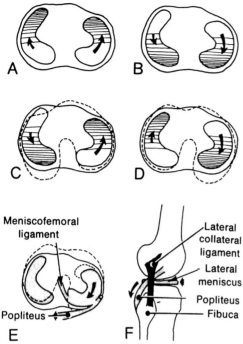

Figure 7.10. *A* through *D*, shifts in tibial weightbearing points and passive accommodations of the menisci during flexion-extension and rotation. *Shading* indicates weight distribution. *Arrows* indicate accommodative passive movements of the menisci. *Longer arrows* over the lateral meniscus symbolize its greater mobility. *A*, full extension. *B*, near full flexion. *C*, medial rotation of the femur. *D*, lateral rotation of the femur. *E* and *F*, active accommodations of the menisci during knee movement. During external rotation of the femur, the movement of the meniscofemoral ligament and the contraction of the popliteus muscle pull the lateral meniscus posteriorly and medially.

These retinacula merge with and reinforce the anterolateral and anteromedial aspects of the knee capsule. The retinacula limit the motions of the patella.

The medial collateral ligament extends in two layers from the medial femoral condyle to the medial tibial condyle. The superficial layer is a broad, triangular ligament with its apex extending posteriorly over the posterior aspect of the medial femoral condyle and joint line. The deep layer is a stout structure that blends intimately with the capsule and has an attachment to the medial meniscus. Located on the medial posterior corner is the posterior portion of the tibial collateral ligament or posterior oblique ligament.

The lateral collateral ligament is a cordlike structure with its main attachments extending from the lateral femoral condyle to the fibula; it does not blend with the capsule. Also part of the lateral stabilizing complex is the popliteus tendon, which runs beneath and attaches to the femur in front of the lateral collateral ligament. The arcuate ligament and short external collateral ligament are also on the lateral corner.

The anterior cruciate ligament extends from the anterior intercondylar area of the tibia to the medial aspect of the intercondylar area of the lateral femoral condyle. The posterior cruciate ligament extends from the posterior intercondylar area of the tibia anteromedially to the intercondylar surface of the medial femoral condyle.

Function

Because of the orientation of its fibers and the shape of the condyles, some portion of the medial collateral ligament is tight from extension through flexion. The posterior fibers are taut in extension and the anterior fibers are taut in flexion. The medial collateral ligament is the primary stabilizer to valgus stress at the knee. Acting as secondary stabilizers are the posteromedial capsule and anterior cruciate ligament. Consequently, a valgus force to the knee may first cause injury to the medial collateral ligament, but as this force continues, the anterior cruciate, posterior capsule, and posterior cruciate may be disrupted (Fig. 7.12).

The lateral collateral ligament is taut in extension and relaxed in flexion. The iliotibial tract assists in the range of 5 to 40° of flexion. The lateral collateral ligament is the primary stabilizer to varus stress. Secondary restraint is provided by the posterolateral complex, consisting of the popliteus tendon, short external collateral ligament, and arcuate ligament. A varus force will likely injure the lateral collateral ligament first, the posterolateral complex next, and if large enough, the posterior and anterior cruciate ligaments.

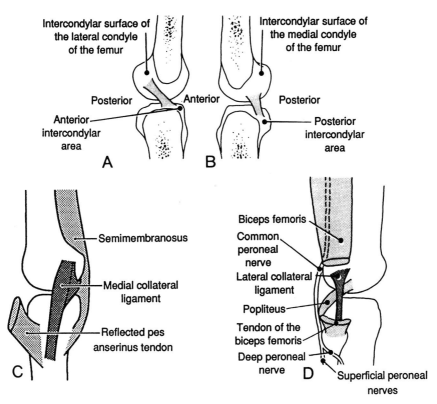

Figure 7.11. Cruciate and collateral ligaments. *A*, medial view of the anterior cruciate ligament. *B*, lateral view of the posterior cruciate ligament. *C*, medial view of the medial collateral ligament. *D*, lateral view of the lateral collateral ligament.

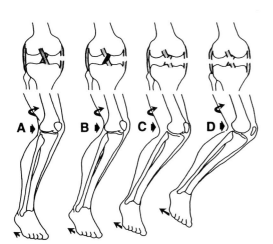

Figure 7.12. Order of vulnerability of ligaments of the knee to a valgus force. *A*, medial collateral ligament. *B*, medial collateral ligament and anterior cruciate. *C*, medial collateral ligament, anterior cruciate, and posterior cruciate. *D*, medial collateral ligament, anterior cruciate, posterior cruciate, and lateral collateral ligament.

The anterior cruciate ligament consists of two bands, the anteromedial and posterolateral. The anteromedial band tightens in flexion; this tightening, along with a twisting of the entire anterior cruciate ligament about the posterior cruciate ligament, controls anterior displacement of the tibia and compresses the joint surfaces. The posterolateral band of the anterior cruciate tightens in extension, maintaining contact. The anterior cruciate restricts anterior translation and resists internal rotation as well as hyperextension. As a secondary stabilizer to varus and valgus forces, the anterior cruciate may be injured as noted previously.

The posterior cruciate also demonstrates two bands: the anterolateral and posteromedial. The posteromedial band is tight in extension and, as the knee flexes, the entire ligament becomes tight. It is the main restraint to posterior displacement of the tibia. A force applied to the front of the tibia is resisted mainly by the posterior cruciate with little restraint from the posterior capsule. The posterior cruciate ligament can be injured in hyperflexion.

MUSCLES CONTROLLING THE KNEE

Extensors

The major extensor of the knee is the quadriceps muscle, which forms the anterior bulk of the thigh. The quadriceps muscle is made up of four parts: the rectus femoris, vastus lateralis, vastus medialis, and vastus intermedius. Illustrated in Figure 7.13 are the origins and insertions.

The vastus medialis lies deep to the rectus femoris proximally and emerges distally to create the medial curve of the distal thigh. The vastus medialis has a special orientation at its distal end. The direction of its fibers applies a medial- and proximal-directed force to the patella during the last 15° of extension. This is important in maintaining patella stability and alignment. Both the vastus lateralis and medialis are in continuity with the knee capsule and can produce knee extension, even in the presence of patella fracture as long as there is not complete disruption of the anteromedial and anterolateral capsule (Fig. 7.14A).

All the extensors are innervated by branches of the femoral nerve, which is derived from the second through fourth lumbar roots.

Flexors

The main flexors of the knee are the gracilis, semitendinosus, semimembranosus, and biceps femoris muscles. Origins and insertions are illustrated in Figure 7.14. The gracilis and semitendinosus along with the sartorius insert into the medial aspect of the shaft of the tibia and anterior to the tibial collateral ligament, just inferior to the attachment of the patellar ligament to the tibial tubercle. This sweep of tendons over the tibial collateral ligament is known as the pes anserinus, or goose's foot.

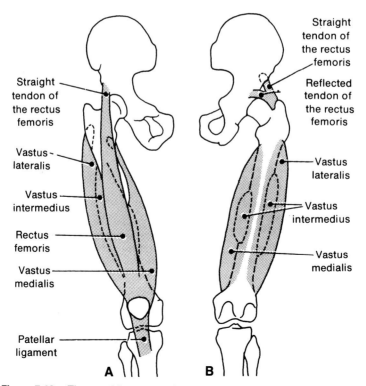

Figure 7.13.   The quadriceps muscle. *A,* anterior view. *B,* posterior view.

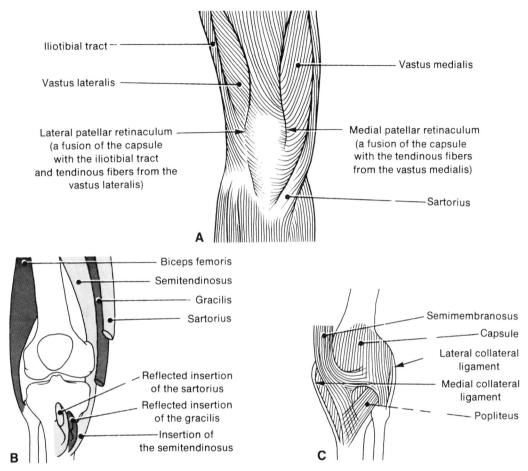

Figure 7.14. Tendinous expansions merging with capsule of the knee joint. *A*, anterior view showing the patellar retinacula. *B*, anterior view showing the tibial insertion of the sartorius, semitendinosus, and gracilis medially, and the fibular insertion of the biceps femoris laterally. *C*, posterior view showing the relationship of the semimembranosus to the capsule medially and posteriorly. The medial head of the gastrocnemius overlies posterior to the semimembranosus tendon (not illustrated).

A bursa is related to the pes anserinus, which is a common site of bursitis, particularly in patients with osteoarthritis of the knee.

The knee flexors have other actions in addition to flexing the knee. With the knee flexed, the flexors can serve as rotators of the leg in which the gracilis, semitendinosus, and semimembranosus internally rotate the leg and the biceps femoris externally rotates the leg. The internal rotators are slightly stronger than the external rotators of the leg.

The popliteus muscle arises on the posterior surface of the tibia. The tendon passes beneath the arcuate ligament and attaches to a depression on the anterior part of the groove

of the lateral condyle of the femur. This muscle unlocks the knee, initiating flexion and rotation.

The sartorius, along with all the anterior muscles of the thigh, is innervated by branches of the femoral nerve. The gracilis, with all the adductors of the hip, is innervated by branches of the obturator nerve, with contribution from the third and fourth lumbar nerve roots. The other three flexors of the knee are innervated by branches of the sciatic nerve.

Fascia Lata

All the muscles of the thigh are enclosed within the fascia, a tough, unyielding covering. The fascia merges medially and laterally with the intermuscular septa. In combination with the fascia, the septa divide the thigh into anterior and posterior compartments. Because this fascial covering will not yield, extravasation of enough blood or edema into either of the two compartments of the thigh may produce a compartment syndrome.

INNERVATION AND BLOOD SUPPLY (FIG. 7.15)

The knee joint receives fibers from both the femoral and sciatic distributions. Because the femoral nerve also innervates the hip, patients with hip disorders may present with knee pain.

The femoral artery gives rise to the deep and superficial femoral arteries in the femoral triangle. The deep artery carries the major blood supply to the muscles of the thigh, and the superficial artery carries the major blood supply to the leg and foot. The deep artery penetrates deep to the adductors and eventually comes to lie between these muscles and the posterior surface of the femur. In this location, the artery and its accompanying veins are vulnerable to injury by the fragments of a fractured femoral shaft. In the distal third of the thigh, the artery passes posteriorly around the femur to lie directly on the popliteal surface of the femur, anterior to the sciatic nerve. In this area, the artery is vulnerable to injury with dislocation of the knee or juxta-articular fractures.

EVALUATION OF THE PATIENT WITH KNEE SYMPTOMS

EXAMINING FOR EFFUSION

Ambulatory patients should first be examined with both knees flexed 90°. Inspect the area on either side of the patellar ligament.

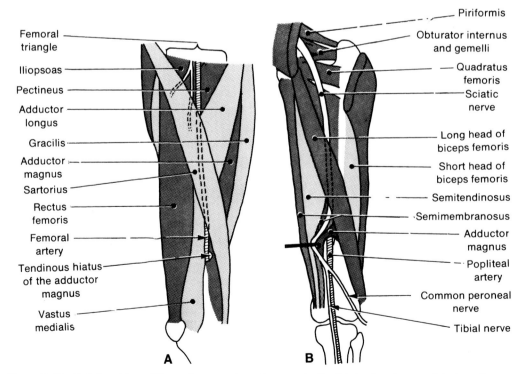

Figure 7.15. Relationships of the major vessels and nerves in the thigh. *A*, anteromedial view. *B*, posterior view.

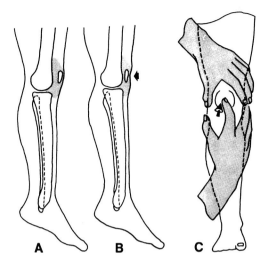

Figure 7.16. Examination for knee joint effusion. *A*, patella forced away from the femur by the effusion. *B*, patella forced downward onto the femur by ballottement maneuver. *C*, illustration of the ballottement maneuver.

Moderate effusions cause a bulging in these areas that is not present in the normal knee.

With the knee fully extended and the extensor apparatus relaxed, compress the knee above and on either side of the patella and attempt to subject the patella to ballottement with a finger. Sufficient effusion forces the patella away from the femur and allows ballottement (Fig. 7.16).

If neither of these observations suggests an effusion, attempt to flex the knee fully, unless a suspected injury to the extensor apparatus contraindicates this. An effusion can interfere with full flexion of the knee.

EXAMINATION OF THE EXTENSOR APPARATUS

Palpate the quadriceps tendon, the body of the patella, and the patellar ligament to look for defects and tenderness. Obtain x-rays if there is evidence of a defect over the quadriceps tendon or the patellar ligament, or if the body of the patella is tender or palpably fractured. A rupture of the extensor apparatus should be presumed if the x-ray reveals a fracture of the body of the patella or avulsion from the superior border or the inferior pole, or if the examination by palpation demonstrates an apparent defect in the quadriceps tendon or patellar ligament. Further examination should be discontinued and orthopaedic referral made.

When no evidence exists of rupture of the extensor apparatus, displace the patella laterally and medially to test for a retinacular tear or strain. Subluxation or dislocation of the patella should be suspected if this type of patella manipulation is associated with apprehension. Displace the patella proximally while forcing it posteriorly into its femoral articulation to test for pain and crepitus associated with chondromalacia patellae.

EXAMINATION OF THE COLLATERAL LIGAMENTS

Test the integrity of the medial and lateral ligaments by applying valgus and varus stress, attempting to open the joint line of the knee with the knee flexed to 30° (Fig. 7.17). If the knee opens in comparison to the opposite knee given the same stress and position, and there is local tenderness and a history of injury, a disruption of the ligament or ligament complex is present. Any opening indicates a complete or third-degree sprain. An opening of 1 to 5 mm is a grade I injury; an opening of 5 to 10 mm is a grade II injury; and an opening

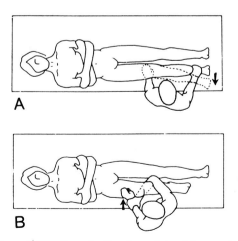

Figure 7.17. Examination for collateral ligament injuries. *A*, applying valgus stress. *B*, applying varus stress.

greater than 10 mm is a grade III injury. With higher grade injuries, the likelihood of injury to the secondary stabilizing ligaments increases. In addition to testing the ligaments with the knee flexed, stress testing should also be done with varus-valgus force with the knee extended. Instability in extension indicates more global ligamentous disruption.

EXAMINATION OF THE CRUCIATE LIGAMENTS

Anterior Cruciate

Perform the **anterior drawer test**. With the knee flexed to 90° and the hip flexed to 45°, the examiner sits on the patient's foot to keep it stabilized and uses both hands to grasp the tibia from behind. Keeping the hamstring relaxed, the pull is straight forward. If the foot is placed in external rotation, this maneuver tests the anterior cruciate ligament and also the secondary stabilizers in the posterior medial corner (Fig. 7.18). The movement of the injured knee is compared with the uninjured knee, as it is for all ligament stability testing.

Perform the **Lachman test** (Fig. 7.19). Place the patient supine and flex the knee to 20°. Stabilize the distal femur with one hand and the proximal tibia with the other. The tibia is moved forward on the femur and the degree of displacement noted. Compare the degree of displacement with the unaffected side.

Perform the **pivot-shift test** (Fig. 7.20). This is pathognomonic of a tear of the anterior cruciate ligament. The test can be performed in many ways, each producing anterior sublux-

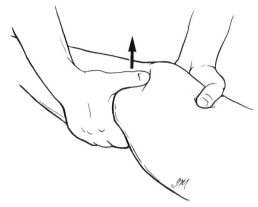

Figure 7.19. Lachman test. The knee is flexed 20°. The proximal tibia is grasped and moved forward while the femur is held with the other hand. (Adapted from Torg JS, Conrad W, Kalen V. Clinical diagnosis of anterior cruciate ligament instability in the athlete. Am J Sports Med 1976;4:84–93.)

ation of the lateral tibial condyle and subsequent relocation, which produces the "pivot shift." One good method is for the examiner to place the patient's ankle beneath the examiner's arm with the patient's hip in abduction. The hands support the proximal tibia, exerting a valgus internal rotation and anterior translation force. With this combination of forces applied in relative extension, subluxation of the tibia occurs. As the knee is further flexed from this position, the tibia falls backward to anatomic position, producing a shifting sensation. This sensation reproduces the feeling of "giving way" that the patient experiences functionally. The pivot-shift test may be difficult to perform in both the acute and chronic stages. In the acute stage, the patient may be unable to extend the leg because of swelling and pain. In the chronic stage, the patient has learned to prevent subluxation by activating the quadriceps muscle because the shifting is uncomfortable.

Posterior Cruciate

Prepare to perform the **posterior drawer test** (Fig. 7.21). The patient's leg is positioned in a fashion similar to the anterior drawer test, with the knee flexed to 90° and the foot on the examining table. In this position, the in-

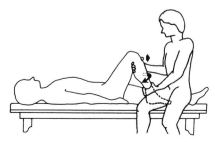

Figure 7.18. Examination for laxity of the anterior cruciate ligament.

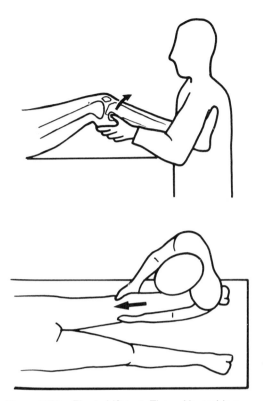

Figure 7.20. Pivot-shift test. The ankle and leg are held under the axilla. The leg is abducted and the knee extended. The hands are under the proximal tibia applying gentle anterior and internal rotation force. The tibia will subluxate forward and, as pressure is applied in line with the leg, the tibia will flex and reduce.

jured leg should be examined and compared with the opposite leg. A posterior "sag" of the injured tibia relative to the femur may occur. This is an important observation and is pathognomonic of posterior instability. Recognizing this also avoids misinterpreting "pseudo" anterior laxity of the knee in which the tibia begins from a posteriorly displaced position and, consequently, there is increased laxity on anterior drawer. In fact, this represents a posteriorly subluxed tibia.

After making the observation for posterior sag, a posterior force is placed against the proximal tibia. The degree of laxity is compared with the opposite side. A positive posterior drawer test or a sag that occurs with the knee flexed indicates posterior cruciate ligament injury. Laxity may be difficult to detect and quantify. In an isolated injury, an effusion may not occur and the pain may be manifest posteriorly. Ecchymosis present posteriorly should suggest posterior cruciate injury. The presence of varus or valgus laxity in full extension is also suggestive of posterior cruciate ligament injury.

EXAMINATION FOR MENISCUS INJURY

Palpate the joint lines. Shortly after an acute tear or displacement of a chronic tear,

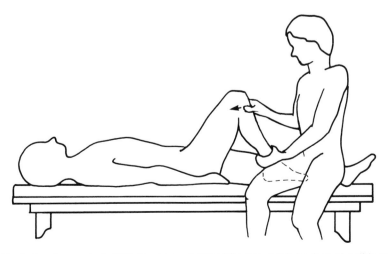

Figure 7.21. Posterior drawer test. With the knee at 90° of flexion, push back on the tibia to see whether there is increased motion or sag compared with the opposite leg.

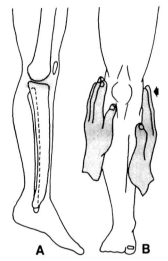

Figure 7.22. Examination for meniscus injury. *A*, area of tenderness. *B*, palpation for tenderness.

the associated joint line will be tender. Palpate the joint lines while rotating the leg back and forth. A torn meniscus may cause a palpable click during this maneuver (Fig. 7.22).

Perform **McMurray's maneuver** (Fig. 7.23). Flex the knee fully, with the leg externally rotated when testing for medial meniscus tear, and internally rotated when testing

for lateral meniscus tear. While maintaining rotation, extend the knee with a firm controlled movement. A painful click in early or midextension is suggestive of a meniscus tear.

Perform **Apley's test** (Fig. 7.24). With the patient lying prone, flex the knee to 90°. While applying upward traction on the leg, rotate the leg internally and externally. Pain during this maneuver is more compatible with ligament injury than with meniscus tear. Repeat the rotation while bearing downward on the leg. Pain during this maneuver is more compatible with meniscus injury.

NONTRAUMATIC CONDITIONS IN ADULTHOOD

AVASCULAR NECROSIS

As in the hip, avascular necrosis can occur in the knee. It most commonly involves the medial compartment, with the femoral condyle more frequently involved than the tibial condyle. In some patients, an associated systemic factor will be noted, such as previous history of alcoholism, steroid therapy, or bone marrow disease. In most patients, avascular necrosis of the knee is idiopathic.

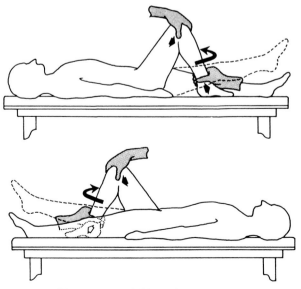

Figure 7.23. McMurray's maneuver.

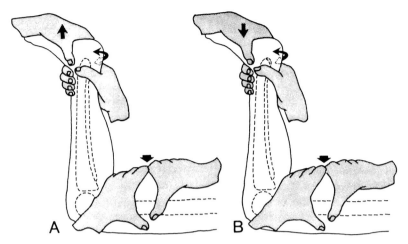

Figure 7.24. Apley's test. *A*, pain is compatible with ligament injury. *B*, pain is compatible with meniscus injury.

Clinical Characteristics

The patient usually presents with an acute onset of pain in the knee, most often on the medial side. Patients are usually over 50 years of age, and women are more commonly affected. A minority of patients have a more subacute onset of pain. The pain initially may be severe, but subsequently is more moderate. Patients often complain of stiffness and swelling, and an effusion is commonly noted.

X-rays taken early in the disease often are negative and the lesion can only be found by bone scan or magnetic resonance imaging. Later in the disease, x-rays become abnormal, usually showing a lucent region of the subchondral bone with surrounding sclerosis. Secondary degenerative changes may occur.

Treatment

The initial treatment of avascular necrosis should be conservative with restricted weight-bearing, anti-inflammatory medication, and analgesics. Many patients will improve with conservative management. For those who continue to have significant symptoms, orthopaedic referral is indicated for possible surgical intervention. Successful treatment usually requires osteotomy or knee replacement.

BURSITIS

Thirteen bursae have been described about the knee (Fig. 7.25). Of these, five are of particular importance to the primary clinician. They are the prepatellar bursa that lies between the patella and the skin; the superficial infrapatellar bursa that lies between the lower end of the patellar ligament and the skin; the deep infrapatellar bursa that lies between the lower end of the patellar ligament and the tibia; the anserine bursa that lies between the medial collateral ligament and the pes anserinus tendon; and the semimembranosus bursa that lies between the semimembranosus tendon and the medial head of the gastrocnemius. This bursa can communicate with the synovial cavity of the knee joint.

Prepatellar and Superficial Infrapatellar Bursitis

The prepatellar and superficial infrapatellar bursae are to the knee what the olecranon bursa is to the elbow. As such, they are exposed and vulnerable to trauma. The chronic form of prepatellar bursitis is classically referred to as "housemaid's knee." Thickening of the bursa is seen in patients whose occupations require kneeling, for example, carpet layers. The thickened bursa may not be symptomatic, but on occasion is sensitive. The bursal thick-

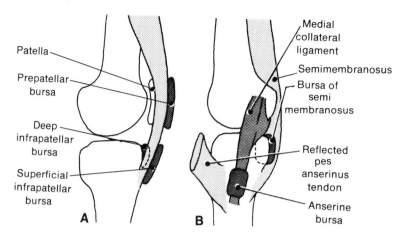

Figure 7.25. Bursae about the knee. *A*, lateral view. *B*, medial view.

enings may be small, firm, and mobile, giving the feeling of nodules or bone chips. Bursal swelling usually is localized to the prepatellar area and not to the surrounding tissue. Often bursal swelling is initiated by trauma, sometimes trivial. When trauma causes a laceration or abrasion over the bursa, differentiating between traumatic or septic bursitis is difficult.

Clinical Characteristics

The patient usually presents with localized pain and swelling in the bursa and tenderness may be present. No effusion of the knee itself is present. Patients with chronic bursitis may have mild swelling but little tenderness, and rarely experience extreme pain. An infected bursa presents with more severe pain, tenderness, and surrounding cellulitis.

Treatment

Chronic forms of bursitis are treated with anti-inflammatory medication. The patient should use padding to avoid repeated trauma. Chronic, recurrent, or persistent bursitis may require excision of the bursa. Acute bursitis is treated with rest, ice, and anti-inflammatory medication. If fluid is present, it can be aspirated. A purulent aspirate indicates a septic bursitis. Both acute and chronic bursitis may respond to cortisone injection, but infection must first be ruled out. Septic bursitis should

be treated by incision, drainage, and antibiotics.

Anserine Bursitis

Individuals who are unaccustomed to lengthy, vigorous, weightbearing exercises may occasionally experience acute inflammation of the anserine bursa.

Clinical Characteristics

Patients usually complain of knee pain, which begins after some traumatic episode or unaccustomed weightbearing exercise. They experience an intense aching pain at rest that becomes worse when resisting extension or flexion. Swelling may be evident, and tenderness is elicited over the pes anserinus tendon or just superficial to its tibial attachment.

Pain and tenderness over the anserine bursa must be distinguished from several other conditions, including medial joint line tenderness associated with meniscal derangement or degenerative arthritis of the medial compartment. In the latter conditions, tenderness is localized to the joint line, whereas anserine bursitis causes tenderness below the joint line in the region of the bursa. Avascular necrosis of the tibial plateau or stress fracture of the tibia may be more difficult to distinguish because pain may be in the area of the anserine bursa. X-ray and bone scan are helpful in distinguishing these conditions. Stress fracture usually occurs in association with a history of recent increase in activity. Finally, patients with fibrositis syndrome may have pain in the anserine bursa area.

Treatment

Instruct the patient to minimize weight-bearing activities and avoid resisted extension (i.e., no climbing, jumping, running, squatting). The patient should apply ice packs over the inflamed bursa four times daily. Quadriceps-setting exercises can begin as soon as pain subsides. When pain and tenderness are fully remitted, range of motion and full quadriceps exercise can begin. Injecting a depository corticosteroid into the inflamed bursa can result in a dramatic remission. Oral anti-inflammatory agents may be prescribed, but these are less effective than local corticosteroid injection (see chapters 12 and 14).

Baker's Cyst

"Baker's cyst" is a term that is commonly applied to the formation of a swollen bursa posterior to the knee joint. This is most often caused by fluid distention of the bursa between the semimembranosus and medial gastrocnemius, but other posterior bursae can be associated with a Baker's cyst. Because these bursae can communicate with the synovial cavity of the knee joint, they often form because of inflammation and effusion in the knee secondary to intra-articular disorders. Because of this, the physician must rule out medial meniscal tear, degenerative joint disease, and rheumatoid or other arthritides.

Clinical Characteristics

Patients complain of a mass behind the knee that may or may not be slightly tender. If there is an underlying meniscal tear or arthritis, additional symptoms will be present. A fluctuant mass is palpable on the medial side of the popliteal fossa when the patient lies prone with the knee extended. Clear serous fluid is readily aspirated from the cyst, causing the cyst to collapse. X-rays may show evidence of degenerative arthritis.

Treatment

Aspiration not only confirms diagnosis, it removes the mass and usually relieves the patient's symptoms. Patients are often fearful that these masses are malignant tumors. To search for the cause of a chronic knee joint effusion, the examiner must obtain more detail about knee symptoms. Take note of range of motion, test patellar and tibiofemoral stability, examine for meniscus tear, and obtain x-rays for evidence of degenerative arthritis. The physician should perform a review of systems and a general orthopaedic examination, and obtain an erythrocyte sedimentation rate if any points of the history suggest an inflammatory arthritic disorder.

When the underlying disorder is obvious and its treatment is within the limits of primary practice, proceed appropriately. When no underlying disorder can be found or conservative treatment is ineffective, orthopaedic referral should be made.

TENDONITIS

Tendonitis is tendon degeneration without inflammation or with peritendinous inflammation, usually at the area of insertion or at the musculotendinous junction. This condition is probably related to microscopic tears that lead to pain. Repeated tearing results in tendon degeneration and scarring, and the scarred tendon is weaker and subject to rupture. Tendonitis is a common overuse syndrome in athletes.

Patellar Tendonitis

Patellar tendonitis, or "jumper's knee," is a common problem for athletes involved in sports that require jumping. Pain occurs during activity but often not enough to curtail the activity. Pain is also present after activity, usually after sitting for a long period. Tenderness is noted at the inferior pole of the patella.

Quadriceps Tendonitis

Quadriceps tendonitis involves the superior pole of the patella at the tendon junction. This type of tendonitis is common for athletes involved in sports that require running, jumping, and acceleration-deceleration activities. Pain and tenderness are noted over the superior pole of the patella.

Iliotibial Tract Tendonitis

The iliotibial tract is a condensation of some of the fibers of the fascia lata. It attaches to Gerdy's tubercle and overlies the lateral epicondyle and fibular collateral ligament. Pain develops from friction between the underlying structures and the iliotibial tract. This is most commonly seen in runners and in patients with an abnormally tight iliotibial tract. The examination reveals tenderness in the lateral epicondylar area that is amplified by pressure over the area as the knee goes through a range of motion.

Popliteus Tendonitis

The popliteus tendon attaches to the lateral aspect of the lateral femoral condyle and runs beneath the fibular collateral ligament. Tendonitis often develops with excessive downhill running, but also can occur with excessive squatting activities. Tenderness in this area must be differentiated from lateral joint line tenderness associated with lateral meniscus injury.

Treatment

Treatment of tendonitis is nonoperative and should begin with a period of rest. Ice after activity is helpful because it reduces inflammation, and anti-inflammatory medication is also helpful. After pain is relieved by the above methods, the patient should begin to gently stretch the scar tissue, then follow a graduated strengthening program. Cortisone injection into tendon sheaths to reduce inflammation is acceptable, but cortisone injection into the tendon causes tendon weakness and subsequent rupture.

Traumatic Disorders of the Knee

INJURIES TO THE EXTENSOR APPARATUS (FIG. 7.26)

The quadriceps muscle and tendon, patella, patellar ligament, and patellar retinacula constitute the extensor apparatus. Direct and indirect forces can disrupt the extensor apparatus at the knee.

Direct Impact Forces

These forces are typically generated in injuries that occur when an individual falls onto the knee or the knee is otherwise struck.

Direct blows to the quadriceps muscle result in varying degrees of injury. Some hemorrhage always occurs within the muscle. Tenderness and ecchymosis develop and associated knee effusion may occur. Tenderness is localized to the area of impact. Contusions of the quadriceps tendon at its insertion on the patella or at the site where it merges with the patellar retinacula are fairly uncommon because the area is not as exposed to

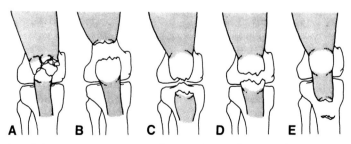

Figure 7.26. Injuries of the extensor apparatus. *A*, comminuted fracture of the patella. *B*, avulsion of the quadriceps tendon. *C*, avulsion of the patellar attachment of the patellar ligament. *D*, transverse fracture of the patella. *E*, avulsion of the tibial attachment of the patellar ligament.

impact. These injuries present with an indistinctly circumscribed swelling above the patella, which may be associated with fluctuation if bleeding into the suprapatellar bursa has occurred. Pain may inhibit active extension.

Direct blows to the patella can contuse the patellar cartilage or fracture the patella. Such fractures are usually comminuted and may or may not be displaced. The prepatellar bursa is always contused when these injuries occur, causing a hemorrhage into the bursa. Therefore, impact injuries to the patella present with circumscribed swelling over the patella and variable pain on lateral compression and manipulation of the patella. Pain may inhibit active extension.

Direct blows to the insertion of the patellar ligament contuse the superficial infrapatellar bursa and the patellar ligament at its attachment to the tibial tubercle. These injuries present with an indistinctly circumscribed swelling and tenderness over and just above the tibial tubercle. Pain may inhibit active extension.

Indirect Distracting Forces

When extension is applied with abrupt violence, as can occur when kicking or jumping, the resultant force may strain or rupture the extensor apparatus. Strain is suggested when tenderness is present over the quadriceps tendon or patellar ligament and the anatomy is palpably intact. Rupture is indicated by one of the following clinical pictures.

The quadriceps tendon may be avulsed from its patellar insertion and from its merger with the patellar retinacula. Such an injury is rare and presents with a depression just above the patella, a fluctuant mass about the depression reflecting hemorrhage into the suprapatellar bursa, and an inability to actively extend the knee without a significant extensor lag.

More commonly, the patella may be fractured. The inferior pole may be avulsed with the patellar ligament, or the patella may fracture into two fairly equal pieces. The injury presents with a fluctuant swelling, a palpable disruption of the patella, and an inability to actively extend the knee fully.

The patellar ligament may be avulsed from the inferior pole of the patella. This injury presents with a distinctly circumscribed swelling about the patellar ligament, an elevated patella, a palpable tendon defect when the knee is flexed to 90°, fluctuation above the tibial tubercle when hemorrhage has occurred into the deep infrapatellar bursa, and an inability to actively extend the knee fully.

Any complete disruption of the extensor mechanism, whether patella, ligament, or tendon, prevents full active extension of the knee. However, the patient may be able to lift the leg or have limited extension to −30° even with the rupture.

As soon as injury to the extensor apparatus is suspected, x-ray of the knee should be obtained to rule out fracture. This will prevent the examiner's converting an undisplaced fracture to a displaced fracture that may require operative treatment. A tangential view of the patella may show a vertical fracture line, often missed by standard AP and lateral views. However, a tangential view should not be requested if the injury is suspected to have occurred from distraction forces. This view requires that the knee be markedly flexed, which may complete the displacement partially produced by distraction forces.

Treatment

A simple contusion or strain may be treated symptomatically with rest, immobilization, and ice packs until active extension and range of motion are nearly painless. Quadriceps exercises (Fig. 7.27) and weightbearing exercises to the point of tolerable pain can then begin and progress as pain recedes. When the prepatellar bursa is swollen and fluctuant, the bursa should be aspirated.

An undisplaced fracture of the patella with injury to the patellar cartilage should be immobilized in a cylinder cast for 4 to 6 weeks. Weightbearing as tolerated is allowed while the extremity is immobilized. When the immobilization is removed, only partial weightbearing is allowed. The patient should be instructed in active quadriceps exercises, and active range of motion exercises are begun.

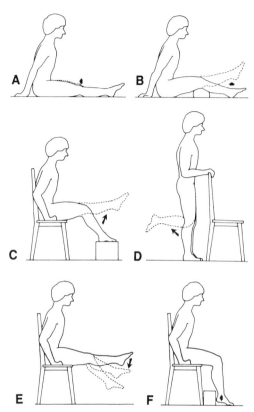

Figure 7.27. Restorative knee exercises. *A,* isometric quadriceps exercise. *B* and *C,* isotonic quadriceps exercises. *D,* gravity-resisted isotonic flexion exercise. *E,* gravity-assisted isotonic flexion exercise. *F,* isometric flexion exercise.

Progressive weightbearing is allowed as range of motion and quadriceps strength are restored. Full weightbearing is permitted when the patient can walk without pain or a limp.

When the extensor apparatus has been ruptured, either through the quadriceps tendon, through the patella, or by an avulsion of a patellar ligament from the inferior pole of the patella, the knee should be splinted in extension, and the patient should be referred to an orthopaedist for definitive treatment. Operative repair usually is required.

MENISCAL INJURY

Meniscal injury occurs when rotation of the femur on the tibia exceeds the normal physiologic range, when the normal synchronous internal rotation with flexion or external rotation with extension does not occur, or when excessive axial compressive loads exceed the meniscus strength. For example, consider the fall that occurs with the foot fixed in external rotation. As the individual falls, the knee flexes. Physiologically, this requires internal rotation, but the tibia is held in external rotation. The femoral condyle pushes the meniscus backward. The meniscus is held forward, however, by the medial collateral ligament. The meniscus is subjected to excessive stress and may be torn.

The medial meniscus is injured more frequently than the lateral meniscus because of its anatomy. The medial meniscus is trapped within the concavity of the medial tibial plateau and has more ligamentous tethers. The lateral meniscus is more mobile and can slide posteriorly more easily, thus avoiding the weightbearing of the condyle. The pattern of injury is also different for the medial and lateral menisci, with the medial more likely to sustain longitudinal tears and the lateral more likely to sustain radial tears (Fig. 7.28).

After the age of 40 years, a different type of injury occurs to the meniscus. A horizontal splitting occurs as a result of a lifetime of bending, squatting, turning, and twisting. The horizontal lesion is seen in a large percentage of people over the age of 55 years and is not necessarily symptomatic. This injury is more common in the medial meniscus and usually occurs at the junction of the mid and posterior one-third.

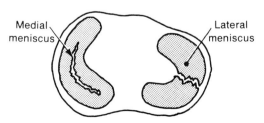

Figure 7.28. Characteristic orientation of meniscus tears.

Clinical Characteristics

Patients complain of pain at the time of injury that usually persists and interferes with weightbearing activity. Symptoms may subside initially, but recurrent episodes with minor stress are common. The pain is usually medial and often posteromedial in the case of the medial meniscus tear. Lateral meniscal pain is usually along the lateral joint line, but may be referred anteriorly or medially.

Effusion may develop, which may be minimal and noted as a feeling of tightness in the knee. If the joint communicates with one of several posterior bursae, swelling may be present in the back of the knee (see "Baker's Cyst"). Cystic swelling at the joint line with meniscal tear is more likely to develop on the lateral side because of the opening of the popliteus recess. Cystic swelling on the medial joint line is rare.

The patient often describes pain or inability to extend the knee fully, which is sometimes termed "locking." It is not true locking in the sense of not being able to move the knee at all, but is the lack of full extension. Because of the interposition of meniscus or the interference of the torn meniscus with normal rotation, there is no external rotation in extension. Therefore, the leg does not come into full extension and is considered "locked."

Many patients report a feeling of "giving way," describing a sense that the knee is going to collapse. Although this "giving way" feeling may occur as a result of a torn meniscus with interposition of meniscal tissue preventing normal rotation, it is a nonspecific symptom. This symptom can also result from pain or from various instabilities of the knee if the femorotibial or patellofemoral surfaces are moving abnormally.

In longstanding meniscal derangement, quadriceps atrophy is common because the pain and swelling inhibit motion of the quadriceps muscle.

Treatment

The knee should be immobilized if there is pain with motion. Painless knee motion does not require immobilization. Crutches should be used if there is swelling and weightbearing is painful. Quadriceps exercises may be initiated, and anti-inflammatory medication or analgesics should be provided. A tense effusion should be aspirated. If the knee is locked, manipulation may be attempted with adequate analgesia; rotation in flexion with a valgus stress may unlock the knee. However, it is not always necessary to attempt a manipulation. Spontaneous "unlocking" often occurs with immobilization and the use of analgesics.

Although most meniscal tears do not heal, a peripheral tear often does. The knee with a peripheral tear may be immobilized for 4 weeks by medial and lateral splints with the knee flexed at 15 to 20°, or a limited motion brace set to allow motion between 20 and 60°. If the knee remains locked or symptoms of pain, giving way, and swelling persist, orthopaedic referral should be made to consider surgical removal or repair. This can be accomplished arthroscopically. Meniscal injuries with symptoms that can be successfully eliminated by modifying activity and avoiding activities that produce effusion, catching, or giving way do not require surgery. Patients must accept limited activity because return to full activity may reactivate symptoms. If return to activity after symptoms have abated does not cause recurrence of symptoms, then patients may proceed with the activity.

LIGAMENT INJURY

The ligaments are subject to external forces as well as those generated by muscular force. Contact forces occur in sporting events, in vehicular accidents, and at work. The history of the injury and the exact mechanism involved are helpful in the evaluation.

Clinical Characteristics

The degree of injury depends on the amount of force and the circumstances of support by muscles. A first-degree sprain is a tear of the fibers of the ligament with no demonstrable instability or laxity. A second-degree sprain is a tear of ligamentous fibers with some loss of function but still no noticeable laxity.

A third-degree sprain is a gross disruption of the fibers with demonstrable laxity. Within this third-degree injury, there are grades I, II, and III laxity. In grade I third-degree sprain, there is a less than 5 mm opening of the joint surface with applied stress. In grade II, there is a less than 10 mm opening. In grade III, there is a greater than 10 mm opening.

All patients complain of pain at the time of injury. With first-degree, second-degree, and grade I third-degree injuries, patients are able to walk or even resume activities. The morning after injury, moderate stiffness is present. The physical examination will detect tenderness in the area of the ligament. Either the attachment site or the area along the line of the ligament is tender. Stressing the ligament will cause pain in all these injuries and slight laxity in the grade I third-degree injuries.

Patients with grade II third-degree injuries manifest more difficulties and are not likely to continue with their activities. They may have an effusion, which suggests that some of the capsule as well as some of the ligament has been stretched. Patients will have more laxity on ligament testing.

Grade III third-degree injuries have gross and easily detectable laxity, usually with accompanying effusion. The development of ecchymosis in the area of the ligaments suggests a moderate tear with gross laxity. In this case, one should suspect that more than one ligament is involved. Patients may have a knee dislocation if they have grossly unstable ligaments with multidirectional laxity and a history of violent injury. A large percentage of knee dislocations are accompanied by popliteal artery injuries; therefore, vascular consultation and angiography are recommended. X-rays will show no evidence of injury, but occasionally will show a small avulsion fragment from the site of ligament attachment.

Medial Collateral Ligament Injury

The medial collateral ligament usually is injured by a valgus force applied to the lateral aspect of the knee with the foot fixed. This ligament may also be injured by a twisting mechanism. Tenderness is present along the line of the ligament or at points of attachment, and grade I, II, or III laxity is present in the third-degree injuries. In the evaluation of a patient with medial or lateral collateral ligament injury, it is important to assess the presence of injury of the anterior or posterior cruciate ligaments. If cruciate ligament injury is suspected, orthopaedic referral should be obtained. It is also important to recognize that patients with medial (or lateral) instability in extension probably do not have an isolated ligament injury and these patients should also be referred for further evaluation and treatment.

Treatment

Isolated grade I and II injuries, without instability in extension, and without cruciate ligament injury, can be treated nonoperatively. The injured knee should be immobilized with commercially available immobilizers or medial-lateral plaster splints. This lessens pain and reduces strain on the ligament. Immobilization may continue for 7 to 14 days, depending on the degree of injury and pain. As pain subsides, the knee should be mobilized because mobilized ligaments heal with greater strength than continuously immobilized ligaments.

The patient should be placed on crutches with weightbearing as tolerated. Crutches are discontinued when there is no limp with ambulation. Aspiration may be required if a tense effusion is present. Ice should be used to reduce swelling and analgesics prescribed as necessary. When pain subsides and motion is full, whirlpool and bicycling are encouraged. Straight leg raising in the immobilizer is encouraged, followed by the use of weights when motion returns. The symptoms of a grade I injury may decrease rapidly and be at a point of strengthening in 2 weeks. A more severe injury will take at least 6 weeks before strength returns and the knee gains functional stability.

Grade III injuries can be treated nonoperatively; however, because it is often difficult to detect associated injury, an orthopaedic consultation is recommended to assess the need for surgical intervention for these injuries.

Lateral Collateral Ligament Injury

The lateral collateral ligament is injured by a varus force from the medial side of the knee. Because the peroneal nerve travels around the fibular head, any force applied to the inner aspect of the knee may cause stretch of the peroneal nerve. Therefore, with suspected lateral collateral ligament injuries, the function of the peroneal nerve should be assessed at the time of initial examination.

Treatment

Isolated grade I and II third-degree injuries can be treated nonoperatively. As in the case of the medial collateral ligament, however, a grade III injury is best handled by the orthopaedic surgeon. Treatment of grade I and II injuries is the same as for medial collateral ligament injury, with initial immobilization, crutches, and analgesics, followed by motion and weightbearing to a point of strengthening.

Anterior Cruciate Ligament Injury

The anterior cruciate ligament may be injured by either varus or valgus force that stretches the medial or lateral ligaments. An anterior cruciate ligament tear can result from a noncontact injury. The history will include a twisting injury accompanied by a pop or a tearing feeling and a subsequent effusion. With this history and the finding of a hemarthrosis, there is approximately a 70% chance of injury to the anterior cruciate ligament.

The anterior cruciate is the major restraint to anterior translation of the tibia on the femur. The quadriceps muscle antagonizes this restraint as the leg goes into extension. Strain is in the ligament in the last 20° of extension. A violent pull of the quadriceps, as in turning quickly or jumping, may rupture the anterior cruciate ligament. The ligament tightens in internal rotation; therefore, when the leg is forced into internal rotation strain is on the anterior cruciate. Strain is also in extreme valgus and external rotation, as occurs in skiing, and the anterior cruciate may be injured along with the medial collateral ligament. Hyperextension, as might occur when stepping in a hole, forces the anterior cruciate against the intercondylar notch, which may result in a tear.

Clinical Characteristics

The patient with an incompetent anterior cruciate ligament falls into one of three categories. The first group is made up of individuals who function satisfactorily without the ligament. This group, which includes some competitive athletes, is small, however, comprising less than 20% of the individuals.

Most individuals fall into a second category that requires modification of activities. High-risk activities that involve jumping are not usually possible. Volleyball and basketball are given up, but racquetball and tennis may be played. If the activities of tennis are difficult, the person may further limit activity to a level of bicycling, swimming, and jogging. Routine activities of daily living are done with little difficulty. The patient may have a giving way episode once or twice a year. With increased activity, there is a high likelihood of injuring a meniscus, and at some point a giving way episode may be followed by meniscal symptoms that require meniscal surgery. Some patients will be able to move up in the activity category by using a stabilizing brace.

In the last category are those individuals who cannot function well without the ligament. These patients are bothered by multiple giving way episodes in the course of daily activities and are significantly limited in sports. A brace may be tried, but does not provide adequate stability and is difficult to use for daily living activity.

After the initial injury, most people fall into one of these categories within 1 to 2 years.

Anterior Cruciate Ligament Examination (see also "Evaluation of the Patient with Knee Symptoms")

With a moderate degree of spasm and effusion, the detection of anterior cruciate ligament laxity can be difficult. The Lachman test is more sensitive than the anterior drawer test because the anterior drawer may be negated by the pull of the hamstrings or spasm about the knee. The pivot-shift test is difficult to elicit in the acutely injured, and even in follow-up examination if the patient learns to protect the knee and use the muscles to prevent subluxation of the tibia. X-rays usually do not provide evidence of injury; however, the finding of avulsion from the lateral tibial plateau (Segond fracture) is pathognomonic of an anterior cruciate ligament tear.

Treatment

Because of the difficulty in detecting anterior cruciate ligament injuries, in separating symptoms of instability from meniscal symptoms, and in determining need for reconstruction, the treatment of these injuries should be supervised by an orthopaedist. The treatment of acute anterior cruciate injury depends on the severity of injury. Patients with suspected injury or partial tear, i.e., hemarthrosis and consistent history but without significant demonstrable instability, may have a tense hemarthrosis requiring aspiration. The knee may be immobilized for comfort. Crutches should be used for nonweightbearing, or partial weightbearing if tolerated without pain. Follow-up examination should be at 5 to 7 days, and if laxity secondary to anterior cruciate ligament injury is not detected quadriceps exercises may be initiated and the knee and leg rehabilitated. For patients with demonstrable instability but without associated meniscal, collateral ligament, or posterior cruciate ligament injury, the knee should be immobilized for comfort and crutches provided for the patient. Because the torn anterior cruciate ligament is not likely to heal, quadriceps setting may be initiated. Patients with associated ligament injury or meniscal injury should be referred immediately to an orthopaedist because surgical intervention may be necessary.

To rehabilitate the leg with anterior cruciate injury, quadriceps exercises are initiated first. More vigorous exercises, with progressive strengthening of the quadriceps and hamstring muscles, are initiated when swelling subsides and range of motion returns. Recovery from an initial episode may take 6 to 8 weeks. If recovery is not sufficient in this time to allow the patient to ambulate, or if swelling is not reduced, the patient should be examined for meniscal injury. Meniscal symptoms may develop in the first 6 months after injury; meniscus injury will require treatment.

If a patient successfully rehabilitates with strength equal to or better than the uninjured leg, a brace may be applied. The patient is allowed to return to sports, and will then find the appropriate level of activity and make necessary modifications according to lifestyle.

The patient who continues to have difficulties in the activities of daily living and is not engaged in any sport activity, and the patient who has difficulties in the brace with absence of any meniscal disorder, become candidates for reconstruction of the ligament. Those persons who are professional or competitive athletes may not want to wait for 1 year to find the category into which they will fall, and should be considered for immediate reconstruction.

Posterior Cruciate Ligament Injury

The posterior cruciate ligament is often injured by a force that is applied to the anterior portion of the tibia, as in a dashboard injury. The ligament may also be injured from medial or lateral forces that injure other ligaments.

Treatment

The posterior cruciate is considered a prime stabilizer of the knee; early operation on gross instability of the posterior cruciate ligament, particularly if accompanied by medial or lateral collateral ligament injuries, yields better results than nonoperative management. Avulsion of the ligament with a bony fragment is best treated by open reduction and fixation. Isolated grade I and II third-degree injury is compatible with normal life activities and can usually be treated nonoperatively. Because of the significant instability, the knee should be evaluated by an orthopaedic surgeon.

It is important to rehabilitate all knee injuries, particularly those that will not require surgery, which may be meniscal or minor ligament injuries. Often, persistent symptoms are related to weakness as a result of the initial injury rather than to any significant intra-articular or extra-articular disorder. Patients will continue to have symptoms of aching and soreness in the knee. Extreme weakness may even result in swelling. The symptoms from weakness may increase the indications for surgery even though it may not be necessary. Improvement in muscle strength is an indication of a healing condition, whereas persistent weakness may indicate an operative condition.

Therapy may be accomplished either by the individual or under the care of a physical therapist. Motivation is a factor in successful rehabilitation and should be monitored either by the therapist or the physician.

FRACTURES

Fractures of the Shaft of the Femur

Fractures of the shaft of the femur are life-threatening injuries. They are typically accompanied by considerable bleeding into the thigh and hypovolemia. The violent forces required to produce them may impact directly on the surface of the thigh, or may apply torque or angulation to the thigh. Like hip dislocations, femur fractures occur most commonly in motor vehicle accidents. These fractures are nearly always complete and markedly displaced, with over-riding, angulation, and rotation of the distal segment on the proximal. Fractures may be transverse, oblique, spiral, or comminuted, and may be simple or compound.

Clinical Characteristics

Patients with fractures of the shaft of the femur often have other injuries. They may develop evidence of circulatory insufficiency shortly after injury. These patients do not move the extremity and, if conscious, complain of intense thigh pain that usually refers throughout the extremity. The thigh is swollen, and the portion of the extremity below the fracture site may be rotated and angulated. Tenderness, false motion, and crepitation are evident at the fracture site. Anteroposterior and lateral x-rays of the thigh will identify the fracture.

Treatment

The patient must be quickly assessed for other injuries. Hypovolemic circulatory failure must be treated (see Chapter 1). The fracture must be splinted, preferably with a "Thomas"-type splint (see Chapter 11). Traction improves alignment and stability. An orthopaedist should be responsible for definitive treatment of the fracture.

Fractures of the Tibial Condyles (Fig. 7.29)

The same forces that tear the collateral ligaments can fracture the contralateral tibial plateau, as well as tear the ipsilateral meniscus. The lateral tibial plateau is fractured more commonly than the medial. Until they tear, the stressed ligaments act as a tension band directing compressive forces onto the opposite tibial plateau. If the bone is less resilient than the ligaments, it will fracture before the ligaments tear. Osteoporotic individuals are more likely to suffer plateau fractures than torn ligaments, and commonly, they are women who fall from steps or ladders.

Clinical Characteristics

All patients with fractures of the tibial condyle complain of pain immediately at the time of injury. Pain persists and prevents weight-bearing. Within the first few hours after injury, the joint capsule becomes tense with a hemarthrosis. The fractured condyle is tender and any manipulation that compresses that side of the joint causes an increase in pain. Ligaments on the opposite side of the joint may or may not be tender. X-ray will reveal the plateau fracture. A neurovascular examination should be performed because fractures of the tibial plateau may be associated with neurovascular injury. The peroneal nerve is particularly vulnerable. This injury is often associated with a fracture of the proximal fibula accompanying a tibial plateau fracture.

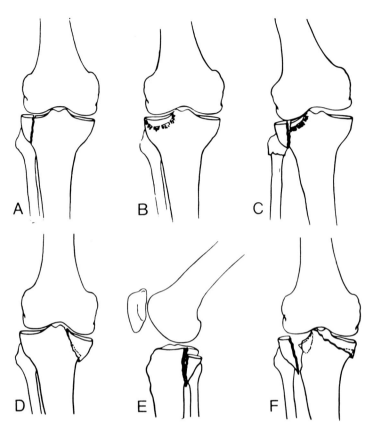

Figure 7.29. Hohl classification of fractures of the condylar end of the tibia. *A*, undisplaced. *B*, local compression. *C*, split compression. *D*, total condylar compression. *E*, split. *F*, comminuted. (Reprinted with permission from Hohl, M. Tibial condylar fractures. J Bone Joint Surg [Am] 1967;49A:1455–1467.)

Treatment

Initial treatment should include arthrocentesis if there is a tense hemarthrosis. Fractures should be splinted in full extension. If the patient is not comfortable in full extension, however, this position should not be forced. Orthopaedic referral is recommended for definitive evaluation and treatment of these intra-articular fractures.

If this is unavailable, minimally displaced fractures can be managed by the experienced primary practitioner. Nonoperative treatment can be considered if there is no significant depression of the joint surface, less than 3 mm of separation or depression at the fracture line, and no associated collateral or cruciate ligament rupture. A variety of treatment methods are appropriate for these minimally displaced fractures. In reliable patients, a long-leg splint can be applied in full extension. The patient is placed on crutches and continues nonweightbearing until healing is evident. Isometric exercise can be carried out in the splint, then at 10 to 14 days, the splint can be discontinued for active range of motion exercise. For less reliable patients, a long-leg or cylinder cast is applied for 3 weeks, then range of motion is begun. Another method is to apply a cast brace primarily. This protects the fracture from compressive force but allows range of motion to the knee. (See Chapter 11 for details of cast technique.) In these injuries, healing usually occurs in 8 to 12 weeks. Weightbearing should be delayed until that time.

If the fracture line is displaced or depressed more than 3 mm, orthopaedic referral should be obtained for definitive evaluation and treatment. These fractures often require open reduction. The goal of treatment is to restore an anatomical joint surface, repair ligament injuries, and progress with early range of motion. Successful accomplishment of these goals reduces the risk of posttraumatic arthritis.

The intimate anatomic relationship between the condylar ends of the femur and tibia and the sciatic nerve and popliteal vessels exposes these neurovascular structures to injury when there is juxta-articular fracture of the knee. In addition, these fractures superficially resemble any of the other causes of a hemarthrosis. Thus, the primary practitioner must consider this injury whenever evaluating a traumatic hemarthrosis because an unwary manipulation could result in displacement of an undisplaced fracture or neurovascular injury.

Fractures of the Condylar End of the Femur (Fig. 7.30)

These fractures usually result from an axial compression force with or without an angulatory force. The fractures in adults are of four kinds. Figures 7.30A and 7.30B show fractures of the medial or lateral femoral condyle. The axial compression force, when accompanied by an angulatory force, usually fractures the condyle on the side of the angulation. Figures 7.30C and 7.30D show T-shaped or Y-shaped intracondylar fractures of the femur. Straight axial compression forces may fracture both condyles at once, driving them proximally to each side of the femur. Figure 7.30E shows a comminuted fracture.

Clinical Characteristics

Except in the severely osteoporotic patient, the injuring forces are violent. Patients with these fractures complain of pain immediately at the moment of injury and are unable to bear weight. All patients with these injuries present with a tense hemarthrosis; some present with shortening or an angular deformity. The condylar end of the femur is severely tender. Firm palpation will often elicit bony crepitation. Evidence of neurovascular injury may be present. Anteroposterior and lateral x-rays of the knee will identify the fracture.

Treatment

The reduction must be precise. Any disturbance of the normal orientation of the condyles to one another will disrupt the joint mechanism, thus decreasing range of motion and increasing wear on the articular surfaces. Vascular injury requires immediate repair to avoid ischemic necrosis below the knee. An orthopaedist and perhaps a vascular surgeon must assume responsibility for treatment. The primary practitioner should facilitate the treatment goals as follows. Assume every hemarthrosis is a fracture of the condylar end of the femur (or tibia) until proven otherwise. Examine sciatic nerve and vascular function whenever the distal end of the femur is tender or crepitant. If a neurovascular injury is evi-

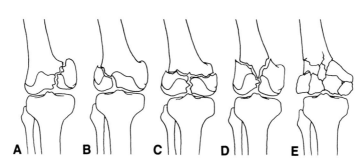

Figure 7.30. Fractures of the condylar end of the femur. *A,* fracture of the medial condyle. *B,* fracture of the lateral condyle. *C,* "T-shaped" intracondylar fracture. *D,* "Y-shaped" intracondylar fracture. *E,* comminuted fracture.

dent, notify a vascular surgeon or an orthopaedist at once, and begin preparations for surgery. When neurovascular function is intact, admit the patient to an orthopaedist and apply a long-leg splint (see Chapter 11). Ensure that neurovascular function is monitored until arrival of the orthopaedist.

Epiphyseal Fractures

Children and adolescents may sustain fractures of the distal femoral or proximal tibial epiphyses. These fractures may present as stable or unstable injuries. Injuries that produce ligament damage in the mature person may produce epiphyseal injury in the immature person. Fractures occur because the epiphysis is weaker than the ligament. Therefore, when stressing ligaments during an examination, be aware that opening may take place at the epiphyseal line and not as the result of ligament laxity. Stress x-ray will determine whether this is a ligamentous injury or a displacement through the epiphysis. Displaced fractures at either epiphysis may have accompanied popliteal artery injury. These injuries should be referred to an orthopaedist.

INJURY OF THE PATELLOFEMORAL ARTICULATION

To support body weight in the many activities of bipedal locomotion, tremendous force is exerted through the extensor mechanism of the knee. The patella is a sesamoid bone embedded in the quadriceps tendon. It enlarges the surface area of the tendon and increases the patella's efficiency by shifting the line of pull of the muscle anteriorly. This improves leverage of the quadriceps in extending the knee. The patella also provides a cartilage-on-cartilage low coefficient of friction for a smooth glide of the quadriceps and maintains the tendon in a centralized track.

The large force needed to attain upright stance produces a large reaction force between the patella and its femoral articulation (Fig. 7.31). The patellofemoral joint reaction force increases as the knee is flexed and is least at full extension. The force across the patellofemoral articulation in stair climbing may be three to five times body weight, and a tremendous force is generated in squat exercises with heavy weights on the shoulder. To meet these demands, the articular cartilage on the under-

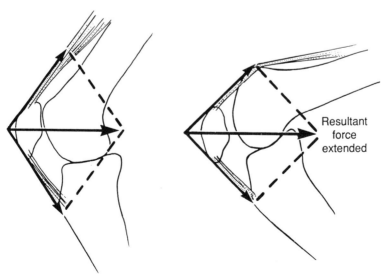

Figure 7.31.   Reaction force across the patellofemoral joint increases with knee flexion. (Adapted from Ficat RP, Hungerford DS. Disorders of the Patello-Femoral Joint. Baltimore: Williams and Wilkins, 1977:24.)

surface of the patella is the thickest in the body.

The patella does not track in a straight line or have contact on the same surfaces throughout the range of motion. At full extension, the patella lies above the trochlea. Within 10 to 30° of flexion, the normal tibial internal rotation pulls the patella into the trochlea. By 60°, the midportion of the patella and midportion of the trochlea are in contact, and at 90°, the proximal portion of the patella and the distal portion of the trochlea are in contact (Fig. 7.32).

These dynamic relationships also accommodate the normal valgus vector of the extensor mechanism. Because of the position of the hips, upright stance requires a valgus position of the knee joint. As a result of this angulation, there is a valgus vector to the muscles. The force of the body tends to bow the knee outward and this is resisted by the lateral musculature and the architecture of the trochlea and patella: the vastus lateralis muscle is stronger than the medialis, and the lateral portion of the trochlea and the lateral segment of the patella are larger than the medial.

The common problems with the patellofemoral mechanism result when these normal relationships and biomechanics are disturbed (Fig. 7.33). These problems can be subdivided into problems of stability, in which there is muscle insufficiency or exaggeration of the normal valgus alignment with excessive lateral pull; problems in which there is excessive force

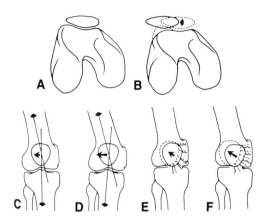

Figure 7.33. Anatomic peculiarities predisposing to recurrent patellar dislocation. *A,* normal, distal end of femur. *B,* flat anterior eminence of the lateral condyle. *C,* normal lateral vector during active extension. *D,* excessive lateral vector. *E,* normal medial retinaculum. *F,* lax medial retinaculum.

across the patellofemoral joint; or a combination of the above.

Examination of the Patellofemoral Articulation

When examining an injured patellofemoral articulation, it is important to differentiate the areas of pain. The pain associated with patellar problems usually is caused by peripatellar synovitis or synovial plica; this pain must be differentiated from medial joint line pain. Often, anterior swelling and inflammation extends to the anterior portion of the meniscus and may create symptoms mimicking meniscal derangement. This occurs when the swelling impinges on the anterior meniscus as the knee is extended. Lateral knee pain also may be present, which is caused by lateral synovitis, extension of the anterior swelling laterally, or hypertrophy of the lateral patellofemoral ligament. Palpable hypertrophy often is present at the lateral patellotibial ligament. This ligament may be tender or there may be tenderness at the insertion of the vastus lateralis at the superior patella. Some patients will have atrophy or actual dysplasia of the vastus medialis.

As noted previously, the alignment of the femur and the arrangement of the muscle at-

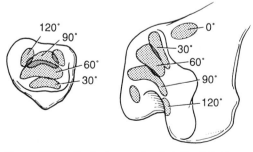

Figure 7.32. Contact areas from extension to flexion. (Adapted from Aglietti P, Insall JN, Walker PS, Trent P. A new patella prosthesis: design and application. Clin Orthop 1975;107(Mar–Apr):175–187.)

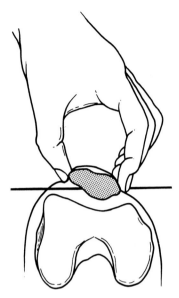

Figure 7.34. Testing for lateral tightness. (Adapted from Rosenberg TD, Kolowich PA. Complications of lateral retinacular release. In: Sprague NF III, ed. Complications in Arthroscopy. New York: Raven Press, Ltd., 1989:146.)

taching to the tibia through the patella have a valgus angle. This is the quadriceps angle (Q angle). The Q angle is determined by measuring the angle formed by a line through the center of the patella and femur and a line from the center of the patella through the tibial tubercle (Fig. 7.33). This angle does not exceed 15° in the normal individual.

Tightness in the lateral retinaculum can be demonstrated by attempting to lift the patella by the lateral edge. Inability to level the patella suggests tightness (Fig. 7.34). With the lateral structure held taut, palpate the lateral patellotibial and lateral patellofemoral ligaments (Fig. 7.35).

Observe the tracking of the patella from extension to flexion with the patient sitting. Normally, the patella is positioned laterally in extension and at 10° of flexion; by 30° of flexion the patella should have moved medially into the trochlear groove. A patella that stays lateral through flexion is abnormal. A patella that starts laterally, becomes medial, then goes back to lateral (a C-shaped route) also is abnormal. When the patella goes from flexion

to extension, there is a gentle lateral excursion at the end; an abrupt lateral excursion suggests abnormality. Swelling may be evident in the peripatellar soft tissue, but effusion is rare except in dislocation. In patients with recurrent subluxation or dislocation, there is apprehension with patellar motion, especially if a lateral push is applied to the knee cap.

Confusion can result when differentiating patellar tendonitis and fat pad synovitis. Direct pressure over the tendon will also contact the fat pad. Isolating the tip of the patella is helpful by pressing on the superior patella and quadriceps tendon (Fig. 7.36), thereby lifting the inferior pole of the patella and palpating the patella at adjacent tendons rather than exerting pressure down on the fat pad.

X-rays in the lateral and skyline (tangential) projection are helpful in evaluating patellofemoral problems. On the lateral view, patella alta, a patellar tendon that is longer than the patella, can be determined by measuring the length of the patellar tendon and comparing this to the length of the patella. Any value over a 1.2 : 1 ratio may be considered patella alta (Fig. 7.37A). Skyline x-rays should be taken at 15°, 30°, 45°, and 60° to see the relationship between the patella and femur in varying degrees of flexion, because abnormal tracking may be missed on a single view (Fig. 7.37B). These views will demonstrate lateral subluxation or abnormal tilt of the patella and also dysplasia of the patella or trochlear groove. Various measurements are determined to demonstrate abnormal patella tilt or an incongruent articulation (Figs. 7.37 C and D).

Instability of the Patella

Instability of the patellofemoral mechanism usually is associated with excessive lateral pull. In the mildest forms, this excessive pull may produce occasional momentary subluxation of the patella. In its most severe form, chronic recurrent or persistent dislocation of the patella may be seen. There is another group of patients with a mild degree of pull in whom it is not possible to diagnose clear subluxation or malalignment, although many

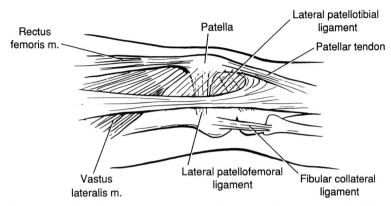

Figure 7.35. The lateral side of the knee. It is important to palpate the lateral patellotibial and patellofemoral ligament and the insertion of the vastus lateralis for their presence, tightness, and possible source of pain.

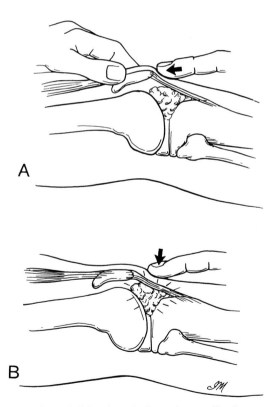

Figure 7.36. *A,* holding the patella and tilting it up isolates the patellar ligament and inferior pole of the patella from fat pad and synovium that may be tender. *B,* direct pressure over the ligament may elicit pain that is from the synovium and not the ligament.

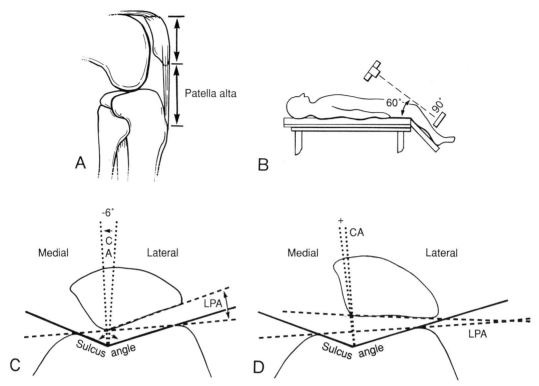

Figure 7.37. *A*, patella alta. *B*, X-ray beam directed across the top of the patella with varied angles to view the patella and trochlea. (Adapted from Carson WG Jr, James SL, Larson RL, Singer KM, Winternitz WW. Patellofemoral disorders: physical and radiographic evaluation. Part II. Radiographic examination. Clin Orthop 1984;185:178–186.) *C* and *D*. The lateral patellofemoral angle (LPA) is formed by a line on the femoral sulcus and a line on the lateral facet. An angle open laterally is normal (*C*) and a parallel or angle open medially suggests subluxation (*D*). The congruence angle (CA) is determined by a line bisecting the sulcus and a line drawn from the lowest point on the patella. The normal CA is $-6° \pm 11°$ (*C*). The sulcus angle is the angle of the trochlear surface measured from the highest point on the medial and lateral trochlea to the lowest midtrochlear point. The normal sulcus angle is 137° (*C*). (Adapted from Merchant AC, Mercer RL, Jacobsen RH, Cool CR. Roentgenographic analysis of patellofemoral congruence. J Bone Joint Surg [Am] 1974;56A:1391–1396; and Laurin CA, Levesque HP, Dussault R, Labelle H, Peides JP. The abnormal lateral patellofemoral angle: a diagnostic roentgenographic sign of recurrent patellar subluxation. J Bone Joint Surg [Am] 1978;60A:55–61.)

of these patients have other characteristic clinical signs that indicate their anterior knee pain is in fact secondary to functional instability of the patella.

Dislocation of the Patella

Some patients have dislocation of the patella as a result of a major acute injury, such as a direct impact on the patella, driving it laterally. These patients may have no underlying anatomic abnormalities. Many patients, however, have one or more anatomic abnormalities that predispose to patella dislocation.

Certain patients with patellar dislocation have Q angles in excess of 20°. Some individuals, however, have Q angles greater than 20° and an otherwise normal mechanism and alignment and may function well. The presence of a Q angle greater than 20° accompanied by excessive external rotation at the tibia and increased internal rotation at the hip is generally referred to as malicious malalignment, and patients with this condition more commonly have patellar dislocation. In patella alta, the increased length of the patellar tendon is inherently unstable because it allows the patella greater medial-lateral translation. It also allows the patella to ride high in the trochlea, where it is somewhat flatter, or even above the trochlea of the femur. Patients with a shallow trochlear groove or small, flat patella have substantially increased chance of dislocation. Finally, atrophy or dysplasia of the vastus medialis muscle also increases the relative strength of the lateral musculature, which can predispose to lateral subluxation.

Clinical Characteristics

Dislocation is manifested during a sudden motion, usually creating a valgus external rotation force. The patella slides over the lateral femoral condyle. Also, the patella may spontaneously reduce or may be reduced by gradual extension of the leg. Accompanying moderate hemarthrosis occurs. If the patient presents with a relocated patella and a moderate hemarthrosis, the history and appearance may suggest an anterior cruciate ligament injury, and medial tenderness may suggest medial collateral ligament injury. Tenderness that is localized to the medial or lateral patella and apprehension with lateral patella push should suggest patella dislocation. Anteroposterior and varus/valgus instability is absent. X-rays may show avulsion fractures from the medial patella, which usually do not require surgery. Lateral femoral condylar fractures also may be present and should be referred to an orthopaedic surgeon.

Treatment

A tense hemarthrosis should be aspirated and the leg immobilized. With dislocation, quadriceps atony is common; however, it is difficult to begin quadriceps setting and isometric exercise until 1 to 2 weeks after injury. Immobilization for 2 weeks allows for some early healing of the medial retinaculum. After 2 weeks, quadriceps setting can be initiated, and motion out of the immobilizer can be started if no pain occurs with motion. Patients will continue to need the immobilizer for support because the quadriceps usually will not gain sufficient strength for independent activity until 6 weeks. Thereafter, quadriceps de-

velopment is important. An acute dislocation does not require surgery unless the patella cannot be maintained in an anatomic position or loose bodies are present that could cause derangement of the joint.

Subluxation of the Patella

Subluxations occur with the same mechanism as dislocations. They are accompanied by a pop and some swelling, but not as severe as with a dislocation. Symptoms are compatible with continued activities or at least with walking. Treatment is the same as with dislocations; however, rehabilitation is shorter, swelling subsides after 1 week, and quadriceps strength returns by 4 to 6 weeks.

Some patients with history of subluxation or dislocation and x-ray findings of patella dislocation may develop degeneration. This type of degeneration is called permanent subluxation. The patient experiences lateral knee pain when sitting and climbing stairs. Examination shows lateral patellar tenderness and tightness, and may show evidence of malalignment. X-ray will show degenerative changes in addition to changes of subluxation. Definitive treatment requires surgical intervention. In some patients, adequate symptomatic relief can be achieved with relief of aggravating activity and the use of anti-inflammatory medication.

Anterior Knee Pain Without Subluxation

The same valgus forces that produce subluxation may in some patients simply produce peripatellar knee pain. This has a more insidious onset and usually is related to athletic activities that involve turning, twisting, or running.

Clinical Characteristics

Pain usually occurs after the event or during the event, but allows the athlete to continue playing. The history may consist of the athlete having difficulties for long periods, but not enough to stop participation. An acute episode may occur in a quick turn. Often the symptoms are intermittent or only related to a certain sport. Effusion is uncommon, but the feeling of swelling medially in the patella and fat pad area may be present.

Pain with these episodes is related to the pull on the medial soft tissues by the lateral force, resulting in inflammation. In many instances, there is an associated synovial plica that is trapped between the patella and femur or against the medial femoral condyle. In other instances, the fat pad attached to the plica is pinched in the same area. The episode may not require medical treatment, but the condition may progress. The patient can continue to participate in sports after a brief period of rest.

Occasionally, symptoms are present with activities of daily living. Patients manifest difficulties in going up and down stairs, kneeling or squatting, and occasionally turning and twisting. They have crepitus in the knee and giving way. Crepitus in these instances usually comes from the swollen soft tissue. These patients may have some of the characteristics of dislocation. Also, they may have hypermobility, some degree of vastus medialis dysplasia or underdevelopment compared with the lateralis, or tightness in the lateral retinaculum.

In those patients whose anterior knee pain and soft tissue swelling are caused by a direct blow, as in a fall or dashboard injury, there may be no manifestation of malalignment or dysplasia.

Treatment

Ice should be used after athletic events, and anti-inflammatory medications may be used for moderate symptoms. A period of rest is advisable if the patient has difficulty participating in sports. Patients should avoid activities that cause irritation, such as bending, squatting, and stair climbing. They should initiate a period of stretching the hamstrings and quadriceps muscles, especially when the symptoms occur at the time of the adolescent growth spurt. Quadriceps muscle strengthening exercises are important for developing the medialis and maintaining a better muscular balance for the patella. This program is usually successful. Patellar bracing providing pressure to resist lateral subluxation may also be helpful. If after 6 months of nonoperative treatment or a long period of intermittent problems the patient still has pain with daily activity and is not able to participate in sports or exercise, evaluation by arthroscopy is indicated. Orthopaedic referral should be made.

Chondromalacia

As noted previously, there can be a large force across the patella in activities such as running or stair climbing. Cartilage that is subject to too much or too little force is likely to soften, producing the lesion known as chondromalacia. Chondromalacia can occur as the result of a direct blow, when a plica rubs against the medial inferior patella, or when high pressure is generated by doing squats with heavy weights. Chondromalacia can also occur in association with recurrent subluxation or dislocation or as a result of an isolated dislocation with damage to the cartilage surface. The softening may produce crepitus. The pain of chondromalacia is related to soft tissue inflammation and is usually peripatellar. Pain involving the patella itself does not become manifest until the cartilage is completely worn and bone-to-bone apposition occurs between the patella and trochlea.

Excessive Lateral Pressure Syndrome

People who do not have full excursion of the patella can develop a lateral tightness that holds the patella tightly in the trochlea. Degeneration develops laterally on the patella and trochlea with no evidence of subluxation. This syndrome is called excessive lateral pressure syndrome.

This condition is characterized by lateral knee pain when sitting and climbing stairs. Females are more commonly affected. Examination shows lateral patellar tenderness and tightness. X-ray changes will show lateral sclerosis and narrowing. As pain increases, the quadriceps weaken and degeneration extends into the medial and lateral compartments, resulting in complete degeneration.

Treatment of Chondromalacia and Excessive Lateral Pressure Syndrome

The problems occurring from chondromalacia or excessive lateral pressure syndrome may be alleviated by removing the source of pressure. This may be accomplished by discontinuing heavy weightlifting, or modifying the work environment to avoid climbing stairs and squatting. If symptoms persist despite force modification and use of anti-inflammatory medication, the patient should be referred to an orthopaedist.

ANTERIOR KNEE PAIN

Patients, especially young individuals, often complain of pain in the anterior portion of the knee. The problems related to patellar biomechanics have been described previously. However, there are other reasons for complaints in this area. The common term for anterior knee pain has been chondromalacia patellae. This is based on the finding that as a person ages, his or her patellar cartilage or articular surfaces become more irregular. The rough surfaces are equated with noise. With the advent of arthroscopy, there have been cases of crepitus that have been related to soft tissue swelling and not to the softening of the cartilage. Therefore, we cannot blame all pain or crepitus across the front of the knee on chondromalacia.

It is helpful to be specific about the area of pain. Several areas have to be considered (Fig. 7.38). First, the medial synovial plica can be related to patellar instability. The medial soft tissues may be pulled laterally by the patella and thereby injured by the mechanics of the patella. The patellar tendon must be evaluated as discussed previously. Laterally, the lateral patellar tibial ligament, the lateral retinaculum, and the area of the insertion of the vastus lateralis must be evaluated. The patella surface must evaluated for bursitis. Lastly, saphenous neuritis is a mimic that causes anterior knee pain that can confuse the evaluation.

Neuritis can be related to problems within the knee but can occur as a separate factor, making us believe that the knee is the cause

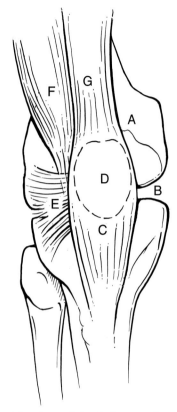

Figure 7.38. *A,* medial soft tissue—plica. *B,* anterior joint line—meniscus. *C,* patellar tendon. *D,* prepatellar bursitis. *E,* lateral retinaculum. *F,* insertion of lateralis vastus. *G,* quadriceps tendon.

of symptomatology. Table 7.1 reveals the numerous factors, both direct and indirect, that can produce saphenous neuritis.

Diagnosis of saphenous neuritis is made by the history and physical examination. Neuritis pain tends to be a steady pain and is not related

Table 7.1. Causes for Saphenous Neuritis

1. Direct
    Direct blow
    Cutting—by incision
    Stretch—posterolateral instability
2. Indirect
    RSD
    Fibromyalgia
    Lumbar disc disease
    Degenerative joint disease
    Medial meniscal pathology

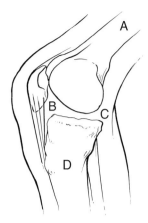

Figure 7.39. *A,* adductor canal. *B,* medial to patella and patellar ligament. *C,* posterior medial joint line. *D,* medial tibial plateau.

to any mechanical activities. The pain occurs even into the night. Often, patients can perform their daily activities. However, by evening when the patient returns home from work, the pain becomes intense, requiring medication. Heat may have a more beneficial effect than ice.

The physical aspects of neuritis are never noted specifically by the patient and must be elicited by the examination. This should be part of all examinations around the knee. The four-point saphenous sensitivity tests, as shown in Figure 7.39, places pressure on the four points. The first is approximately four finger breadths above the epicondyle at the adductor canal. The other points are medial patella and patella ligament, the posterior aspect of the medial joint line, and the medial

tibial plateau. It is obvious that this is a mimic for meniscal pathology because point 3 makes the physician believe that the patellar ligaments or medial soft tissues are involved. Point 2 at the medial joint line suggests the diagnosis of meniscal injury. Indeed, medial meniscal injuries can produce the neuritis, thus providing a strong diagnostic challenge to differentiate between the two conditions. MRI is often helpful. If the MRI is negative, the medial meniscus is not the cause of the neuritis. Likewise, pressure over palpable pain of the medial tibial plateau can suggest pes anserine bursitis, when the pressure may be related to the neuritis. Four-point saphenous testing is an important part of the examination, because neuritis can be the cause of unnecessary or repeat surgery about the knee. If the saphenous test is positive and there is no mechanical cause such as posterolateral rotatory instability or meniscal injury, other causes for the neuritis should be considered (see Table 7.1).

Diagnostic block of the saphenous nerve at the adductor canal can help in the differential diagnosis. The block also may be therapeutic.

SUGGESTED READINGS

Ewing JW, ed. Articular Cartilage and Knee Joint Function: Basic Science and Arthroscopy. New York: Raven Press, 1988.
Fulkerson JP, Hungerford DS. Disorder of the Patellofemoral Joint. Baltimore: Williams & Wilkins, 1990.
Insall JN. Surgery of the Knee. New York: Churchill Livingstone, 1984.
Muller W. The Knee—Form, Function, and Ligament Reconstruction. Berlin: Springer-Verlag, 1982.

CHAPTER 8

Leg and Ankle

Anthony K. Teebagy, M.D.

ESSENTIAL ANATOMY

BONES, JOINTS, AND LIGAMENTS

Tibia and Fibula and Their Articulations

The tibia and fibula are bound together proximally through a synovial joint called the tibiofibular articulation. This joint is located approximately 1 cm distal to the posterolateral joint line of the knee. The joint is reinforced by strong anterior and posterior ligaments.

Distally, the tibia and fibula are joined through the tibiofibular syndesmosis. This is a ligamentous complex made up of the anterior inferior tibiofibular ligament and the posterior inferior tibiofibular ligament with the interosseous membrane (Fig. 8.1). These ligaments allow slight motion at both joints. The interosseus membrane joins the tibia to the fibula throughout the entire length of the fibula. The two bones, along with the interosseus membrane, form the anatomic barrier that separates the posterior compartments of the leg from the anterior and lateral compartments.

Ankle Joint

The distal tibia and fibula form a boxlike frame, which is commonly termed the "mortise." Following this carpentry terminology, the anatomic tenon is the dome of the talus, which fits into the mortise made up of the fibula and tibia (Fig. 8.2). Unlike a wooden mortise and tenon joint, the ankle is not rigidly stable throughout its range of motion. Because the talus is wider anteriorly than posteriorly, the ankle is more stable in dorsiflexion than in a plantar flexion. An important x-ray view of the ankle joint is the so-called "mortise

view." This x-ray is done with the ankle in slight internal rotation and most clearly demonstrates the boxlike configuration of the ankle joint (Fig. 8.3). The ankle joint is surrounded by a fibrous and synovial capsule.

The ankle has several important stabilizing ligaments. The syndesmotic ligamentous complex, which has been described above, is responsible for maintaining the width of the mortise. When these ligaments are torn, the fibula can separate from the tibia, the mortise widens, and the talus becomes unstable. The deltoid ligament is a strong fan-shaped ligament medially. There are three lateral ligaments: the anterior and posterior talofibular ligaments and the calcaneofibular ligament (Fig. 8.1). The degree to which these ligaments are torn determines the degree of talar instability. Motion within the ankle joint is mainly dorsiflexion and plantar flexion. With disruption of specific ligaments, the ankle becomes unstable. This can be demonstrated by abnormally increased motion to abduction (eversion), adduction (inversion), or anterior stress.

Growth of the leg occurs at both ends of the tibia and fibula. Approximately 75% of the growth of the lower leg occurs at the proximal end of the bone and the remaining 25% at the distal end (Fig. 8.4). Any abnormality or injury that involves the growth plates should be referred to an orthopaedic surgeon, as angular or length deformities may result.

NEUROMUSCULAR ORGANIZATION

Muscle Compartments of the Leg

The bones and muscles of the leg are surrounded by a strong fascial sheath called the

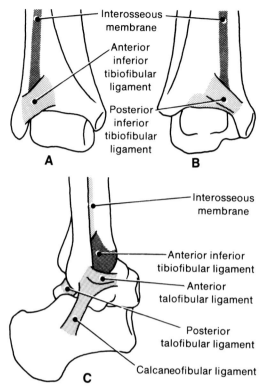

Figure 8.1. Distal tibiofibular joint and tibiotalar joint. *A,* anterior view. *B,* posterior view. *C,* lateral view.

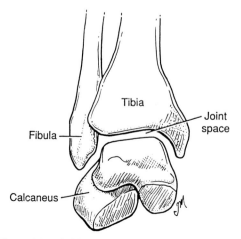

Figure 8.2. Ankle mortise. The talus fits into the frame comprised of the tibia and fibula.

crural fascia. This fascial sheath is densely adherent to the tibia anteromedially and loosely adherent to muscles posteriorly. Fibrous septi, which extend inward from the crural fascia, along with the interosseus membrane, divide the leg into four compartments: the anterior compartment, the lateral compartment, the deep posterior compartment, and the superficial posterior compartment (Fig. 8.5). Contained within these compartments are various muscles, nerves, and blood vessels (Fig. 8.6). These compartments are relatively closed, and because of the stout fascial envelope, increased pressure within these compartments caused by bleeding or posttraumatic edema can lead to necrosis of the structures within the compartment.

Nerves of the Leg

The sciatic nerve divides into two major nerve trunks above the popliteal fossa: the common peroneal nerve and the tibial nerve. The common peroneal nerve travels across the lateral head of the gastrocnemius and along the medial border of the biceps tendon, then curves laterally below the head of the fibula across the fibular neck. At about that point, the common peroneal nerve divides into the superficial and deep peroneal nerves. The common peroneal nerve is securely fixed as it comes around the neck of the fibula. This fact, combined with its superficial location, render the peroneal nerve prone to injury by a variety of mechanisms, including trauma to the proximal leg, especially on the lateral side, and pressure from tight casts or bandages around the knee. After branching, the superficial peroneal nerve travels to the lateral compartment and the deep peroneal nerve to the anterior compartment. The tibial nerve passes medially between the two femoral attachments of the gastrocnemius muscle and continues distally into the deep posterior compartment. After branching, these nerves share the cutaneous innervation of the leg and foot (Figs. 8.7 and 8.8).

Muscles of the Leg and Their Innervations

The muscles of the anterior compartment are the dorsiflexors of the ankle and toes. They

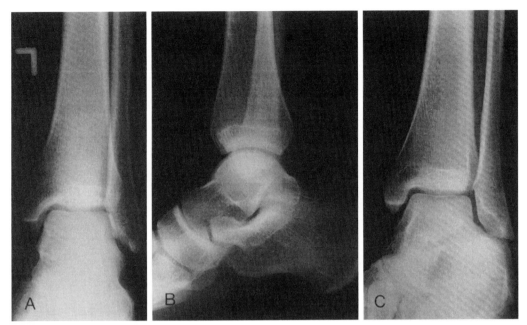

Figure 8.3. *A,* anteroposterior view of the ankle; overlap on the lateral aspect is a normal appearance. The lateral process of the talus is well seen. *B,* lateral view of the ankle; note the congruency of the distal tibia and the talar dome. *C,* mortise view of the ankle; note the symmetry of the joint space and the frame formed around the talus by the tibia and fibula. This film is taken with the ankle internally rotated 15°. An asymmetric joint space is abnormal and may represent injury to the ankle ligaments, arthritis, or other pathologic conditions.

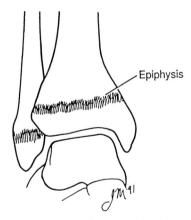

Figure 8.4. Location of the growth plate at the distal tibia and fibula. Any suspected injury to the growth plate should be referred to an orthopaedic surgeon.

are all innervated by the deep peroneal nerve. These muscles include the tibialis anterior, the extensor hallucis longus, the extensor digitorum longus, and the peroneus tertius. The tendon of the tibialis anterior crosses the ante-romedial aspect of the ankle to insert on the plantar surface of the medial cuneiform and base of the first metatarsal. This tendon functions as a powerful dorsiflexor of the ankle. The tendon of the extensor hallucis longus crosses the ankle just lateral to the tendon of the anterior tibialis and passes distally to insert on the dorsal base of the distal phalanx of the great toe. As its name implies, it extends the distal phalanx of the great toe. The extensor digitorum longus and the peroneus tertius share a common origin and separate as they become tendinous. They cross the anterolateral aspect of the ankle together. The peroneus tertius inserts on the dorsum of the base of the fourth and fifth metatarsals and acts as a weak ankle extensor. The extensor digitorum longus divides into four tendons, one to each of the lesser four toes, and functions to extend the distal phalanx of the lesser toes (Fig. 8.9A).

The muscles of the lateral compartment are the peroneus longus and peroneus brevis.

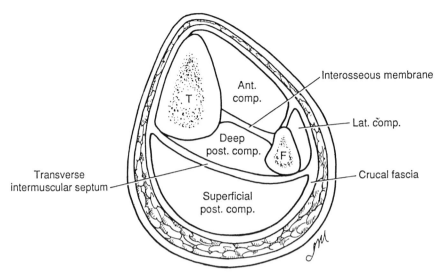

Figure 8.5. Cross section of the leg. The crural fascia and septa divide the leg into four compartments.

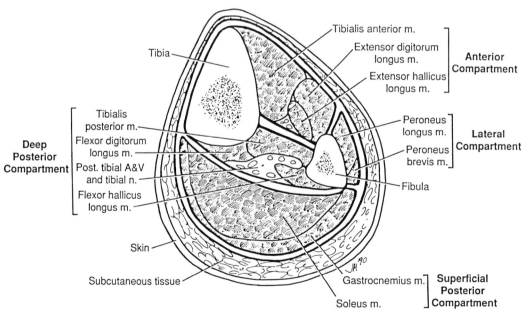

Figure 8.6. Cross-sectional anatomy of the leg.

They are pronators of the foot and evertors of the hindfoot. Both the peroneus longus and peroneus brevis are innervated by the superficial peroneal nerve. They originate from the lateral surface of the fibula and pass as separate tendons behind the lateral malleolus. The peroneus brevis inserts on the base of the fifth metatarsal. The peroneus longus passes around the cuboid and crosses the plantar aspect of the foot to insert on the medial cuneiform and base of the first metatarsal (Fig. 8.9B).

The three long muscles of the deep posterior compartment are all innervated by the

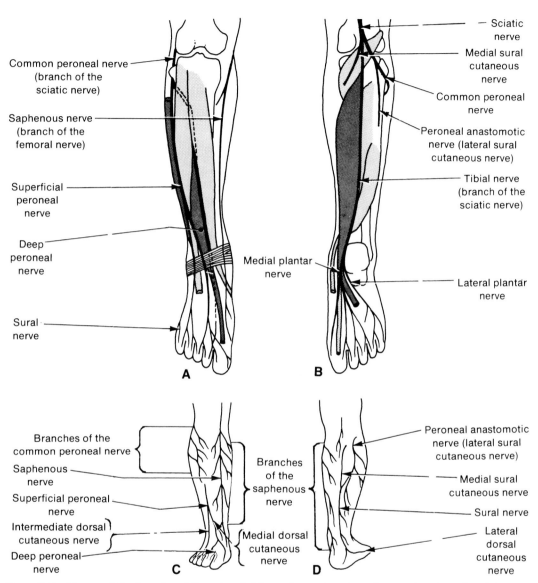

Figure 8.7. Nerves of the leg. *A* and *B,* major divisions. *A,* anterior view. *B,* posterior view. *C* and *D,* cutaneous nerves of the leg. *C,* anterior view. *D,* posterior view.

tibial nerve. The flexor hallucis longus originates from the posterior surface of the fibula and passes behind the medial malleolus through the plantar aspect of the foot to insert on the base of the distal phalanx of the great toe. The flexor hallucis longus flexes the distal phalanx of the great toe. The flexor digitorum longus originates from the posterior aspect of the tibia and passes under the medial malleolus

just behind to the posterior tibialis tendon. It then divides into four tendons that pass through the plantar aspect of the foot to insert in the bases of the distal phalanges of the four lateral toes. These four tendons act to flex the distal phalanx of the lesser toes. The tibialis posterior muscle originates between the two flexor muscles from the tibia, fibula and interosseus membrane. The tendon of the tibi-

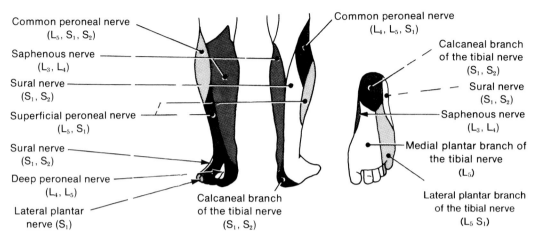

Common peroneal nerve
(L₅, S₁, S₂)

Saphenous nerve
(L₃, L₄)

Sural nerve
(S₁, S₂)

Superficial peroneal nerve
(L₅, S₁)

Sural nerve
(S₁, S₂)

Deep peroneal nerve
(L₄, L₅)

Lateral plantar
nerve (S₁)

Common peroneal nerve
(L₄, L₅, S₁)

Calcaneal branch
of the tibial nerve
(S₁, S₂)

Sural nerve
(S₁, S₂)

Saphenous nerve
(L₃, L₄)

Medial plantar branch of
the tibial nerve
(L₅)

Lateral plantar branch
of the tibial nerve
(L₅ S₁)

Calcaneal branch
of the tibial nerve
(S₁, S₂)

Figure 8.8. Distribution of the cutaneous nerves of the leg.

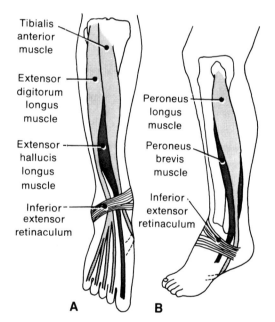

Tibialis anterior muscle

Extensor digitorum longus muscle

Extensor hallucis longus muscle

Inferior extensor retinaculum

Peroneus longus muscle

Peroneus brevis muscle

Inferior extensor retinaculum

A   **B**

Figure 8.9. *A*, muscles of the anterior compartment. *B*, muscles of the lateral compartment.

alis posterior muscle passes behind the medial malleolus and inserts on the medial and plantar surface of the navicula, the plantar surfaces of the cuneiform bones, and bases of the second, third, and fourth metatarsals. This mus-

cle is a powerful invertor and supinator of the foot (Fig. 8.10A).

The large muscles of the superficial posterior compartment are the strong plantar flexors of the ankle, the gastrocnemius, and the soleus. The more superficial of the two, the gastrocnemius, originates from two attachments (one from each femoral condyle), and the deeper soleus originates from its broad attachment to the upper third of the tibia and fibula. These two muscles merge to form the Achilles tendon, which inserts on the calcaneus. It should be recognized that the gastrocnemius originates above the knee joint and therefore crosses the knee and the ankle as well as the subtalar joint. The plantaris muscle and its long narrow tendon crosses the soleus and gastrocnemius muscles from its origin on the femoral condyle to its insertion with the fibers of the Achilles tendon. The muscles of the deep and superficial posterior compartments are all innervated by branches of the tibial nerve (Fig. 8.10B).

Retinacula of the Ankle

Across the ankle joint are thickenings of the crural fascia called retinacula. These structures hold the long tendons to the ankle and foot in positions of mechanical advantage as they cross the ankle joint, preventing bowstrings as the muscles contract (Fig. 8.11).

RADIOGRAPHIC EVALUATION OF THE PATIENT WITH LEG OR ANKLE SYMPTOMS

When patients complain of difficulties in the leg or ankle, it is standard practice to include a radiographic examination in the patient's overall evaluation.

The standard radiographs for the leg are the anteroposterior (AP) and lateral views, with the knee and ankle included on the same film. Abnormalities of the bone structure and alignment can be evaluated with these x-rays, and the angular relationship between the knee and ankle also can be visualized. Soft tissue abnormalities often can be noted and can be represented by soft tissue swelling or defects or both.

Standard ankle radiographs include the AP, lateral, and mortise views. The importance of the mortise view was discussed in the section "Bone, Joints, and Ligaments."

NONTRAUMATIC CONDITIONS OF THE LEG AND ANKLE

A variety of congenital torsional and angular deformities of the leg, ankle, and foot can occur. Also, a variety of congenital aplasias can occur in which complete bones or sections of bones are absent or hypoplastic; these have associated soft tissue deformities. This group of conditions will be discussed in the pediatric section of this text.

In the adult, the normal lower extremity is a mechanical axis aligned so that a straight line can be drawn from the center of the femoral head, through the midportion of the knee, to the center of the talus, and into the second ray of the foot. The knee normally has 5 to 8° of anatomic valgus, and the tibia is relatively straight, although a few degrees of varus, or less often, valgus alignment may be normal for

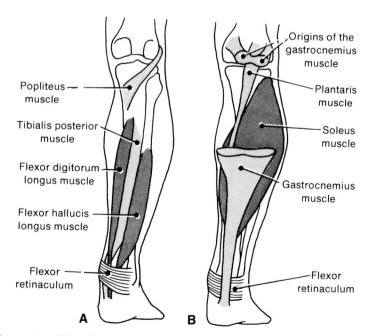

Figure 8.10. *A*, muscles of the deep posterior compartment. *B*, muscles of the superficial posterior compartment.

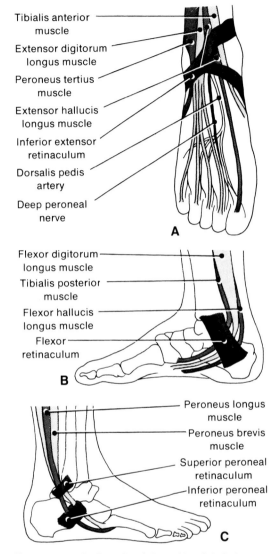

Tibialis anterior muscle
Extensor digitorum longus muscle
Peroneus tertius muscle
Extensor hallucis longus muscle
Inferior extensor retinaculum
Dorsalis pedis artery
Deep peroneal nerve

A

Flexor digitorum longus muscle
Tibialis posterior muscle
Flexor hallucis longus muscle
Flexor retinaculum

B

Peroneus longus muscle
Peroneus brevis muscle
Superior peroneal retinaculum
Inferior peroneal retinaculum

C

Figure 8.11. Retinacula of the ankle. *A*, inferior extensor retinaculum. *B*, flexor retinaculum. *C*, superior and inferior peroneal retinacula.

relatively greater amount of internal rotation compared with the adult.

TRAUMATIC DISORDERS OF THE LEG AND ANKLE

Traumatic disorders may be the result of a single major traumatic event or of repetitive minor trauma, often designated as overuse or overdemand syndromes. Some conditions,

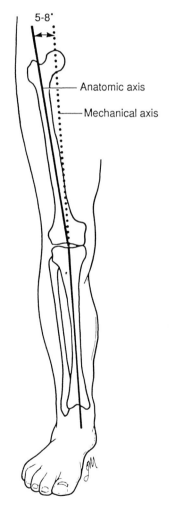

5-8°

Anatomic axis
Mechanical axis

Figure 8.12. Anatomic axis depicts an angle of 5 to 8° between the shaft of the femur and the shaft of the tibia. The mechanical axis is usually a straight line from the femoral head, through the center of the knee joint, to the middle of the ankle. Weightbearing is along the mechanical axis. Reconstructive surgery uses the anatomic axis.

some individuals (Fig. 8.12). The alignment of the foot relative to the leg or the thigh-foot angle has a wide range of normal values from approximately 5° of internal rotation to 15 to 20° of external rotation. Postures that significantly exceed these "normal limits" are considered deformities.

In the infant, it is common to have more varus through the knee and tibia. The alignment of the foot to the leg also may have a such as compartment syndrome, may be associated with either category of trauma.

OVERUSE SYNDROMES

Shin Splints

Shin splints is a term that many people use, perhaps inappropriately, to refer to any pain in the leg occurring during or soon after exercise. Similar to the term internal derangement of the knee, the term shin splints can refer to a number of different pathologic problems in the leg.

In many cases, specific diagnosis is difficult. Certain muscular activity or stretching is associated with muscle pain of varying severity and persistence. Shin splints can be applied to this type of pain and is usually described as pain along the tibia with a varying location when the muscles of the anterior or deep posterior compartments are overstressed. Visible evidence of inflammation suggests that the pain syndrome represents myositis, periostitis, or musculotendinous strains or tears. Also included in the differential diagnosis are stress fractures, exertional compartment syndrome, and tenosynovitis.

Clinical Characteristics

The patient complains of pain over a muscle compartment of the leg. Pain may be referred to the foot or into the knee. Movements that stretch or work the affected muscle increase the pain. Palpation over the affected muscle group or the adjacent tibia will reveal tenderness. Slight swelling and redness may be visible over the affected muscle and its origin.

These symptoms often occur in athletes who change their running surfaces or types of shoes, alter their techniques, or participate in intensive hard training. These symptoms also may be noted in nonathletes who perform activities to which they are unaccustomed, such as walking up a large hill or numerous stairs.

The evaluation of a patient who complains of shin splints is an attempt to confirm a specific diagnosis. Plain radiographs may be normal, reveal periosteal elevation, show soft tissue swelling, reveal a linear lucency, or even in a rare instance, reveal a neoplastic condition.

Periosteal elevation is a reaction to bony stress of any source, including fractures, infection, or neoplasia. A linear lucency usually represents a fracture. A large defect or unorganized bone production may represent infection or neoplasia.

Technetium bone scanning frequently is performed for periostitis or if stress fractures are suspected when the radiographs are negative. Periostitis often is revealed as diffuse uptake along the tibia, whereas intense local uptake usually is seen with a stress fracture.

An MRI also can be performed to evaluate abnormalities with the bones as well as the soft tissue structures. Exercise compartment pressure measurements are performed to confirm the diagnosis of exertional compartment syndrome.

Treatment

Minor stress myalgias can be treated with ice and anti-inflammatory medications. When pain is intense or inflammation is visibly evident, the provoking activity should be avoided until recovery is well advanced. Ice is the safest applied analgesic during the first 2 or 3 days. Thereafter, heat or ice may be used, whichever is more comforting. Stretching and mild exercise may begin as soon as visible evidence of inflammation has subsided. The provoking activity should be resumed gradually.

In some cases foot abnormalities, such as excessive pronation as seen in patients with flatfeet (pes planus), may be the cause of shin splints, and orthotics may be beneficial in these patients.

Stress Fractures

Stress fractures may occur in either the tibia or the fibula. They usually will occur after prolonged and repeated loading, as in long distance or cross country running or repeated jumping. Many times, the individual is not properly conditioned before participating in the inciting activity. Tibial stress fractures typically occur in the upper two-thirds of the bone, although they may occur at the junction of the middle and distal third as well. Fibular stress fractures usually occur in the lower 5 to 7 cm above the tip of the lateral malleolus.

Clinical Characteristics

During or soon after the repeated load, the patient typically complains of pain in the affected leg, which subsides with rest after a variable length of time. Upon feeling well again, the patient (often an athlete) will resume the activity, which will again produce symptoms. Local tenderness and some swelling are noted over the fracture site.

Differential diagnosis includes shin splints, exertional compartment syndrome, and tenosynovitis. Radiographs will often be negative when initially performed. Technetium bone scanning or an MRI confirms the diagnosis before radiographs become positive.

Treatment

Treatment of tibial stress fractures consists of cessation of the inciting activity for approximately 6 to 8 weeks, and then gradual return at a pace that is below the level that causes pain. Patients who have pain even with walking or who will not comply with the required decreased level of activity should be placed in a short-leg walking cast or functional walking brace for 4 to 6 weeks, allowing healing to progress. After that time, a progressive return is allowed, as described previously.

A bone scan or an MRI can be used in those patients who require an expeditious diagnosis or who do not seem to be progressing as expected. Follow-up radiographs should be obtained. Nonunion of the fracture is an unusual occurrence but can result in those patients who persist in running "through the pain." This may present treatment problems that require consultation with an orthopaedic surgeon.

Stress fractures of the fibula can be treated effectively in the same fashion.

Compartment Syndrome

Compartment syndrome is the result of increased volume within one or more compartments of an extremity caused by increased blood flow or swelling. The anatomic compartments are surrounded by dense fascial layers that have little capacity for stretch. Consequently, bleeding or edema that would increase the potential volume of the tissue within the compartment will lead to increased pressure rather than actual distention of the compartment, which rapidly reaches its limit because of the inelasticity of the fascial envelope. Compartment syndromes of the lower extremity may be the result of acute trauma or may be chronic and related to exertion.

Acute Compartment Syndrome

Acute compartment syndromes may result from a single traumatic event to the lower leg, including fractures and crush injuries. They may also result from disruption of arterial blood flow as seen in vascular injuries. These are surgical emergencies, and the diagnosis must be sought in any extremity that is subject to trauma. Evaluation for compartment syndrome involves a motor, sensory, and circulatory examination of the extremity.

Clinical Characteristics   The early and most dramatic characteristics of acute compartment syndrome are severe pain in the leg, tense swelling of one of more compartments with associated tenderness, and extreme pain with passive motion and stretching of the musculotendinous units in the involved compartment.

Acute compartment syndrome includes pallor, paresthesia, pain with passive motion, paralysis to active motion, and pulselessness. The absence of a pulse, however, is a late finding and is not a dependable finding in the early stages of an acute compartment syndrome. Pallor or a whitish discoloration of the skin is also related to blood flow and is also a late finding. Paresthesia and anesthesia of the skin are frequently seen, and the patient will often be unable to discriminate a pinprick from a dull sensation. Severe pain with passive motion of the toes and paralysis or inability to voluntarily move the toes or ankle are significant findings in the diagnosis of an early acute compartment syndrome.

If presented with a patient with an acute compartment syndrome or if the diagnosis is difficult to determine, immediate referral is required for pressure measurements and/or surgical decompression by fasciotomy.

Chronic Exertional Compartment Syndrome

Chronic exertional compartment syndromes are often more difficult to diagnose than the acute syndrome and usually do not present as surgical emergencies.

Clinical Characteristics   Symptoms of exertional compartment syndrome are not unlike the symptoms of other stress-induced problems in the lower leg. These include pain in the lower leg when running or during repeated jumping. Some patients may even have pain with fast walking. As muscles are exercised, they increase their volume and blood flow. This results in increased pressure that may actually decrease blood flow, leading to a relative lack of oxygenation, increased lactic acid production, and further swelling. Subsequently, pain of a dull quality develops and will usually resolve with a few minutes of rest; other symptoms include a feeling of weakness and paresthesia. The location of symptoms will help define which compartment is affected, with the anterior compartment being the most common. Occasionally, the patient will have a history of blunt trauma to the soft tissues or a previous fracture of the affected extremity.

Treatment   The diagnosis as well as the treatment of true exertional compartment syndrome are invasive, and therefore, it is worthwhile to initially treat the patient with conservative measures. This first treatment consists of conditioning the muscles to the increased demand with stretching and strengthening, and a slow progression to the desired activity. If these prove to be ineffective, a bone scan to rule out stress fracture and periostitis is performed and will be normal in the case of exertional compartment syndromes. The diagnosis is confirmed with pressure measurements of the compartments during exercise and the "cool-down" period. Specific criteria have been elaborated for the diagnosis. If these criteria are met, surgical release is indicated. Because the measurements and treatment are invasive, referral to an orthopaedist is recommended when conservative measures fail to relieve symptoms. Rarely, a patient with exertional compartment syndrome will unknowingly attempt to "run through the pain." This can result in an acute compartment syndrome in which the symptoms do not resolve with rest, and immediate referral is required as emergency decompression may be necessary.

Tenosynovitis

The long tendons to the foot and their synovial sheaths are vulnerable to irritation where they pass under the retinacula at the ankle. Activity that requires prolonged repetitive movement of a tendon is most likely to provoke its inflammation. The tibialis anterior and posterior, and the peronei longus and brevis are most commonly involved.

It is important to note that, occasionally, patients with systemic disease such as rheumatoid arthritis or a collagen vascular disease will present with a localized tendosynovitis as a manifestation of their generalized illness. When evaluating a patient, this fact must be considered in a differential diagnosis.

Clinical Characteristics

Pain is felt over the affected tendon and may refer into that portion of the foot distal to it, as described here: tibialis anterior—anteromedial aspect of the ankle and dorsum of the foot; tibialis posterior—posteromedial aspect of the ankle and medial plantar aspect of the foot; and peronei—posterolateral aspect of the ankle and lateral aspect of the foot. Tenderness to palpation, visible fullness, and often a creaky crepitation are evident over the tendon where it passes beneath the retinaculum. Movement or action of the tendon usually causes pain. This includes passive stretching of the tendons as well as active function of the inflamed tendons.

Treatment

Specific treatment depends on the severity of the symptoms. In general, rest, ice, and anti-inflammatory agents are used. Although mild ambulation may continue, activities requiring prolonged repetitive motions should be avoided. Any activity that causes the symptoms should be avoided. When symptoms are so severe that even level walking produces symptoms, or if mild symptoms continue beyond 2 to 3 weeks, a 4- to 6-week period with a short-leg walking cast or functional walking brace may be used to provide complete rest of the tendon. Ice may be used until the visible signs of inflammation have disappeared, and oral anti-inflammatory agents can be helpful in relieving the tenderness.

As symptoms are resolving, a physical therapy program consisting of stretching and strengthening the involved tendons should be employed to avoid recurrence.

POSTERIOR HEEL AND ANKLE PAIN

The primary practitioner will likely encounter three distinct areas of posterior heel or posterior ankle pain. These include the Achilles tendon, posterior calcaneal area, and retrocalcaneal area.

Achilles Tendon

The diagnosis includes tendinitis, paratendinitis, partial Achilles tendon rupture, or intrinsic degeneration of the Achilles tendon. The loose connective tissue surrounding the Achilles tendon then becomes irritated whenever the Achilles tendon is subjected to uncustomary repetitive stress, such as hiking or jogging. Although commonly known as Achilles tendinitis, the inflammation more frequently involves the paratendon surrounding the Achilles tendon. In severe or chronic cases, the tendon itself can become inflamed. The physical findings and treatment of tendinitis or paratendinitis are identical. The inflammation can present from running or competing in shoes with heels lower than street shoes or training shoes. In addition, flatfooted patients with hyperpronating feet are at increased risk

for developing Achilles tendinitis or paratendinitis. Partial tears of the Achilles tendon and intrinsic degeneration present as Achilles tendinitis. An MRI is helpful to differentiate chronic cases that do not respond to conservative management.

Clinical Characteristics

The patient complains of pain in the back of the heel and leg that worsens when the Achilles tendon is stretched or worked. Tenderness and swelling will be noted approximately 3 to 4 cm above the tendon's insertion on the calcaneus.

Treatment

Treatment is directed toward reducing the inflammation, reducing the stress on the Achilles tendon, and increasing the flexibility of the gastrocsoleus complex. Specifically, oral anti-inflammatories, a heel lift of ¼ to ½ inch, and a stretching and strengthening physical therapy program are prescribed. Often, complete rest by way of a short-leg walking cast or functional walking brace for 4 to 6 weeks is initially necessary to reduce the inflammation. A soft orthotic with a navicular pad and a 1/8-inch medial wedge can be of benefit in those patients whose feet tend to hyperpronate and who have recurrent symptoms. In chronic cases, an MRI may reveal areas of degeneration or evidence of a partial tear. Surgical treatment to excise these areas is warranted in recalcitrant cases.

Retrocalcaneal Area

Retrocalcaneal bursitis and Haglund's disease are two common causes of pain and tenderness located in front of the Achilles tendon, but posterior to the calcaneus.

Haglund's disease is a prominence of the posterior superior aspect of the calcaneus and may impinge on the Achilles tendon when the ankle is dorsiflexed (Fig. 8.13). The retrocalcaneal bursa is located between the upper one-third of the calcaneus and the Achilles tendon. This bursa is prone to inflammation following activities that require repetitive ankle dorsiflexion and plantar flexion. Haglund's disease may be associated with an inflammatory arthritis such as rheumatoid arthritis and can, on occasion, show erosive changes in the upper one-third of the posterior calcaneus (Fig. 8.14).

Clinical Characteristics

The patient complains of heel pain worsened by dorsiflexion of the ankle. Tenderness is present just anterior and superior to the insertion of the Achilles tendon on the calcaneus. Swelling and redness may be evident in this location or at the Achilles tendon insertion itself. X-rays may reveal the promi-

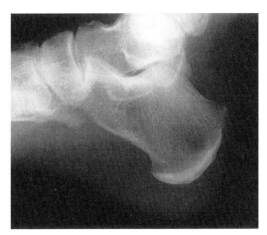

Figure 8.13. Haglund's disease. Note the prominence at the superoposterior aspect of the calcaneus.

nence of Haglund's disease or the erosive damage of inflammatory arthritides.

Treatment

Weight bearing is minimized, and when necessary, a ¼- to ½-inch elevation of the heel is used to decrease the tension of the Achilles tendon. Hot or cold compresses may provide some relief. Oral anti-inflammatories and, occasionally, steroid injection may speed the remission. In chronic or recurrent cases, orthopaedic referral should be considered for surgical treatment, which may include excision of the prominent tubercle and removal of the retrocalcaneal bursa (Fig. 8.15).

Posterior Calcaneal Area

The three distinct causes of posterior heel pain in the adult are insertional Achilles tendinitis, calcific insertional Achilles tendinitis, and posterior calcaneal bursitis. In the child, Sever's disease is a cause, which will be covered in the pediatric chapter.

Clinical Characteristics

Insertional Achilles tendinitis consists of pain and tenderness posteriorly at the insertion of the Achilles tendon. This may be accompanied by redness or swelling, and the deformity is usually minimal. Calcific insertional tendinitis has a similar presentation; however, redness and swelling are usually

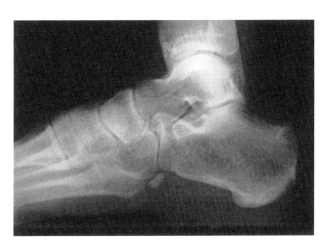

Figure 8.14. Erosions of the calcaneus from inflammatory arthritis affecting the retrocalcaneal bursa.

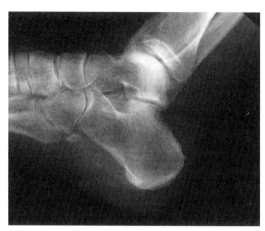

Figure 8.15. Note the removal of Haglund's disease with resection of the calcaneal superoposterior prominence.

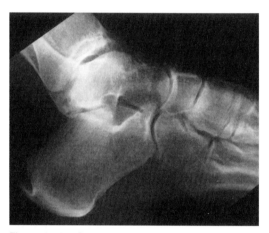

Figure 8.16. Spurs at the insertion of the Achilles tendon on the calcaneus.

more prominent, and a bony prominence of various degrees generally is in this location. A radiograph will reveal bony spurs at the insertion of the Achilles tendon (Fig. 8.16). Posterior calcaneal bursitis, sometimes called a pump bump, is an inflammation of the sub-cutaneous bursa superficial to the insertion of the Achilles tendon. These three conditions are caused by the friction of the upper border of the heel counter of the shoe. They can result from laceless shoes and loafers that must fit closely to the heel or from high-heeled shoes.

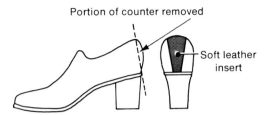

Figure 8.17. Insertion of soft leather into the back of the heel counter.

Treatment

Ideally, open-heeled shoes or sandals should be used until the inflammation sub-sides. Local injection of the bursa with corti-costeroid is not recommended in these situations as it may weaken the tendon. Oral anti-inflammatories can be used to decrease the inflammation. When shoes with heel counters are again worn, the counter should be less convex and its upper border should be soft. A posterior wedge can be cut away from the posterior counters of the shoe and soft leather sewn across the defect (Fig. 8.17). Alternatively, a U-shaped pad can be placed between the heel and the counter to relieve the irritated prominent area. In chronic or recurrent cases, orthopaedic referral is indicated for possible surgical treatment, which might include ostectomy of the prominent tubercle, osteotomy of the calcaneal, resection of the spurs, or excision of the painful bursas.

TENDON DISRUPTIONS

Tendon disruptions of the leg and ankle are relatively uncommon events. The disruption may be caused by a direct laceration, a sudden force applied to the tendon, or a gradual intrinsic degeneration of the tendon. In the first instance, the diagnosis should be made at the time of evaluation of the laceration. The patient will demonstrate weak and usually painful motion when testing the action of the specific tendon involved. Following a sudden force, the patient will again demonstrate painful and weak action of the specific tendon, and a palpable gap may be noted along the course of the tendon if examined before significant swelling occurs. Gradual disruption may be more difficult to diagnose. The patient will complain of ankle and foot fatigue, and a progressive foot or ankle deformity may be noted.

The posterior tibialis tendon disruption is most commonly the result of gradual deterioration. Disruption of the anterior tibialis tendon is usually the result of a laceration because of its anterior and relatively vulnerable position. Disruption of the peroneal tendons is occasionally caused by either trauma or deterioration. The etiology of Achilles tendon ruptures is most commonly the result of a sudden force applied to the plantar-flexed ankle.

Disruption of the Achilles tendon will be discussed in this chapter; the other tendon disruptions will be discussed in Chapter 9, "Foot."

Achilles Tendon Rupture

Rupture of the Achilles tendon is usually the result of forced dorsiflexion against a plantar-flexed foot.

Clinical Characteristics

The typical patient is over 25 years old and sustained the injury during an athletic event. The athlete notices a snap in the back of the heel, often stating that it felt as if a stick may have struck the back of the ankle or lower leg. Activities in which this most often occurs are diving, racquet sports, and basketball. Any activity in which the patient may suddenly "toe off" or land on his toes after a jump can cause the excessive load.

In addition to the typical history, the diagnosis is made on the basis of three diagnostic signs on physical examination. The first is a palpable defect noted between 2 and 6 cm above the Achilles insertion on the calcaneus. The second is weak active plantar flexion against resistance. The third and pathognomonic finding is a positive Thompson-Doherty squeeze test. This test is performed with the patient prone and the knees bent at 90°. Squeezing the calf will produce a definite plantar flexion of the ankle in the normal extremity; however, in the extremity with the ruptured Achilles tendon, plantar flexion will be significantly less distinct or absent. Comparison with the normal side is important to

convince the examiner of the difference. Occasionally, radiographs can delineate the tendon rupture or may demonstrate a bony avulsion from the os calcis. The diagnosis, however, can be made clinically by history and physical examination (Fig. 8.18).

Treatment

Treatment of Achilles tendon rupture is controversial. There are many advocates for both nonoperative treatment and operative treatment. Nonoperative treatment consists of the application of a long-leg cast with the knee in 45° of flexion and the ankle in gravity equinus. Gravity equinus is the amount that the ankle will naturally assume when the knee is bent over the edge of a table. This is continued for 4 weeks followed by a short-leg cast with the ankle in gravity equinus for another 4 weeks. Following this, the patient obtains a 1-inch heel lift that is gradually decreased by 1/4-inch per week for the next 4 weeks. Braces that can adjust plantar can be used in lieu of heel lifts. During the period in a heel lift, a physical therapy program, including active dorsiflexion and gentle resistive plantar flexion, is begun and continued until the ankle regains normal strength. If nonoperative treatment is chosen, it is much more successful if treatment is begun within 3 to 5 days of injury.

Operative treatment consists of surgical approximation of the disrupted tendon. The postoperative treatment is identical to the nonoperative treatment.

Surgical treatment has the benefit of slightly increased resistance to fatigue and slightly decreased rate of rerupture. The risks of surgery include anesthesia, infection, and wound problems. Recommending surgery in active individuals who wish to remain active is probably appropriate.

Rupture of the Gastrocnemius Muscle or the Plantaris Tendon

Included in the differential diagnosis of Achilles tendon rupture is a partial tear of the gastrocnemius muscle, usually at the medial muscle aponeurotic junction. The patient may have the same history as the patient with

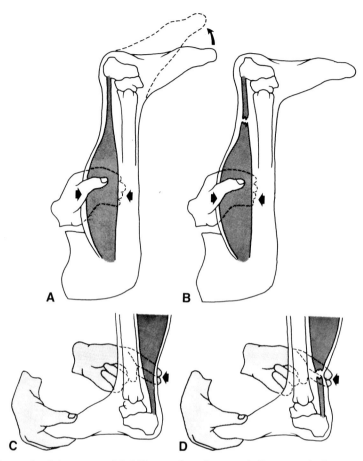

Figure 8.18. Diagnosis of the ruptured Achilles tendon. *A*, normal. *B*, ruptured. *C*, normal. *D*, ruptured.

Achilles tendon rupture, but the classic physical findings will be absent, and the tenderness will be noted medially about midway between the knee and ankle. A partial tear of the gastrocnemius can be treated with an elevated heel after the tenderness has resolved. Care should be taken to assure that no compartment syndrome develops.

Rupture of the plantaris has a similar history and physical examination as the partial tear of the gastrocnemius and is treated in a similar manner.

MAJOR TRAUMATIC INJURIES TO THE LEG AND ANKLE

The prognosis of lower extremity injuries depends heavily on the integrity of the circulation. Patients with pre-existing arterial or venous insufficiency are at much higher risk for infection, as well as poor soft tissue and bone healing. This increased risk is also seen in patients with diabetes, especially if a peripheral neuropathy is present. This contingency bears emphasis because inexperienced clinicians may have a tendency to overlook these facts in their preoccupation with the details of the injury. It is also important to note that the presence of an acute vascular injury or compartment syndrome significantly worsens the patient's prognosis. The neurologic and circulatory status of any injured extremity must be evaluated, and patients with compromised vascular or neurologic function should be referred to an orthopaedist immediately.

In addition, the following injuries should

be referred whether obvious arterial, venous, or neurologic injury has occurred: (*a*) extensive muscle contusion, (*b*) unstable sprains and dislocations, and (*c*) compound (open) fractures and avulsions of the integument.

Evaluation and treatment of specific injuries will be described.

CONTUSIONS OF THE LEG

Anterior Compartment

Because the crural fascia is tough and tense over the anterior compartment, severe contusion and crush injuries such as a lower extremity caught between the bumpers of two cars can result in a compartment syndrome. Bleeding and edema into the confined anterior compartment can increase the tissue pressure to such an extent that ischemic necrosis of the muscle occurs. Because the skin over the anterior aspect of the leg is tightly bound to the crural fascia, it also tolerates swelling poorly, and contusions of the anterior skin commonly lead to necrosis of the central zone of the contused skin. The clinician must minimize swelling and closely watch for signs of anterior compartment muscle ischemia.

Treatment

Any associated abrasions must be scrubbed as free of ground dirt as possible, under local anesthesia using a surgical scrub brush. The extremity must be elevated moderately above heart level. Too little elevation will allow the swelling to continue; too much elevation will decrease the hydrostatic pressure of the arteriovenous gradient. Toe gripping exercises should be repeated every few minutes to encourage venous and lymphatic return. Ice packs should be applied over the injury for the first 24 to 48 hours. The leg should not be bound with a circular bandage because this will increase compartment pressure externally. Dorsiflexion of the ankle and extension of the toes should be attempted every 30 minutes for the first 12 hours and several times daily thereafter. Any decline in apparent strength or significant increase in pain with the effort suggests muscle ischemia. Pain alone can inhibit extensor tone, but many patients who are made aware of the importance of the test will generate a stronger movement with a well-perfused muscle than with an ischemic muscle. The inability to discriminate a sharp point from a dull touch over the dorsum of the foot can also suggest increased compartment pressure because of the pressure on the nerves. If at any point muscle ischemia or nerve compression is suspected, an orthopaedist must be consulted to evaluate the patient for compartment measurements or to consider fasciotomy. As swelling and pain subside, active stretching and working exercises of the anterior compartment are begun. The patient should avoid ambulation during the first 48 hours, except for bathroom needs, and then ambulation should be nonweightbearing with crutches. Partial weightbearing may begin when nonweightbearing ambulation and active exercises have been performed for 24 hours without an increase in pain or swelling.

Posterior Compartment

Contusions to the posterior compartment are less subject to the danger of muscle ischemia, and restorative treatment can proceed more rapidly. However, the principles above must be kept in mind. In the posterior compartment, the muscles to observe closely are those that plantar flex the ankles and toes. Active working and stretching exercises and weightbearing as tolerated can usually begin after 24 to 48 hours of ice and elevation.

Vigorous running and exposure to further contusion should be avoided until healing is complete, because repeated intramuscular bleeding can cause myositis ossificans.

FRACTURES OF THE SHAFTS OF THE TIBIA AND FIBULA

The tibia is fractured more frequently than any other long bone. Fractures of the tibia and fibula can occur anywhere along the length of the bones. Fractures may be open (compound) or closed (simple), displaced or undisplaced, angulated or not angulated, stable or unstable.

Fractures of the tibia and fibula can be associated with acute compartment syndromes, and diligent monitoring of the neurovascular condition, as noted above, is mandatory. It is important to categorize tibia and fibula shaft fractures with each of the above descriptions to help with treatment decisions and to communicate information to a consulting orthopaedist.

A closed fracture is a fracture in which the skin of the lower leg is not broken. An open fracture is classified according to the degree of skin disruption and whether or not there is periosteal stripping, soft tissue loss, blood vessel disruption, or gross contamination (Table 8.1). It must be understood that the open fracture does not decompress compartments and, therefore, does not preclude the danger of compartment syndrome. Open fractures should be covered with an antiseptic solution such as povidone-iodine (Betadine) and a bulky sterile dressing, splinted, and transferred to the care of an orthopaedic surgeon. The wound and fracture ends will then be thoroughly irrigated and debrided, and the fracture will be treated with casting, external fixation, or open reduction and internal fixation. A vascular surgeon will be consulted if vascular injury is present. Displacement of less than 50% in either anteroposterior or lateral planes is adequate reduction, and angulation of less than 10° in the anteroposterior plane or less than 5° in the lateral plane is usually acceptable. Shortening of the extremity less than 2 cm is also acceptable.

Stability of the reduction is a function of the configuration of the fracture, the degree of comminution, and extent of periosteal disruption. A useful definition of an unstable fracture is one in which acceptable position and length cannot be easily maintained with a well-applied cast immobilizing the joint above and below the fracture. Usually, short oblique fractures are less stable than transverse fractures. Comminuted fractures are often unstable. Unstable fractures should be referred to an orthopaedic surgeon.

Careful neurovascular evaluation must be performed and repeated at frequent intervals on all extremities that have sustained a tibial or fibular fracture. An acute compartment syndrome can result in loss of function of the extremity. Compartment syndromes can occur in any or all of the four compartments of the lower leg, and evaluation as previously described in the section on "Contusions of the Leg" is mandatory. If any question of compartment syndrome exists, immediate referral to an orthopaedist is required because a fasciotomy may be indicated.

Role of the Primary Practitioner

The primary practitioner should evaluate and describe the injury. A neurovascular examination should be performed initially and repeated frequently. Open wounds should be dressed, the limb placed in a splint without tight circular bandages, and ice applied to the injured extremity. Prompt consultation with an orthopaedic surgeon should be the routine.

Table 8.1. Open Fracture Classifications[a]

Grade	Wound	Comment
I	<1 cm	This is usually a low-energy injury in which the skin defect is frequently caused by the bone piercing the skin from inside to outside, rather than from penetrating trauma.
II	>1 cm but <10 cm	Moderate energy trauma, without gross contamination.
III	>10 cm	High-energy trauma; this grade is also attributed to injuries with any size wound where there is marked skin loss, periosteal stripping, gross contamination (as in farm injuries), vascular compromise, or segmental bone injury.

[a]Adapted from Chapman MW. The role of intramedullary fixation in open fractures. Clin Orthop 1986;212:27; and from Gustilo RB, Anderson JT. Prevention of infection in the treatment of one thousand and twenty-five open fractures of long bones: retrospective and prospective analyses. J Bone Joint Surg 1976;58A:453–458.

In some cases, it is appropriate for an experienced practitioner to definitively treat tibial shaft fractures. These would include noncomminuted, closed fractures in which a satisfactory position is present initially or in which a stable acceptable position can be obtained with closed manipulation and cast application. The extremity must have a normal neurovascular examination. Acceptable position and angulation are noted above.

A long-leg cast is applied with the knee in 30 to 45° of flexion. Radiographs taken after reduction must confirm acceptable position. The patient is admitted to the hospital, and the limb is elevated with ice packs over the fracture site. Frequent neurovascular examinations are performed to ensure that no compartment syndrome is developing. After 48 hours, the patient may begin nonweightbearing ambulation. The long-leg cast is kept on for 4 to 6 weeks and is followed by a patellar tendon bearing cast for the next 4 to 6 weeks. The patient can often be at a partial weightbearing status at this point. A short-leg cast is then applied for an additional 4 to 6 weeks with weightbearing as tolerated. If healing has not occurred by this time, referral to an orthopaedist is recommended. Should a compartment syndrome start to develop after the cast is applied, the cast is split along the medial and lateral sides, and the top half is discarded, effectively leaving a posterior splint. If the examination does not rapidly improve, prompt referral is mandatory.

Fibular shaft fractures in the proximal two-thirds of the bone are most commonly the result of a direct blow. Uneventful healing is the usual case. The ankle should be included in the radiographs and clinical examination to ensure that there is no injury or displacement of the talus within the mortise. Also, careful examination for a compartment syndrome is performed. If no ankle injury is evident by examination and by x-ray, and the neurovascular examination is normal, a short-leg walking cast or functional walking brace is applied mostly for comfort. The fracture will usually heal even without the cast. The patient should be instructed to keep the extremity elevated for at least 48 hours with ice packs, frequently move the toes and check them for color and sensation, and return if any problems develop. The cast or brace is kept on for 4 to 6 weeks.

ANKLE INJURIES

Ankle Sprains

Ankle sprains are common injuries seen in every emergency department. They occur in both athletes and nonathletes. Ankle sprains are commonly misunderstood and underestimated by both the patient and many physicians.

The most common mechanism of injury that produces ankle sprains is a supination or inversion force. This occurs when the foot turns under the ankle after walking or running on uneven surfaces, during an athletic event when the upper body is twisted over the planted foot, or when landing on the inverted foot after a jump. The result is stretching or tearing of the ligaments of the lateral side of the ankle. The most common ligament injured is the anterior talofibular ligament, followed by injury to the calcaneofibular ligament, and rarely, the posterior talofibular ligament. The fibulocalcaneal ligament is also more commonly injured if the ankle is in the dorsiflexed position at the time of injury (Fig. 8.19).

Clinical Characteristics

Examination of a patient with an ankle sprain reveals a variable amount of swelling and tenderness over and around the lateral malleolus. The severity of the injury can often be estimated by the history. Mild sprains will allow the patient to walk soon after the injury, whereas severe injuries will be such that the patient cannot walk immediately. The amount of swelling is often an indication of the severity of the injury as well. If a person is examined within a few minutes of the injury, location of the tenderness over the specific ligament can help the examiner determine which ligaments have been injured (Fig. 8.20). In most instances by the time the patient is examined, the swelling and tenderness are diffuse, and

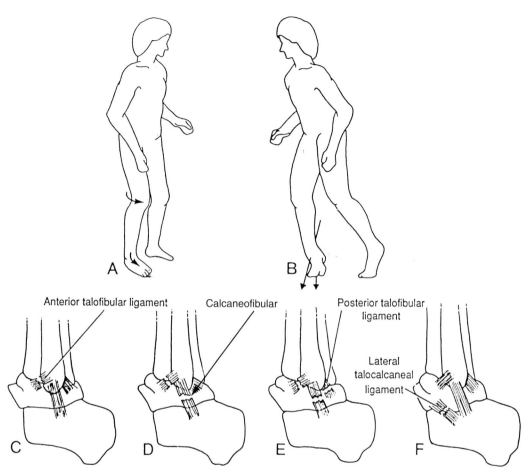

Figure 8.19. *A* and *B*, modes of injury. *A*, by convention, deformities are measured from distal as related to proximal. Therefore, in this supinated foot, as the leg internally rotates on the planted foot, the foot is relatively externally rotated. Thus, this is a supination external rotation injury. *B*, plantar flexed foot is forced into supination. *C* through *E*, sequence of injury to the ligaments based on severing of the force producing the injury. *F*, the lateral talocalcaneal ligament also may be injured and can contribute to subtalar instability, which may follow ankle sprains.

determination of the specific ligaments injured is more difficult.

Tests for ankle instability, such as the anterior drawer and varus stress tests, can assist in determining the severity of ligamentous disruption if performed before the onset of severe swelling or soon after the swelling has diminished (Figs. 8.21A, and 8.21B).

Radiographic studies are necessary to rule out fractures of the malleoli, talus, and foot. In reviewing the ankle radiographs, it is important to specifically look for certain bony injuries that can occur after the inversion stress. These include osteochondral fracture of the talus, fractures of the lateral process of the talus, fractures of the posterior tubercle of the talus, fractures of the anterior process of the calcaneus, and fractures of the base of the fifth metatarsal. Treatment of these injuries will be discussed in Chapter 9, Foot (Fig. 8.22).

Treatment

If radiographs are negative, initial treatment is aimed at controlling the swelling and pain about the ankle. This is accomplished by splinting the foot and ankle in a neutral position. A simple posterior plaster splint often breaks down within a day or two and is not recommended. A U-shaped, short-leg stirrup splint extending around the ankle, heel, and midfoot, over a bulky compressive dressing, provides comfortable, sturdy immobilization. The foot is wrapped with a cotton roll, if available, and cotton padding as if a cast were to be applied. A splint is then made of 4- or 5-inch plaster, depending on the patient's size, and applied in a stirrup fashion using 10 to 12 thicknesses of plaster. This is held in place by an elastic bandage applied without excessive tension around the entire dressing (Fig. 8.23).

Ice is then applied for 20 minutes every 4 hours, and elevation above the heart is observed. The patient is encouraged to move the toes in the dressing. Three to five days after the injury, the patient returns and the dressing is removed. Usually, the swelling has resolved substantially, and a re-examination is performed in an attempt to localize the ligaments injured and to reassess the stability of the ankle.

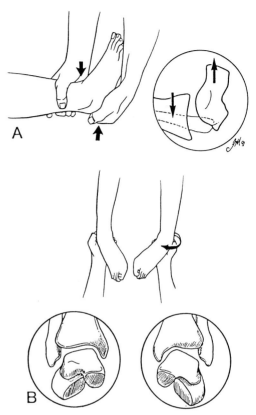

Figure 8.21. *A,* anterior drawer test. While holding the tibia steady, the heel is grasped and directed forward. A lateral radiograph is taken and will show 3 mm or greater anterior displacement if positive. *B,* varus (inversion) stress test. Both heels are grasped and a supination force is applied. Mortise radiographs are taken of both ankles. A difference in the tibiotalar joint angle of 10° or greater is an indication of significant lateral ligament injury.

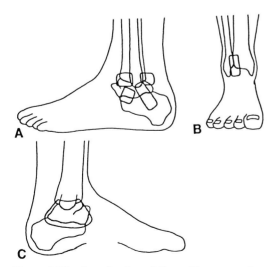

Figure 8.20. Examination of the ankle: zones of tenderness of the individual ligaments. *A,* the lateral ligaments. *B,* the anterior-inferior tibiofibular ligament. *C,* the deltoid ligament.

The treatment of ligamentous disruptions is controversial. Some practitioners recommend symptomatic treatment and suggest range of motion exercises and ambulation "as tolerated" with a stirrup ankle brace. The other extreme is routine operative repair of injuries involving several ligaments. Most ankle sprains can be treated successfully with nonoperative measures. The exception would be the grossly unstable ankle, either at the time of injury or on subsequent follow-up. Obvious instability of the ankle is present to inversion or anterior stress. Operative repair

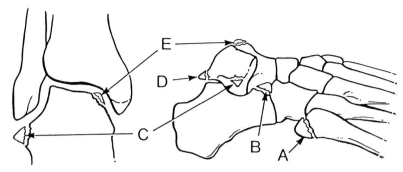

Figure 8.22. Schematic of fractures occasionally missed during a twisting injury to the ankle. *A*, base of the fifth metatarsal. *B*, anterior process of the calcaneus. *C*, lateral process of the talus. *D*, posterior tubercle of the talus. *E*, osteochondral fracture of the talus.

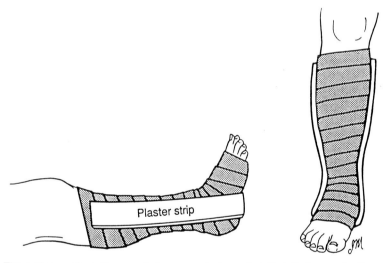

Plaster strip

Figure 8.23. The author prefers stirrup splint over posterior splint. Details for application are noted in the text.

is especially considered in the competitive or serious recreational athlete.

After removal of the initial dressing, if the ankle is still markedly tender and range of motion is painful, the patient is placed in a short-leg walking cast for 2 to 4 weeks. Physical therapy follows with range of motion exercises, peroneal strengthening, and proprioceptive training. Once range of motion is normal and ankle strength returns, the patient may return to normal activities.

For many patients, return to activity can be hastened by physical therapy after the initial dressing is removed. The competitive or serious recreational athlete is usually willing to devote the time and effort to such therapy, which consists of early range of motion exercises, the use of electrical stimulation to decrease swelling, and sequential compressive dressings. Once the swelling is under control and range of motion approaches normal, peroneal strengthening is begun. This is followed by proprioceptive training, and the use of a stirrup brace is begun to start the return to athletics. The athlete can progress with rehabilitation as comfort allows. A return to athletic activity is allowed when the patient feels the ankle is at least 90% recovered and is able to perform the usual demands of the activity.

In milder ankle sprains in which the patient can walk soon after the sprain, a more progressive return is indicated. Rather than splinting, protection can be provided with prefabricated plastic stirrups with an air or gel bladder. Patients who have sustained ankle sprains should

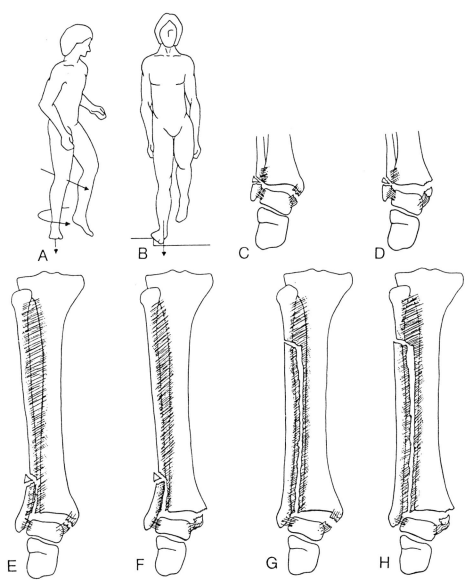

Figure 8.24. Pronation injuries of the ankle. *A* and *B*, modes of injury. *A*, extremity rotates internally on the fixed foot. *B*, the foot is forced into pronation by weight taken on the lateral aspect of the forefoot. *C* and *D*, the medial injury may be ligamentous or involve a fracture of the medial malleolus. The fibular fracture is frequently comminuted. *E*, *F*, *G*, and *H*, the fibular fracture can occur at any level, with an accompanying tear of the interosseous membrane up to the level of the fracture. Note that the medial injury can be either ligamentous or bony.

be advised that residual tenderness, a propensity to swell after activity, and pain on inversion of the injured ankle commonly persist for 6 to 12 weeks and may be present for 6 or more months after the injury.

Patients who have continued pain after 3 months or problems with ankle instability should be referred to an orthopaedist for evaluation and possibly reconstructive surgery.

Eversion ankle sprains are much less common than inversion injuries. These will present with medial tenderness and involve injury to the deltoid ligament. Eversion injuries are frequently accompanied by injuries to the syndesmotic ligament or fractures of the fibula, and these must be carefully evaluated. The treatment philosophy is similar to inversion injuries, in which control of swelling is followed by immobilization and physical therapy.

Fractures of the Ankle

Fractures of the ankle are common injuries. The fracture pattern is the result of the forces applied to the ankle at the time of injury. Fractures may involve the distal fibula alone, or occur in combination with a fracture or ligamentous injury of the medial ankle. Fractures that involve the medial malleolus alone are uncommon, and a careful search for additional injury on the lateral side of the ankle must be performed. This should include radiographs of the entire leg, because a fibular fracture may occur anywhere along the length of the bone. Also, a tear of the interosseous ligament will often occur in certain fracture patterns, especially those with a more proximal fibular fracture and a medial malleolar fracture.

Clinical Characteristics

The examination of a patient who has sustained an ankle fracture includes a thorough examination of the skin and the neurovascular status of the injured extremity. The location of the tenderness and the areas of swelling will give clues to which portions of the ankle have sustained either bony or ligamentous injury. Any gross deformity in the alignment of the ankle can be a sign of a fracture or

dislocation, and severe displacement should be reduced immediately if the skin or neurovascular structures are at risk.

Radiographs are necessary and should include AP, lateral, and an internal oblique view to visualize the ankle mortise. In cases in which there is a medial fracture but no obvious lateral fracture or, in cases in which there is lateral tenderness but no lateral fracture, radiographs of the entire leg should be per-

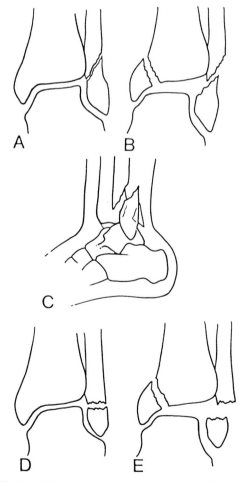

Figure 8.25. *A* and *B*, supination injury with external rotation produces a spiral fibular fracture with or without an accompanying fracture of the medial malleolus. *C*, lateral view of supination, external rotation injury. *D* and *E*, supination injury with the foot in adduction results in an avulsion fracture of the fibula with or without a fracture of the medial malleolus.

formed to check for a more proximal fibular fracture.

The specific pattern of injury at the ankle is largely a function of the direction of forces applied to the ankle and foot at the time of injury. Pronation injuries may be associated with an abduction force or an external rotational force. Those associated with an abduction force produce either a ligamentous tear of the deltoid ligament or an avulsion fracture of the medial malleolus. The fibular fracture is often comminuted and appears as a crush-type injury. Those associated with an external rotational force produce a similar medial lesion, but the interosseous ligament is often torn and the fibular fracture is often spiral with the spike of the distal fragment noted anteriorly (Fig. 8.24).

Supination injuries may be associated with an adduction or an external rotational force. In adduction injuries, the medial fracture is often vertical, and the fibular fracture is avulsed. In external rotational injuries, the medial malleolus is often avulsed, and the fibula sustains a spiral fracture usually at the joint line and with the spike of the distal fragment noted posteriorly (Fig. 8.25).

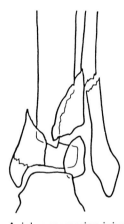

Figure 8.26. Axial compression injury produces severe disruption and fragmentation of the distal tibia. These injuries are difficult to treat. (Adapted with permission from Mast J. Reduction Techniques in Fractures of the Distal Tibial Articular Surface. Techniques in Orthopaedics. Vol 2. Frederick, MD: Aspen Publishers, Inc, 1987:30.)

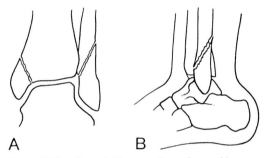

A   B

Figure 8.28. Acceptable reduction of an ankle fracture results in virtually an anatomic position on the mortise radiograph and less than 3 mm displacement of the nonarticular portion of the fibula; fracture on the lateral view.

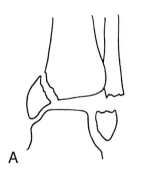

A

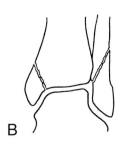

B

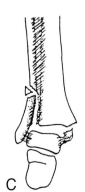

C

Figure 8.27. Weber classification of ankle fractures. *A,* fibular fracture is below the ankle joint line. *B,* fibular fracture begins at the ankle joint line. *C,* fibular fracture is above the ankle joint line.

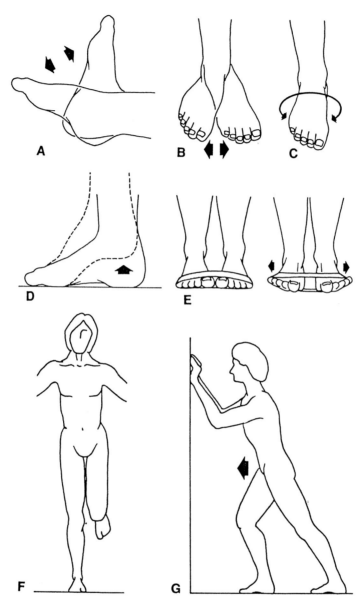

Figure 8.29. Range of motion and strengthening exercises of the foot and ankle. *A*, active movement of the tibiotalar joint by alternate dorsiflexion and plantarflexion. *B*, active movement of the subtalar, intertarsal, and tarsometatarsal joints by alternate supination and pronation. *C*, active movement of the tibiotalar, subtalar, intertarsal, and tarsometatarsal joints by circling the foot. *D*, repeated elevation onto the toes when standing. *E*, pronation and abduction against elastic resistance. *F*, balancing on one foot. *G*, heel cord stretching.

Axial compression forces can produce dramatically comminuted fractures of the tibial plafond (Fig. 8.26) and are referred to as pylon fractures.

Classification systems range from simple to complex. These classifications are used not only for communication purposes but also as complex systems to infer mechanisms of injury, for probable structures injured, and for prognostic purposes. The Weber classification is simple and useful when communicating to an orthopaedist. This classification describes the location of the fibular fracture, as shown in Figure 8.27.

Treatment

A displacement of 1 to 2 mm of the talus within the mortise reduces the area of contact force between the tibia and talus by 42%. Consequently, this dramatically increases the degree of force on the remaining articular joint. These abnormal stresses can predispose to traumatic arthritis over time. Because of this predisposition, anatomic restoration of displaced fractures or dislocations of the ankle is a routine goal of treatment. Fortunately, the techniques of open reduction and internal fixation have improved substantially, and if closed treatment cannot provide anatomic reduction, it can now be safely and almost routinely achieved by surgical means.

An anatomic result is one in which the subchondral plate of the tibia is continuous and does not show more than 1 mm of step-off or displacement on any radiographic view of the ankle. The subchondral margin of the fibula likewise should show less than 1 mm of step-off or displacement. The joint space between the talus, and the tibia and fibula should be symmetrical on the mortise view, and the displacement of the nonarticular portion of the fibula less than 3 mm on the lateral radiograph. Any result of a closed reduction that does not meet these criteria should be referred to an orthopaedist for possible internal fixation (Fig. 8.28).

From a practical standpoint, this means that all fractures or fractures with ligamentous injury that occur on both sides of the ankle joint are best managed by consultation with an orthopaedist. Closed treatment of bimalleolar injuries requires a specific reduction and casting technique, and subsequent displacement often occurs.

When a fracture apparently involves the fibula alone, it is important to be sure that there is no medial tenderness or widening of the medial joint space, which indicates a deltoid ligament injury. When there is no medial injury and the displacement of the nonarticular portion of the fibula is less than 3 mm on the lateral view, the fracture can be treated with a short-leg cast for 6 weeks. A follow-up radiograph should be obtained at 2 weeks to ensure that no displacement occurs. To achieve range of motion and strengthening, physical therapy should follow the removal of the cast (Fig. 8.29).

SUGGESTED READINGS

D'Ambrosia R, Drez D Jr. Prevention and Treatment of Running Injuries. Thorofare, New Jersey: Charles Slack, Inc., 1982.

Lovell WW, Winter RB, eds. Pediatric Orthopedics. Vol 2. 2nd ed. Philadelphia: JB Lippincott, 1986.

Mann RA: Surgery of the Foot. 5th ed. St. Louis: CV Mosby Co., 1985.

Rockwood AR Jr, Williams KE, King RE. Fractures in Children. Vol 3. Philadelphia: JB Lippincott, 1984.

Rockwood CA Jr, Green DR. Fractures in Adults. Vol 2. 2nd ed. Philadelphia: JB Lippincott, 1984.

Torg JS, Vegso JJ, Torg E. Rehabilitation of Athletic Injuries. Chicago: Yearbook Medical Publishers, 1987.

Foot

Thom A. Tarquinio, M.D.

ESSENTIAL ANATOMY

BONES, JOINTS, AND LIGAMENTS

In this discussion, the foot will be divided into the hindfoot, midfoot, and forefoot. The hindfoot consists of the talus, the calcaneus, and the articulation between them called the subtalar joint. The midfoot includes the navicular, cuboid, and three cuneiforms. The forefoot is composed of the metatarsals and phalanges of the toes. The seven bones of the hindfoot and midfoot are collectively referred to as the tarsal bones (Figs. 9.1 and 9.2).

Hindfoot

The talus is divided into the larger posterior portion called the body and the rounded anterior end called the head, joined by the neck of the talus (Fig. 9.2). Because the talus is largely covered with articular cartilage, vascular supply has limited access. The main blood supply to the body of the talus enters at the level of the neck. Therefore, a fracture through the neck of the talus may cause loss of blood supply to the body, resulting in avascular necrosis of the talus. The body of the talus articulates with the ankle mortise above and the calcaneus below at the subtalar joint. Anteriorly, the head of the talus articulates with the navicular at the talonavicular joint.

The largest bone of the foot is the calcaneus (Fig. 9.2), which articulates with the talus above and the cuboid at its anterior end. The calcaneus has a large posterior portion called the tuberosity, which serves as the site of insertion of the Achilles tendon. The superior surface of the calcaneus is covered by three areas of articular cartilage, forming the posterior,

middle, and anterior facets of the subtalar joint. The subtalar joint is a stable articulation because of the corresponding irregular bony surfaces of the calcaneus and talus, plus the strong talocalcaneal interosseous ligaments. On the anterolateral aspect of the hindfoot, just in front of the lateral malleolus, is a sulcus between the calcaneus and talus called the sinus tarsi. The plantar, medial, and lateral surfaces of the calcaneus serve as the site of origin of several intrinsic muscles of the foot. The plantar aspect of the calcaneus also serves as the origin for the strong plantar ligaments of the foot, including the long plantar ligament, plantar calcaneocuboid ligament, and plantar calcaneonavicular (spring) ligament. These plantar ligaments are under tension during weightbearing and aid in maintaining the longitudinal arch. Although the calcaneus sits beneath the talus in the posterior aspect of the subtalar joint, the anterior ends of the talus and calcaneus diverge. Because of this divergence, the anterior end of the talus lies medially and slightly superiorly to the anterior end of the calcaneus.

Midfoot

The proximal surface of the navicular is cup-shaped to articulate with the head of the talus. Distally, the navicular articulates with the three cuneiform bones. The navicular sits at the apex of the medial longitudinal arch and is supported in this position by the strong spring ligament (calcaneonavicular ligament) and the posterior tibial tendon. The importance of the posterior tibial tendon in supporting the midfoot medially is demonstrated by the severe flatfoot deformity that may develop after rupture of this tendon, as discussed in a

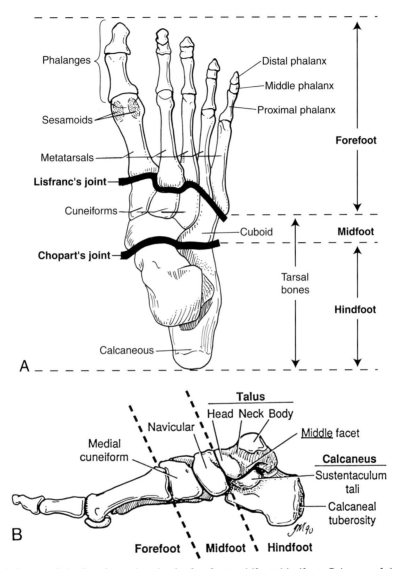

Figure 9.1. *A*, bones of the foot (superior view)—forefoot, midfoot, hindfoot. *B*, bones of the foot (medial view).

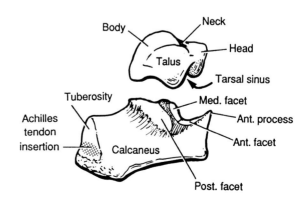

Figure 9.2. Lateral view of the hindfoot.

later section. The cuboid articulates proximally with the anterior end of the calcaneus on the lateral side of the midfoot and distally with the bases of the fourth and fifth metatarsals. The calcaneocuboid joint and the talonavicular joint together form the transverse tarsal joint, also referred to as Chopart's joint. Because of the obliquity between the subtalar joint and the transverse tarsal joint, the midfoot is flexible in pronation and becomes rigid (stable) in supination. The importance of this will be discussed in the section "Biomechanics of Gait."

The three cuneiform bones are called the medial, middle, and lateral cuneiforms, or the first, second, and third cuneiforms, respectively. Cuneiforms provide the articulation for their correspondingly numbered metatarsal bases. The relatively transverse tarsometatarsal joints are collectively referred to as the Lisfranc joint. The second metatarsal base extends slightly more proximally than the remaining metatarsal bases and is the keystone

of the Lisfranc joint, providing increased stability across the tarsometatarsal joint complex.

Forefoot

The five metatarsals are each composed of a base that articulates with a tarsal bone, a shaft, and an enlarged rounded distal end called the metatarsal head. The distal end of the metatarsal head provides the articular surface for the proximal phalanx of the toe, and the plantar surface of each metatarsal head is a major weightbearing surface of the foot. Beneath the first metatarsal head are the medial (tibial) and lateral (fibular) sesamoid bones, which are incorporated into the flexor hallucis brevis tendon. Transverse metatarsal ligaments connect the metatarsal heads. The relative lengths of the individual metatarsals are variable. Because of the plantar declination of the metatarsals as seen from the lateral view, a longer metatarsal will project further toward the plantar and may be subjected to greater weightbearing forces. Therefore, the ana-

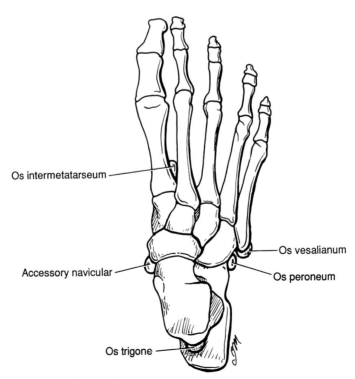

Figure 9.3.   Accessory ossicles of the foot.

tomic variability in the length of the metatarsals may cause or contribute to metatarsalgia. The great toe has only two phalanges (proximal and distal), whereas the second, third, and fourth toes have three phalanges (proximal, middle, and distal). The fifth toe may have either two or three phalanges.

Accessory Ossicles of the Foot

The foot has several accessory ossicles or separate ossification centers, which can be symptomatic or may be mistaken for a fracture (Fig. 9.3). The os trigonum and the os vesalianum are present in approximately 10% of adolescents and may be misdiagnosed as avulsion fractures. An accessory navicular bone may cause a painful prominence on the medial side of the midfoot. These ossicles may fuse to their adjacent bone in adulthood.

Muscles of the Foot

Active motion of the joints of the foot and active support of the foot during stance and gait are provided by the extrinsic muscles of the leg and intrinsic muscles of the foot. The extrinsic muscles (Fig. 9.4), described in Chapter 8, arise in the leg, and their tendons insert on the tarsals, metatarsals, and phalanges. The long extensor tendons (anterior tibial, extensor hallucis longus, extensor digitorum longus, and peroneus tertius) can be palpated individually on the dorsum of the foot and occasionally may be affected by pathologic conditions such as tendinitis, ganglion cysts, or tendon rupture. The extrinsic flexors include the posterior tibialis; the flexor digitorum longus and flexor hallucis longus tendons, which course behind the medial malleolus; and the peroneal longus and brevis tendons, which curve around the posterior aspect of the lateral malleolus. The posterior tibialis is the major supinator of the foot and is largely responsible for the dynamic support of the arch of the foot. This important tendon can be palpated at the posterior edge of the medial malleolus and then along the medial side of the hindfoot and midfoot. The posterior tibialis and the peroneal tendons are the most common sites for tendinitis in the foot.

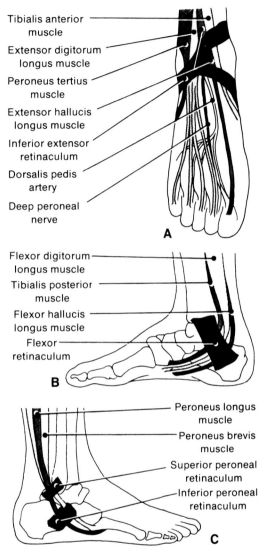

Figure 9.4. Extrinsic tendons of the foot. *A*, dorsal view. *B*, medial view. *C*, lateral view.

The intrinsic extensor muscles of the foot include the extensor digitorum brevis (which dorsiflexes the proximal phalanges of the middle three toes and occasionally the small toe), the extensor hallucis brevis (which dorsiflexes the proximal phalanx of the great toe), and the four dorsal interossei. The plantar intrinsics of the foot function as a group to provide flexion of the metatarsophalangeal joints and extension of the interphalangeal joints of the toes. Therefore, if plantar intrinsic function is lost,

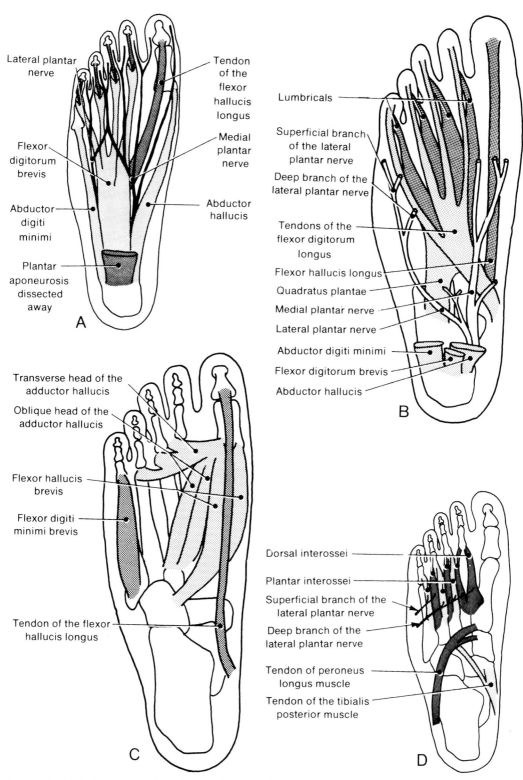

Figure 9.5. Intrinsic muscles of the foot. *A,* first layer (most superficial). *B,* second layer. *C,* third layer. *D,* fourth layer (most deep).

the metatarsophalangeal joints will extend and the interphalangeal joints will flex due to extrinsic tendon pull, causing a hammertoe or claw toe. The intrinsic muscles on the plantar aspect of the foot are arranged in layers along with the tendons of the long extrinsic flexors. These layers of the foot have significance for surgical procedures on the foot and are shown in Figure 9.5.

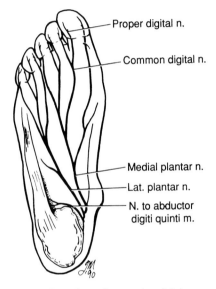

Figure 9.6. Branches of posterior tibial nerve on plantar aspect of the foot. (Adapted from Baxter DE, Thigpen CM. Heel pain — operative results. Foot Ankle 1984;5(1):16–25.)

INNERVATION AND BLOOD SUPPLY

The posterior tibial nerve courses behind the medial malleolus and then gives off one or more medial calcaneal branches, which supply sensation to the heel. The posterior tibial nerve then continues deep to the abductor hallucis muscle, dividing into the medial and lateral plantar nerves (Fig. 9.6). These nerves innervate the plantar intrinsic muscles and supply sensation to the remaining sole of the foot. The first branch of the lateral plantar nerve innervates the abductor digiti minimi, and compression of this nerve may cause plantar-medial heel pain.

The medial plantar nerve supplies sensory innervation to the medial half of the sole of the foot as well as the medial three and one-half toes, whereas the lateral plantar nerve supplies the lateral portion of the sole of the foot and the lateral one and one-half toes. Also, the medial plantar nerve supplies the innervation to the following intrinsic foot muscles: abductor hallucis, flexor hallucis brevis, flexor digitorum brevis, and first lumbrical. The lateral plantar nerve innervates the following intrinsic foot muscles: quadratus plantae, flexor digiti minimi, adductor hallucis, all interossei, and lateral three lumbricals. The sensation to the remainder of the foot is provided by the sural, saphenous, superficial peroneal, and deep peroneal nerves, as indicated in Figure 9.7.

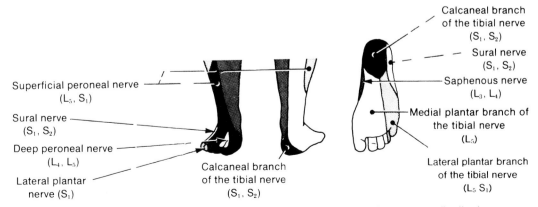

Figure 9.7. Sensory innervation of the foot by peripheral nerve and nerve root distribution.

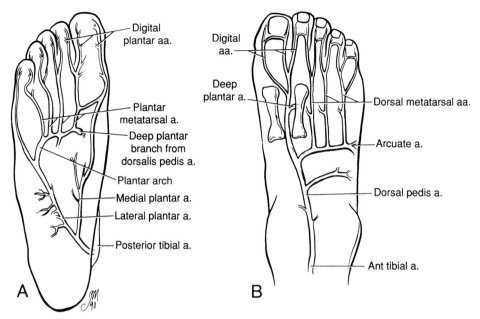

Figure 9.8. Circulation of the foot. *A,* branches of posterior tibial artery. *B,* branches of anterior tibial artery.

Circulation to the foot is derived from the posterior tibial artery and anterior tibial artery. The posterior tibial artery (Fig. 9.8A) curves behind the medial malleolus and then courses deep to the abductor hallucis muscle, where it divides into the smaller medial and larger lateral plantar arteries. The lateral plantar artery yields the plantar metatarsal arteries, which terminate in the common and digital arteries to the toes. The anterior tibial artery (Fig. 9.8B) becomes the dorsalis pedis artery just distal to the ankle joint, at which level it lies just laterally to the extensor hallucis longus tendon. The dorsalis pedis artery gives rise to the deep plantar artery and the arcuate artery, and then terminates as the first dorsal metatarsal artery.

BIOMECHANICS OF THE FOOT

DEFINITIONS OF FOOT POSTURE (FIG. 9.9)

The hindfoot is said to be in equinus when the talus and calcaneus are plantar flexed, e.g., heel cord tightness. The hindfoot is said to be in a calcaneus position when the talus and

the calcaneus (the bone) are dorsiflexed, e.g., loss of gastrocsoleus function after polio. Viewing the heel from behind, the hindfoot is in varus or inversion if the heel is inclined so that the heel pad is medial to the ankle. The hindfoot is in valgus or eversion when the heel is inclined so that the heel pad is lateral to the ankle.

Several terms are used to describe the position of the forefoot. When viewing the foot from the bottom, the metatarsals are normally in line with the hindfoot. Forefoot adduction means the metatarsals are angled medially toward the midline of the body when compared with the hindfoot. Metatarsus primus varus refers to adduction of the first metatarsal only, thereby increasing the angle between the first and second metatarsal shafts. Forefoot abduction means that the metatarsals are deviated laterally when compared with the hindfoot. If the forefoot is rotated around its long axis so that the sole of the foot is turned toward the midline of the body with the first metatarsal head higher than the fifth, the forefoot is said to be in varus, or supination. If the sole of the foot is rotated around its long axis so that the

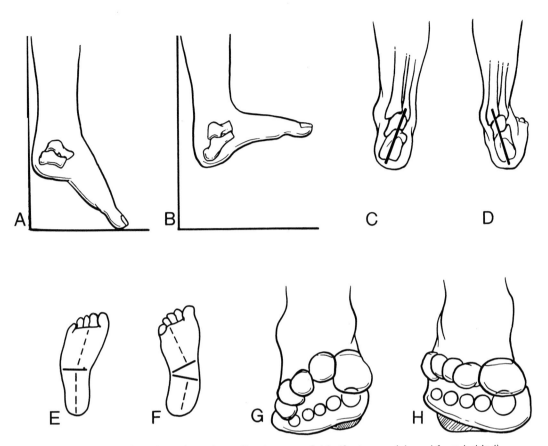

Figure 9.9. Postures of the foot. *A*, equinus. *B*, calcaneus. *C*, hindfoot varus (viewed from behind). *D*, hindfoot valgus (viewed from behind). *E*, metatarsus adductus (viewed from sole of foot). *F*, metatarsus abductus (viewed from sole of foot). *G*, forefoot supination (varus). *H*, forefoot pronation.

sole of the foot is turned away from the midline of the body with the first metatarsal head lower than the fifth, the forefoot is said to be in valgus, or pronation.

Motions of the ankle, hindfoot, midfoot, and forefoot are all interconnected. As the normal foot goes into plantar flexion at the ankle, the hindfoot goes into varus and the forefoot supinates and adducts. As the ankle dorsiflexes, the hindfoot goes into valgus and the forefoot pronates and abducts. Metatarsus adductus may occur alone or in association with forefoot varus (supination). In the sagittal plane, the foot is in a cavus position when the forefoot is plantarflexed excessively relative to the calcaneus (Fig. 9.10).

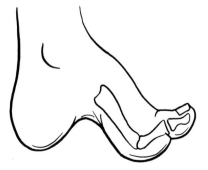

Figure 9.10. Cavus (high arch) foot. This deformity may be caused by calcaneus position of the hindfoot (see Fig. 9.9B) or equinus position of the forefoot.

BIOMECHANICS OF GAIT

The gait cycle during normal walking is divided into the stance phase and swing phase for each foot. Each foot is in stance phase for 62% of the cycle and swing phase for 38% of the cycle. Stance phase is further subdivided into three phases: (*a*) heel strike to foot flat, (*b*) period of foot flat, and (*c*) heel raise to toe-off. At the beginning and the end of each stance phase, there is a brief period of double limb support, during which time both feet are in contact with the floor.

First Phase (Heel Strike to Foot Flat)

As the heel strikes the ground, the anterior tibial and long toe extensors are active, allowing controlled plantar flexion and preventing foot slap. As the body weight progresses over the foot, the foot is loaded and passively pronates. The posterior tibial and the foot intrinsics are silent during this phase and provide no support for the foot. As previously mentioned, the transverse tarsal joints are flexible in the pronated position, allowing the foot to adapt to the ground during the first phase of stance. Although some pronation is normal during stance phase of gait, excessive pronation may cause foot pain.

Second Phase (Foot Flat to Heel Raise)

During the second phase of gait, the foot is flat on the ground, and the ankle passively dorsiflexes as the tibia passes forward over the fixed foot. The gastrocsoleus complex fires at this point to limit the forward motion of the tibia, which allows the knee to passively extend. At this time, the posterior tibialis and the foot intrinsics begin to function actively, causing the foot to supinate and the heel to invert. This supinated position of the foot provides stability to the foot in preparation for push-off. In a patient with an equinus contracture, the ankle cannot dorsiflex, so pressure is increased beneath the forefoot during this phase of gait, which may result in metatarsalgia or forefoot plantar callus formation. If the posterior tibial tendon is not functioning (because of paralysis or tendon rupture), the foot cannot actively be converted to the stable supinated position. Push-off then occurs with the foot in the flexible pronated position, resulting in foot strain and pain.

Third Phase (Heel Raise to Toe Off)

During the third phase of gait, the heel raises off the ground as body weight is progressively increased on the forefoot. The posterior tibialis and the foot intrinsics progressively supinate the foot to provide a more rigid structure for push-off. The windlass effect of the plantar fascia also assists in supination of the foot and elevation of the plantar arch during push-off as the metatarsophalangeal joints passively extend when the patient "walks over" the metatarsophalangeal joints (Fig. 9.11). The triceps surae, peroneals, and long toe flexors all actively fire at this point to assist in push-off. During this phase of gait, the vertical load on the forefoot is 20% greater than body weight.

BIOMECHANICS OF RUNNING

The gait cycle, as just described for walking, is altered when running. However, there is no period when both feet are on the ground, and instead, there is a period of time when both feet are off the ground. The pronation to supination seen during walking still occurs, but this change in position occurs much more rapidly when running. Also, the peak vertical loads when running can reach many times body weight. Because of the rapid change of position of the foot, increased vertical loads, and the repetitive nature of running, patients may develop symptoms in the foot not seen during normal walking.

EVALUATION OF THE PATIENT WITH FOOT SYMPTOMS

PHYSICAL EXAMINATION

The examination of the foot may vary slightly when evaluating a toddler for intoeing, a young adult after a specific trauma, or a geriatric patient with chronic foot pain. However, important basic principles should

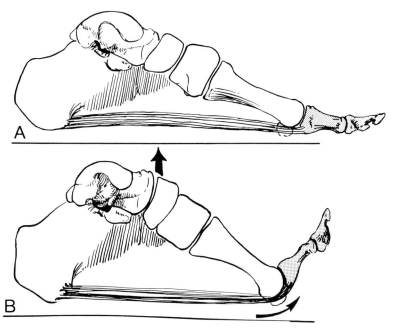

Figure 9.11. Windlass mechanism. When toes are dorsiflexed, the plantar aponeurosis becomes tight. This raises longitudinal arch and assists in creating a stable supinated foot for push-off. (Reprinted with permission from Mann R, ed. Surgery of the Foot. 5th ed. St. Louis: The CV Mosby Co, 1986:11.)

be understood for any foot examination. The foot must always be examined in non-weightbearing (sitting), standing, and walking positions.

For most clinical problems, the examination begins by observing the feet with the patient sitting and the feet hanging over the side of the examination table. Observation may reveal swelling, color change, fixed deformity such as rigid flatfoot, or evidence of superficial infection. The skin is examined for changes such as corns and calluses, plantar warts, or areas of ulceration. Temperature and pedal pulses are evaluated by palpation or Doppler studies, if clinically indicated. Next, each range of motion of the ankle, subtalar joint, midtarsal joints, and metatarsophalangeal joints and toes is evaluated. The motor, sensory, and deep tendon reflex examination is performed while the patient is sitting. Careful palpation will reveal areas of tenderness, and accurate location of tenderness based on a knowledge of anatomy is extremely important.

The patient is asked to stand and the overall alignment of the legs evaluated. Leg length is evaluated by checking for a level pelvis during stance. Thigh and calf atrophy may be observed during stance. As the patient stands, the amount of heel varus or valgus and the height of the plantar arch are observed.

Next, the patient is asked to perform toe raises, and the foot is observed to make sure that normal varus of the heel and supination of the foot occur. The patient is then asked to walk, and any limp is evaluated. The examiner also checks for in-toeing or out-toeing. The examiner should try to determine whether the foot normally pronates during initial stance phase and then supinates at push-off.

Many foot deformities may result in unusual patterns of shoe wear and, therefore, the patient's shoes should be evaluated.

RADIOGRAPHIC EVALUATION

Some foot complaints may be evaluated adequately without x-rays, but the primary care physician should be aware of certain radiographic studies that often are helpful in evaluating foot symptoms. Routine radiographs are satisfactory in the evaluation of most foot disorders (Fig. 9.12). Anteroposterior (AP), lateral, and oblique views are necessary for evaluating trauma, suspected osteomyelitis, or tumors. Standing AP and lateral radiographs provide valuable information in disorders such as flatfeet, hallux valgus, and some congenital abnormalities. The Harris axial view of the heel is useful in the evaluation of the calcaneus and talocalcaneal coalition. Technetium bone scans may be useful in suspected cases of osteomyelitis or stress fractures when plain radiographs are normal or equivocal. Computed tomography (CT) scan of the hindfoot often provides more information about the os calcis, talus, ankle joint, and subtalar joint than can be obtained with plain radiographs. MRI is useful in evaluating soft tissue disorders such as tendinitis or tendon rupture, bone and soft tissue tumors, and osteomyelitis.

NONTRAUMATIC CONDITIONS IN ADULTHOOD

Pain and deformity are the most common complaints in adults presenting with a nontraumatic foot problem. The patient will usually relate symptoms to the hindfoot, midfoot, or forefoot and toes, and this section of the chapter will be subdivided on this basis. After the history is obtained, examination of the foot is performed following the principles previously described. At this point, a differential diagnosis is established and further evaluation and treatment planned. Radiographic evaluation, e.g., routine x-rays, bone scan, CT scan, or MRI, may then be appropriately ordered. For some foot disorders, blood tests may be helpful. Certain systemic diseases, such as diabetes or inflammatory disorders, may affect the foot and will be discussed separately.

HINDFOOT PAIN

One of the most common foot complaints is heel pain. The pain will usually be localized to the posterior aspect or the plantar surface of the heel. Less frequently, the medial or lateral side of the heel may be symptomatic. Common causes of posterior heel pain, such as Achilles tendinitis and calcaneal bursitis, were discussed in the previous chapter. Pain on the plantar aspect of the heel is usually caused by plantar fasciitis. Pain on the medial side of the heel may arise from the subtalar joint or the posterior tibial tendon. Lateral-sided heel pain may arise from subtalar joint pathology or a disorder of the peroneal tendons. A differential diagnosis of heel pain may therefore be developed by history alone, based on the location of the pain. Several common causes of heel pain are discussed next.

Plantar Fasciitis

An extremely common complaint is plantar heel pain secondary to plantar fasciitis. The patient typically will localize the pain to the distal medial aspect of the plantar surface of the heel pad at the site of origin of the plantar fascia. The pain is usually most severe when the patient first stands up in the morning or stands after prolonged sitting during the day. Pain may gradually worsen toward the end of the day and is usually relieved when the patient lies down at night.

The most dramatic physical finding is tenderness to palpation on the plantar aspect of the heel in the anteromedial aspect of the heel pad at the site of origin of the plantar fascia (Fig. 9.13). An x-ray may be normal or may show a plantar calcaneal spur. In addition to plantar fasciitis, other terms used to describe this syndrome include heel spur syndrome or plantar heel pain syndrome. The pain may result from inflammation or microtearing of the origin of the plantar fascia from the os calcis, or in some cases this syndrome is caused by entrapment of the nerve to the abductor digiti minimi on the plantar surface of the os calcis. The plantar calcaneal spur is more likely to be a radiographic result of the trauma and inflammation rather than the cause of the pain. This distinction is important because some patients falsely believe the pain is caused

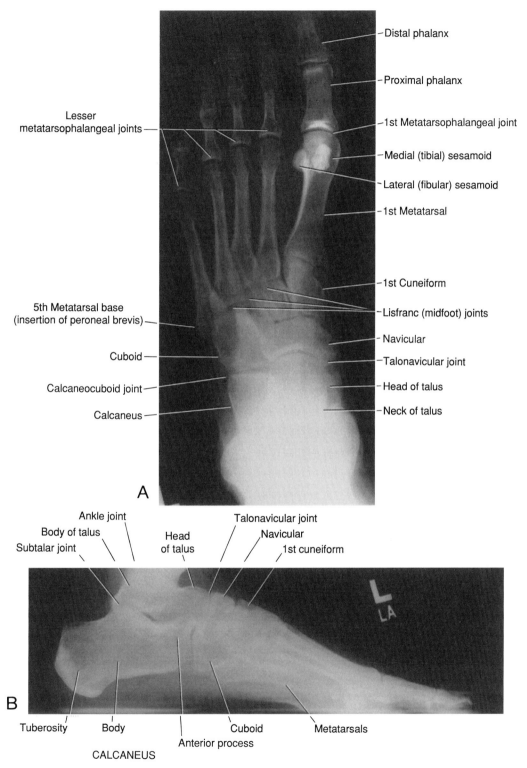

Figure 9.12. X-rays of the feet in a standing position. *A,* AP view. *B,* lateral view.

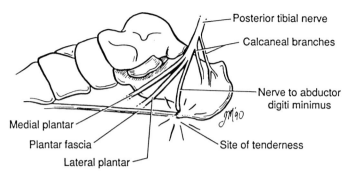

Figure 9.13. Plantar fasciitis. Note site of tenderness on plantar aspect of the heel at origin of plantar fascia off calcaneus. Also note course of nerve to abductor digiti minimi. (Adapted from Baxter DE, Thigpen CM. Heel pain—operative results. Foot Ankle 1984;5(1):16–25.)

by the spur and therefore can only be relieved by surgical excision of the spur. In actuality, the pain of plantar fasciitis will often be improved with passive stretching exercises, non-steroidal anti-inflammatory drugs (NSAIDs), rest, heel pads, heel cups, or inexpensive over-the-counter arch supports. As shown in Fig. 9.14, passive stretching exercises performed by the patient are more effective than physical therapy in relieving the pain of plantar fasciitis. The patient forcibly dorsiflexes the foot and the first metatarsophalangeal joint while simultaneously massaging the plantar fascia. The exercises must be done three times per day, but only for 2 to 3 minutes each time. If the patient has continued significant pain after the above conservative treatment modalities, the judicious use of steroid injection can be considered. Although steroid injection has been implicated as possibly contributing to rupture of the plantar fascia, one or two injections into the area of maximum tenderness on the plantar medial heel may be useful in severe cases of plantar fasciitis. The skin on the plantar aspect of the heel may be anesthetized with ethyl chloride spray to minimize the discomfort of the injection. Night splints that maintain the foot and ankle in maximum dorsiflex-

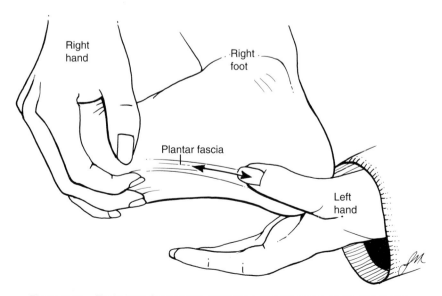

Figure 9.14. Technique for passive stretching and massage of plantar fascia.

ion may also decrease the pain of plantar fasciitis.

With the above conservative treatment measures, at least 90% of patients will have satisfactory pain relief. The small remaining group of patients require orthopaedic referral for consideration of surgery. Several different operative approaches used in treating this disorder include simple plantar fascial release, excision of the heel spur, neurolysis of the nerve to the abductor digiti minimi, or a combination of these procedures.

Subtalar Joint Pathology

Hindfoot pain or pain in the tarsal sinus anterior to the lateral malleolus, should alert the physician to carefully evaluate the subtalar joint on physical examination and radiographic studies. By allowing inversion and eversion of the heel, subtalar joint motion allows the foot to accommodate to uneven ground. Therefore, a patient being evaluated for hindfoot pain should be specifically questioned about pain or difficulty walking on uneven ground. If such history is present, subtalar joint pathology should be suspected. When asked to localize the pain, the patient with subtalar joint pathology will often grasp the heel from behind with the thumb and index finger below both malleoli. The pain may be felt medially or laterally, or on both sides of the hindfoot. On physical examination, the range of motion of the subtalar joint will be decreased or painful. Subtalar joint motion is examined with the ankle in dorsiflexion to lock the talus into the ankle mortise. The heel is grasped by the examiner's hand and rocked into varus and valgus. The symptoms and signs of pathology involving the subtalar joint are nonspecific and may be seen with inflammatory arthritis, posttraumatic arthritis, loose bodies, tumors, or tarsal coalitions. In addition to routine radiographs, the Harris axial view of the calcaneus and CT scanning are helpful in evaluating the subtalar joint.

Posterior Tibial Tendon Dysfunction

Posterior tibial tendon (PTT) dysfunction includes tenosynovitis, partial tendon rupture, complete tendon rupture, or avulsion of the insertion of the tendon into the navicular. Disorders of the posterior tibial tendon may result in pain anywhere along the course of the tendon, from above the medial malleolus, to the posteromedial side of the ankle, to the medial side of the midfoot. Partial or complete rupture of the posterior tibial tendon often occurs secondary to degeneration of the tendon, with an insidious onset, unlike the acute onset seen with Achilles tendon tear. The diagnosis of a ruptured posterior tibial tendon is rarely made at the time of rupture, and the primary care physician should be aware of the existence of this entity and the typical physical findings (Fig. 9.15). Frequently, a posterior tibial tendon tear is misdiagnosed as a "medial" ankle

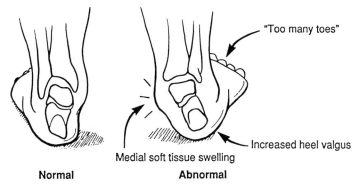

Figure 9.15. Physical findings in posterior tibial tendon rupture. Note soft tissue swelling behind medial malleolus and increased heel valgus. Because of forefoot abduction, "too many toes" will be visible on the affected side compared with the normal side when both feet are viewed from behind.

sprain. In addition to pain, there may be soft tissue swelling along the course of the tendon. When the posterior tibialis does not function, the foot loses its active supination at time of heel rise during gaits, and a flatfoot deformity may develop. The patient is unable to stand on tiptoes on the affected side or can do so only with pain. Normally, the heel will actively invert when the patient stands on tiptoes, but with PTT dysfunction, the heel will remain in valgus when the patient stands on tiptoes. With rupture of the posterior tibial tendon, the forefoot may also abduct or deviate laterally. When viewing the standing patient from behind, the examiner will see more toes on the affected foot than on the normal foot, the positive "too many toes" sign. Although posterior tibial tendon dysfunction initially causes pain on the medial side of the foot, the secondary deformity of hindfoot valgus and forefoot abduction may result in lateral foot pain, especially over the sinus tarsi. Active inversion of the foot against resistance will be decreased in PTT dysfunction, although the anterior tibialis and the long toe flexors may combine to give the appearance of active function of the posterior tibial tendon. Routine foot x-rays may be normal, although weight-bearing x-rays may show subtle malalignment of the foot, including loss of the plantar arch and lateral deviation of the forefoot. MRI of the foot may show abnormalities such as fluid around the posterior tibialis tendon or a tear of the tendon. However, the diagnosis is usually evident by history and physical examination, and it is usually unnecessary to obtain an MRI for PTT dysfunction.

Conservative treatment for mild posterior tibial tendinitis includes nonsteroidal anti-inflammatory medications, physical therapy, and the use of an ankle brace or an orthotic device. If partial or complete rupture of the posterior tibial tendon is suspected or if the symptoms do not resolve with the above treatment, referral should be made to an orthopaedic surgeon for further treatment. A delay in referral may have negative effects on the outcome in patients with posterior tibial tendon dysfunction if the patient develops a more complete tear or a more severe foot deformity. Further treatment might include a cast, although PTT dysfunction will often require surgical treatment such as tendon repair, tendon transfer, or fusion to correct the foot deformity.

MIDFOOT PAIN

Pain restricted to the area of the midfoot is relatively uncommon compared with pain in the hindfoot or forefoot. An accessory navicular (Fig. 9.3) may cause pain from shoe pressure or from stretch of the posterior tibial tendon as it passes around the accessory navicular. In addition to local tenderness over the accessory navicular, the foot may show increased pronation. An orthotic and nonsteroidal anti-inflammatory medication may relieve symptoms related to stress on the posterior tibial tendon. Steroid injections around the insertion of the posterior tibial tendon are generally contraindicated because of the increased risk of tendon rupture. A short-leg walking cast for 3 to 4 weeks may relieve the pain of a symptomatic accessory navicular. If conservative treatment does not relieve symptoms, surgical excision of the accessory navicular may be indicated.

Another cause of pain in the midfoot is a tarsal boss, which is an osteophyte or bone spur on the dorsum of the midfoot. This osteophyte is usually small but easily palpated on the dorsum of the foot and may be tender on palpation. The tarsal boss may be painful from direct shoe pressure or may lead to extensor tendinitis from irritation of the extensor tendons by the osteophytes. Shoes with a softer, well-padded tongue may be successful in relieving the pain from the dorsal osteophytes. Surgical excision of a tarsal boss is occasionally necessary.

The dorsolateral aspect of the midfoot is a common site for ganglion cysts, which are another cause of midfoot pain. The soft tissue mass can be aspirated, yielding the typical jellylike material of a ganglion cyst, thereby confirming the diagnosis. After aspiration of the cyst, it can be injected with a small amount of steroid preparation. Injection with steroids may decrease the recurrence rate after aspiration of a ganglion. Aspiration will result in resolution of approximately 50% of foot ganglions. An asymptomatic ganglion cyst does not necessarily need to be surgically excised, but a symptomatic ganglion cyst can usually be excised under local anesthesia.

Plantar fibromatosis is a locally aggressive, frequently bilateral process that occurs as a painful nodule or multiple nodules involving the plantar fascia. Initially, tenderness may be present along the entire course of the plantar fascia, and the patient may be seen before development of palpable nodules. As the process continues, however, one to several soft tissue masses develop along the course of the plantar fascia. Although not a malignant process, plantar fibromatosis may recur after surgical excision. Because of this high rate of recurrence, simple excision of the nodule is not recommended. The incidence of recurrence is decreased by surgically excising a large margin of normal plantar fascia rather than simply excising the individual fibrous nodules. However, small plantar fibromas often become painless and need no active treatment.

FOREFOOT PAIN

Pain in the forefoot, with or without deformity, is one of the most common foot complaints for which patients will seek medical attention. Several common disorders involving the metatarsals, metatarsophalangeal joints, and toes will be seen by the primary care physician.

HALLUX VALGUS

The major cause of pain and deformity on the medial side of the forefoot is hallux valgus, which is a deviation of the great toe toward the lateral side of the foot (Fig. 9.16). This angular deformity occurs at the level of the metatarsophalangeal joint and is usually associated with an exostosis or prominence of the medial aspect of the first metatarsal head. An overlying bursa also may become inflamed. The combination of the angular deformity of

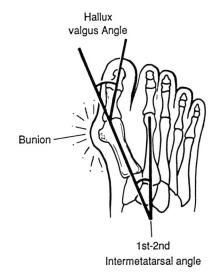

Figure 9.16. Hallux valgus. Lines demonstrate the hallux valgus angle and the first-second intermetatarsal angle.

the great toe and the medial prominence of the first metatarsal head is often referred to as a bunion. Metatarsus primus varus refers to angulation of the first metatarsal shaft away from the second metatarsal shaft, which predisposes to the development of the hallux valgus and a bunion. Hyperpronation of the foot also may predispose the patient to the development of hallux valgus. Hallux valgus is much more common in females, and there is often a positive family history. Extrinsic pressure by shoes undoubtedly also contributes to the development of hallux valgus.

Hallux valgus may be painful because of the development of bursitis or soft tissue inflammation over the bunion caused by shoe pressure. Conservative treatment for hallux valgus, therefore, begins with shoe modification. Many women prefer to wear "fashionable shoes," which often have high heels and a pointed toe. The pointed toe of the shoe forces the great toe into further valgus, and the high heel causes the body weight to be borne more directly by the already symptomatic forefoot. In addition to pain over the bunion, hallux valgus may cause a secondary painful deformity of the second toe. The valgus position of the great toe may result in an overriding second toe. The second toe is therefore pushed up against the inside of the shoe and may become symptomatic.

Treatment of hallux valgus begins with educating the patient about proper shoe shape and fit. The toe box of the shoe should be rounded rather than pointed, and the heel should be of minimum height. The shoe should be made of soft leather without seams over the bunion. If the patient has increased pronation, the shoe should have a good arch support or an orthosis should be added to the shoe to decrease pronation. Exercises and night splints are not helpful in the treatment of hallux valgus. Patients who have significant symptoms from hallux valgus in spite of shoe modifications should be referred to an orthopaedic surgeon for evaluation for surgical correction. Several different surgical procedures are used in the treatment of hallux valgus, depending on such factors as age of the patient, severity of the angular deformity, and associated foot deformities.

Hallux Rigidus

Hallux rigidus, an uncommon but sometimes very painful disorder of the great toe, is an unusual type of degenerative joint disease isolated to the first metatarsophalangeal joint. Unlike degenerative joint disease of other joints, hallux rigidus is often seen in young adults and may even occur in teenagers. Hallux rigidus, more common in male than female patients, usually occurs spontaneously, although there may be a history of a specific injury. Examination reveals palpable, tender osteophytes dorsally on the first metatarsophalangeal head (Fig. 9.17), rather than medially as in a bunion. The range of motion of the first metatarsophalangeal joint is decreased, and dorsiflexion is especially limited and painful. X-rays show osteophytes on the first metatarsal head as well as on the base of the proximal phalanx and varying degrees of sclerosis and loss of the joint space of the first metatarsophalangeal joint. Rest, nonsteroidal anti-inflammatory medications, and a stiff-soled shoe with a high toe box may provide some relief, but often surgical treatment is

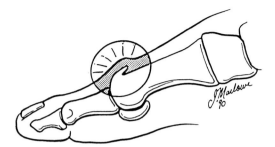

Figure 9.17. Hallux rigidus. Prominent dorsal osteophyte on first metatarsal head seen on lateral radiographic view.

required. Surgical options include cheilectomy (removal of the osteophytes), osteotomy, or fusion of the first metatarsophalangeal joint.

Lesser Metatarsal Pain

Pain in the area of the second through the fifth metatarsals (the so-called lesser metatarsals) is common and may have many causes. The term metatarsalgia is sometimes used nonspecifically to describe any pain in the area of the lesser metatarsals. However, this author prefers to use the term metatarsalgia specifically to describe pain beneath the metatarsal heads that is caused by abnormal weight distribution among the metatarsal heads. Common causes of lesser metatarsal pain include stress fractures, metatarsalgia, Morton's neuroma, Freiberg's infraction, and synovitis of the metatarsophalangeal joints.

Stress Fracture

Stress fractures, also called fatigue fractures or march fractures, may occur if a bone is mechanically weakened secondary to osteoporosis or other disease states, or when a bone is subjected to mechanical stresses of unusual severity. These severe mechanical stresses may occur in an individual who starts a new exercise program or rapidly increases his or her exercise level. Stress fractures are common in the lesser metatarsals, although they also occur in the calcaneus, tibia, fibula, and femur. Metatarsal stress fractures are more common in females than males. Bone will remodel in response to the increased mechanical demands, but a stress fracture may occur before the bone can adequately reinforce itself. If a patient presents with pain, swelling, and tenderness over the shaft or neck of one of the lesser metatarsals, a stress fracture should be suspected. X-rays may show periosteal new bone formation, sclerosis across the metatarsal shaft, a radiolucent fracture line, or the x-rays may be normal. If a stress fracture is suspected and x-rays are normal, repeat x-rays may show a stress fracture in 2 to 3 weeks. A technetium bone scan is the most sensitive technique for early diagnosis of a stress fracture, and a bone scan will often be "hot" before x-ray changes are seen. A stress fracture of a lesser metatarsal may be treated with crutches and decreased activities, but if symptomatic, the patient should be placed in a short-leg walking cast or removable boot walker for 3 weeks. Once the cast is removed, it is important that the patient be advised to return to the prior activity level on a very gradual basis. Orthotics also may be helpful in balancing metatarsal weightbearing.

Metatarsalgia

If one or more metatarsal heads are subjected to increased weightbearing stress, pain may occur beneath those metatarsal heads. This may occur if one metatarsal is longer or more plantar flexed than adjacent metatarsals. A hammertoe may cause metatarsalgia because the top of the shoe will press the toe down, which will secondarily depress the metatarsal head (Fig. 9.18), and the involved toe will not share the weightbearing function with the metatarsal head. Other causes of metatarsalgia include a tight heel cord and the habitual use of high-heeled shoes that may cause pain under several metatarsal heads. If one metatarsal head bears more than its fair share of weight over a long period, the skin beneath the metatarsal head may become thickened and hyperkeratotic, resulting in a corn or callus, also called a plantar keratosis (Fig. 9.19).

It is critical to understand that a corn or a callus beneath the metatarsal head is a re-

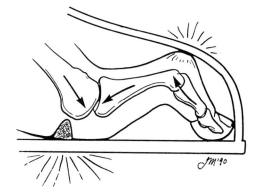

Figure 9.18. Hammertoe causing pain over top of proximal interphalangeal joint of the toe and beneath the metatarsal head. Either area also may develop a hyperkeratotic lesion (corn or callus). (Adapted with permission from Mann R, ed. Surgery of the Foot. 5th ed. St. Louis: The CV Mosby Co, 1986.)

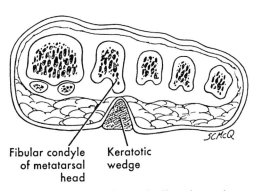

Fibular condyle   Keratotic
of metatarsal   wedge
head

Figure 9.19. Plantar keratosis. Hyperkeratotic lesion (corn) develops secondary to abnormally high weightbearing pressure by underlying metatarsal head. (Reprinted with permission from Crenshaw AH, ed. Campbell's Orthopaedics. 7th ed. St. Louis: The CB Mosby Co, 1987.)

sponse to increased pressure under the metatarsal head rather than a primary disease process. Therefore, to permanently cure a patient's pain by shaving or removing the callus is not possible. Unless something is done to distribute weightbearing more equally, the callus will always recur. However, temporary relief of symptoms can be obtained by carefully shaving down the plantar keratosis with a scalpel, stopping before bleeding occurs. Corn plasters with acid should be avoided because they can cause ulcerations. Modifications of the shoe with an orthosis, metatarsal pads, and lower heels may be the only treatment required for mild metatarsalgia. In severe cases, surgical realignment of the metatarsal may be required to balance the weightbearing among the metatarsal heads.

Morton's Neuroma

A common cause of forefoot pain is an interdigital neuroma, called a Morton's neuroma, which begins as an entrapment of the common digital nerve between the metatarsal heads (Fig. 9.20). The most common locations are between the third and fourth metatarsal heads or between the second and third metatarsal heads. This entrapment of the nerve will lead to an inflammatory process, and with time edema, perineural fibrosis, and demyelinization of the nerve will occur. The patient commonly complains of pain on the plantar aspect of the forefoot, beneath the metatarsal heads, or at the distal portion of the fat pad at the base of the toes. The pain is often poorly localized and may radiate to the toes or, occasionally, proximally up the foot. The patient may complain of a sensation of catching or clicking between the metatarsal heads and tingling or paresthesias of the toes. Patients with interdigital neuromas also frequently note that they feel like they have a "lump" or prominence under the ball of their foot.

The symptoms of a Morton's neuroma are usually worse with shoe wear and weightbearing and are relieved by shoe removal or rest. The key to the diagnosis is tenderness between the metatarsal heads, rather than directly beneath the metatarsal head as seen in metatarsalgia. Routine x-rays are normal, although in rare cases an MRI or ultrasound may be helpful in diagnosing a Morton's neuroma. Treatment includes shoes with a wider toe box and a soft sole, metatarsal pads or an orthosis, nonsteroidal anti-inflammatory medications, and steroid injections. The injec-

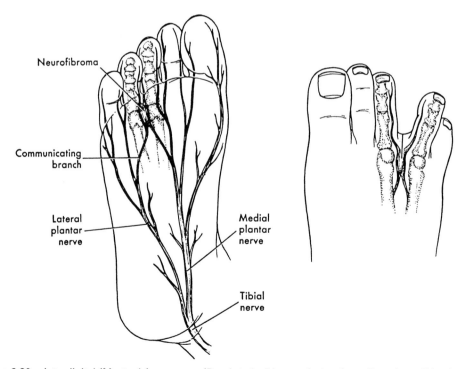

Figure 9.20. Interdigital (Morton's) neuroma. (Reprinted with permission from Crenshaw AH, ed. Campbell's Orthopaedics. 7th ed. St. Louis: The CV Mosby Co, 1987, and redrawn from McElvenny RY. J Bone Joint Surg 1943;25:675.)

tion is given through a dorsal approach between the involved metatarsal heads. The needle is passed between the metatarsal heads, and the steroid preparation is infiltrated in the plantar aspect of the foot. If severe symptoms persist, surgical excision of the neuroma may be performed, although reported rates of persistent pain after surgery have ranged from 10 to 30%.

Osteochondrosis of the Second Metatarsal Head (Freiberg's Infraction)

For unknown reasons (perhaps akin to Legg-Perthes) the head of the second metatarsal may undergo aseptic necrosis in adolescence. The young person will complain of forefoot pain, worsened by weightbearing or extreme movements of the second metatarsophalangeal joint. Examination reveals tenderness of the second metatarsal head and often swelling over the dorsum of the metatarsal head. X-ray confirms the necrotic process within 2 to 3 weeks of the onset of symptoms. Initially, fracture and fragmentation of the metatarsal head occurs, followed by new bone formation, resulting in a second metatarsal head that is flattened and enlarged with osteophytes.

If the pain is significant, the foot may be immobilized in a short-leg walking cast, in which the plantar surface extends beyond the toe. When the cast is removed, the patient should be taught range of motion and strengthening exercises for the ankle and foot. An orthosis or metatarsal pad may decrease the pain, although surgical treatment may be necessary.

Synovitis of the Metatarsophalangeal Joint

The second metatarsophalangeal joint (and less frequently, the third metatarsophalangeal joint) may develop synovitis, which presents as pain and swelling in the area of the involved metatarsophalangeal joint, sometimes with swelling of the involved toe. The patient may or may not have a history of a preexisting hammertoe of the involved toe. Physical examination will reveal tenderness directly over the metatarsophalangeal joint and pain with range of motion of the joint. The affected toe may be unstable if dorsal force is applied on examination. X-rays may be normal or may show joint space widening initially, but subsequent x-rays may show subluxation or complete dislocation of the metatarsophalangeal joint. Nonsteroidal anti-inflammatory medications and metatarsal pads may be helpful. If the joint progresses to subluxation or dislocation, surgical correction will usually be necessary.

Lesser Toe Pain

Other than pain radiating into the toes from a Morton's neuroma, pain in the lesser toes is usually caused by shoe pressure on a deformed toe. Common deformities are hammertoes, claw toes, and mallet toes, which may be dynamic (occurring only during gait) or fixed deformities (Fig. 9.21). These toe deformities have a variety of etiologies, including muscle imbalances, cavus feet, excessively pronated feet, arthritis, and improper shoe wear;

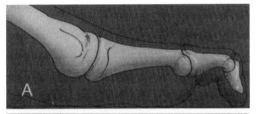
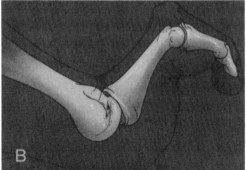

Figure 9.21. *A*, mallet-toe. Flexion deformity of DIP joint. *B*, clawtoe. Accentuated hammertoe deformity with hyper-extension at metatarsophalangeal joint and flexion at PIP and DIP joints. (Reprinted with permission from Johnson KA. Surgery of the Foot and Ankle. New York: Raven Press, 1988.)

however, they also may be idiopathic. Initially, skin changes may be absent, but eventually the patient will develop corns over the dorsum of the proximal interphalangeal (PIP) or distal interphalangeal (DIP) joint, or at the tip of the toes. Corns at the tips of the lesser toes are often painful and may cause skin breakdown and osteomyelitis. A toe crest pad (Fig. 9.22) may successfully relieve the pain of these "end corns." As mentioned in the section "Metatarsalgia," hammertoes and claw toes also may result in calluses beneath the metatarsal heads.

The most effective form of conservative treatment of these toe deformities is a change in shoe wear. The toe box should be rounded rather than pointed and high heels should be avoided. Extra depth shoes provide increased height of the toe box so that the deformed toes do not strike the inside of the shoe. If

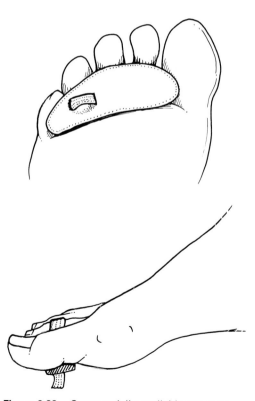

Figure 9.22. Commercially available toe crest pad is useful in treating painful end corns of lesser toes.

the toe deformity is not rigid, metatarsal pads or an orthosis may provide relief of symptoms. The corns over the toes may be treated by the patient with a pumice stone after bathing or may be shaved with a scalpel by the physician. "Donut pads" with a hole in the center often aid in the relief of symptoms when applied over the corn on the toe. Foot pads with chemical agents to dissolve the corn are to be avoided because of the possibility of skin breakdown. Because these corns develop in response to shoe pressure on the deformed toe, they cannot be surgically excised without a recurrence unless the shoe is changed or the toe deformity is corrected. Surgical treatment of these toe deformities, including resection of underlying bony prominences and surgical realignment of the toes, is indicated when conservative treatment fails.

Another cause of pain in the lesser toes is an interdigital corn, or soft corn. As already mentioned, corns are caused by pressure on the skin from underlying bone. In soft corns, there is pressure between bony prominences of adjacent toes. The corn that subsequently develops becomes softened by moisture between the toes and may macerate or ulcerate. The most common location for a soft corn is in the proximal part of the web space between the 4th and 5th toes, caused by pressure between the medial side of the 5th toe PIP joint and the lateral side of the base of the proximal phalanx of the 4th toe (Fig. 9.23). Once the soft corn macerates, it may also become secondarily infected. Soft corns are much more painful than the more common hard corns on the dorsum of the toes. Conservative treatment with lamb's wool or pads between the toes is often unsatisfactory. Surgical excision of the underlying bony prominence will result in spontaneous resolution of the soft corn and relief of pain.

Onychocryptosis (Ingrown Toenail)

Onychocryptosis, commonly called ingrown toenails, usually involve the nail of the great toe. On rare occasions, this process can involve the lesser toes. Either the medial or lateral (or both) nail plate becomes deeply em-

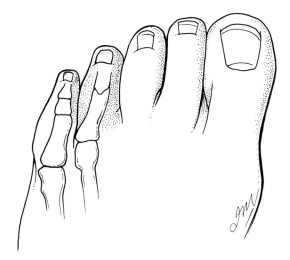

Figure 9.23. Painful soft corns are most common between the 4th and 5th toes.

bedded into the nail fold. A secondary infection may ensue, although the process can be painful even without infection. It is often assumed that the nail plate has "grown down into the nail margin," but often the problem is swelling of inflamed soft tissue up and over the nail plate. The irritation of the embedded nail causes more soft tissue swelling, and the process will worsen. Onychocryptosis is more common with improper trimming of the toenail, or if the normal convexity of the nail is exaggerated. Toenails should be cut straight across and the corners of the nail allowed to extend beyond the nail groove. If the distal corner of a nail is trimmed back, the nail groove may swell over the nail in response to the dependent position of the feet and the upward pressure caused by weightbearing. With growth of the nail plate, the distal edge will cut into the swollen nail groove. Infection may occur, resulting in a paronychia. Efforts to trim the corners of an embedded nail plate inevitably create a deep spicule, which then hooks into the nail groove and prevents the nail margin from clearing the end of the toe distally.

In mild cases, warm soaks, elevation, and antibiotics may be successful. The edge of the nail groove is gently pressed down off the underlying nail plate, and a small piece of cotton is placed beneath the nail edge. This may make it possible for the distal end of the embedded nail margin to grow beyond the end of the nail groove.

In more severe cases, surgical treatment is necessary. The basis of surgical treatment is to remove the embedded nail plate under block anesthesia at the base of the toe (Figs 9.24A and 9.24B). A small straight hemostat is gently placed under the embedded edge of the nail. The nail edge is then grasped with the hemostat, rotated out of the nail margin, and cut off with heavy scissors. The exposed matrix is covered with bacitracin ointment so that the dressing will not be adherent when it is changed. The patient begins dressing changes at 24 hours. The swelling and tenderness usually resolve rapidly, and daily dressing changes and warm soaks are performed at home. Although the simple removal of the embedded nail edge will usually provide prompt relief of symptoms, the patient must be advised that the nail will grow back and that the problem may recur.

If the nail has a deep convexity or in recurrent cases, it is necessary to ablate the edge of the nail matrix so that the nail plate does not grow back. (Fig. 9.24 C through E). This results in a narrower and less convex toenail that is less likely to become embedded. Ablation of the matrix can be performed either surgically or chemically. The surgical proce-

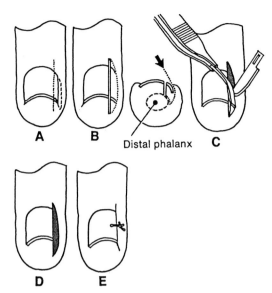

Figure 9.24. Surgical treatment of onychocryptosis. *A* and *B,* partial excision of the nail plate (nail matrix left intact). *C* through *E,* permanent ablation of the nail edge by surgical excision of the nail matrix. (Reprinted with permission from Johnson KA. Surgery of the Foot and Ankle. New York: Raven Press, 1988:121–128.)

dure consists of removal of a wedge-shaped segment of nail matrix and underlying soft tissue down to the periosteum of the distal phalanx. It is imperative that the germinal matrix at the proximal end of the nail is completely removed. The wound can then be dressed open with a nonadherent dressing, or the free skin edge may be loosely reapproximated to the remaining edge of the toe nail. Some physicians remove only the nail plate surgically and then ablate the nail matrix chemically with phenol.

FOOT MANIFESTATIONS OF SYSTEMIC DISEASES

Many systemic disease processes, including diabetes, rheumatoid arthritis, gout, psoriasis, and Reiter's syndrome, frequently affect the foot. Diabetes mellitus can result in severe limb-threatening and life-threatening complications in the foot. The diverse clinical problems of these disorders, as well as the diagnosis

and medical treatment, are beyond the scope of this chapter. However, the important manifestations of the foot secondary to these diseases will be discussed.

Diabetes Mellitus

Complications of diabetes mellitus in the foot are extremely common, disabling, expensive in terms of medical care and lost wages, and sometimes limb-threatening. Most patients with diabetes will eventually develop a peripheral neuropathy, and neuropathic ulcers on the foot can occur with trivial trauma or without a history of trauma. Foot ulcers in a diabetic patient may quickly progress to deep abscess formation, osteomyelitis, and gangrene, even with proper treatment. The best treatment with regard to neuropathic ulcers is prevention. The diabetic patient must be taught the importance of proper foot care and proper foot hygiene. The patient should visually inspect the feet on a regular basis and must never walk barefoot or wear shoes without socks, even for short distances. New shoes must be broken in gradually. Heat sensation is lost early in diabetic neuropathy. Soaking the feet in hot water or exposure to heat from a radiator can cause devastating burns in a diabetic patient with a peripheral neuropathy. Corns or calluses should never be trimmed by the patient with a razor, and proper nail care is critically important. The patient should notify the physician immediately if a skin breakdown or evidence of infection occurs.

If a diabetic foot ulcer occurs, a team approach, including the primary care physician, orthopaedist, vascular surgeon, and orthotist, may be necessary for successful treatment. Systemic antibiotics based on deep cultures, surgical debridement when indicated, protection from weightbearing, and local wound care may all be necessary to promote healing of a diabetic ulcer. Protection of the ulcer from weightbearing is extremely important when trying to heal a diabetic ulcer. Absolute nonweightbearing with bedrest or full-time use of crutches or a walker may be necessary. However, the orthopaedist may treat a diabetic foot ulcer with a total contact cast that redistributes weight off of the ulcer while still allowing the patient to ambulate. If pedal pulses are not palpable, then segmental Doppler pressures or a vascular surgical consultation should be obtained. Superficial neuropathic ulcers that have not progressed to osteomyelitis or deep abscess will usually heal with this conservative approach. Custom-molded shoes with soft accommodative inserts may prevent recurrence of the ulcer, although surgical correction of a bony deformity may be necessary to prevent recurrence.

If deep abscess or osteomyelitis is present, aggressive surgical debridement and drainage is needed. This should be performed in the operating room with adequate anesthesia, because failure of treatment often occurs with attempted drainage or local debridement at the bedside. If gangrene is present, at least partial amputation will be necessary. If vascular evaluation reveals a treatable lesion, revascularization may promote healing of the ulcer; or if amputation is necessary, revascularization may allow a more distal amputation level.

In addition to neuropathic ulcers, diabetic patients may develop a Charcot arthropathy of the foot. Early diagnosis of a Charcot foot is difficult but important, because early treatment is much more successful than late treatment. Because of the diabetic peripheral neuropathy, subluxation of joints with collapse and fragmentation of bone may occur. This process usually involves the midfoot, although the hindfoot and forefoot may be affected, and may result in a severely deformed, stiff foot with bony prominences. The bony prominences and the stiff, deformed foot make shoe fitting and ambulation difficult. The deformity may often cause skin ulceration and deep infection.

It is imperative for the primary care physician to be aware of this complication, because early treatment may prevent the progressive deformity. The early manifestations of a Charcot foot are swelling, erythema, and warmth of the foot, and the clinical presentation may be identical to cellulitis. The initial x-rays are normal, and the patient is often treated for "cellulitis" with bedrest, elevation, and IV antibiotics. The swelling, erythema, and warmth rapidly improve because of the bedrest and elevation, not because of the antibiotics. The patient then returns in 2 to 6 weeks with recurrent swelling at which time new x-rays show severe bony destruction or deformity. Early treatment of a Charcot foot with total contact casting put on before bone destruction occurs may prevent the progressive deformity. Therefore, the author believes that an orthopaedic surgeon should be consulted early in the treatment of suspected cellulitis of the foot in a diabetic patient to rule out an early Charcot foot. Once the deformity has developed, custom-molded shoes with soft inserts or bracing may prevent skin breakdown. However, surgery may be needed at that point to resect bony prominences or to fuse the affected joints.

Rheumatoid Arthritis

The forefoot and the hindfoot are frequently affected by rheumatoid arthritis, which often involves the metatarsophalangeal joint and the subtalar joint. Rheumatoid arthritis may cause severe hallux valgus, with a lateral deviation or valgus deformity of the lesser toes as well. The lesser toes often dislocate dorsally at the metatarsophalangeal joints, causing prominence of the metatarsal heads on the plantar aspect of the foot and distal migration of the plantar forefoot fat pad. This may lead to disabling intractable plantar keratoses and make ambulation painful. Rheumatoid nodules also may develop on the plantar aspect of the forefoot, further adding to the difficulty in weightbearing. The midfoot joints are less commonly involved, but the subtalar joint frequently is affected by rheumatoid arthritis. Inflammation of the subtalar joint causes pain with inversion and eversion and may result in a progressive hindfoot valgus deformity or a painful rigid flatfoot. Inflammatory tendinitis of the tibialis posterior also may be caused by rheumatoid arthritis.

Local treatment of the foot in rheumatoid arthritis includes soft accommodative orthoses to relieve weightbearing beneath the prominent metatarsal heads, ankle bracing for the hindfoot, and local steroid injections into the joints of the foot or into rheumatoid nodules. If severe deformity of the foot is present, surgery may be necessary. Surgery of the hindfoot and midfoot usually involves fusion of the subtalar joint, triple arthrodeses, or localized fusion of involved midfoot joints. Surgery of the forefoot usually includes resections of the lesser metatarsal heads and fusion of the first metatarsophalangeal joint to correct the hallux valgus. Surgical treatment of the rheumatoid foot can be gratifying to the patient, providing decreased pain and improved ambulatory capabilities.

Gout

The diagnosis of gouty arthritis may be obvious when the patient presents with a sudden onset of severe pain and swelling of the first metatarsophalangeal joint, referred to as podagra. However, the presentation of gout in the foot may be subacute and less severe, possibly involving other joints or even tendons. In these cases, the diagnosis of gout may not be entertained. The definitive diagnostic test for gouty arthritis or tenosynovitis is evaluation of joint fluid under a polarizing microscope, where negatively birefringent crystals are seen. X-rays early in the course of gouty arthritis will be normal except for possible soft tissue swelling. With chronic gout, there may be joint destruction, juxta-articular erosions, and tophaceous deposits in the soft tissue. In addition to medical treatment with anti-inflammatory medications and hyperuricemia agents, occasionally, it may be necessary to surgically debride chronic tophaceous deposits, especially if they are spontaneously draining or secondarily infected.

Reiter's Syndrome

Involvement of the foot is common with Reiter's syndrome. The heel is the most commonly affected site in the foot, and patients with Reiter's syndrome may present with pain on the plantar aspect of the heel or posteriorly at the insertion of the Achilles tendon. X-rays may be normal or may show fluffy soft tissue

calcifications on the plantar or posterior aspect of the calcaneus. Inflammation of the metatarsophalangeal joints may also occur in Reiter's syndrome. The clinical findings in the forefoot also include the occurrence of "sausage toes." Local treatment of foot symptoms include oral anti-inflammatory medications, local steroid injections, physical therapy, heel pads, and orthoses.

Psoriasis

Psoriatic involvement of the foot is generally limited to the toes. In addition to the typical psoriatic nail changes, the PIP and DIP joints of the toes are most frequently affected. The radiographs may show severe destruction of these joints, often with a great deal of bone resorption.

TRAUMATIC DISORDERS OF THE FOOT

The foot is subject to a variety of injuries, including contusions, sprains, fractures, dislocations, and lacerations, many of which can be definitively treated by the primary care physician. In any case of trauma with open fracture or neurovascular compromise, immediate referral to an orthopaedic surgeon or vascular surgeon is necessary. The discussion that follows is based on the assumption of an intact neurovascular status to the foot.

CONTUSIONS

Any type of blunt trauma may result in a contusion of the foot. If the patient has a history of significant trauma, or if severe swelling and pain are present, then x-rays are indicated to rule out a fracture or dislocation. If the x-rays are normal, the initial treatment is ice, elevation, and a compression dressing. Within 2 to 3 days, at least partial weightbearing should be possible and activity level can be progressed as tolerated. Physical therapy is helpful if significant stiffness of the foot occurs after a contusion. After severe crushing injuries to the soft tissue, prolonged disability is possible, and intensive physical therapy and anti-inflammatory medications may be necessary. If pain out of proportion to the extent of injury persists, especially if accompanied by hyperesthesia of the skin and changes in the color and temperature of the foot, then the possibility of reflex sympathetic dystrophy should be considered. Reflex sympathetic dystrophy will require more intensive and more prolonged treatment, including possible referral to a pain clinic or to an anesthesiologist for local or lumbar nerve blocks.

SPRAINS

The bony configuration and strong ligaments make sprains of the foot uncommon compared with sprains of the ligaments of the knee or ankle. When a sprain of the foot occurs, it usually involves the tarsometatarsal (Lisfranc) joints. The patient presents with a history of a weightbearing, twisting injury to the foot, and pain across the midfoot. Examination will reveal soft tissue swelling and tenderness to palpation across the top of the midfoot. Although the initial x-rays may be normal, there is the potential for subtle subluxation of the tarsometatarsal joints after a sprain of the ligaments of Lisfranc's joints. Because of this potential for joint subluxation and chronic pain, any patient with a "sprain" of the midfoot should be referred to an orthopaedic surgeon for further evaluation and treatment.

DISLOCATIONS

Dislocations of the foot are relatively uncommon. A subtalar (or peritalar) dislocation occurs when the talus remains within the ankle joint, but the calcaneus and the rest of the foot are displaced either medially or laterally off the talus. The foot is markedly deformed clinically, and the skin may be disrupted or stretched tightly over the convex side of the deformed foot. Immediate reduction may be necessary to prevent skin necrosis and it will also decrease pain. If an orthopaedic surgeon is not readily available, the primary care physi-

cian may have to attempt the closed reduction under intravenous sedation and analgesia. The hip and knee are flexed, and then longitudinal traction is applied to the forefoot and heel. The physician then tries to reposition the foot out of its medially or laterally displaced position. If reduction of the subtalar joint can be obtained, it is usually stable because of the complex bony configuration of the subtalar joint. The ankle and foot are immobilized in well-padded splints. The patient should be referred to an orthopaedic surgeon for evaluation for associated fractures and for follow-up care.

Dislocations through the level of the tarsometatarsal joints generally do not occur without fractures. This so-called Lisfranc fracture-dislocation will be discussed in the section "Fractures."

Dislocations of the metatarsophalangeal joints and interphalangeal joints of the toes are relatively uncommon. They are treated with closed reduction by longitudinal traction in the same fashion as when these dislocations occur in the corresponding joints in the hand. Occasionally, a dislocated metatarsophalangeal joint will be irreducible by closed methods, and referral to an orthopaedic surgeon will be necessary for an open reduction.

FRACTURES

Fractures of the Talus

Twisting injuries to the foot may result in a variety of fractures of the talus. Talar dome fractures and lateral process fractures (Fig. 9.25) clinically appear similar to ankle sprains, but their treatment is significantly different from the treatment of an ankle sprain. If these talar fractures are small and nondisplaced, they should be treated with nonweightbearing in a short-leg cast for 4 to 6 weeks followed by a short-leg walking cast for an additional 4 weeks. Follow-up x-rays are necessary to ensure that the fracture heals. If these fractures are large or displaced, patients should be referred to an orthopaedic surgeon, because immediate surgical fixation or removal of the fracture fragment may be indicated.

Fractures through the neck of the talus (Fig. 9.26) are serious injuries because they may interrupt the blood supply to the body of the talus and may lead to avascular necrosis of the talus. Therefore, all fractures of the neck of the talus should be referred immediately to an orthopaedic surgeon.

Fractures of the Calcaneus

The calcaneus is subject to avulsion fractures on the lateral side and fractures of the anterior process (Fig. 9.27), both of which clinically may appear identical to ankle sprains. Nondisplaced avulsion fractures can be treated in a short-leg walking cast for 3 to 4 weeks, followed by a rehabilitation program. Nondisplaced fractures of the anterior process of the calcaneus are treated in a short-leg cast, with nonweightbearing for 4 weeks, followed by a short-leg walking cast for 4 weeks. Displaced fractures of the anterior process should be referred to an orthopaedic surgeon for treatment.

Much more serious than the small avulsion fractures are fractures of the calcaneus occurring through the tuberosity and the articular surface of the subtalar joint (Fig. 9.28). These fractures usually occur in a fall from a height or, occasionally, in a motor vehicle accident. The fracture is often comminuted and is accompanied by severe pain and marked swelling. These fractures often yield a poor clinical result and historically have been treated by elevation and casting. However, it is now well accepted that many of these fractures will have a better outcome if treated by open reduction and internal fixation. Therefore, patients with these severe fractures of the os calcis should be placed in a well-padded splint

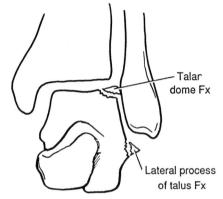

Figure 9.25. Talar dome fracture and lateral process fracture of talus can both clinically mimic an ankle sprain.

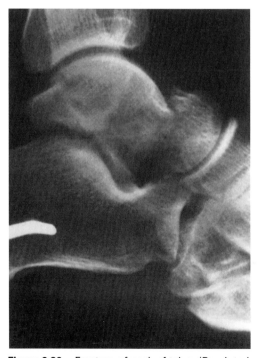

Figure 9.26. Fracture of neck of talus. (Reprinted with permission from Rockwood CA, Green DP. Fractures of the Talus in Fractures in Adults. Vol 2. Philadelphia: JB Lippincott Co, 1984:1737.)

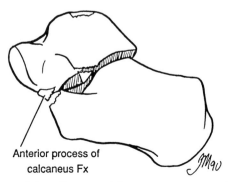

Figure 9.27. Fracture of the anterior process of the calcaneus can clinically appear identical to an ankle sprain.

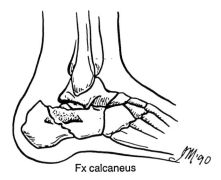

Fx calcaneus

Figure 9.28. Intra-articular fracture of the calcaneus.

with the lower extremity elevated and referred to an orthopaedic surgeon for initial treatment.

Fractures of the Midfoot

Acute fractures of the navicular, cuboid, and cuneiform bones are uncommon. They usually are small avulsion fractures from twisting injuries and can be treated in a short-leg walking cast for 3 to 4 weeks. Stress fractures may occur in the navicular, although much less commonly than in the metatarsals. A bone scan or CT scan may be necessary for the diagnosis of a navicular stress fracture. Rarely, a crush-type injury or high-energy trauma may result in a complete fracture through the body of one of the mid tarsal bones. These are more serious injuries that may be associated with subtle subluxations or dislocations of the tarsometatarsal joints; they should be splinted and referred to an orthopaedic surgeon.

Fractures of the Forefoot

Fractures of the metatarsals and toes are frequent, and many can be definitively treated by the primary care physician. An isolated fracture of the shaft of a single metatarsal is rarely displaced significantly and can be treated in a short-leg walking cast for 3 to 4 weeks. Fractures of the shafts of two or more metatarsals may be unstable and may require operative treatment. Therefore, orthopaedic

consultation should be obtained when multiple metatarsals are fractured. A common fracture is an avulsion fracture of the base of the fifth metatarsal caused by an inversion injury to the foot. Some textbooks suggest that this fracture may simply be treated in a comfortable shoe, but the author has found that patients with these fractures have much less pain if they are placed in a short-leg walking cast or boot walker. In rare cases, this fracture will result in a painful nonunion, and referral to an orthopaedic surgeon may be necessary. If a fracture of the fifth metatarsal occurs through the proximal diaphysis rather than through the base, called a Jones' fracture, it is much more likely to result in delayed union or nonunion, and therefore, referral to an orthopaedic surgeon is advisable. Particular caution is indicated when treating fractures of the bases of the second, third, and fourth metatarsals. These fractures, especially when multiple, may be associated with dislocation of the tarsometatarsal joints—the so-called Lisfranc fracture-dislocation. This serious injury may at times be difficult to diagnose and is usually difficult to treat. If a Lisfranc fracture-dislocation is present or suspected, referral to an orthopaedic surgeon is necessary.

Fractures of the phalanges of the toes usually are caused by a crush-type injury or by kicking a hard object while barefoot. Fracture of the lesser toes are treated successfully by taping to adjacent toes. Reduction is indicated if marked angular or rotatory deformity is present. This reduction can be performed by traction under a Xylocaine block, and the toe is taped to an adjacent toe. Taping is usually continued for 2 to 3 weeks. Nondisplaced fractures of the great toe are best treated by a short-leg walking cast with a toe plate or a boot walker for 3 to 4 weeks. Displaced fractures of the great toe and fractures of the great toe that extend into the metatarsophalangeal joint or interphalangeal joint should be referred to an orthopaedic surgeon. In these fractures, open reduction and internal fixation is sometimes necessary to decrease the chance of posttraumatic degenerative arthritis.

SUGGESTED READINGS

Crenshaw AH, ed. Campbell's Operative Orthopedics. St. Louis: The CV Mosby Co, 1987.

Jahss M. Disorders of the Foot and Ankle. Philadelphia: WB Saunders Co, 1991.

Mann R, ed. Surgery of the Foot. 5th ed. St. Louis: The CV Mosby Co, 1986.

Tachdjian MO. Pediatric Orthopedics. 2nd ed. Philadelphia: WB Saunders Co, 1990.

Wu KK. Foot Orthoses. Baltimore: Williams & Wilkins, 1990.

CHAPTER 10

Mechanical Therapeutics (Casts, Splints, Traction)

John J. Monahan, M.D.

Orthopaedic treatments are essentially mechanical, whether done to a patient or by a patient. They apply forces to support, stabilize, or reconstruct disrupted structures or to mobilize and strengthen stiffened, weakened structures. Details of manipulation and exercise for each area of the body are described in the regional chapters. This chapter presents general principles of treatment with specific attention to reduction of displaced injuries, application of casts and splints, traction, and rehabilitation.

CLOSED TREATMENT OF FRACTURES AND DISLOCATIONS

TIMING OF REDUCTION

All dislocations must be reduced as soon as possible, otherwise pain remains intense. Neurovascular injury is more likely the longer the joint is allowed to remain dislocated. Open fractures and dislocations always require immediate irrigation, debridement, reduction, and immobilization to minimize the risk of infection. Closed fractures do not constitute an emergency unless there is neurovascular injury or impending skin breakdown. Fractures should, however, be reduced as soon as possible because swelling of the extremity increases for hours after the fracture. This hemorrhage and transudate makes the muscle tissue indurated and inelastic. The longer reduction is delayed, the more difficult the reduction. If reduction cannot be accomplished relatively promptly, it is sometimes better to delay reduction for several days

rather than to attempt manipulation of a severely swollen, edematous extremity that will be difficult to reduce and for which external immobilization will be difficult to maintain. During this waiting period, the extremity should be elevated and carefully monitored (i.e., neurovascular integrity).

STANDARDS OF REDUCTION

No reduction is required if no significant displacement has occurred or if the displacement is of little consequence. Avulsion fractures usually do not require reduction.

Any displacement is unacceptable when it threatens skin or neurovascular structures, disrupts the continuity of a joint surface, or delays healing. For example, displaced tibial fractures threaten the tight overlying skin. A significant number of all elbow and knee fractures or dislocations are associated with neurovascular complications. Displaced ankle fractures or dislocations can threaten adjacent neurovascular structures and skin integrity.

The degree of acceptable axial displacement varies with the nature of the injury, the age of the patient, and the bone involved. In an adult with a tibia and fibula fracture, an attempt should be made to correct more than 1 cm of shortening. In a child's fractured long bone, it is desirable to allow some axial shortening. This compensates for the usual accelerated growth of the fractured bone. Unless the long bone is shortened by axial displacement, the extremity will ultimately grow undesirably longer than the uninjured extremity. Therefore, for children it is reasonable to allow 1 cm of overriding for tibial or humeral fractures, and 1 to 1.5 cm for femoral fractures. In other instances, axial displacement should be corrected because it may delay healing or alter muscle balance and can create subluxation at joints between paired bones.

Angular deformity in mature bone has limited "remodeling" potential. Mild deformity, i.e., 5 to 10°, in a long bone is generally acceptable. Angular deformity near a joint in the plane of the major joint motion is more acceptable than a similar deformity at the midshaft of the bone. For example, in an elderly patient with a fractured neck of the humerus, 30° of varus deformity can be accepted. Thirty degrees of deformity in a fracture of both bones of the radius and ulna in the same patient would not be acceptable. Angulation of long bones changes the orientation of the articular surfaces of adjacent joints. In weightbearing extremities, the angulation may create shearing forces across the joint and will burden a portion of the surface as well as the investing ligaments of the joint with abnormally high stresses. Posttraumatic instability or arthritis may develop. In nonweightbearing extremities the arc of motion may change. The shoulder joint can adjust to posttraumatic deformities of the humerus because of the wide range of motion and degrees of freedom within the joint. The elbow is less accommodating.

Translational displacement of fractures is relatively unacceptable when the expected remodeling is unlikely to restore a fairly normal appearance to a subcutaneous bone or when the degree of displacement is severe enough to impair bone healing. As a general rule, when translational displacement does not exceed half the width of the bone, position is acceptable.

Growing bones can correct a significant degree of nonrotational displacement. Greater remodeling potential exists if the fracture is close to an epiphysis and if the angulation is in the plane of the adjacent joint. Rotational deformity does not remodel well in growing or mature bone, and significant deformity should be corrected by reduction.

Because the criteria for "acceptable reduction" differs significantly with the patient and the injury, it is recommended that the reader consult the details for management of specific injuries in the regional chapters. A primary care physician who is not experienced in the management of these injuries should freely consult the orthopaedist for help in the evaluation and management of these patients.

DIRECTION OF FORCES OF REDUCTION

Most reductions are accomplished by manually applying a gentle, sustained traction force to the fragment that can be controlled. Apply the force in line with the long axis of the part to gain the necessary length. Then, to achieve satisfactory anatomical alignment, apply appropriate angular or rotational forces to reverse the deformity and usually the mechanism of injury that produced the fracture or dislocation. Traction forces sometimes must be strong and persistent (but always controlled and gradual in application) to overcome muscle spasm and friction forces that bind impacted fractures. Angular and rotational forces are applied gently and more briefly.

Traction is effective in gaining a reduction only if the bone ends are connected with sufficient soft tissues. These tissues usually survive the injury by their location in the concavity of the deformed bone or joint. By using this natural tension band or hinge, the bone ends can be manipulated into a stable or relatively stable position. If there is no soft tissue tension band, a stable reduction is more difficult to achieve by closed manipulation. Although the length can be restored, displacement and angulation may persist (Fig. 10.1).

FORCES APPLIED TO DISLOCATIONS

Good analgesia or anesthesia will greatly diminish muscle resistance and often make the difference between success and failure when manipulating dislocations of the larger joints. The manipulator should await evidence that the patient is relaxed and then begin with fairly gentle traction, e.g., merely the weight of the

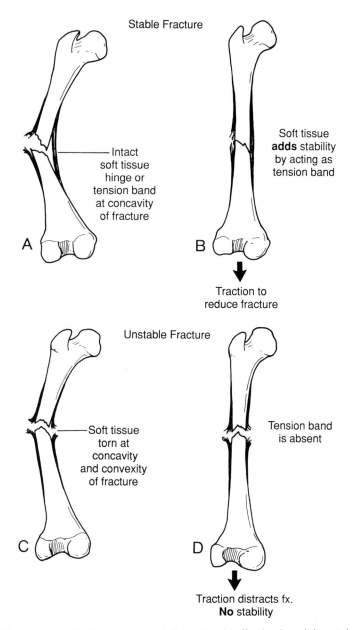

Figure 10.1. Stable and unstable fractures. *A* and *B*, traction is effective in gaining stable reduction of a fracture when the soft tissue tension band or hinge is intact (shown at the concavity of the fracture). *C* and *D*, traction is ineffective in gaining stable reduction when the soft tissue is torn from the concavity and convexity of the fracture.

dependent arm when manipulating an anterior dislocation of the shoulder. Gentle rotational and angular forces are then applied, as described in the regional chapters, stopping when mechanical resistance is encountered.

Forceful angular and rotational forces have caused fractures during efforts to reduce large joint dislocations. When these gentle maneuvers fail, stronger traction should be applied for many minutes before the appropriate rotational and angular forces are gently applied again. At times, a dislocation will be "irreducible." In certain dislocations, the bone end has "buttonholed" through the capsule and ligaments and may be entrapped by these structures or adjacent tendons. In these circumstances, traction may not be beneficial, thus, orthopaedic consultation should be obtained. In addition, a dislocation may not be reducible because better muscle relaxation or pain relief is necessary. Caution should be exercised in the use of increasing doses of analgesics or relaxants. When one cannot gain a reduction under usual and customary doses of such medication, a regional anesthesia or general anesthesia under an anesthesiologist's direction should be considered.

FORCES APPLIED TO FRACTURES

Unless the operator is uncommonly strong, impacted and overriding fractures are more readily reduced by weighted traction. This can outlast the strongest patient, is usually not very painful, and leaves the operator free to apply well-controlled angular and rotational forces to the fracture fragments. The angular and rotational forces needed rarely require more strength than what abides in the hands and wrists alone. Various gripping forces that bridge the fracture site are typically all that are required to complete the reduction of most forearm, wrist, hand, and ankle fractures. Modest arm forces are required to complete the reduction of shaft fractures of the tibia and fibula consisting of one hand gripping above and the other below the fracture site. Angular and rotational forces are initiated gently and increased smoothly until the desired position is achieved.

Having gained a satisfactory reduction, immobilization in a splint, a cast, or continuous traction is required. Radiographs should be taken to confirm maintenance of reduction. The injured extremity should be elevated and ice applied to the injury site. Appropriate neurovascular checks of the extremity are always mandatory.

Exceptions to the general principles of reduction outlined in the preceding text are considered in the regional chapters.

PRINCIPLES OF IMMOBILIZATION

Immobilization techniques include casts, splints, and weighted traction. Two types of cast and splint materials will be discussed: plaster of Paris and fiberglass.

Plaster of Paris rolls are muslin impregnated with starch and the hemihydrate of calcium sulfate. This material has a long, successful track record in that it is strong, rigid, moldable, porous (allows the skin to "breathe"), absorbent (absorbs any drainage from a wound), relatively inexpensive, and accessible. The disadvantages of plaster of Paris include a prolonged curing (hardening) period, which delays weightbearing for 36 hours. Also, the material is destroyed by moisture and is relatively radiopaque.

Fiberglass materials are available as an alternative. Fiberglass is durable, radiolucent, and light weight; it allows immediate weightbearing, and is stronger than plaster of Paris (less material required). However, it is more expensive, less available, less moldable, and harder to cut and trim than plaster of Paris. Fiberglass occasionally causes skin irritation and is therefore less useful on fresh fractures. Although fiberglass provides an advantage because it tolerates wetness much better than plaster, this, in practice, is of limited benefit. A patient still must keep the underlying skin clean and dry. If a fiberglass-casted extremity is immersed in water, there is potential for skin maceration. Consequently, these extremities need to be protected from moisture in a fashion similar to extremities casted in plaster of Paris.

SPLINTING

Indications

A splint usually is chosen for temporary immobilization of an injury while the patient is awaiting definitive treatment, or for immobilization of an injury that needs protection but not great stability. In emergent situations, any material that can safely provide stability or protection to the injured part may be used, e.g., magazines, cardboard, padded wood, plastic, prefabricated air/plastic or metal splints, and traction splints for femur fractures. In the emergency or outpatient departments, however, plaster or fiberglass splints are preferred. Splints are useful for joints affected by acute arthritis and periarticular pain syndromes when rest to the painful structures is indicated and when splinting can provide comfortable stability in the context of the person's expected activities.

The five splints that are often used by primary clinicians for the upper extremities are as follows:

1. The volar forearm splint is used to temporarily immobilize forearm, wrist, and hand fractures; to protect wrist sprains and strains; and to rest an acutely arthritic wrist.
2. A volar splint with a thumb extension is used to immobilize an ulnar collateral ligament tear at the first metacarpophalangeal joint.
3. An ulnar or radial gutter splint is used to treat stable fractures and dislocations of the wrist and hand after reduction. For sprains and strains, the gutter splint protects involved metacarpals and phalanges while freeing the uninvolved portions of the hand for function.
4. The dorsal forearm splint is used for protection of fractures at the base or shaft of metacarpals two through five as an alternative to the ulnar or radial gutter splint. The dorsal splint also is used to rest inflamed flexor tendons associated with carpal tunnel syndrome.
5. The long-arm splint is used for temporary immobilization of fractures, dislocations, and sprains and strains of the forearm, elbow, and distal humerus. It is also used to protect contusions, infections, or inflammatory processes of the upper extremity.

Splints for the lower extremity include the following:

1. The short posterior leg splint is used for temporary immobilization of ankle and foot injuries until swelling subsides and proper evaluation for stability can be conducted. It also is used to rest an arthritic ankle or foot joint or to immobilize sprains, strains, and fractures of the foot.
2. The long posterior leg splint is used for temporary immobilization of injuries of the extensor apparatus and potentially or obviously unstable injuries of the collateral or cruciate ligaments of the knee. This splint is used to immobilize fractures of the shaft and proximal condyles of the tibia and, if a traction splint is not available, the condyles of the femur. The long posterior splint also is used to protect a stable knee sprain or fracture and to rest the arthritic knee.
3. The traction splint is best used to splint femur fractures, i.e., the "Thomas" splint, which is one of the many modifications (Fig. 10.2). The force of the traction splint

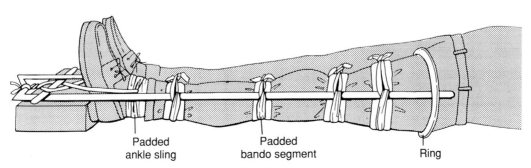

Padded ankle sling   Padded bando segment   Ring

Figure 10.2.   Traction splint.

is applied distally to the foot while proximally, the padded ring, or half ring, is secured to the thigh and hip area. Wide soft bandages are then tied at intervals along the splint to support the limb. Distal circulation and neural function should be monitored frequently before and after application of the splint. Femoral fractures should be referred to an orthopaedic surgeon for management after immobilization.

Technique (Fig. 10.3)

Depending on the mass of the extremity, the splint must be 8 (upper extremity) to 16 (lower extremity) plaster strips (or 6 to 8 fi-

berglass strips) in thickness. Such splints are made by stacking precut plaster splints on top of one another then cutting the whole to the desired length, or by rolling out strips of the desired length back and forth from a plaster roll. The width of the plaster is chosen so that approximately half the girth of the extremity will lie within the splint. The length varies: a short-arm splint to include finger fractures would extend from the fingertips to a point two finger breadths distal to the antecubital crease, or 2 cm from the biceps tendon in the antecubital space with the elbow at a right angle. Arm splints are shaped at one end to fit around the thenar eminence and to parallel

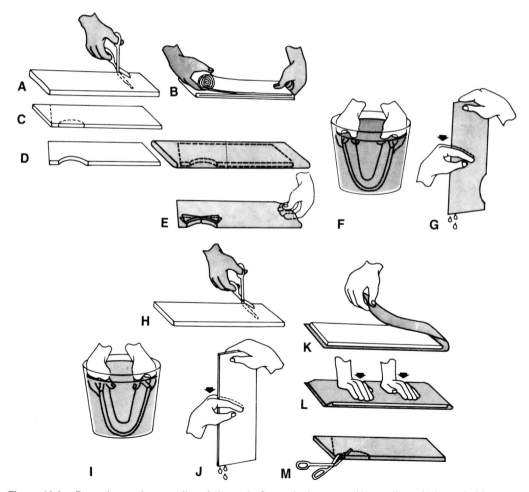

Figure 10.3.   Preparing a plaster splint. *A* through *G*, employing a stockinette liner. *H* through *M*, employing a cast padding liner.

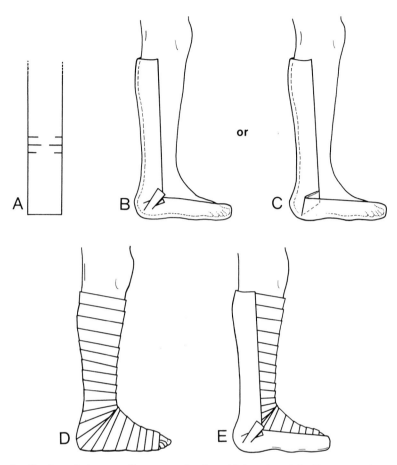

Figure 10.4. Application of plaster splints around a flexed joint. *A* and *B*, slits are made at right angles to the long axis of the splint and overlapped smoothly; or *C*, the redundant material is tucked and smoothed at the angles. *D* and *E*, a thick layer of cast padding is wrapped on the extremity and a posterior splint is applied over the padding.

the distal palmar crease. Other splints are left square at the ends. Where the plaster must round a flexed joint, slits are made in the sheets of plaster-impregnated muslin at right angles to the long axis of the splint to allow a smooth overlap at the turns or angles (Figs. 10.4A and 10.4B), or careful tucks are taken to avoid skin pressure (Fig. 10.4C).

An alternative method would be to wrap a thick layer of cast padding to the extremity and apply the water-soaked splints directly to the cast padding, overwrapping with wet gauze or a layer of padding plus Ace bandage (Figs. 10.4D and 10.4E). This often gives a better contouring than the "complete splint application" method.

The plaster is immersed in warm water until thoroughly wet, stripped of excess water, and laid on three or four layers of cast padding. The plaster is then covered with an additional strip or two of padding to prevent the Ace bandage or gauze (that will be applied over the plaster to hold the material in place) from sticking to the surface of the plaster, which would interfere with rewrapping. The splint then is applied to the extremity and firmly wrapped and molded into place using wet Kling or gauze. As the plaster or fiberglass hardens, the extremity is held in the desired position while the splint is molded to the contours of the extremity. Direct pressure over bony prominences should be avoided. When the plaster is hardened, the circulation is evaluated. If circulation is normal, the Kling, along the margins of the splint, is cut through to prevent a tourniquet effect on the extremity if further swelling occurs. The Kling is cut approximately 2 to 2-1/2 inches at a time, beginning distally and working proximally, while an assistant begins to roll an Ace bandage distally without added tension to maintain the splints in place. Care must be taken not to lose the position of reduction while rewrapping the splints. Always check neurovascular status after rewrapping and elevate the extremity to lessen swelling.

CAST IMMOBILIZATION

Indications

Casts immobilize by rigidly enveloping the unstable injured extremity and effectively producing soft tissue compression (a positive hydraulic force) that maintains apposition and alignment of the bone ends. In addition, a cast can provide a three-point force to maintain the position of a fracture, as seen in Figure 10.5. Avoid excessive point pressure over bony prominences, especially the fracture site, because this could cause skin necrosis. Rather, disperse the force over a larger surface area.

In certain circumstances, the cast also must maintain a distracting force necessary to prevent overriding or angulation of the fracture fragments. Casts are less efficient in maintaining distraction, however. With the elbow flexed to 90°, and with snug molding of the hand and wrist, a long-arm cast may maintain the necessary distraction force on oblique and spiral fractures of the forearm. With the knee in 90° of flexion, a long-leg cast may maintain the necessary distraction force on oblique and spiral fractures of the tibia. A similar effect can be achieved using gravity, such as long-arm "hanging cast" that applies a gentle distracting force to an overridden fracture of the humerus. It must be emphasized that casts alone can rarely safely maintain strong distractive forces without skin problems.

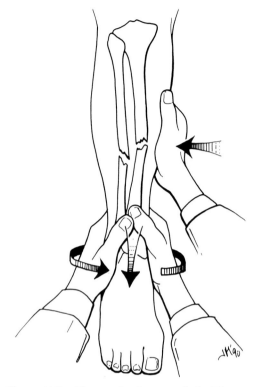

Figure 10.5. Three-point force applied while molding the cast to hold the position of a fracture with an intact soft tissue tension band.

The six basic casts often used by primary clinicians are as follows:

1. The short-arm cast is used in appropriate forms for stabilization of finger splints and for immobilization of metacarpal fractures, carpal fractures, reduced carpal dislocations, and distal third of the forearm fractures.

2. The long-arm cast is used in appropriate forms for immobilization of upper and middle-third forearm fractures. It is used for immobilization of reduced elbow dislocations and condylar and supracondylar fractures of the humerus after the circulatory response to injury has stabilized and swelling has subsided. The long-arm cast also is used for carpal and distal-third forearm fractures when swelling, muscle mass, or obesity prevent the well-molded short-arm cast from adequately limiting rotation.

3. The hanging arm cast (the cast is suspended by a strap connecting a collar about the neck and a cuff about the wrist) provides traction immobilization of humeral shaft and humeral neck fractures.
4. The short-leg cast is used in appropriate forms for immobilization of unstable ankle sprains, stable ankle fractures, fractures of the proximal phalanges of the great toes, metatarsal fractures, minimally displaced fractures of the tarsus and calcaneus, and subluxations of the peroneal tendons.
5. The long-leg cast is used for immobilization of fractures of the ankle, fractures of the shaft of the distal femur, tibia, or fibula, undisplaced fractures of the tibial condyles, injury to the extensor apparatus of the knee, unstable ligament injuries of the knee, and for treatment of Achilles tendon ruptures.
6. The patellar tendon weightbearing cast (PTB) is preferred to the long-leg cast for immobilization of stable reduced transverse fractures of the lower extremity when weightbearing is to begin. This cast prevents rotation while allowing knee motion.

Technique

Position the extremity with the fracture reduced as much as possible. Final adjustment is made as the cast is setting up. The practitioner usually needs assistance to control the limb. The position of the extremity and the areas of the cast that require special molding are unique to each injury and cast and are described in the regional chapters. Small wads of padding may be placed between the toes or fingers to provide adequate space in the cast for these members. The stockinette may be applied in stable injuries to cover the upper and lower ends of the cast. These should be of an approximate size to fit firmly without wrinkles (Fig. 10.6). In unstable injuries, the additional manipulation required for placement of the stockinette is not worth the extra step.

Cotton padding is then applied as smoothly as possible from the distal to the proximal end of the limb. Each layer is overlapped approxi-mately 60% to achieve a uniform two-layer padding (minimal padding feasible). The roll is held a few inches from the limb and pulled slightly as one circles the limb in a direction oblique to the long axis of the limb. Slight bagging of the lower edge of the cotton padding will occur as one proceeds from distal to proximal. These areas are simply torn away and the remaining edges smoothed into place. The cotton padding surfaces must be wrinkle-free to avoid wrinkles in the plaster that can cause skin irritation or breakdown. The layers of padding vary. If considerable swelling is expected, an extra layer or two should be added. Also, extra layers should be added over and about bony prominences. Excessive padding should not be used, however, because it lessens control of the fracture fragments.

The width of the plaster roll depends on the size of the extremity. Five- to 6-inch rolls can be used for the adult thigh, 4- to 5-inch rolls for the lower leg, and 2- to 4-inch rolls for the wrist and forearm. The widest rolls that can be conveniently controlled allow the most rapid delivery of plaster to immobilize the part, giving the physician more time to mold and manipulate the fracture. The roll of plaster is thoroughly immersed in water with the end free so that it can be easily identified after soaking. Wearing gloves is optional when working with plaster of Paris but mandatory for fiberglass. The water temperature should be as cool as possible to retard the setting time and allow more time to apply, mold, and manipulate. In addition, as casts set, they give off heat, and using warm water can increase the overall temperature and lead to superficial burns. The plaster should be left in water until all the bubbles stop rising. The ends of the roll are squeezed to force plaster into the body of the roll (Fig. 10.6).

Plaster should be applied wet. The plaster is rolled obliquely onto the limb, in the same direction as the cotton padding, keeping the roll on the surface and using the fingertips to control the unrolling of the plaster (Fig. 10.6). The roll should be kept moving at all times and should not be lifted off the extremity or pulled. The loose lower border is controlled

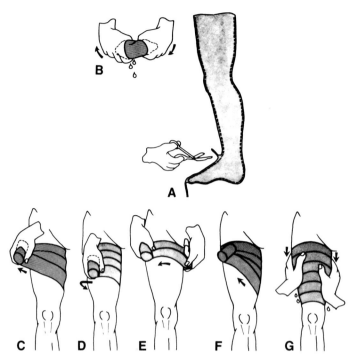

Figure 10.6. Application of roll plaster. *A,* applying and fitting the stockinette. *B,* pinching the ends of the wet plaster roll. *C* and *D,* plaster must not be pulled on as in *C,* but rolled on as in *D. E* and *F,* directing the lie of the plaster. *F,* the contour of the extremity guides the plaster in a wrong direction. *E,* by pleating, the plaster can be guided as desired. *G,* stroking the plaster to fuse the layers and smooth the surface.

by taking tucks and smoothing them into position to avoid wrinkles in the plaster. When using fiberglass, use slightly narrower rolls to offset the stiffer and thicker material. This prevents ridges in the cast when taking tucks around prominences or changes in diameter of the extremity. Each turn should be overlapped by 50% to ensure a uniform thickness. (Uneven application creates stress risers in the finished product, which cause breakage.) A second pass with additional rolls of plaster will result in a uniform four-layer cast approximately 1/8-inch thick, which is adequate for the upper extremity. A 3/16-inch cast is adequate for most lower extremity fractures. These casts can be reinforced with additional longitudinal splints across the concavity of the elbow, wrist, knee, or ankle joints to lessen the overall weight of additional rolls of plaster. Avoid reinforcing splints over the convexity

of joints because they are mechanically less effective.

The plaster is rubbed and smoothed constantly, adding water as necessary, to mold the cast to the contours of the limb. This avoids irregular ribs and depressions that cause skin damage and also prevents air and water from being trapped between the layers of plaster, which creates weak spots that can cause early breakage. This rubbing motion is done with the entire palm for large surfaces and the thenar and hypothenar eminences and the fingertips for smaller surfaces. Direct point pressure is never applied over a bony prominence. Instead, the plaster is shaped around the prominence. Avoid manipulation of the cast during the late stages of hardening. Motion at this stage will cause cracks and subsequent weakening of the cast. If this occurs, additional plaster must be added.

With experience, casts can often be made to the appropriate length and require little trimming. Before a practitioner becomes experienced, however, casts usually should be made longer than necessary and trimmed after they harden. This is most easily and safely done using a cast saw once the cast is hardened. A cast knife or scalpel can be used before full hardening of the cast. The handle of the knife or scalpel is gripped with all four fingers and steady counterpressure maintained on the cast with the thumb. Pull the margin of the cast to be trimmed up into the knife blade with the opposite hand, rather than incising downward into the plaster surface and risking cutting the patient. A special hardened saw blade is necessary to trim or cut fiberglass.

In routine long-leg or short-leg casts, the plantar aspect of the cast may be extended beyond the toe tips to protect them from injury. The metatarsophalangeal joint is kept at neutral by molding with the fingertips along the plantar aspect of the foot piece at the metatarsophalangeal joint level, while the toes are molded down into a neutral position. Hyperextension of these joints must be avoided. The extra padding previously placed between the toes is removed to afford adequate toe space for active motion. (This also applies for hand casts: removal of the padding in the web space allows the fingers to be comfortable and not compressed.) A walking plaster cast cannot support weightbearing until the cast has completely dried, usually 24 to 36 hours.

IMMOBILIZATION BY CONTINUOUS TRACTION

Weighted Traction While at Bedrest

Indications

Weighted traction in bed is a distracting force exerted parallel to the axis of the extremity or trunk. It maintains the length, alignment, stability of a fractured extremity or stability of the axial skeleton. Weighted traction is specially effective if the soft tissue tension band is intact. It allows joint motion while maintaining length, alignment, and control of the extremity. With the patient at bedrest,

weighted traction supplements immobilization of a painful joint while lessening the protective muscle spasm, providing relief of pain and swelling and allowing minimal motion of the affected joint. The primary care physician will be involved in the use of skin traction techniques. Traction techniques using transcutaneously placed skeletal pins also are widely used by orthopaedic surgeons when larger forces must be exerted.

Technique

Commercial skin traction boots/sleeves, when available, or moleskin traction tapes backed with sponge rubber are applied over an unshaved lower extremity with appropriate felt or cotton padding to prevent pressure over bony prominences or on superficial nerves. The straps are held in place by elastic bandages that are wrapped distally to proximally. Do not apply the bandages too tightly. They are rolled on—not pulled under tension. The proximal end of the straps must be well anchored. A distal-to-proximal pressure gradient is produced to prevent a tourniquet effect on the limb. This is done by wrapping the distal slightly tighter than the proximal extremity. Distally, each turn is overlapped by three-fourths of the width of the bandage. The overlap is gradually lessened proximally so that the proximal wrap overlaps one-third of the width. Moleskins are attached to a spreader, and through this to a rope, which passes through pulleys to an attached weight. The amount of traction that can be applied is a function of the surface area of skin. In a child, usually 4 lb of traction can be applied to the lower extremity, whereas an adult can tolerate approximately 8 lb. The traction straps must be rewrapped at least three times a day. The skin must be inspected and wiped with alcohol to cleanse and toughen before rewrapping.

Types of Skin Traction

Buck's Traction (Fig. 10.7)

This type of traction is used to relieve pain, inflammation, and muscle spasm about the knee and hip. Traction tapes (as previously described) are applied to the lower legs, from immediately proximal to the malleoli to below the knee. Pads are placed over the malleoli and about the proximal fibula over the peroneal nerve. This prevents skin breakdown over the malleoli or damage to the peroneal nerve, which runs subcutaneously two finger breadths distal to the head of the fibula. For comfort, pillows are placed under the knees, and the head of the bed is raised. An example of the use of Buck's traction is for toxic synovitis of the hip in a child. Four to 5 lb of weight are required, and intermittent heat to the involved hip is used three to four times a day. The child is removed from traction for gentle active-assistive range of motion exercises three to four times a day.

Split Russell Traction (Fig. 10.8)

This type of traction is used for the same conditions as Buck's traction, but allows better control of rotation and some active motion of

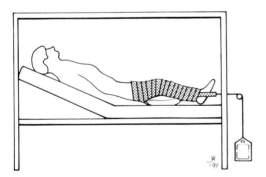

Figure 10.7. Buck's traction.

the knee and hip. Traction straps are applied as for Buck's traction. A soft felt sling is placed under the knee. This sling attaches to a spreader, then by a rope to an overhead pulley, it is placed over the knee, and finally over the foot of the bed, through a second pulley, to a weight at the end of the bed. Weight is selected according to the patient's age and size. Typically, the axial traction is 3 to 5 lb, and 3 to 5 lb is used for the knee sling. This usually provides comfort and support to an acutely inflamed hip or knee. Traction could be coupled with ice massage or moist hot packs and gentle active-assistive range of motion as tolerated.

Pelvic Traction (Fig. 10.9)

A corsetlike lined canvas is wrapped about the waist. Straps with rope extension extend from the corset at its midlateral points, through pulleys, to the bottom of the bed, and to weights. Adults can tolerate 20 to 30 lb of weight. The foot of the bed is elevated, and body weight acts as counter-traction. Traction is applied for 1 to 3 hours four to six times per day, with intermittent heat for 20 minutes three times per day. This amount of weight is really not enough to cause any significant distraction through the lumbar or lumbosacral spine. Much larger forces are necessary to provide true distraction but cannot be tolerated in any type of corset or skin traction arrangement.

Cervical Traction (Fig. 10.10)

A head halter or a soft head harness is commercially available to apply traction to the

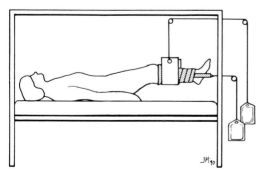

Figure 10.8. Split Russell traction.

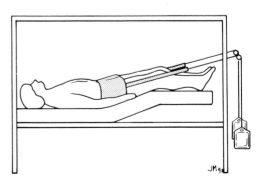

Figure 10.9. Pelvic traction.

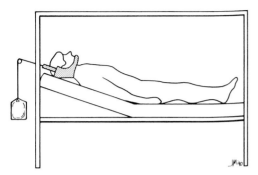

Figure 10.10. Cervical traction.

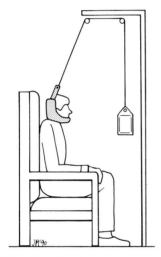

Figure 10.11. Over-the-door arrangement for cervical traction.

mandible and occiput. Avoid excessive pressure on the mandible by positioning the occipital strap to accept most of the load, or use a bite plate or mouth piece to minimize the pressure on the temporomandibular joint, which can precipitate the temporomandibular (joint) syndrome. The halter is attached to a spreader bar above the head. A rope is attached to the spreader and is carried through a pulley at the head of the bed to a weight. The patient is usually positioned comfortably with the neck in slight flexion. Cervical traction can also be effectively performed with the patient sitting using an over-the-door arrangement, demonstrated in Figure 10.11. Treatment begins with about 5 lb of weight, which is gradu-

ally increased to 10 to 15 lb as tolerated. The patient's comfort is used as a guide. The traction is used intermittently for 20 minutes to 1 hour, four to six times per day. Cervical traction requires appropriate skin care to avoid skin breakdown over the chin or occiput. This therapy is useful for neck pain associated with degenerative conditions and secondary to muscular strain or cervical sprains without instability.

COMPLICATIONS

Complications of immobilization techniques include tight cast, cast sores or burns, joint stiffness, thrombophlebitis, compartment (cast) syndrome, soft tissue contracture, allergic reaction to fiberglass, pressure ulcers, and nerve palsies secondary to traction apparatus. Three of the most common cast complications, compartment (cast) syndrome, skin necrosis, and joint stiffness, will be discussed.

The Compartment (Cast) Syndrome

The extremities are comprised of soft tissue compartments bounded by rigid fascial envelopes oriented along the long axis of the extremity. The muscles, nerves, and vessels of the extremity traverse these compartments. The fascial envelopes have little compliance and are anchored to the supporting bone (Fig. 10.12). Injury to the contained bone or associated soft tissues that traverse the compartment results in bleeding or swelling in the compartment, which may increase intracompartment pressure. If the acutely injured extremity has been wrapped in a rigid cast, the compliance of the leg is further reduced, which, in turn, may further increase the compartment pressure. If the compartment pressures exceed the venous pressure, the venous system collapses. Secondary failure of the capillary circulation occurs and then subsequent collapse of the arteriole circulation, resulting in ischemia of the soft tissues in the compartment. The ischemia, in turn, causes more edema. This further increases the fluid and, consequently, pressure within the compartment, further worsening the syndrome. Thus, a vicious cycle is trig-

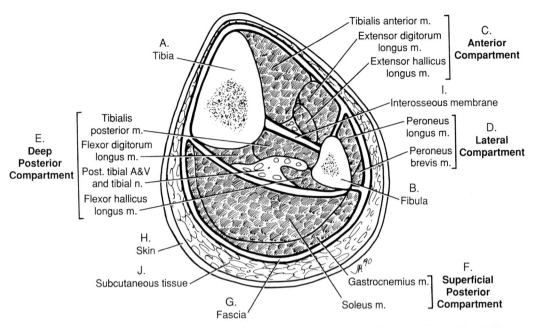

Figure 10.12. Compartments of the lower leg shown in a cross section of the midcalf. *A*, tibia. *B*, fibula. *C*, anterior compartment. *D*, lateral compartment. *E*, deep posterior compartment. *F*, superficial posterior compartment. *G*, fascia. *H*, skin. *I*, interosseous membrane. *J*, subcutaneous tissue.

gered which, unless treated, will continue until it effectively strangles the soft parts.

The key to prevention or successful treatment is early recognition. The earliest sign of an impending compartment syndrome is severe pain that is of greater magnitude than one would ordinarily expect in an extremity that is well supported subsequent to an injury. One of the earliest signs is increased pain on passive stretching of the muscles within the affected compartment. Paresthesia and paralysis are later findings. It should be noted that the distal pulses are usually present. The first step in treating compartment syndrome is to split the cast medially and laterally along the midlateral and midmedial lines, respectively (Fig. 10.13). All wrappings should be cut down to the skin so that the limb can be fully decompressed. Compartment pressures diminish 65% after bivalving and spreading the cast. Cutting the padding and removing the cast further decreases the compartment pressure by a small amount. The extremity should be elevated a few inches above the heart. Avoid excessive elevation because this might impair

arterial circulation. Following elevation, the patient should be observed closely for signs of improvement.

If the syndrome persists, that is, the signs and symptoms do not return to normal, one assumes that the findings are related not only to the tight cast, but to a developing compartment syndrome. At this point, an emergency orthopaedic referral should be made. Time is of the essence: any delay in this communication could be disastrous. Prolonged ischemia, greater than 6 hours, may result in irreversible tissue injury and significant sequelae.

If there is an obvious compartment syndrome, the orthopaedist may proceed directly with fasciotomy of the extremity. If there is any question, direct measurement of the compartment pressure can be performed. This is often the only means of making the diagnosis in an equivocal situation. Patients with fractures frequently have severe pain and, because of the damage to muscular tissue or slight movement of the fracture, may have increased pain with passive stretch. Assessing these patients clinically is often difficult and it be-

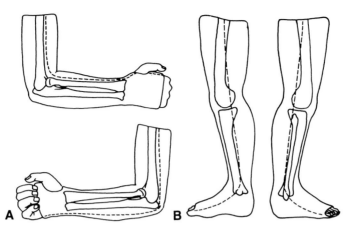

Figure 10.13. Splitting casts. The *dotted line* indicates where the cast is split. *A,* long-arm cast. *B,* long-leg cast.

comes more difficult if the patient is heavily medicated. In the unconscious patient, only direct inspection of the involved compartment and compartment pressure measurement can be used to detect an early compartment syndrome. Measurement of compartment pressure is a fairly simple procedure that the orthopaedist can perform using commercial kits or a large bore needle, IV tubing, 3-way stopcock, and manometer. When the compartment pressure is measured to be above 30 mm Hg in a normotensive patient, the diagnosis of compartment syndrome is confirmed. Once this diagnosis is made, a fasciotomy is indicated on an emergent basis.

Because of the potential for increased swelling in an injured extremity that has been immobilized in a circumferential cast, patients must be carefully instructed and observed following cast application. Individuals who are stable and deemed at low risk for such complications may be treated on an ambulatory basis but must be instructed to be aware and observe their extremity for signs of circulatory or neurologic impairment. The following should be explained as possible danger signs: coolness or sluggishness of capillary refill in the fingers or toes, cyanosis or pallor of the fingers or toes, tingling of the fingers or toes, and increasing pain, particularly with passive stretch. The patient is instructed to return promptly if these conditions develop. Patients who are

judged to be at high risk for compartment syndrome should be hospitalized and observed for at least 24 to 48 hours until their conditions stabilize.

Skin Necrosis

A constant point of pressure will cause local cutaneous ischemia, and slight axial movement occurring under a cast will in time cause erosions over bony prominences and beneath the irregularities on the undersurface of the cast. To avoid these problems, the padding must fit snugly without wrinkles. The plaster must be applied smoothly over the padding and must be separated from the skin over bony protrusions by padding and careful molding.

In addition to the circulatory precautions taught to patients, the following skin precautions are also taught. Patients are to return immediately if they experience burning pain inside a cast or any other sensation that they interpret to feel like an abrasion or a boil. When faced with any such complaints, the primary clinician is obliged to window the cast over the area of concern or split the cast and remove one-half of the cast at a time to better examine the extremity.

If a cutaneous injury is evident, the injured area is cleansed and dressed with a nonadherent dressing. Several layers of padding are applied over the dressing, the window of the cast is replaced and held in place with tape, or the bivalve is reapplied and held in position with cast straps. If the window is left open, tissue will swell up through the window, causing erosions at the margin of the window or possibly impairing circulation to the skin of that area (window edema).

Joint Stiffness

The stiffness that results after immobilization is proportional to the length of time immobilized. The main factor in the production of this contracture is shortening of the surrounding musculature; changes in the joint capsule contribute to a lesser degree. During immobilization, the normal pumping action that is generated by motion and produces the flow of tissue fluids out of an extremity is prevented. Tissue capillaries congest, and the capsules, ligaments, and tendons they serve also congest and become thickened and, consequently, shortened. (Forces that stretch a viscoelastic material in one dimension will at the same time shorten it in the perpendicular direction.) Intra-articular changes also occur that can result in thinning of the cartilage, fibrosis, or bony ankylosis.

No joint should be immobilized unnecessarily. Certain injuries do not require rigid immobilization. For example, fractures of the shaft of the femur can be managed in traction, which allows controlled knee motion as well as isometric and limited isotonic exercises. Salter introduced the concept of continuous passive motion (CPM), which utilizes an apparatus that supports the injured extremity while passively moving the joint through a carefully controlled arc of motion at a specific rate to avoid pain. This alleviates pain, preserves joint range of motion, and may enhance healing in both articular and ligamentous injuries.

The benefits and hazards of prolonged immobilization must be weighed before initial treatment is chosen, and a regimen of mobilization as well as strengthening must follow the period of immobilization. Treatment with a cast and discharge before monitoring the patient through a well-guided rehabilitation program is incomplete treatment. Each regional chapter describes exercises used to mobilize and recondition stiffened extremities.

RADIOGRAPHIC MONITORING

At least two views at right angles to one another should be taken of any suspected fracture. At times, special views, such as obliques, spot views, stress films, tomograms, or computed tomography scans, are required to adequately visualize the injury. These have been discussed appropriately in the regional chapters.

Once the diagnosis is made and treatment accomplished, an x-ray should be obtained after manipulation and casting or splint to assess the accuracy of reduction and the maintenance of position. The extremity should then be x-rayed at 5 to 7 days to detect any change in position of unstable injuries. This should be repeated at an interval of another 5 to 7 days. In fractures that heal rapidly, another x-ray is appropriate in 2 to 4 weeks, when the fracture should be assessed clinically and radiographically for progress in healing. An x-ray should always be done when the fracture is considered clinically stable and immobilization is going to be discontinued. This provides information about the degree of healing and, consequently, the degree of further protection necessary. Another x-ray should be obtained when it is thought that remodeling of the fracture is fairly mature to assess the integrity and form of the final structure. X-rays should be done during treatment if further injury to the extremity occurs, if the cast becomes grossly loose or breaks, or if increased pain is present at the fracture at a time remote from injury.

The exact timing of x-ray examination depends on many variables, including the nature and location of the fracture as well as the age of the patient. For example, the time course of fracture healing of the femur can be 3 to 5 weeks in a 3-year-old, 8 to 10 weeks in an 8-year-old, 12 to 14 weeks in a 12-year-old, and 20 to 24 weeks in an adult. A developing deformity in an unstable fracture must be recognized before healing becomes too advanced for remanipulation to correct the malposition.

The practitioner consequently must be aware of which fractures heal rapidly, and carefully follow unstable injuries in the initial phase. For example, a metaphyseal fracture of the distal radius in a 6-year-old will be stable by 2 weeks, and there is little chance of progressive deformity. Recurrent deformity must be recognized before 2 weeks postinjury to correct the deformity by remanipulation. Fractures that heal more slowly must have a longer period of close follow-up. A midshaft tibial fracture in an adult can change position 2 to 4 weeks after reduction.

REHABILITATION FOLLOWING MUSCULOSKELETAL INJURIES

Rehabilitation efforts begin in the emergency department when the patient is admitted. The goals for the patient's recovery include regaining full range of motion of the involved joints; regaining full strength, endurance, and power in the affected motor groups in the extremity; gradually increasing functional activity of the injured parts to promote healing; and, finally, returning to as near a normal state as possible. The specific rehabilitative regimens are outlined in the regional chapters. It is best to use the resources of the acute physical rehabilitation services at the hospital or in the community to ensure optimal recovery.

BASIC PRINCIPLES

Muscle strengthens in proportion to load moved. It is usually safe and effective to choose a resistance that will fatigue the muscles, but not precipitate pain, within 20 repetitions. To increase muscle strength, it is necessary to make a muscle contract with maximum power every day without overloading. To increase muscle endurance, use repetitions of lighter loads, stopping short of fatigue. Strength of a muscle contraction is proportional to the starting length of the muscle. Therefore, fully extend the muscle before exercising. Avoid overstretching of muscles because this retards healing. Weak or partially innervated muscles should be protected from overstretching.

The three basic types of exercise routines are isometric, isotonic, and isokinetic. The routines are prescribed by the physician in specific situations. Warm towels should be placed on the muscle group for 5 to 10 minutes before the workout to promote relaxation and warm-up.

Isometric exercises strengthen muscle groups by contracting the muscle (producing tension) but not moving the affected joint or changing the length of the muscle. This is the best way to develop strength if joint motion is painful and there is secondary muscle inhibition. For example, quadriceps isometrics or "setting" involves maintaining the knee in a fixed position and contracting the muscle in rhythmic, gentle, gradual fashion to avoid pain. The contraction is sustained for 5 to 10 seconds and then relaxed for an equal period. This is repeated 10 to 20 times per "set," followed by a 5-minute rest period. The sets are repeated two to three times to the patient's fatigue point tempered by pain. The routine may be repeated two to three times per day as tolerated. Again, pain and fatigue are the controlling end points.

In isotonic exercises, the joint and muscle group move an applied load through a range of motion. This is probably the best way to regain motion, strength, and endurance when the joint is not painful. A useful technique to enhance the effects of isometric and isotonic programs is progressive resistance exercises, in which the load is increased progressively as strength increases, thereby enhancing strength, power, and endurance.

Isokinetic exercises control the rate of joint motion while the resistance varies with the strength of the subject's muscular effort. For example, patients may push or pull as little or as much as they wish, but the cadence is unchanged. Therefore, muscle power, which is the amount of work accomplished over a unit of time, may be increased by exercising at a higher rate even if the loads are smaller. Exercising at a higher rate also increases endurance. The isokinetic machine can also measure torque; thus, it is a simple matter to graph the actual motor strength and power generated. The physician, therapist, and patient can see the results and hence gauge progress or lack of progress in the therapy program. Joints begin to mobilize when moved regularly, barely through the point of pain. Active exercise is preferred to passive exercise because it is independent, strengthens while it mobilizes, and is less likely to do harm than passive movements. Gentle active-assistive exercise is necessitated by weakness, timidity, harmful incoordination, or a pain process that is worsened by active movement, e.g., traumatic hemarthrosis or acute arthritis. As discussed in "Complications," congestion is relieved by movements that rhythmically compress the congested structures. Joint movement to the mechanical limit of motion or the onset of pain (whichever occurs first) will apply such compression. This technique can be useful at the outset of a rehabilitation program, when pain, stiffness, and patient reluctance are greatest. Often, after a single session, the patient is capable of performing a therapeutically beneficial range of motion.

Wet heat is more analgesic than dry heat. Heat can burn, hence the heat source must be tested on the volar forearm of the therapist before applying to the patient. The heat source must not be applied to insensitive or ischemic skin. If the skin is prevented from cooling by the patient's position or a covering, a continuous source of heat must not be applied. For example, a common and blistering error is to lie upon a heating pad. Wet heat is best applied as a local bath, but may be applied as a hot wet towel kept hot with a heating pad that has been insulated in plastic. Note that local heating, e.g., immersion of the injured part alone, is more effective than total heating, e.g., immersion of the whole body, because the part can be kept hotter longer without harm to the patient. Usually, heat applications are limited to 10 or 15 minutes, three or four times a day. If exceeded, this tends to produce a hyperemic state in the local area, which causes more local inflammation and congestion and attendant pain and tenderness.

Cold is less likely to congest an area than heat, and it can be analgesic. The analgesic benefit is more likely to be appreciated after, rather than during, the application. Cold is unequivocally preferred to heat during the first 36 to 72 hours after injury. After that initial period of cold applications, heat or cold may be applied symptomatically on a trial basis.

Cold can be effectively applied in several ways. Water can be frozen in a paper cup, then the ice, held in the cup or a washcloth, can be massaged over the painful areas. To avoid thermocutaneous injury, the ice must be kept moving throughout the treatment. Five to 10 minutes of massage is usually effective. The patient will suffer a burning pain before the analgesic effect is achieved. Alternatively, a bath towel can be folded to the size of the area to be treated, dampened thoroughly but not dripping, and chilled. The chilled or "soft-frozen" towel may then be applied to the painful area for 5 or 10 minutes. To prevent an ice burn, a damp towel must be placed between the "soft-frozen" towel and the disordered part. For example, the individual with a painful disorder of the low back can lie with his back on a damp towel over a chilled towel. Finally, an ice bag or pack are effective means of cooling an injured part. To avoid injury, the skin must not be in direct contact with the ice. The application should be for 5 to 10 minutes and the part should be allowed to return to normal temperature before reapplying the cold application.

Painfully reactive muscle tone must be kept at a minimum. Any manipulation or motion, active or passive, which is followed by an increase in painfully reactive muscle tone must be avoided, or its harmful influence on muscle tone somehow neutralized. Topical and systemic analgesics facilitate a decrease in painfully reactive muscle tone. Topical analgesics include heat, cold, and gentle massage. Systemic analgesics include drugs such as salicylates and nonsteroidal anti-inflammatories. Fatigue must be recognized, relieved, and subsequently avoided when it appears to augment pain. Anxiety and depression must be recognized and relieved.

THE MEASUREMENT OF JOINT MOTION

Although a qualitative sense of joint motion is often adequate for diagnostic and planning purposes, a quantitative measure provides a more objective assessment of the effect of therapy and a better documented report of disability. Joint motion is most accurately measured with a goniometer. One limb, the static limb, of the goniometer is aligned with a reference axis along the body part just proximal to the joint; the other limb, the dynamic limb, of the goniometer is aligned with the moving axis along the body part just distal to the joint. The joint motion is measured from a position as close in line with the reference axis as the moving axis can attain, to a position as far from the reference axis as the moving axis can attain, within the intended plane of motion. The reference axis is always designated 0°. With experience, the examiner can fairly accurately estimate the degrees of joint motion without a goniometer.

Figures 10.13 through 10.28 name the motion and the plane of its measurements, designate the reference axis, and show the proper alignment of the goniometer for each measurement.

MUSCLE STRENGTH GRADING

The strength of individual muscles may be indicated by functional grades (Table 10.1).

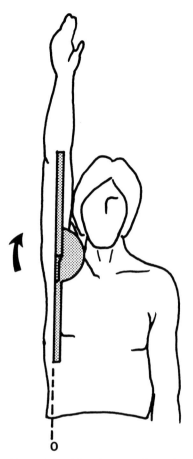

Figure 10.15. Shoulder elevation through abduction. Measurement is made in the frontal plane of the trunk.

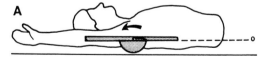

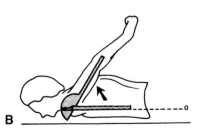

Figure 10.14. *A*, shoulder elevation through flexion. Measurement is made in the sagittal plane of the trunk. *B*, shoulder extension. Measurement is made in the sagittal plane of the trunk.

Table 10.1. Muscle Strength Grading

Grade	Characteristics
Normal (5)	Full active range of motion against gravity and normal resistance
Good (4)	Full active range of motion against gravity and good resistance
Fair (3)	Full active range of motion against gravity
Poor (2)	Full active range of motion with gravity eliminated
Trace (1)	Muscle contracts but no joint motion
None (0)	No muscle contraction

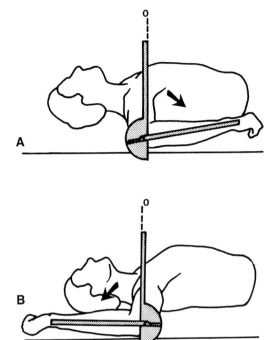

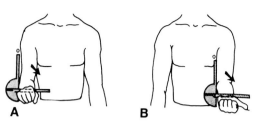

Figure 10.18. *A*, forearm pronation with the elbow at 90° flexion, with the forearm in the sagittal plane of the trunk. Measurement is made in the frontal plane of the trunk. *B*, forearm supination with the elbow at 90° flexion, with the forearm in the sagittal plane of the trunk. Measurement is made in the frontal plane of the trunk.

Figure 10.16. *A*, internal rotation of the shoulder at 90° abduction. Measurement is made in the sagittal plane of the trunk. *B*, external rotation of the shoulder at 90° abduction. Measurement is made in the sagittal plane of the trunk.

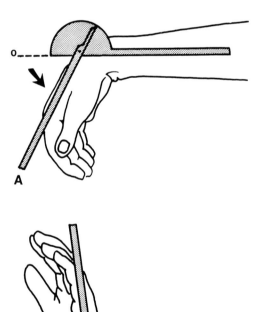

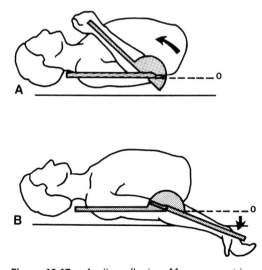

Figure 10.17. *A*, elbow flexion. Measurement is made in the sagittal plane of the arm. *B*, elbow extension. Measurement is made in the sagittal plane of the arm.

Figure 10.19. *A*, wrist flexion. Measurement is made in the sagittal plane of the forearm. *B*, wrist extension. Measurement is made in the sagittal plane of the forearm.

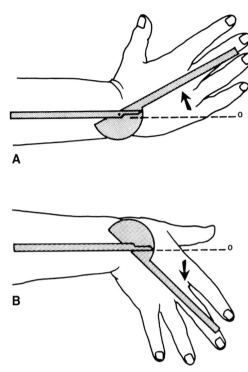

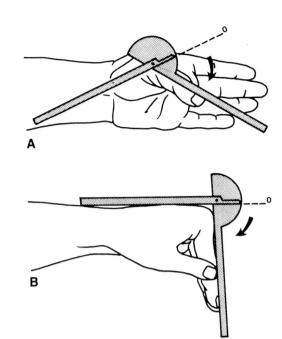

Figure 10.20. *A*, radial deviation of the wrist. Measurement is made in the frontal plane of the forearm. *B*, ulnar deviation of the wrist. Measurement is made in the frontal plane of the forearm.

Figure 10.21. *A*, flexion of the first metacarpophalangeal joint. Measurement is made in the frontal plane of the forearm and hand. *B*, flexion of the second, third, fourth, and fifth metacarpophalangeal joints. Measurement is made in the sagittal plane of the forearm and hand.

AMBULATION AIDS AND GAIT TRAINING

Patients with injuries to the lower extremities usually require some form of ambulation aid (crutches, canes, walkers) to protect the injured parts. Before this step, as soon as possible after injury and definitive care, prepare the patient for ambulation by regaining full range of motion, strength, endurance, balance, and control of the trunk and uninjured extremities. The most important muscles for assisted walking using aids are the abdominal and paraspinous muscles of the trunk; the shoulder abductors, depressors, adductors, flexors, and extensors; the elbow extensors; the forearm rotators, wrist extensors, and finger flexors in the upper limbs; and the antigravity muscles of the uninjured lower extremity. Isometric exercises are used first, followed by isotonic and isokinetic exercises as described earlier. Patients must be taught a proper gait pattern using support. They begin standing in the parallel bars with their feet slightly apart to get their balance. Next, they transfer their weight front-to-back and side-to-side to attain balance on each foot. They are then taught to use crutches, a cane, or a walker.

Crutches

Crutches should be adjusted for the patient so that there are three fingers between the "axillary" pad of the crutch and the axilla when the tip of the crutch is located slightly lateral and anterior to the tip of the shoe with the feet side by side. The "axillary" pad is designed to take pressure on the lateral side of the upper chest, and not in the axilla where the brachial plexus could be injured. The hand piece should be positioned so that the elbow is flexed comfortably (approximately 10 to 20°) while bearing weight. The tip of the crutch should be covered with a wide rubber crutch tip to add traction and stability.

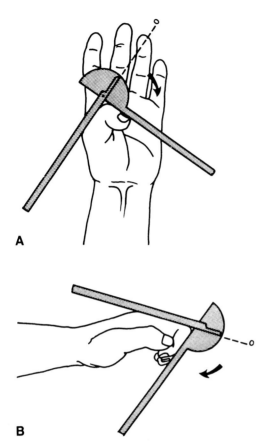

B

Figure 10.22. *A,* flexion of the first interphalangeal joint. Measurement is made in the frontal plane of the hand. *B,* flexion of the second, third, fourth, and fifth interphalangeal joints. Measurement is made in the sagittal plane of the hand.

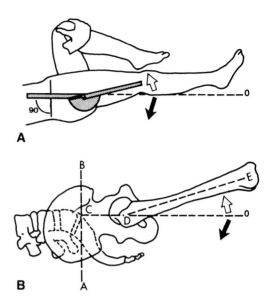

Figure 10.23. *A,* skeletal landmarks used to orient the goniometer when measuring hip extension and flexion. The 0° axis is perpendicular to a line connecting the point of the anterior-superior iliac spine with the point of the posterior iliac spine. *B,* hip extension. Measurement is made in the sagittal plane of the trunk. The example illustrates limitation of extension to a point short of the 0° axis (open arrow).

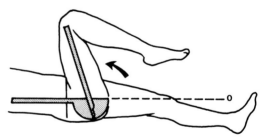

Figure 10.24. Hip flexion. Measurement is made in the sagittal plane of the trunk.

Crutch Gaits

The simplest gait is the swing-through gait, in which both crutches are placed forward and the patient swings the body and both lower extremities through both crutches so that the feet end up ahead of the crutch tips. Weight can be borne on both feet or on the well foot with the injured foot nonweightbearing. This is a nonphysiologic gait but is quick and easy to learn.

The three-point gait is a smoother gait biomechanically. In this method, the two crutches are advanced and followed closely by the injured extremity, so that the crutch tips are firmly planted just before the injured ex-

tremity strikes the ground. The degree of weightbearing to the injured extremity is controlled by the weight borne on the upper extremities, and is expressed as a three-point, partial weightbearing crutch gait. The desired weight (or none) to be borne on the injured extremity is specifically prescribed by the physician.

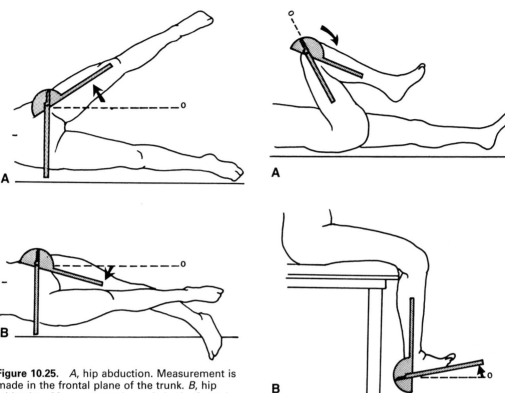

Figure 10.25. *A*, hip abduction. Measurement is made in the frontal plane of the trunk. *B*, hip adduction. Measurement is made in the frontal plane of the trunk.

Figure 10.27. *A*, knee flexion. Measurement is made in the sagittal plane of the thigh. *B*, ankle dorsiflexion. Measurement is made in the sagittal plane of the leg.

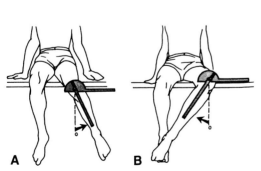

Figure 10.26. *A*, internal rotation of the hip. Measurement is made in the transverse plane of the thigh. *B*, external rotation of the hip. Measurement is made in the transverse plane of the thigh.

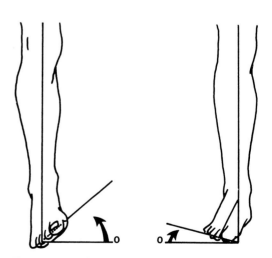

Figure 10.28. Supination and pronation of the foot. Supination is measured in the transverse plane of the foot. Pronation is measured in the transverse and frontal planes of the foot.

Canes

Canes are fitted by having the patient hold the cane in the hand opposite to the injured lower extremity. The length should be such that the elbow is flexed approximately 20° while the rubber cane tip rests on the ground 3 to 4 inches laterally to and slightly ahead of the tip of the ipsilateral shoe. Canes are less cumbersome and easier to use than crutches, but they are much less effective in unloading an extremity. Patients advance the cane with the normal alternating swing of the upper extremity, e.g., the right hand swings forward with the left foot. The cane and the heel of the injured limb should strike the ground simultaneously. At contact, the elbow should be flexed 10 to 20°, and the tip of the cane should be slightly outside the progression of the swing phase of the normal extremity and opposite the midfoot of the injured extremity. The requirements for muscle strength are similar to those for crutches. The cane is a useful intermediate device when weaning a patient from crutches to full weightbearing.

Walkers

A walker is more stable than a cane or crutches and offers an alternate device for protected weightbearing that is particularly useful for patients who do not have the strength, agility, or coordination to use crutches or a cane. Walkers are fitted to the patient while the patient stands with both hands on the handles of the walker and flexes the elbows 20 to 30° (handle bars approximately at the level of the greater trochanter). Patients should be instructed to stand in the embrace of the walker in a comfortable position with the necessary weight on the handles of the walker to protect the injured part. They then advance the walker for the length of their arms and set it firmly on the ground. Patients then shift their weight to the handles and walk into the bars of the walker. This provides a partial or nonweightbearing gait, much like the three-point or four-point crutch gait. The walker is particularly useful for elderly patients after hip fracture.

SUGGESTED READINGS

Nickel VL, ed. Orthopedic Rehabilitation. New York: Churchill Livingstone, 1982.

Rockwood CA Jr, Green DP, eds. Fractures in Adults; Vol. 1, 2. 2nd ed. Philadelphia: JB Lippincott Co., 1984.

Rockwood CA Jr, Wilkins KE, King RE, eds. Fractures in Children. Vol. 3. Philadelphia: JB Lippincott Co., 1984.

Salter RB. Textbook of Disorders and Injuries of the Musculoskeletal System: An Introduction to Orthopaedics, Fractures and Joint Injuries, Rheumatology, Metabolic Bone Disease and Rehabilitation. 2nd ed. Baltimore: Williams and Wilkins, 1983.

Southmayd W, Hoffman M. Sports Health: The Complete Book of Athletic Injuries. New York: Quick Fox, 1981.

Staff, Prosthetics and Orthotics. Lower-Limb Orthotics. New York: New York University Postgraduate Medical School, 1986.

Staff, Prosthetics and Orthotics. Lower-Limb Prosthetics. 1990 revision. New York: New York University Postgraduate Medical School, 1990.

Staff, Prosthetics and Orthotics. Upper-Limb Prosthetics. New York: New York University Postgraduate Medical School, 1982.

Turek SL. Orthopaedics: Principles and Their Application. 4th ed. Philadelphia: JB Lippincott Co., 1984.

Aspiration and Injection Techniques: Joints, Bursae, and Local Anesthesia

Carlton M. Akins, M.D., and W. Thomas Edwards, Ph.D., M.D.

During the evaluation of orthopaedic disorders, the clinician may introduce a needle for a variety of reasons: (*a*) aspiration for diagnosis of joint or bursal effusion, (*b*) evacuation of painful hemarthrosis or other effusion, (*c*) injection of corticosteroid into the joint or bursa, or (*d*) local anesthesia. An understanding of both general and local principles is important in the safe and effective use of these techniques. These local principles are concerned with specific applications and are described and diagramed later in this chapter.

ASPIRATION AND INJECTION TECHNIQUES

GENERAL PRINCIPLES

Aspiration is performed as part of the evaluation of a joint or bursal effusion (see Chapter 12) or to relieve the painful pressure of a tense effusion. Aspiration also facilitates further clinical examination. Corticosteroids may be injected into an inflamed bursa or joint once it has been established that the inflammation is not secondary to an infection. The clinician is most likely to use these techniques in the following areas for the conditions listed: injuries with effusion—knee, elbow, ankle, shoulder; degenerative joint disease with synovitis—trapeziometacarpal joint of the thumb, knee and metatarsophalangeal joint of the great toe, ankle; rheumatoid arthritis—knee, metacarpophalangeal and interphalangeal

finger joints, wrist, ankle; bursae—subacromial, greater trochanteric, olecranon, prepatellar, and pes anserine. The following general technique is recommended (Fig. 11.1):

1. Identify joint or bursal landmarks by fingertip palpation and define the site of needle insertion. (Specific sites are designated later in this section.)
2. Cleanse the area with povidone-iodine solution. Drape the site with sterile drapes.
3. Create a 1% lidocaine wheal at the site of needle entry using a small (25- to 27-gauge) needle and sterile gloves.
4. For joint or bursal aspiration, use an 18- or l9-gauge needle (smaller sizes are often ineffective) and syringe appropriate to the site. For the knee, ankle, shoulder, elbow, and wrist, use a 20-mL syringe; and for smaller joints and bursae, a 5- or 10-mL syringe.
5. For corticosteroid injection, after aspiration, use the same needle for both. For injection alone, use the narrowest gauge needle of appropriate length. For the shoulder, elbow, wrist, knee, and ankle, a 1 ½-inch 22-gauge needle usually suffices; finger and toe joints can usually be injected with a ¾-inch 25-gauge needle.
6. Draw the corticosteroid preparation from the vial into a small syringe, using an 18- or 20-gauge needle; then exchange the needle, using sterile technique, for the needle

intended for the injection. The volume of corticosteroid to be injected depends on the size of the joint or bursa: in finger and toe joints, 0.25 mL; elbow, wrist, and ankle, 0.5–1.0 mL; shoulder, hip, knee, and associated bursae, 1.0 mL.

7. Continue to use sterile technique for the process of needle insertion. Introduce the needle with a steady thrust, not an abrupt push. Hold the syringe like a pencil, and use only the force of the fingers and wrist to introduce the needle. The opposite hand may be used to steady the syringe hand, stabilize the area, or to compress the joint if necessary.

8. When aspirating a joint or bursa, the syringe may have to be detached from the needle hub and emptied several times, leaving the needle inserted. Use a hemostat to hold the needle back while twisting off the syringe and when replacing it.

Specific Applications

Figures 11.2 through 11.12 identify the landmarks and proper site of needle insertion for aspiration or injection.

LOCAL ANESTHESIA

GENERAL PRINCIPLES

Remember that the most common cause of serious problems in the performance of any

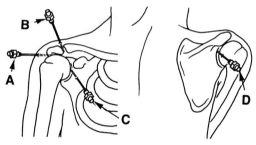

Figure 11.2. Placing a needle into the shoulder joints. *A*, into the subacromial bursa. *B*, into the acromioclavicular joint. *C*, into the glenohumeral joint. Anterior approach. *D*, into the glenohumeral joint. Posterior approach.

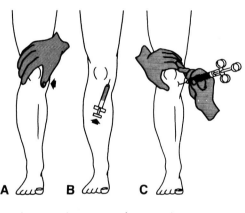

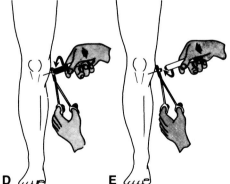

Figure 11.1. Aspirating the knee. *A*, identifying the joint space. *B*, anesthetizing the skin. *C*, passing the needle. *D*, removing the filled syringe. *E*, replacing the emptied syringe.

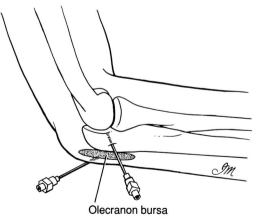

Olecranon bursa

Figure 11.3. Placing a needle into the elbow joint or the olecranon bursa from the radial aspect.

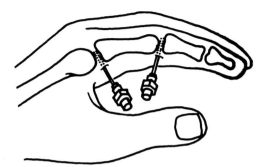

Figure 11.6. Placing a needle into the metacarpophalangeal and interphalangeal joints.

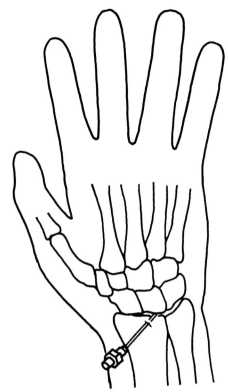

Figure 11.4. Placing a needle into the radiocarpal joint through the dorsal aspect of the wrist.

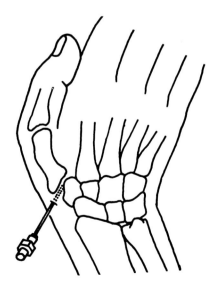

Figure 11.5. Placing a needle into the trapeziometacarpal joint.

local anesthetic procedure is related to the toxic effects of local anesthetic agents. These toxic effects can occur because of accidental intravascular injection of the appropriate amount of the drug, injection of an overdose of the drug into the appropriate tissue space, toxic reactions to drugs with which a local anesthetic agent is compounded, or allergic reaction to the local anesthetic drug or any substance with which it is prepared. Put simply, these can be remembered as the following: (*a*) right amount of drug in the wrong place; (*b*) wrong amount of drug in the right place; (*c*) right drug in the right place, wrong adjunct; and (*d*) right drug, right place, unexpected reaction.

These problems can be avoided by taking some simple precautions in choosing drugs and dosages as well as being prepared to deal with unexpected outcomes. In general, every local anesthetic administration should follow these simple principles:

1. Always be familiar with the drugs you are administering, especially with the maximum safe dose of all drugs contained in the agent you are using.
2. Expect the unexpected and be prepared. Be sure your office is equipped to deal with the consequences of toxic and allergic reactions.
3. Have the necessary resuscitation equipment and drugs at hand when you administer local anesthetics. At the minimum, these include the following: equipment to

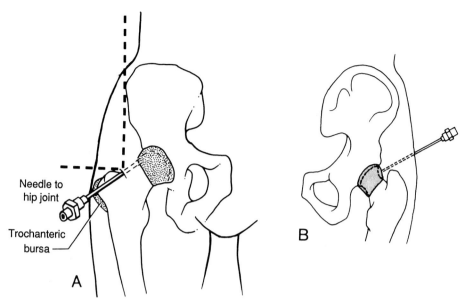

Figure 11.7. Passing a needle into the hip joint or trochanteric bursa. *A*, anterior approach. *B*, lateral approach.

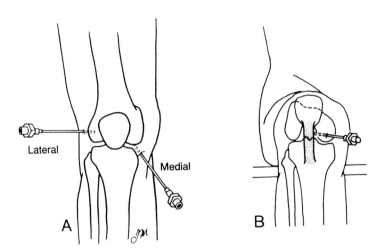

Figure 11.8. Passing a needle into the knee joint. *A*, medial or lateral. *B*, anterior approach, with the knee flexed at 90°.

establish intravenous line and intravenous fluids; oxygen and the appropriate equipment for its administration; appropriate airway support equipment including suction, oral and nasal airways, endotracheal tube, laryngoscope, and hand resuscitator (Ambu bag); and drugs for cardiovascular support in the event that advanced cardiac life support techniques need to be instituted.

LOCAL ANESTHETICS — DRUGS, AGENTS, ADJUNCTS

The author distinguishes the local anesthetic drug (such as lidocaine) from the agent

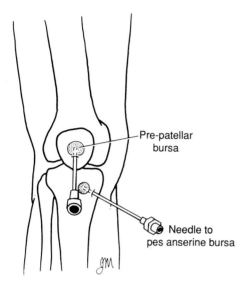

Figure 11.9. Passing a needle into bursae of the knee.

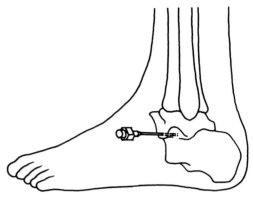

Figure 11.11. Passing a needle into the subtalar joint by way of the sinus tarsi. Note the position relative to the lateral malleolus. The depression of the sinus tarsi is palpable there, especially when the ankle is inverted.

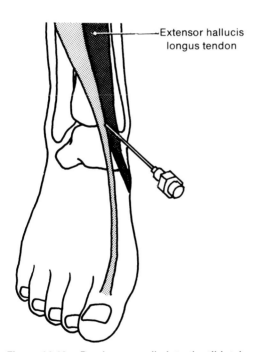

Figure 11.10. Passing a needle into the tibiotalar joint.

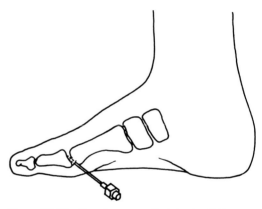

Figure 11.12. Passing a needle into the first metatarsophalangeal joint.

used for local anesthesia. The agent includes the drug, its concentration, all adjunctive agents and their concentrations, as well as the total volume of the solution administered to produce anesthesia. For example, the agent for a digital block might be 4 mL of 1% plain lidocaine (Xylocaine). A complete statement of the agent used can give an indication of why a problem has occurred.

A bewildering array of local anesthetics is commercially available. Five drugs are in common use today: cocaine, chloroprocaine, lidocaine, mepivacaine, and bupivacaine. For practical purposes, it is advisable that the physician become familiar with a limited number of drugs and use only these.

Cocaine is available in a 5% solution and is used only for application to mucosal surfaces of the upper airway to produce topical anesthesia. Higher concentrations are available but the toxicity can be profound. Chloroprocaine is available in 1 to 3% solutions. The use of concentrations between 1 and 2% for routine office practice is recommended. This drug is the most rapidly acting of all injectable local anesthetics and generally has the lowest systemic toxicity. As with cocaine, chloroprocaine is a member of the group of ester local anesthetics that are hydrolyzed in the circulation by plasma pseudocholinesterase. Procaine and tetracaine are other available esters but are not particularly useful in the office setting. This group of local anesthetics has been associated with a measurable incidence of allergic phenomena.

Lidocaine (Xylocaine and others), mepivacaine (Carbocaine and others), and bupivacaine (Marcaine and others) are the three commonly used amide-type local anesthetics. A new local anesthetic, ropivacaine (Naropin), has recently been introduced, and clinical experience is still being gained with this drug. All are metabolized in the liver, and the degradation products are excreted in the urine. Speed of onset is roughly the same with all of these. Duration of action is in the following order: lidocaine *less than* mepivacaine *less than* bupivacaine = ropivacaine, but this is dependent in part on the total dose administered. Amide-type local anesthetics have not been associated with true allergic phenomena. Recommended concentrations and maximum total doses are listed as follows:

1. Chloroprocaine (plain) 1–2% (10–20 mg/mL); not to exceed 10 mg/kg.
2. Lidocaine (plain) 0.5–1.5% (5–15 mg/mL); not to exceed 5 mg/kg.
3. Lidocaine (with epinephrine) 0.5–1.5% (5–15 mg/mL); not to exceed 7 mg/kg.
4. Mepivacaine (plain) (0.5–1.5%) (5–15 mg/mL); not to exceed 5 mg/kg.
5. Mepivacaine with epinephrine is not commercially available and not particularly useful.
6. Bupivacaine (plain) 0.25–0.5% (2.5–5 mg/mL); not to exceed 2.5 mg/kg.
7. Bupivacaine (with epinephrine) 0.25–0.5% (2.5–5 mg/mL); not to exceed 3.5 mg/kg.

8. Ropivacaine (Naropin, Astra) (plain) 0.5–1.0% (5–10 mg/mL); not to exceed 4.0 mg/kg (Although studies indicate that ropivacaine is less toxic than bupivacaine, the maximum allowable dose presented here is extrapolated from those comparisons and has not been determined with the accuracy of that for older drugs.)

Epinephrine (adrenaline) is commonly added to local anesthetics to extend the duration of action and to decrease blood flow in the region being blocked. Solutions containing epinephrine in a concentration greater than 1:200,000 (5 g/mL) cannot be recommended. The commercial preparations of lidocaine containing 1:100,000 epinephrine do not offer any particular advantage to practitioners of office anesthesia. Other agents found in commercially prepared local anesthetic solutions include preservatives designed to retard growth of molds in multidose vials and agents needed to adjust the pH to keep the local anesthetic in solution. Because all local anesthetic agents are weak bases, the pH is adjusted to an amount below their pKa. Solutions of lidocaine and mepivacaine may have a pH as low as 2.5 to 3.0. This may explain in part why these drugs are painful to inject.

PREVENTION OF TOXIC REACTIONS

Before administering the medication, calculate the maximum allowable volume of the agent to be used. Remember to adjust downward the maximum allowable dose for elderly patients by 10 to 30%, depending on each patient's general state of health. If a field block with 1% lidocaine with 1:200,000 epinephrine is planned, and the patient is a healthy 25-year-old person weighing 60 kg, 420 mg or 42 mL of this solution should not be exceeded. In addition, all resuscitation equipment should be immediately available, i.e., not in the next room. The following rules should also be observed:

1. Take a careful history. Patients who state that they are allergic to local anesthetics rarely are, but more likely they have had a

toxic reaction. You may be able to identify the type of reaction from the history. Some of these reactions are simple "faints" or vasovagal reactions. Some are reactions to an overdose of a vasoconstrictor, usually epinephrine, and are characterized by a pounding sensation in the head followed by rapid heartbeat and, sometimes, by loss of consciousness. Occasionally, these reactions are examples of intravascular injection of local anesthetic with vasoconstrictor and may have been followed by convulsion. These types of problems are commonly seen during dental blocks. An episode that is characterized by the onset of buzzing in the ears, numb mouth or tongue, blurred vision, and loss of consciousness is probably an episode of an overdose of local anesthetic (wrong amount of drug, right place). A question should arise in the physician's mind if a patient has been told that he or she is allergic to lidocaine because of the low incidence of true allergy to amide local anesthetics.

2. Monitor carefully during injection. Pulse and blood pressure monitoring during the performance of a block may be most helpful in preventing toxic reactions, because intravascular injection can usually be noted immediately, particularly if an epinephrine-containing solution is being used. It is heralded by rapid increase in heart rate followed quickly by increase in blood pressure. Monitor the patient's sense of well-being and frequently ask questions about "funny feelings in the head" or tingling around the mouth.

3. Perform all local anesthetic injections in a "fractionated" manner. Inject no more than 5 mL, wait one circulation time (15 to 30 seconds), inject another 5 mL, wait another 15 seconds, etc. It is rare to miss the onset of a toxic reaction from intravascular injection, although it will still be mild if this technique is used regularly.

4. Recognize the early warning signs. (Toxic reactions are described in preceding text.) Be aware that if one stops injection at the earliest sign of toxicity and a fractionation technique has been used, it is unlikely that the worst will happen. This may not be true for bupivacaine, however, so this drug should be chosen with due appreciation for its tendency to produce high-grade ventricular arrhythmias as a first manifestation of toxicity. These can degenerate rapidly into ventricular tachycardia and fibrillation that may be refractory to treatment. With almost *all other drugs*, the usual progression of symptoms and signs when toxicity occurs is tinnitus → circumoral numbness → dizziness and excitation → unconsciousness and seizures → cardiovascular collapse → cardiopulmonary arrest. Each of these sets of events happens at definable blood levels of local anesthetic. Thus, with all commonly used local anesthetics (with the exception of bupivacaine), careful monitoring can identify the onset of a toxic reaction before it becomes serious.

What to do if the worst happens:

1. Stop the injection.
2. Administer oxygen.
3. Remember the "ABCs" of cardiopulmonary resuscitation:
   a. open the airway;
   b. breathe for the patient if spontaneous ventilation has stopped;
   c. support circulation as indicated by external cardiac massage and principles of basic life support (and advanced cardiac life support if necessary).
4. Convulsions that follow toxic reactions to most local anesthetics are brief. Intubation of the trachea may not be needed and will only protect against aspiration if it is performed correctly. The airway must be kept open and oxygenation sustained by administration of oxygen by mask. Diazepam 5 mg or Midazolam 3 to 5 mg may help suppress a seizure but usually are not needed.

REGIONAL BLOCKS

The use of regional blocks is advantageous because relatively large areas of the body can

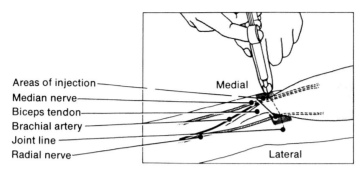

Figure 11.13. Block of the radial and median nerves at the elbow.

be anesthetized (by the injection of local anesthetic agents) in specific areas close to an individual nerve or where bundles of nerves are congregated. The disadvantage of this method is that if the nerves are damaged by the needle, there will likewise be a relatively large area subject to paresthesia or numbness; also, the nerves may lie deep and close to other vital structures (such as lungs or arteries), thus risking possible damage to these areas. Consequently, if local infiltration is sufficient without having to use excessive volumes, the occasional anesthetist should not subject a patient to the potential hazards of these blocks. The goal of regional blocks is to deposit the anesthetic solution as close as possible to the nerve without actually penetrating it. For regional blocks requiring large volumes of solution, the simplest method is to draw up the maximum dose into a 30- to 50-mL syringe with an extension tube and needle attached, to inject the recommended amount after proper location of the needle, and to alternate small increments with repeated aspiration, as described previously. The needle should be a 1-½ inch 22-gauge B-bevel needle.

Blocks of the Forearm and Hand

Elbow Block (Fig. 11.13)

The radial, median, and ulnar nerves can be blocked independently at the elbow and will provide analgesia to their respective areas in the hand. However, this will not be adequate for operations on the forearm, unless a subcutaneous block of the area above the el-

bow is also administered to block the medial cutaneous nerve to the forearm. The arm is flexed 90°, and a line is drawn along the crease of the elbow. The arm is then extended, and injections are made on this line.

Radial Nerve

The needle is inserted approximately 1 cm laterally (radial side) to the biceps tendon, and 5 mL are deposited in a fan-wise manner down to the bone, unless paresthesias are encountered. This injection generally blocks the musculocutaneous nerve as well, because the needle passes through the brachioradialis.

Median Nerve

The needle is inserted medially to the brachial artery until paresthesias are elicited; 5 to 10 mL are injected.

Ulnar Nerve (Fig. 11.14)

The nerve is rolled under the palpating finger proximally to the cubital tunnel behind the medial epicondyle. Two milliliters are injected on either side of the nerve. Do not inject directly into the sulcus, because the nerve may be impaled against the bone and could possibly suffer from compression.

Medial Cutaneous of the Forearm

This can be accomplished by superficial injection of the medial half of the arm just above the elbow.

Wrist Blocks (Fig. 11.15)

These blocks are indicated for specific areas in the palm or fingers. Each of the three blocks is made by injection into the volar aspect of the wrist at a level identified by a line drawn between the radial and ulnar styloid processes.

Ulnar

The needle is inserted perpendicularly to the skin immediately radial to the flexor carpi ulnaris tendon and ulnar to the ulnar artery, at the level of the styloid process of the ulna. Four milliliters are injected, with or without paresthesias.

Median

The needle is inserted perpendicularly between the tendons of the palmaris longus and flexor carpi radialis through the flexor retinaculum. Five milliliters are injected at this site.

Radial

The needle is inserted perpendicularly over the radial artery, just proximally to the radial styloid and directly dorsally, injecting 5 mL superficially around the radial aspect of the wrist. The needle must not enter the radial artery. The specific danger with these blocks is nerve damage after needle penetration of a nerve. Intravascular injection is guarded against by repeated aspiration during the injection.

Metacarpal Blocks (Fig. 11.16)

These blocks are useful for operations on the fingers, where digital injections are not suitable by reason of location of the operation, or compromise of blood flow due to compression of finger vessels. The needle is inserted on either side of the adjoining metacarpal, proximally and close to the metacarpophalangeal joint. The solution is injected continuously as the needle is advanced until the tip of the needle can be felt in the palm. If anesthesia is still inadequate after 5 minutes, the needle is reinserted through the same puncture site and advanced distally into each web, close to the designated digit; 1 to 2 mL are injected at each site. Intravascular injection is

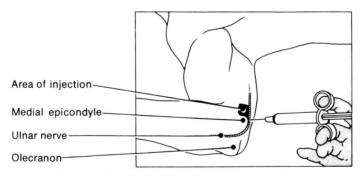

Area of injection
Medial epicondyle
Ulnar nerve
Olecranon

Figure 11.14. Block of the ulnar nerve at the elbow.

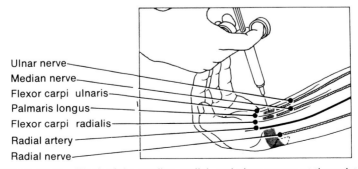

Ulnar nerve
Median nerve
Flexor carpi ulnaris
Palmaris longus
Flexor carpi radialis
Radial artery
Radial nerve

Figure 11.15. Block of the median, radial, and ulnar nerves at the wrist.

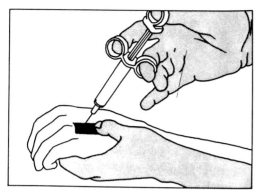

Figure 11.16. Metacarpal block.

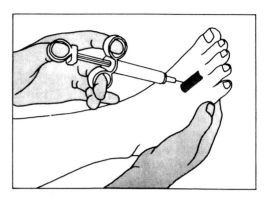

Figure 11.18. The metatarsal block.

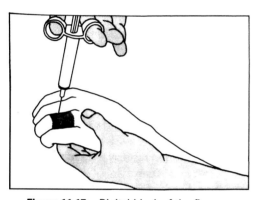

Figure 11.17. Digital block of the finger.

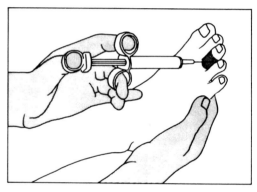

Figure 11.19. Digital block of the toe.

guarded against by repeated aspiration during the injection.

Digital Blocks (Fig. 11.17)

These blocks are indicated for operations on the distal portion of the finger or nail. The needle is inserted from the dorsal aspect on each side of the finger, and 2 mL are injected at each site as the needle is advanced toward the volar surface. A specific danger of digital blocks is the swelling of the proximal phalanx with solution that can result in impaired circulation to the remainder of the finger. Epinephrine should not be used with either the metacarpal or the digital block.

Foot Blocks

The anterior tibial (deep peroneal) and posterior tibial nerves can be blocked individually, and the saphenous, sural, and terminal cutaneous branches of the superficial peroneal nerve may be blocked by circumferential subcutaneous infiltration proximal to the ankle joint. Metatarsal and digital blocks (Figs. 11.18 and 11.19) are performed as are the metacarpal and digital blocks of the hand.

Anterior Tibial Block (Deep Peroneal Block, Fig. 11.20)

A line is drawn across the front of the ankle between the two malleoli. The needle is inserted laterally to the tendons of the tibialis anterior and extensor hallucis longus and advanced until a paresthesia is elicited; 5 mL are then injected. Risk of injection into the anterior tibial artery that may lie on either side of the nerve can be minimized by intermittent aspiration during the injection.

Posterior Tibial Block (Fig. 11.21)

The needle is inserted midway between the medial malleolus and the Achilles tendon. The nerve is posterior and lateral to the artery. The needle is advanced until a paresthesia is elicited, and 5 mL are then injected. If no paresthesia is elicited, the needle is withdrawn and a fan-wise injection is made.

Block of the Saphenous, Sural, and Terminal Branches of the Superficial Peroneal

This block is accomplished by circumferential posterior subcutaneous infiltration of 10 to 15 mL proximal to the ankle joint.

Intravenous Regional (Bier Block)

This is suitable for most operations on the upper limb but has a limited application to the lower limb because of the huge volume of solution required. A double tourniquet is recommended. It should be reiterated that an intravenous infusion must be set up in the other arm and the patient's vital signs monitored. The double tourniquet is positioned in the upper arm and connected to the inflator, which should not be not turned on. The pressure is set at approximately twice the systolic blood pressure, generally in the area of 300 mm Hg.

A small plastic cannula, 22-gauge, is inserted into a vein on the dorsum of the hand. Following aspiration of blood, it is flushed with 2 mL of saline, preferably with a heparin-type lock. The cannula is taped in position. The arm is then raised vertically and exsanguinated by means of an Esmarch's bandage. The distal cuff is inflated and then the proximal cuff; after satisfactory inflation of the proximal cuff, the distal cuff is then released. It is important to check the tourniquet by palpation to see if it is inflated, and not simply rely on the pressure gauge. Forty milliliters of 0.5% lidocaine *without epinephrine* are now injected, making sure that the lidocaine is not

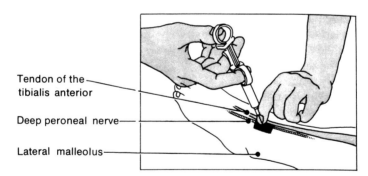

Figure 11.20. Block of the deep peroneal nerve at the ankle.

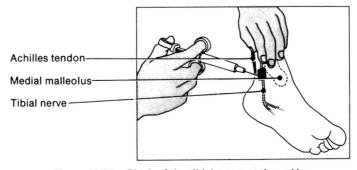

Figure 11.21. Block of the tibial nerve at the ankle.

infiltrating. The cannula is then withdrawn and pressure maintained over the puncture site for approximately 3 minutes. Anesthesia develops within approximately 5 minutes and will last for 60 to 70 minutes.

If the operation lasts over 15 minutes and the patient is complaining of tourniquet pain, the distal tourniquet is then inflated, and after 1 minute, the proximal tourniquet released. By this time, the agent will have anesthetized the arm under the distal cuff. It is important not to release the tourniquet completely until a minimum of a ½ hour has elapsed after injection, because it takes that long for the bulk of the anesthetic to diffuse out of the vasculature into the tissue fluid. If the operation finishes before then, the tourniquet is kept inflated for the required time. If deflated sooner, the amount of anesthetic remaining in the vasculature can be enough to cause a toxic reaction. After deflation, the patient should be carefully monitored for a further ½ hour to make sure no toxic reaction develops.

Specific Dangers

1. Inadequate or noninflation of the tourniquet before administrating the agent will result in a failed anesthetic as well as a bolus dose injection of the local agent into the circulation.
2. Premature release of the tourniquet will result in a similar effect. Complications of local anesthetic toxicity are treated with administration of oxygen, up to 5 mg of intravenous diazepam, and intravenous fluids. If seizure occurs, follow the ABCs described earlier in this chapter.

3. Administration of an epinephrine-containing solution will result in hypertension, arrhythmias, and possible cardiac arrest.

Local Infiltration of Fracture Sites

This is a relatively easy procedure and consists of the injection of approximately 10 mL of 1% lidocaine into the hematoma of the fracture site. An intradermal wheal is raised over the fracture site with a 1-inch 25-gauge needle, and following this, a 1½-inch 22-gauge needle is attached to the syringe and inserted into the fracture site. After aspiration of blood, 10 mL of 1% lidocaine are injected. This procedure has the theoretic disadvantage of converting a simple fracture into a compound one. Consequently, surgical preparation of the area is necessary. In addition, there are the dangers of intravascular absorption of the agent with its consequent effect. For a Colles' fracture, it will be necessary to inject not only the radial fracture site but the styloid process of the ulna as well, in the event that this is fractured.

SUGGESTED READINGS

Akins CM. Aspiration and Injection of Joints, Bursae, and Tendons. In: Vander Salm TJ, ed. Atlas of Bedside Procedures. Boston: Little, Brown and Co, 1988: 451–464.

Pfenninger JL. Injections of joints and soft tissue: part I. general guidelines. Am Fam Physician 1991;44:1196–1202.

Pfenninger JL. Injections of joints and soft tissue: part II. guidelines for specific joints. Am Fam Physician 1991;44:1690–1701.

Saunders S, Cameron G. Injection Techniques in Orthopaedic & Sports Medicine. Philadelphia: WB Saunders, 1998.

Nontraumatic Arthropathies

David F. Giansiracusa, M.D., and Steven L. Strongwater, M.D.

Common nontraumatic arthropathies include osteoarthritis (OA), rheumatoid arthritis (RA), systemic lupus erythematosus (SLE), crystal-induced arthritis (gout, calcium pyrophosphate, and hydroxyapatite), the spondyloarthropathies (ankylosing spondylitis, psoriatic arthritis, Reiter's syndrome, and arthritis associated with inflammatory bowel disease), fibrositis, and Lyme disease.

ANATOMY, INNERVATION, AND JOINT FUNCTION

Two types of joints are commonly affected by nontraumatic arthropathies: (*a*) diarthrodial or synovial joints, which move freely and are lined by a synovial membrane; and (*b*) amphiarthrotic or fibrocartilaginous joints, which have a more restricted range of motion. Diarthrodial joints (knee, wrist, shoulder, etc.) may be affected by a wide range of disorders such as OA, RA, SLE, and crystal-induced arthritis. The fibrocartilaginous joints, including the pubic symphysis, sacroiliac (SI) joints, and intervertebral disks, are frequently involved in the spondyloarthropathies.

Diarthrodial joints consist of two or more bones or bone ends with opposing surfaces covered by extremely low friction hyaline cartilage. The joint is lubricated by synovial fluid produced by the synovial membrane and surrounded by the capsule, ligaments, and often tendons adjacent to the capsule. The articular cartilage is composed of type II collagen fibers, which form the structural skeleton of the cartilage; between these fibers is ground substance composed of aggregates of large proteoglycan molecules that contain negatively charged sulfate branches. These branches generate a strong osmotic force, facilitate the flow of nutrients from synovial fluid into the cartilage, and contribute to the expansile properties of cartilage. The collagen fibers and proteoglycans are synthesized by chondrocytes present in the cartilage. Cartilage is devoid of blood vessels and depends on diffusion of nutrients for its nutrition. This process is facilitated by the normal compression and decompression of the cartilage during joint use.

Articular cartilage is bathed in synovial fluid (SF), which serves several functions: it nourishes cartilage; it helps maintain a low coefficient of friction due to a protein called lubricin; and it contains a number of proteins and other substances important in the regulation of inflammatory joint processes.

In contrast to articular cartilage, the synovium has a well-developed vascular, lymphatic, and nerve supply. Nerve fibers arise from roots supplying muscles that span the joint. Irritation of nerves in one joint may cause pain referred to surrounding muscle and adjacent joints. The synovium shares the same blood supply as the joint capsule and juxta-articular bone. Fenestrations in the microvasculature allow diffusion of small solutes from the plasma and interstitial spaces into the joint. If, as in the case of chronic rheumatoid synovitis, the microcirculation is compromised, the delivery of nutrients (glucose and oxygen) may be significantly impaired.

The synovium is composed of two types of lining cells. Type A lining cells are derived from monocytes and resemble macrophages. Type B cells synthesize hyaluronic acid and other synovial fluid proteins. Other cellular components include antigen-presenting "dendritic" cells, mast cells, and white blood cells, which are important in regulating inflammatory conditions.

The composition of synovial fluid proteins is the result of diffusion from blood vessels, synthesis by synovium, articular consumption, and removal via lymphatic channels. Proteins passively diffuse from the microcirculation into the synovial interstitium and synovial fluid. The rate of diffusion is inversely proportional to the molecular size. Consequently, large molecules, such as IgG, are found in lower concentrations in synovial fluid than in plasma, whereas small proteins are more abundant. Hyaluronic acid, which gives synovial fluid its viscosity and lubricates the contact surface between the synovium and articular cartilage, is synthesized by the synovial membrane.

Several factors provide stability throughout a joint's range of motion. Joint shape enhances a close, congruous fit of the articular surface during weightbearing. Ligaments maintain the relationship of opposing articular surfaces and guide joints through normal range of motion, preventing excessive movement or movement into an unstable position. Muscles and tendons are particularly important in conferring dynamic stability while facilitating polyplanar motion, as in the shoulder where the rotator cuff muscles and tendons are essential. Synovial fluid facilitates the sliding motion of articular surfaces and resists distraction of the joint. This stability is lost when the normal film of synovial fluid is replaced by a "pathologic" joint effusion.

Any disorder that causes a joint effusion ultimately interferes with the normal synthetic activity or physical characteristics of synovial fluid, synovial lining cells, articular cartilage, ligaments, tendons, or subchondral bone. Reflex changes affect the function of the neuromuscular apparatus so that joint protection is limited. In the process, pain, joint instability, and functional impairment develop.

OSTEOARTHRITIS

Osteoarthritis (OA) is the most common nontraumatic arthropathy. Its prevalence increases with age and it is present in almost everyone by the age of 65. Physical demands, anatomic abnormalities of joints, and genetic factors predispose to OA. OA is characterized pathologically by progressive injury to and loss of articular cartilage, accompanied by reactive changes at joint margins and in subchondral bone. Clinically, OA is characterized by slowly progressive pain, stiffness, loss of joint motion, and bony joint enlargement. An inflammatory process involving the synovium may occur, associated with flares of joint symptoms (inflammatory variant of OA).

PATHOGENESIS AND PATHOPHYSIOLOGY

Osteoarthritis is initiated by biomechanical, biochemical, inflammatory, or immunologic insults that stimulate chondrocytes to release enzymes that break down articular proteoglycans and collagen. Biomechanical factors potentiate disruption of collagen and cause microfractures into subchondral bone. Loss of the stress-absorbing properties of cartilage and subchondral bone leads to progressive joint injury, prompting reparative responses that include bony proliferation (osteophyte formation), chondrocyte proliferation, and chondrocyte synthesis of smaller proteoglycan subunits that are less effective in supporting the normal function of cartilage. Locally produced prostaglandins augment the inflammatory response while immune complexes and T lymphocyte responses, directed against proteoglycan components, accelerate cartilage damage.

Pathologically, OA is characterized by thinning, fissures, and focal erosions of articular cartilage. As the disease progresses, the erosions become deeper and more confluent, causing complete loss of cartilage in stress-bearing areas. Osteoarthritic spurs form at joint margins. Microfractures in subchondral bone lead to sclerosis and cyst formation. In advanced stages of disease, inflammatory reactions may cause flares of pain and joint effusions.

CLINICAL CHARACTERISTICS

Early in the course of OA, pain is aggravated by weightbearing and relieved with rest;

transient morning stiffness may occur. As the disease progresses, pain may occur even at rest. Nocturnal pain and prolonged morning stiffness may develop as a result of progressive irritation of nerves within subchondral bone, periosteum, joint capsules, ligaments, tendons, and muscles. Cracking, popping, or grinding with joint motion, called crepitus, often occurs because of joint destruction and intra-articular fragments of bone or cartilage. Joint motion becomes progressively restricted. An inflammatory synovitis may develop from microcrystals of calcium pyrophosphate dihydrate, apatite, or monosodium urate. Cartilage fragments or minor trauma exacerbate this process.

Several clinical subsets of OA have been defined as follows: (a) primary OA of weight-bearing joints (knee, hip, first metatarsophalangeal [MTP]); (b) nodal OA of the distal (DIP) and proximal (PIP) interphalangeal finger joints and thumb carpometacarpal joints; (c) erosive inflammatory OA; (d) ankylosing hyperostosis (also called Forestier's disease or diffuse idiopathic skeletal hyperostosis [DISH]); and (e) secondary OA.

The various clinical presentations of OA of the weightbearing joints will be found in the pertinent regional chapters of this text. Patients present with pain, swelling, stiffness, and crepitation. On examination, tenderness, contracture, deformity, and swelling are demonstrable.

Primary OA of the hands, often referred to as nodal OA, is an autosomal dominant trait that tends to affect women. Distal interphalangeal and PIP joint involvement results in bony proliferation, termed Heberden's and Bouchard's nodes, respectively. The carpometacarpal joint of the thumb and the metatarsophalangeal joint of the great toe are commonly affected. In most patients, the disease begins insidiously and progresses slowly. Pain and erythema, if present, may be severe early in the course of the disease. Later, low-grade aching and stiffness, limited flexion, deviation of the fingers, and the nodular appearance of the joints predominate. Mucinous cysts resembling ganglions may develop over the Heberden's or Bouchard's nodes.

Inflammatory OA represents another OA subset and, like nodal OA of the hands, involves the interphalangeal joints of the fingers and can involve other joints as well, including the carpometacarpal joints of the thumbs, the first toe metatarsophalangeal, the hips, and the knees. It is characterized by acute bouts of inflammation leading to erosive joint disease. Radiographically, the margins and central aspect of the joint are destroyed, resulting in deformities and, occasionally, ankylosis of bone. This arthropathy may be confused with mono- or oligoarticular forms of arthritis, such as psoriatic arthritis, which is another form of erosive disease that affects the DIP joints.

The subset of OA termed ankylosing hyperostosis, also called diffuse idiopathic skeletal hyperostosis (DISH) or Forestier's disease, may affect the spine. Manifestations include stiffness, loss of motion, and ossification of the anterolateral aspect of the vertebral bodies with preservation of intervertebral disk spaces (in contrast to primary OA in which disk height is reduced). Patients with DISH may also produce proliferative spurs at sites of tendon and ligament attachments and heterotopic bone after joint surgery.

Primary OA most often affects the knees, hips, and cervical and lumbar spine. It tends to spare the metacarpophalangeal (MCP), wrist, elbow, and shoulder joints. Osteoarthritic involvement at these sites should raise concern of some other joint insult. Secondary causes of OA include mechanical joint injury, after a treated inflammatory arthropathy, deformity from congenital or developmental disease (congenitally dislocated or dysplastic hip, slipped capital femoral epiphysis, Legg-Calve-Perthe's, etc.), metabolic abnormalities of cartilage (hemochromatosis and acromegaly), neurologic diseases causing neuropathic arthropathy (diabetes, tabes dorsalis), or repetitive bleeding within the joint (hemophilia).

Laboratory and Radiographic Features

Laboratory studies in OA are generally normal, including erythrocyte sedimentation rate (ESR), complete blood count, and other acute phase reactants. Synovial fluid when present is noninflammatory (Table 12.1).

Table 12.1. Classification of Synovial Effusions

Characteristic	Normal	Noninflammatory (Type I)	Inflammatory (Type II)	Septic (Type III)
Color	Clear, straw-colored	Straw to yellow	Yellow	Variable
Clarity	Transparent	Transparent	Translucent	Opaque
Viscosity	High	High	Low	Variable
WBC (mm^3)	< 200	200–2000	2000–75,000	> 100,000
Polys (%)	< 25	< 25	> 50	> 75+
Culture	Negative	Negative	Negative	Often positive
Mucin clot	Firm	Firm	Friable	Friable
Glucose	Near blood	Near blood	< 25 mg/dL lower than blood	> 25 mg/dL lower than blood

Synovial fluid may contain calcium pyrophosphate, monosodium urate, hydroxyapatite crystals (see "Crystal-Induced Rheumatic Diseases"), or cartilage fragments and have mildly inflammatory features.

X-rays reveal joint space narrowing (indicative of cartilage loss), which in the knees and hips is best demonstrated by weightbearing views. Also seen are joint effusions, increased density of subchondral bone (termed sclerosis or eburnation), subchondral cysts, and osteophytes. Radionuclide bone scans reveal discrete areas of increased uptake and are more sensitive in detecting early disease.

TREATMENT

The patient should be instructed to minimize stress to the affected joints. This includes weight loss, avoidance of activities producing a high load across the joint, judicious rest, splinting, and the use of assistive devices such as a cane for patients with hip or knee disease. Other modalities include heat; ice; exercise; analgesic and anti-inflammatory agents (Table 12.2), a number of which are now available over-the-counter; along with selective use of injectable steroid preparations. Topical capsaicin may also help relieve joint pain. When pain becomes severe, symptoms are unresponsive to conservative measures, and joint dysfunction leads to inability to perform activities of daily living, surgery should be considered.

RHEUMATOID ARTHRITIS

Rheumatoid arthritis (RA) is a chronic, inflammatory immunologic process that affects joints and may also involve visceral structures (Table 12.3). The incidence of RA is highest in women (two to three times that of men) ages 30 to 50, with an overall incidence of 0.3 to 1.5%. The HLA-DR4 haplotype confers susceptibility in most ethnic groups; however, only a minority of individuals with this haplotype develop rheumatoid arthritis.

PATHOGENESIS

Although the etiology of rheumatoid arthritis is unknown, two immune mechanisms are important. The first immune mechanism is that within the synovial fluid, immune complexes form as a result of interaction of antibodies with self immunoglobulin (Ig) molecules. These Ig-anti-IgM complexes are called rheumatoid factors. Antibodies are also generated to constituents of damaged articular cartilage. These immune complexes activate the complement cascade, producing an inflammatory reaction with attendant microvascular injury, increased vascular permeability, and formation of subsynovial edema. Polymorphonuclear leukocytes, which are chemotactically attracted, ingest immune complexes and, in the process, release injurious oxygen radicals, hydrolytic enzymes (collagenases, elas-

Table 12.2. Nonsteroidal Anti-Inflammatory Drugs[a,b]

Class Generic Name	Brand Name(s)	Tablet Size (mg)	Daily Dose
Salicylates Acetylsalicylic acid	ASA, aspirin	325	8–12/day
Nonacetylated Choline salicylate Choline magnesium salicylate	Arthropan Trilisate	500 mg/tsp 500, 750, 1000	1–2 tsp qid 1000 mg tid 1500 mg bid
Salsalate	Disalcid	500, 750	1000 mg tid 1500 mg bid
Propionic Acids Ibuprofen	Advil, Nuprin, Motrin	200 400, 600, 800	400–8000 mg tid
Naproxen	Naprosyn	250, 375, 500	250 mg bid to 500 mg tid
Fenoprofen	Nalfon	300, 600	300–600 mg qid
Ketoprofen	Orudis	50, 75	50–75 mg tid
Flurbiprofen	ANSAID	50, 100	100–150 mg bid
Indolacetic Acids Indomethacin	Indocin	25, 50, 75 SR	75–150 mg/day
Sulindac	Clinoril	150, 200	150 mg bid to 200 mg bid
Tolmetin sodium	Tolectin	200, 400	1200–2000 mg in divided doses
Fenamic Acid Mefenamic acid	Meclomen	50, 100	200–400 mg in three to four divided doses
Oxicam Piroxicam	Feldene	10, 20	10–20 mg/day
Phenylacetic Acid Diclofenac sodium	Voltaren	25, 50, 75	50–75 mg bid

SR, sustained release.
[a] Indications for use—see text.
[b] Common adverse side effects include the following: gastrointestinal intolerance (dyspepsia, nausea, vomiting, diarrhea, bleeding); impairment of renal function; inhibition of platelet function (minimal inhibition by nonacetylated salicylates); and central nervous system effects (headache, tinnitus, depersonalization).

tases), and arachidonic acid metabolites (prostaglandins). The second immune mechanism is that infiltrates of lymphocytes, macrophages, and dendritic cells liberate interleukin-1, which stimulates antibody production and proliferation of synovial lining cells, chondrocytes, and osteoclasts. Granulation tissue, termed pannus, is formed from synovial tissue and erodes bone and cartilage. Osteoclasts release destructive substances that erode cartilage and bone and contribute to periarticular injury of ligaments, tendons, and joint capsules. Vascular engorgement, thrombosis, perivascular hemorrhage, proliferation of macrophage-like (synovial type A) and fibrocyte-like (synovial type B) cells can be seen. Collections of mononuclear cells, predominantly lymphocytes and plasma cells, locally produce rheumatoid factor and other antibodies.

CLINICAL CHARACTERISTICS

The severity of RA is variable. It may affect one or many joints for a few months or may be widespread, symmetrical, and destructive, with associated extra-articular manifestations. Rheumatoid arthritis characteristically be-

Table 12.3. Extra-Articular Manifestations of Rheumatoid Arthritis

SKIN:
Subcutaneous nodules
Vasculitic lesions (leg ulcers, medium vessel vasculitis)
Ecchymoses and thin skin

RESPIRATORY TRACT:
Lung (pleural effusions, pleural thickening; pneumonitis and interstitial lung disease; rheumatoid nodules; necrotizing bronchiolitis)
Upper airway (dryness secondary to Sjogren's syndrome; laryngeal obstruction secondary to cricoarytenoid arthritis)

CARDIOVASCULAR:
Pericarditis
Rheumatoid nodules of myocardium/valves conduction system
Interstitial myocarditis
Coronary arteritis

NERVOUS SYSTEM:
Mononeuritis Multiplex Secondary to Arteritis
Peripheral Nerve Entrapment (carpal tunnel syndrome, ulnar nerve entrapment at the elbow (cubital fossa), tarsal tunnel syndrome, popliteal cyst compression of posterior tibial nerve)
Compressive myelopathy—cervical subluxation
Stroke

EYE:
Dryness due to keratoconjunctivitis sicca (Sjogren's syndrome)
Episcleritis or scleritis

gins insidiously over weeks to months. Prolonged morning stiffness (one or more hours), fatigue, malaise, and gelling (stiffness after immobility) may be prominent symptoms. Joint stiffness improves with activity only to be limited by afternoon fatigue and pain. Periarticular and diffuse muscle aching, low grade fevers, malaise, weight loss, and depression are not infrequent symptoms. Although RA may remit (10% or less), the majority of patients have progressive disease. Joint involvement is typically symmetrical and involves the PIP and MCP joints of the hands, wrists, elbows, shoulders, cervical spine, hips, knees, ankles, subtalar, tarsal, and metatarsophalangeal joints. Less frequently, the temporomandibular, cricoarytenoid, and sternoclavicular joints are affected.

Synovitis of the hands results in symmetric fusiform swelling, most prominently affecting the second and third MCP and PIP and the wrist joints of the dominant side. With soft tissue injury to ligaments and tendons, the fingers deviate laterally at the MCP joints (so-called ulnar deviation). Soft tissue injury to the MCP and interphalangeal joints may cause a swan-neck deformity, which is a flexion contracture of the MCP and DIP joints with hyperextension of the PIP joint. A boutonniere deformity may also develop as a result of a flexion contracture of the PIP and hyperextension of the DIP joints. For the details of finger and wrist involvement by rheumatoid arthritis, see Chapter 5.

Elbow involvement may cause flexion contractures, occasionally in the absence of pain. Synovial proliferation and effusion may be palpated at the joint line between the lateral epicondyle and the tip of the olecranon process. Synovitis at the elbow in the ulnar (cubital) groove may cause a compressive neuropathy of the ulnar nerve.

Cervical spine disease causes pain, stiffness, and muscle spasm. Erosion of the transverse ligament of C-1 may allow the odontoid process to compress the spinal cord during neck flexion caused by anterior subluxation of C-1 on C-2. Another cause of compressive cervical myelopathy is "stair-case" subluxation of multiple cervical vertebral units.

Like OA, rheumatoid hip disease tends to be felt as pain in the groin, buttock, medial or anterior thigh, or knee. In contrast to OA, pain may be significant even with nonweightbearing. Motion of the hip is globally restricted.

Knee synovitis is readily apparent. Because the true knee joint is almost always continuous with the suprapatellar bursa, swelling is appreciated above, medial, and lateral to the patella. A firm or cystic swelling behind the knee in the medial popliteal space indicates the presence of a popliteal or Baker's cyst.

Foot and ankle involvement cause considerable morbidity because of difficulty standing and walking. Tibiotalar arthritis is manifest by swelling adjacent and anterior to the malleoli, with restricted dorsiflexion and plantar flexion. Tenderness anterior and inferior to the lateral malleolus and pain on inversion and eversion of the ankle are indicative of subtalar joint disease. With progression, the ankle develops a valgus deformity and the foot becomes flattened. Patients walk by rolling off the inner aspect of a flattened foot. Involvement of the metatarsophalangeal joints may also cause subluxation, forcing patients to walk on tender metatarsal heads. If subluxation of the phalanges occurs superiorly, claw or hammer-toe deformities develop.

Laboratory Features

Rheumatoid factor is present in 75 to 80% of patients. Normochromic, normocytic anemia develops as a result of chronic disease. Low-grade gastrointestinal bleeding caused by nonsteroidal anti-inflammatory drugs (NSAIDs) may cause hypochromic anemia. White blood cell counts are generally normal unless the patient has either systemic-onset (Still's) disease, in which a marked leukocytosis may be evident, or Felty's syndrome, manifested by leukopenia (generally granulocytopenia) and splenomegaly. Nonspecific markers of inflammation, including thrombocytosis and elevation of the ESR, reflect the degree of inflammatory activity. Synovial fluid is classified as type II, inflammatory (Table 12.1).

Radiographic Features

Early radiographic features of RA consist of fusiform soft tissue swelling, joint effusions, and periarticular demineralization. Ligamentous and tendon laxity result in joint subluxations, which on x-ray reflect the clinically apparent deformities previously described. With disease progression, erosions of articular cartilage and bone occur. Uniform joint space narrowing reflects irreversible and global injury to cartilage. Erosions occur earliest at the margins of subchondral bone, at so-called bare areas of bone where bone is not protected by articular cartilage. Erosions also occur at sites of ligamentous and tendinous attachments and inflamed bursae. Large subchondral cysts are seen. An important abnormality that may

cause profound neurologic complications is the C-1, C-2 subluxation. Lateral flexion and extension radiographs of the cervical spine will demonstrate this finding.

TREATMENT

Because it is a chronic systemic disease, RA is best managed by an interdisciplinary team consisting of the primary care physician, rheumatologist, orthopaedist, physical and occupational therapists, social worker, nurse, and vocational counselor. Management of each patient must be individualized. Goals of therapy are to relieve pain, stiffness, and muscle spasm; to provide education regarding sexual, marital, and work-related problems; and to maintain or improve joint function, and thereby the quality of life. Adequate rest, including late morning or afternoon naps, may help counteract fatigue. Occupational therapists fashion splints, provide aids to assist with activities of daily living, and instruct patients in exercise to maintain and improve fine motor control.

The NSAIDs are effective first-line agents in the treatment of RA (Table 12.2). When synovitis is not well-controlled by NSAIDs or bony erosions appear, slow-acting disease-modifying drugs should be added. These include antimalarial drugs, gold salts, penicillamine, azathioprine, and sulfasalazine. All of these second-line agents have the potential for causing serious adverse reactions, and regular clinical and laboratory monitoring is necessary.

Periarticular (bursal and tendon sheath) and intra-articular corticosteroid injections may be helpful in suppressing inflammation in one or two particularly painful joints while waiting for a second-line agent to work.

Because of the toxicity of systemic corticosteroids, use of these agents should be restricted. When used, they should be prescribed only in low doses (equivalent to 2.5 to 10 mg of prednisone per day) while waiting for remittent agents to become effective. Higher steroid doses may be required for extra-articular manifestations such as pericarditis, pleuritis, rheumatoid vasculitis, and rheumatoid pneumonitis.

Once the diagnosis of RA has been made, consultation is appropriate if questions arise about the diagnosis, if synovitis is not controlled by conservative measures, if joint damage is evident radiographically or by clinical examination, or if serious extra-articular problems become evident.

Systemic Lupus Erythematosus

Systemic lupus erythematosus (SLE) is a multisystem, chronic inflammatory disease. Although the etiology is unknown, SLE appears to develop as a result of the interaction of genetic, environmental, and hormonal factors. Like RA, SLE most frequently affects women during their child-bearing years. Underlying abnormalities of immune regulation result in the production of autoantibodies, proliferation and alteration of lymphocyte subsets, and activation of the complement system. Autoantibodies to cell membranes cause immune thrombocytopenia, hemolytic anemia, leukopenia, lymphopenia, and some forms of lupus cerebritis; immune complex formation leads to vasculitis, pleuritis, rashes, and glomerulonephritis.

CLINICAL CHARACTERISTICS

Musculoskeletal manifestations of SLE include arthralgias and arthritis (synovitis). Involvement of wrists, finger joints, elbows, and knees in a symmetrical distribution (similar to RA) with morning stiffness, joint pain, and swelling are common. Inflammatory disease of soft tissues, specifically joint capsules, tendons, and ligaments, may cause joint malalignment and subluxation. Although erosive arthritis is rare, reversible ulnar deviation of the fingers, deviation of the toes (termed Jaccoud's arthritis), and tendon rupture may occur.

Other musculoskeletal manifestations include myalgias and, less commonly, inflammatory muscle disease (myositis) and os-

teonecrosis. Myalgias are characterized by aching and, occasionally, muscle tenderness with maintenance of strength. In contrast, myositis causes weakness, particularly of the shoulder and hip musculature, and is associated with elevated muscle enzymes (creatine kinase, aldolase, aspartate aminotransferase) and electromyographic abnormalities.

Osteonecrosis, also termed avascular necrosis or ischemic necrosis of bone, may develop spontaneously in patients with SLE. Predisposing factors are vasculitis, Raynaud's phenomenon (digital vasospasm), and systemic corticosteroid therapy. The femoral head is most often affected, but numerous other bones, including the humeral head, talus, and bones of the knees and wrist, may be affected. Symptoms of osteonecrosis include pain, often sudden in onset, aggravated by weightbearing and use. The diagnosis is made on the basis of symptoms and findings on plain radiographs, bone scans, or magnetic resonance imaging studies.

The diagnosis of SLE requires a constellation of clinical and laboratory abnormalities, which might include malar rash, arthralgias/arthritis, polyserositis, oral ulcerations, photosensitivity, glomerulonephritis, seizures or psychoses, vasculitis, leukopenia, thrombocytopenia, hemolytic anemia, positive ANA, antibodies to double-stranded DNA, Sm antigen, and cardiolipin.

Radiographic Features

Skeletal radiographic abnormalities in SLE develop as a result of ligamentous instability, osteonecrosis, or osteoporosis.

TREATMENT

Lupus tends to have a fluctuating clinical course requiring on-going monitoring and adjustments in therapy. Polyarthralgias, myalgias, and arthritis are treated with NSAIDs (Table 12.2), splints, and physical therapy. Resistant joint or skin disease is treated with antimalarials, generally in the form of hydroxychloroquine (Plaquenil). Severe systemic manifestations, such as pleuritis, pericarditis, lupus pneumonitis, hemolytic anemia, immune thrombocytopenia, cerebritis, transverse myelitis, glomerulonephritis, vasculitis, and severe rash, are treated with high-dose glucocorticosteroids (1 mg/kg of methylprednisolone per day or its equivalent). Consultation with a rheumatologist for management of such serious disease manifestations is recommended. To avoid the toxicities associated with long-term, high-dose steroid therapy, a number of alternative therapeutic regimens employing cytotoxic agents (cyclophosphamide), anti-metabolites (azathioprine), and pheresis (plasmapheresis, lymphapheresis) have been developed.

SPONDYLOARTHROPATHIES

The spondyloarthropathies form a group of rheumatic diseases that includes ankylosing spondylitis (AS), psoriatic arthritis (PsA), Reiter's syndrome (RS), and the arthritis associated with inflammatory bowel disease. Inflammation at sites of ligament or tendon insertion is common. All have a predilection for the SI joints (sacroiliitis), longitudinal ligaments of the spine (spondylitis), facet joints, peripheral diarthrodial joints, ligaments, tendons, and fascia. Additionally, all share a strong association with the class I histocompatibility antigen, HLA-B27.

ANKYLOSING SPONDYLITIS

Ankylosing spondylitis is regarded as the prototype of the spondyloarthropathies. It occurs most frequently in men 20 to 30 years old (three-fold male predominance), with an overall prevalence of 0.1 to 0.2%. Ankylosing spondylitis affects the SI joints symmetrically and the spine in a progressive ascending fashion.

Clinical Characteristics

The earliest manifestations of AS are back discomfort and stiffness that are most severe in the morning and improve over the course of 1 or 2 hours. The back discomfort may return after periods of immobility associated with late afternoon or early evening fatigue.

Sacroiliac joint discomfort is felt in the region of the posterior iliac crest, but may be interpreted as occurring in the hip or down the back of the legs. Occasionally, a peripheral tendonitis occurs, such as Achilles or supraspinatus tendonitis, or plantar fasciitis occurs. In women, bouts of tendonitis or plantar fasciitis may predominate, or they may present with a peripheral arthritis (wrist and hand or ankle arthritis), cervical spine disease, or both, with a paucity of sacroiliac or lumbar involvement.

The physical examination of patients with AS characteristically reveals tenderness of the SI joints on direct palpation and pain with stress of the SI joints. Lumbar motion is restricted, and the reduction may be documented by the Schober index. A mark is made on the skin between the posterior iliac crests and a second mark is made 10 cm cephalad. The patient is asked to touch his or her toes (maximally flex the back with knees extended), and the distance between the two skin marks is remeasured. Normally, the distance in flexion (the numerator) is more than 5 cm greater than the initial 10 cm (the denominator). Therefore, a normal Schober index is greater than 15/10. Chest expansion at the nipple line during full inspiration compared with full expiration also may indicate spondylitis; expansion of less that 3 cm may indicate arthritis of the costovertebral or costochondral joints. Other physical findings include limited motion of the shoulders and hips, synovitis of the knees, plantar fasciitis, and supraspinatus and Achilles tendonitis.

Extra-articular manifestations of AS consist of anterior uveitis (photophobia, difficulty with accommodation, eye redness and soreness, and headache), cardiac abnormalities (aortic insufficiency, aortic dissection, heart block as a result of valvular disease and atrioventricular nodal disease), and fracture of the fused osteopenic spine (most commonly involving the cervical area, which may result in quadriplegia or death). Inflammation of the arachnoid of the lower spine may cause intermittent sciatica and, rarely, a cauda equina syndrome. In less than 1% of patients, interstitial lung disease develops in the upper lobes.

Laboratory Features

Normochromic, normocytic anemia and elevation of the ESR are common in AS. The HLA-B27 antigen can be detected in approximately 80 to 90% of Caucasians with this disease, compared to an incidence of 4 to 8% in the general population.

Radiographic Features

Radiographic features of AS include bilaterally symmetrical sacroiliitis. As the disease progresses, fibrous union followed by eventual ankylosis may occur. Early changes of spondylitis include a "squared" appearance of the lumbar vertebral bodies as a result of erosion of the anterosuperior and inferior margins of the vertebral bodies and deposition of bone in the concave aspect of the vertebral body. Ossification of paraspinal ligaments creates a "bamboo" appearance, and there may be ankylosis of the facet joints. Generalized osteopenia of the spine is common.

REITER'S SYNDROME

The triad of conjunctivitis or uveitis, arthritis, and urethritis represent the classical features of Reiter's syndrome (RS). Sacroiliitis, spondylitis, tendonitis, bursitis, and mucocutaneous disease also occur commonly. Like AS, RS is most common in young men with the HLA-B27 haplotype. Reiter's syndrome has also been referred to as a form of "reactive arthritis" because it often occurs after venereal infection or after an epidemic of dysentery caused by *Yersinia*, *Shigella*, *Salmonella*, or *Campylobacter* species. Infectious agents are regarded as possible triggers of the disease in a genetically predisposed individual.

Clinical Characteristics

Urethritis, manifested by dysuria or a urethral discharge or both, may develop several weeks after venereal exposure or a diarrheal illness. Other genitourinary manifestations include acute and chronic prostatitis, cervicitis, and vaginitis. Development of conjunctivitis or anterior uveitis or both may follow.

The arthritis of RS typically affects less than four peripheral joints in the lower extremities, most commonly the knees and foot joints. Involvement of the periosteum of the phalanges and tendon mechanism may result in a diffusely erythematous and swollen digit, referred to as a "sausage" digit. Tendonitis, particularly of the Achilles tendon and plantar fasciitis, often occur as isolated musculoskeletal manifestations of RS.

Axial joint disease includes sacroiliitis (unilateral or bilateral) and spondylitis. The latter may involve the cervical spine with sparing of the lower spine.

Mucocutaneous manifestations of RS include a hyperkeratotic rash termed keratoderma blennorrhagicum, painless oral mucosal ulcers, circinate balanitis, and nail ridging and pitting. Keratoderma blennorrhagicum may be clinically and pathologically indistinguishable from psoriasis. Other extra-articular manifestations of RS include intermittent fever, weight loss, heart block, aortitis, and amyloidosis.

Laboratory Features

Laboratory abnormalities in RS are similar to those in AS. Joint effusions, when present, tend to have inflammatory characteristics (Table 12.1).

PSORIATIC ARTHRITIS

Approximately 5% of patients with psoriasis develop arthritis that affects the back or peripheral joints. Typically, joints of the upper extremities are involved. Psoriatic arthritis (PA) resembles RS clinically and radiographically. Approximately 20% of individuals with PA have sacroiliitis and spondylitis, and half of these have the HLA-B27 haplotype.

Clinical Characteristics

Psoriatic arthritis affects men and women with equal frequency in their young adult years. Usually, the rash precedes the arthritis, but not infrequently the joint disease precedes or accompanies the onset of psoriasis. In a small fraction of individuals, the arthritis may be present with only subtle evidence of skin disease such as nail pitting or excessive dandruff.

Psoriatic arthritis affects the joints in five distinct patterns. The most common is a peripheral, asymmetric arthritis involving four or fewer joints of the hands. A second subset consists of DIP arthritis involving the fingers or toes, often associated with severe psoriatic nail disease of the same digit. The third form is a symmetric polyarthritis resembling RA but without subcutaneous nodules and rheumatoid factor in the blood. A fourth form, a severe, destructive arthritis termed arthritis mutilans, results in joint erosions and resorption of bone to the degree that the affected fingers and toes become shortened and markedly unstable. A fifth form is sacroiliitis with or without spondylitis, similar to that of RS.

A characteristic pattern of peripheral psoriatic arthritis is the so-called "ray" distribution, in which all the joints of a given digit are inflamed, resulting in the appearance of a "sausage" digit. These findings are similar to the toes of patients with RS.

Laboratory Features

The ESR is frequently elevated. Rheumatoid factor is characteristically absent. Approximately 50% of individuals with psoriatic spondylitis possess the HLA-B27 haplotype.

Radiographic Features

The sacroiliitis of psoriatic arthritis may be unilateral or asymmetric as in RS. Spondylitic involvement may proceed in a progressive, ascending manner as in AS, but may also skip areas of the spine. Syndesmophytes in psoriatic and Reiter's spondylitis may be nonmarginal (originate and join adjacent vertebral bodies some distance from the inferior and superior end plates), in contrast to the marginal syndesmophytes seen in AS or spondylitis of inflammatory bowel disease.

ARTHROPATHIES OF INFLAMMATORY BOWEL DISEASES

Approximately 5 to 10% of individuals with ulcerative colitis and regional enteritis (Crohn's disease) develop either sacroiliitis and spondylitis or peripheral arthritis affecting the large joints of the lower extremities. These forms of spondyloarthropathy have been termed enteropathic or colitic arthritis. The peripheral arthritis may be associated with skin lesions, including erythema nodosum, pyoderma gangrenosum, oral mucosal ulcers, or uveitis. The activity of the peripheral arthritis tends to correlate with that of the bowel disease, whereas the axial arthritis may progress independently.

The laboratory and radiographic features of the spine resemble those of AS, while the peripheral arthritis is generally not erosive.

TREATMENT OF THE SPONDYLOARTHROPATHIES

The major treatment goals for the spondyloarthropathies are to suppress inflammation (Table 12.2), relieve discomfort, and facilitate physical therapy to maintain maximal function. Physical therapy is crucial to minimize joint contractures, maintain optimal posture, and improve joint motion. Exercises as well as participation in sports that emphasize back extension and deep-breathing are valuable. Patients should sleep on firm mattresses, use thin pillows, and sleep or lie prone to minimize the development of flexion contractures of the back.

Referral to a rheumatologist is indicated for the patient with erosive peripheral arthritis associated with psoriasis or RS. The rheumatologist will consider treatment with slow-acting drugs, analogous to the treatment of erosive rheumatoid arthritis with gold compounds, methotrexate, sulfasalazine, or azathioprine.

Local injections of depot corticosteroid preparations are helpful. Systemic corticosteroids aggravate the accelerated osteoporosis associated with these arthropathies and do not improve inflammatory back disease and, therefore, should not be prescribed. Appropriate footwear and orthotics are often prescribed for pain caused by infracalcaneal bursitis or plantar fasciitis.

Extra-articular manifestations of the spondyloarthropathies may require specialized care. This would be necessary for uveitis, cardiac conduction defects, inflammatory bowel disease, and cutaneous manifestations. Nongonococcal urethritis should be treated with a 14-day course of tetracycline, because often the infecting agent is *Chlamydia trachomatis.*

CRYSTAL-INDUCED ARTHROPATHIES

GOUTY ARTHRITIS

Gout occurs as a result of sustained hyperuricemia secondary to uric acid overproduction (defined as a urinary excretion of more than 600 mg/day of uric acid on a purine-restricted diet, or more than 800 mg/day on a regular diet), or excessive intake, and/or diminished urinary excretion of uric acid. Hyperuricemia most commonly occurs as a result of (*a*) diminished renal clearance of uric acid; (*b*) disease states that increase purine turnover, such as psoriasis, sarcoidosis, myeloproliferative and lymphoproliferative diseases, multiple myeloma, and hemolytic anemia; or (*c*) acquired renal disease or drug ingestion, which impairs excretion. Clinically, gouty arthritis manifests as recurrent acute attacks of arthritis or a chronic erosive deforming arthritis (tophaceous gout).

Pathogenesis

During the initial phase of a gouty attack, monosodium urate (MSU) crystals are shed into the synovial fluid. This initiates an inflammatory process leading to formation of a painful swollen joint. Gout characteristically affects "cooler" joints, such as the feet, ankles, knees, hands, and elbows; tophi deposit in the cartilaginous helix of the external ear and the olecranon bursa because of the cooler temperature. Stresses such as twisting an ankle or stubbing the great toe may dislodge urate crystals from otherwise stable sites. Crystal shedding, leading to acute gouty arthritis, can also occur as a result of rapid changes in urate concentration, such as institution of uric acid-lowering therapy or ingestion of alcohol or salicylates.

Clinical Characteristics

Acute gouty arthritis is characterized by the abrupt onset of exquisite pain, tenderness, swelling, and erythema most commonly affecting a single joint, generally after 10 or more years of asymptomatic hyperuricemia. It most frequently affects men in their 4th through 6th decades of life and, less commonly, postmenopausal women. Approximately 50% of patients experience their first attack in the metatarsophalangeal joint of the great toe (podagra). Other peripheral joints are involved in a monoarticular or migratory fashion. Approximately 10 to 15% of patients present with polyarticular gout. Even if untreated, acute attacks are usually self-limited, lasting 3 to 7 days, after which the patient becomes asymptomatic, referred to as the intercritical period. With the passage of time, attacks become more frequent and prolonged, eventually resulting in chronic persistent gout with tophi palpable on examination or erosions visible on radiographs.

Radiographic and Synovial Fluid Features

Radiographically, acute gout is manifest as soft tissue swelling and joint effusions. In chronic or tophaceous gout, cortical erosions that have sharply defined sclerotic margins as a result of tophaceous deposits in the periosteum of cortical bone may be seen, as well as oval-shaped cysts with sclerotic margins in periarticular medullary bone. Joint space preservation, absence of profound periarticular demineralization, and the eccentric location of soft tissue swelling are characteristic of gout.

The diagnosis of gouty arthritis is established by demonstration of needle-shaped MSU crystals within polymorphonuclear leukocytes in synovial fluid aspirated from affected joints. The MSU crystals are readily visualized by polarizing microscopy.

Treatment of Hyperuricemia and Gouty Arthritis

The goals of treatment of gouty arthritis are (*a*) to terminate the acute attack, (*b*) to prevent recurrent attacks, and (*c*) to prevent or resorb tophi. Agents employed are either anti-inflammatory, prophylactic, or urate- (and uric acid) lowering drugs.

The earlier an acute attack of gouty arthritis is treated, the more rapidly the inflamed joints respond. NSAIDs are given in high doses for the first 2 to 3 days (Table 12.2), then tapered to lower doses. If treatment is begun within several hours of onset, 0.6 mg oral colchicine given every hour for a maximum of eight tablets or until gastrointestinal side effects develop, followed by maintenance therapy of 0.6 mg twice daily may be effective. Colchicine may also be given intravenously. Initial infusion is 2.0 to 3.0 mg, followed by 0.5 to 1.0 mg 8 to 12 hours later, not to exceed a total dose of 4.0 mg in 48 hours. Colchicine is extremely irritating to soft tissues and should be diluted in 20 mL of normal saline and infused over 10 to 20 minutes in a well-running IV, with care taken to prevent extravasation. Colchicine is particularly useful in patients requiring oral anticoagulation, or those who have gastrointestinal bleeding or heart failure; however, colchicine should not be used in patients with significant liver or renal disease.

Corticosteroids may be required to treat acute gouty arthritis if contraindications exist to the use of other agents. Systemic or intra-articular administration may be given once joint sepsis has been excluded.

After an acute attack of gout has subsided, chronic maintenance therapy with colchicine (0.6 mg twice daily) or low doses of NSAIDs can be used to prevent subsequent attacks.

Indications for chronic uric acid-lowering therapy are (*a*) repeated attacks of disabling arthritis, (*b*) presence of tophaceous deposits, (*c*) clinical or radiographic signs of chronic gouty joint disease, (*d*) progressive renal impairment, (*e*) recurrent urolithiasis, and (*f*) gross overproduction of uric acid (urinary uric acid excretion > 1000 mg/day). Uric acid-lowering therapy is also used in patients with lymphoproliferative and myeloproliferative disease before cytotoxic therapy to prevent hyperuricemic nephropathy.

Two types of uric acid-lowering agents are available: uricosuric drugs, which increase urate clearance, and xanthine oxidase inhibitors (allopurinol), which block uric acid production. Uricosuric agents are given to patients with near-normal renal function who excrete less than 700 mg of uric acid per day. Probenecid is given initially in a dose of 250 to 500 mg twice daily and increased to 1.5 g twice daily; alternatively, sulfinpyrazone 100 mg twice daily to 400 mg twice daily may be used. An agent to prevent acute gouty arthritis (prophylactic colchicine or a NSAID) should be administered and continued for at least 6 months after the serum urate level is below 6 mg/dL or 6 months after resolution of tophi. Side effects of probenecid include headache, nausea, anorexia, skin rash, and, rarely, nephrotic syndrome, hepatic necrosis, and aplastic anemia. Sulfinpyrazone may cause gastrointestinal irritation and bone marrow suppression.

Allopurinol is used in patients with excessive uric acid excretion (over 1 g in 24 hours), with urolithiasis or tophaceous gout, and in patients with renal insufficiency who require uric acid-lowering therapy. Allopurinol should only be instituted after resolution of an acute attack of gout and with the concurrent prophylactic administration of either NSAIDs or colchicine 0.6 mg once or twice daily. The initial dose is 100 mg/day; this is increased by 100 mg every 2 to 4 weeks to the dose required to depress the serum urate level below 6 to 7 mg/dL, up to a maximum of 300 mg/day. In renal insufficiency, the dose must be reduced considerably (100 mg/day or less). Allopurinol reduces the metabolism of warfarin, 6-mercaptopurine, and azathioprine, and therefore, the dose of these medications must be appropriately reduced. Potential toxicities of allopurinol include a severe allergic reaction, nausea, diarrhea, drug fever, leukopenia, hepatotoxicity, interstitial nephritis, vasculitis, and a rash that may evolve into exfoliative dermatitis or toxic epidermal necrolysis. Serious side effects most commonly occur when allopurinol is prescribed in renal insufficiency, particularly in the setting of concomitant thiazide administration.

If gouty arthritis develops in a patient taking allopurinol or a uricosuric agent, the dose of the uric acid-lowering agent should not be changed until after resolution of the attack.

CALCIUM PYROPHOSPHATE DEPOSITION DISEASE

Calcium pyrophosphate dihydrate (CPPD) crystal deposition disease (pyrophosphate arthropathy) is a crystal-induced disease associated with the deposition of CPPD crystals in and around joints. The deposits may be found in the fibrocartilage, articular hyaline cartilage, and intervertebral disks as well as in tendons, ligaments, synovial membranes, and joint capsules.

Calcium pyrophosphate deposition disease is seen in disorders associated with elevated calcium levels, such as hyperparathyroidism, metabolic disorders characterized by diminished activity of pyrophosphatases (familial hypophosphatasia and hypomagnesemia), familial hypocalciuric hypercalcemia, hemochromatosis, and hypothyroidism. The degeneration of tissue seen with normal aging and osteoarthritic degeneration of cartilage also facilitate CPPD deposition.

Clinical Characteristics

Calcium pyrophosphate deposition disease commonly affects the knees and wrists and, less often, the MCP, ankle, shoulder, and elbow joints. Calcium pyrophosphate deposition is best known for causing "pseudogout." Pseudogout, which mimics gout, most commonly affects elderly women. The joint most often affected is the knee, in contrast to gout, which most commonly affects the first MTP joint.

Calcium pyrophosphate deposition may also be associated with a more subacute, polyarticular presentation similar to RA ("pseudorheumatoid" form), a "pseudo-osteoarthritis" form, and a destructive ("pseudoneuropathic") form. CPPD may be asymptomatic and identified radiographically as articular chondrocalcinosis.

Work-up of the patient with CPPD should include evaluation for underlying medical disorders. Screening laboratory studies should include calcium, phosphorus, albumin, magnesium, thyroid function studies, alkaline phosphatase, iron and total iron binding capacity, and ferritin levels.

Diagnosis

The diagnosis of CPPD deposition disease is suggested by acute arthritis with radiographic articular chondrocalcinosis. The diagnosis is confirmed by joint aspiration and visualization by compensated polarized microscopy of the rhomboid or square-shaped positively birefringent CPPD crystals within synovial fluid leukocytes (blue crystals when parallel to the axis of the red compensator). Synovial fluid should also be cultured and Gram stained to exclude bacterial infection.

Treatment

Like OA, CPPD deposition disease is managed with NSAIDs (Table 12.2), non-narcotic analgesics, joint splinting as appropriate, and range of motion and strengthening exercises. Joint lavage and arthroscopic irrigation may be beneficial. In severe destructive cases of CPPD arthropathy, particularly involving the hips and knees, joint replacement is indicated. Management of CPPD should include treatment of underlying medical disorders.

HYDROXYAPATITE ARTHROPATHY

Calcium hydroxyapatite deposition, now a well-recognized entity, causes an acute or chronic arthropathy as well as periarthritis (formerly termed degenerative calcific tendonitis and bursitis). These disorders range in severity from asymptomatic to severe and cause pain, tenderness, localized edema, and restricted motion. Conditions that may predispose to calcific periarthritis include excessive repetitive motion, diabetes mellitus, thyroid disorders, and chronic renal failure (particularly in patients on chronic hemodialysis). The most familiar form of hydroxyapatite-induced disease is supraspinatus tendonitis or calcific subacromial bursitis.

Synovial fluid is characterized by a paucity of white cells; crystals cannot be easily detected by polarized microscopic examination but can be detected by alizarin red or von Kossa's stains.

Treatment includes analgesics, NSAIDs (Table 12.2), aspiration, local injection of corticosteroids, and physical therapy (application of heat or cold, diathermy, and ultrasound). In recurrent and refractory cases, surgical removal of calcium deposits may be necessary.

Hydroxyapatite crystals may cause acute flares of arthritis in patients with OA in knee and finger joints. Hydroxyapatite crystals also cause a destructive form of arthritis of the shoulders (called Milwaukee shoulder or rotator cuff arthropathy), knees, and hips.

LYME DISEASE

Lyme disease is a tick-borne disorder caused by the spirochete *Borrelia burgdorferi*. It closely simulates other rheumatic disorders in causing arthritis, systemic manifestations, and a tendency for remissions and exacerbations.

The vector carrying *Borrelia burgdorferi* is a tick, typically *Ixodes dammini*, although other strains may carry the spirochete. After inoculation, a rash may develop 3 to 32 days later. The Lyme spirochete invades regional lymph nodes, and in some patients, spreads hematogenously to the eye, heart, joints, central or peripheral nervous system, resulting in clinical symptoms. The spirochete may also remain dormant, particularly in the central nervous system, and later cause organic brain or multiple sclerosis-like syndromes.

CLINICAL CHARACTERISTICS

Common complaints include the development of rash (erythema chronicum migrans), neurologic symptoms (Bell's palsy, meningoencephalitis), carditis, and arthritis. Rash is the earliest manifestation of Lyme disease, whereas other organ system involvement occurs 3 or more weeks post inoculation.

Arthritis affects approximately 60% of patients. In the early phase, joint involvement is generally asymmetric, affecting large joints (e.g., knees) in a migratory fashion. Months later, a destructive, erosive form of arthritis may develop that must be distinguished from the spondyloarthropathies, RA, and crystalline arthritis.

Laboratory Features

The diagnosis of Lyme disease is confirmed by serologic tests (finding of specific IgM and IgG antibodies against the Lyme spirochete) or by the direct identification of a spirochete in tissue samples. IgM antibody titers peak between 3 to 6 weeks after inoculation of the organism. Specific IgG titers rise more slowly and are detectable for months thereafter. A culture is usually unsuccessful. Radiographic findings are nonspecific and depend on the extent of joint destruction.

TREATMENT

Therapeutic decisions are largely based on the extent of organ system involvement. For early disease, tetracycline is the drug of choice. During the latter phases, in the presence of significant joint, cardiac, or neurologic involvement, high-dose parenteral penicillin or ceftriaxone are preferred. (See The Medical Letter, Vol. 39, May 9, 1997, p 48, for Table of Treatment.)

FIBROSITIS

Fibrositis, also referred to as psychogenic rheumatism, myofascial pain syndrome, fibromyalgia, or simply a form of nonarticular rheumatism, is a chronic pain amplification syndrome. It is characterized by diffuse musculoskeletal aching of 3 or more months, localized muscle tenderness (trigger points), a sleep disorder characterized by interrupted and nonrestorative sleep, and morning stiffness. Other somatic complaints and stress-related disorders such as tension headaches, irritable bowel syndrome, primary dysmenorrhea, premenstrual syndrome, and depression are commonly associated.

PATHOPHYSIOLOGY

The etiology of fibrositis is unknown. The possibility of a primary sleep disorder playing a pathophysiologic role is suggested by three observations: (a) disrupted stage IV delta wave sleep in some individuals with fibrositis; (b) development of fibrositic symptoms in healthy subjects deprived of stage IV non-REM sleep; and (c) improvement of sleep and musculo-skeletal symptoms with therapy such as amitriptyline, which raises intracerebral serotonin levels that modulate stage IV non-REM sleep.

CLINICAL CHARACTERISTICS

Pain, stiffness, and easy fatigability are the three most common presenting complaints in primary fibrositis. Perceived but unverifiable joint pain and swelling, muscle weakness, paresthesia, or burning are common symptoms, as is digital vasospasm (Raynaud's phenomenon). A disturbed sleep history may be reflected by not awakening refreshed and by excessive fatigue despite many hours of sleep. This cadre of complaints is often exacerbated by cold damp weather, excessive stress or anxiety, and exercise. Young, healthy, "driven" women are most often affected, comprising nearly 90% of those with the disorder. Men and children may also develop this syndrome.

Physical examination is normal except for the presence of tender points in characteristic locations (Fig. 12.1). Dermatographia and exquisite tenderness to rolling the skin between the thumb and index finger (positive skin rolling tenderness) may be demonstrated over

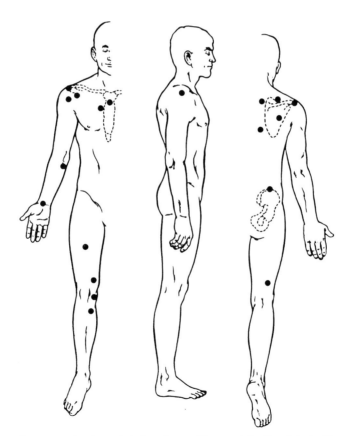

Figure 12.1. Sites of common tender points in primary fibromyalgia. Reprinted with permission from Simms RW, Goldenberg DL, Felson DT, Mason JH. Tenderness in 75 anatomic sites. Arthritis Rheum 1988;31:182–187.

tender points, particularly the upper back. Neurologic and musculoskeletal examinations are otherwise normal.

Laboratory and Radiographic Features

The absence of any radiographic or significant laboratory findings typifies patients with fibrositis. Erythrocyte sedimentation rate is normal. Psychometric testing may, however, be abnormal.

TREATMENT

Fibrositis does not cause weakness or joint destruction and is not progressive despite the many significant problems it causes for the patient. Treatment is symptomatic and begins with patient education. Aerobic training is beneficial despite the initial discomfort that must be endured. Stress reduction programs, mild analgesics or NSAIDs (Table 12.2), massage, applications of moist heat, transcutaneous electrical nerve stimulation, and medica- tion to restore sleep (amitriptyline or cyclobenzaprine) may be of benefit, as may be the serotonin reuptake inhibitors (sertraline hydrochloride, fluoxetine hydrochloride, and paroxetine hydrochloride). Prognosis for the motivated and cooperative patient is excellent despite some episodic exacerbations.

SUGGESTED READINGS

Katz WA, ed. Diagnosis and Management of Rheumatic Diseases. 2nd ed. Philadelphia: JB Lippincott Company, 1988.

Kelley WN, Harris ED Jr, Ruddy S, Sledge CB, eds. Textbook of Rheumatology. 3rd ed. Philadelphia: WB Saunders, 1989.

McCarty DJ, ed. Arthritis and Allied Conditions. 11th ed. Philadelphia: Lea and Febiger, 1989.

Noble J, Greene HL, Levinson W, Modest GA, Young MJ, eds. Musculoskeletal Section VIII. In: Textbook of Primary Care Medicine. 2nd ed. St. Louis: Mosby, 1996.

Schumacher HR Jr, ed. Primer on the Rheumatic Diseases. 9th ed. Atlanta: The Arthritis Foundation, 1988.

Sheon RP, Moskowitz RW, Goldberg VM. Soft Tissue Rheumatic Pain. 2nd ed. Philadelphia: Lea and Febiger, 1987.

CHAPTER 13

Musculoskeletal Infections

Lisa S. Tkatch, M.D., and Nelson M. Gantz, M.D., F.A.C.P.

Despite the widespread availability of antibiotics over the past several decades, osteomyelitis continues to be a common health problem that may result in limb amputation. Similarly, septic arthritis may result in severe limitation of joint function. Early diagnosis is important for successful treatment of bone and joint infection.

ACUTE OSTEOMYELITIS

Acute osteomyelitis occurs by three mechanisms: hematogenous seeding of the bone, contiguous spreading from a nearby focus of infection, or direct inoculation into bone as a result of trauma or surgery. Pathogenesis is multifactorial and poorly understood, but underlying host immune function clearly plays a role. The immune status of the host and the virulence of the organism are important determinants of the severity of infection. A history of previous trauma is an important risk factor because infectious organisms tend to seed sites of previous, often minor, trauma.

HEMATOGENOUS OSTEOMYELITIS

Hematogenous osteomyelitis in children usually involves the appendicular skeleton, whereas in adults, the axial skeleton is more commonly affected (Fig. 13.1). *Staphylococcus aureus* is the causative organism in 50% of cases. Virulence factors secreted by *S. aureus,* expression of collagen-binding proteins that increase the likelihood of *S. aureus* adherence in the area of infection, and production of extracellular proteins, such as enterotoxin and toxic shock syndrome toxin that subvert the immune system, create a milieu in which *S.*

aureus thrives to create an infection. Salmonella is seen frequently in immunocompromised hosts, especially those with sickle cell disease. Gram negative pathogens, such as *Pseudomonas aeruginosa*, are prevalent in injection drug users who dilute their drugs with unsterile water. *E. coli* and *Proteus* species are seen in elderly males who develop vertebral osteomyelitis from the genitourinary tract.

Clinical Manifestations

In children, sudden onset of high fever, systemic toxicity, and restricted painful motion of the involved extremity are typical. In contrast, only one-half of adult patients will have symptoms of pain, swelling, and fever and chills of acute onset (less than 3 weeks duration before seeking medical attention). Other patients experience pain in the affected bone and vague symptoms for 1 or 2 months with few systemic signs of illness.

Pyogenic vertebral osteomyelitis is most commonly seen either in persons over 50 years of age or in injection drug users. Greater than 90% of patients will present with back pain; few will have fever, leukocytosis, or constitutional symptoms. The sedimentation rate is a helpful test because it is usually elevated. Blood cultures or Gram stain and culture of CT-guided needle biopsy of the affected disc space or vertebral body are required for definitive diagnosis.

OSTEOMYELITIS SECONDARY TO CONTIGUOUS SPREAD AND DIRECT INOCULATION

Spread of infection from a nearby source, such as a soft tissue infection or infected teeth

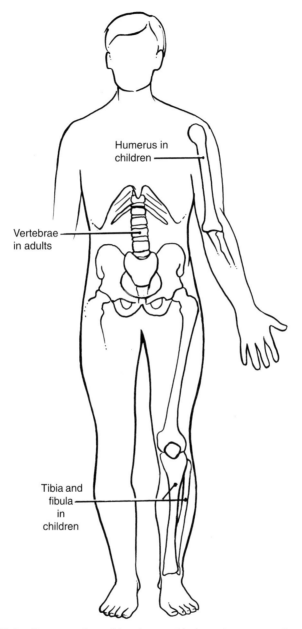

Figure 13.1. Common sites of involvement in hematogenous osteomyelitis.

or sinuses, is the usual route of osteomyelitis caused by contiguous spread. Postoperative infection, such as that after open reduction of fractures or placement of prosthetic joints, and intraoperative contamination of wounds are common precipitating factors. *S. aureus* is the most common infective organism. Gram-

negative organisms are commonly associated with osteomyelitis of the mandible, pelvis, and small bones of the feet. *Pasteurella multocida* is seen as a result of animal bites, and *Pseudomonas aeruginosa*, which thrives in the warm, moist inner soles of sneakers, can be directly inoculated into the deep tissues of the foot after a penetrating injury. Fever, swelling, and erythema are seen in one-half of such cases. During recurrences, few systemic signs occur; sinus tract formation and wound drainage are the common manifestations.

OSTEOMYELITIS ASSOCIATED WITH DIABETIC FOOT INFECTIONS

Underlying osteomyelitis is present in one- to two-thirds of diabetics with moderate or severe limb infections, especially if ulceration of the foot is present. Osteomyelitis develops by contiguous spread from an overlying infective ulcer, generally in the setting of an associated sensory neuropathy and vascular impairment. Infections of diabetic foot ulcers tend to be polymicrobial. Gram-positive organisms, such as staphylococci and streptococci, are the most common pathogens and usually are the cause of monomicrobial infections. Gram-negative bacilli and anaerobes are isolated in 50% of the cases of diabetic foot infections. Culture of bone specimens obtained by percutaneous biopsy that does not transverse the ulcer or by surgical excision are the best methods for establishing and determining the cause of osteomyelitis.

DIAGNOSIS AND TREATMENT

Diagnosis of acute osteomyelitis can be difficult, especially if an overlying soft tissue injury or ulceration is present. The erythrocyte sedimentation rate (ESR), which suffers from low sensitivity and specificity, is often measured. The ESR usually is elevated when osteomyelitis is present; however, an elevated ESR is not diagnostic of osteomyelitis because it can be increased in a variety of inflammatory and infectious conditions. The C-reactive protein is another acute phase reactant that is usually elevated in the presence of osteomyelitis but is also nonspecific. Blood cultures may be positive in up to 50 to 60% of cases. Leukocytosis usually is not seen.

Radiographic imaging modalities available to help diagnose osteomyelitis include conventional radiography, computerized tomography (CT), magnetic resonance imaging

(MRI), and radionuclide studies. Although the least sensitive, the first radioimaging study that should be ordered is a plain film of the affected area to determine whether osteomyelitis or another pathologic condition is present. If obtained early in the course of disease, conventional radiographs may not be helpful because it takes 10 to 21 days for sufficient bone loss to occur before abnormalities may be detected on plain film. In contrast, a bone scan becomes positive within 24 to 48 hours after onset of symptoms because it detects increased osteoblastic activity. The classic findings of osteomyelitis by triple-phase bone scan are increased regional perfusion (seen on the flow phase and blood pool phase) and corresponding increased uptake (seen on delayed images). With cellulitis, only the flow phase shows increased uptake. If the skin or soft tissues overlying the bone are disrupted, the specificity of the bone scan falls to as low as 34%. In these cases, leukocyte scanning has been proposed as a more useful diagnostic test with a sensitivity of 89% and a specificity of 69 to 88%. Gallium scanning is of limited use because of the high rate of false-positive scans. Leukocyte scans are not useful in diagnosing vertebral osteomyelitis because their accuracy is low.

CT has significantly contributed to the evaluation of musculoskeletal pathologic processes. However, MRI has superior resolution of soft tissue versus bone infection and thus is more accurate than CT scanning. MRI is the most sensitive technique available to diagnose osteomyelitis followed by conventional radiography and then bone scans. At present, the high cost of MRI scanning has prohibited this modality from becoming a routinely ordered diagnostic test.

In diabetic patients, probing to bone has been found to be a sensitive (66%) and specific (85%) clinical sign of underlying osteomyelitis in infected pedal ulcers. To perform this maneuver, any overlying eschar should be debrided. The base of the ulcer can then be assessed for the presence or absence of palpable bone using a sterile blunt 14.0 cm 5F stainless steel eye probe. A positive test is consid-

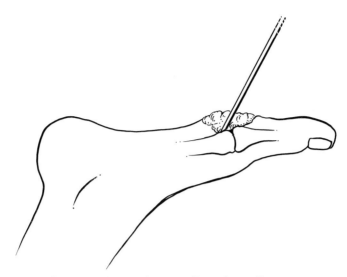

Figure 13.2. Probing to bone using a sterile probe to diagnose osteomyelitis.

ered present when a rock-hard structure is felt at the ulcer base without any intervening soft tissue (Fig. 13.2). The gold standard for diagnosis of osteomyelitis is histopathologic and microbiologic examination of bone obtained from percutaneous core biopsy through uninfected tissue. The presence of neutrophils on histologic examination is consistent with an acute inflammatory response as a result of osteomyelitis; positive cultures confirm the diagnosis and guide appropriate antimicrobial therapy. Sinus tract cultures are most useful if *S. aureus* is isolated as the sole pathogen. Cultures of sinus tract drainage are less helpful when Gram-negative bacilli are isolated. Superficial cultures of diabetic foot ulcers may be helpful in choosing appropriate antimicrobial therapy. Because the infected ulcers are usually polymicrobial, the antimicrobial therapy for the osteomyelitis may be unnecessarily broad.

Antimicrobial therapy should be directed toward organisms obtained from culture of blood or bone tissue. Empiric antibiotic therapy can be chosen based on results of Gram stains of appropriate specimens. If neither cultures nor Gram stains are available, antibiotic therapy should be based on suspected causative organisms. A 6-week course of high-dose parental antibiotic therapy is required to treat acute osteomyelitis. Surgery is indicated if an abscess is present or if there is no clinical response after 72 hours of appropriate antibiotic therapy. When osteomyelitis is secondary to contiguous focus, a result of trauma or direct inoculation, surgery is indicated to drain pus and debride devitalized tissue and sequestra. When adequate debridement of devitalized tissue is followed by several weeks of intravenously administered antibiotics, subsequent oral administration of antibiotics is not needed.

CHRONIC OSTEOMYELITIS

Chronic osteomyelitis refers to recurrence of infection after treatment of the initial episode of osteomyelitis. It is associated with necrotic bone that may serve to sequester bacteria that do not rapidly multiply but remain relatively dormant. In contrast to acute osteomyelitis, high fever, toxicity, and localized tenderness, swelling, and erythema occur less frequently. Localized pain and drainage from a sinus tract are the most common presenting symptoms. A history of pre-existing fracture, injury, or surgery is often elicited. The differential diagnosis can be broad and may include inflammatory soft tissue processes, stress fracture, and bone tumor. The diagnosis of chronic osteomyelitis is aided by the radiographic studies previously discussed. As with acute osteomyelitis, antibiotic therapy depends on the identification of infecting organism(s). More important, however, is surgical intervention to remove dead and devitalized tissue.

When the diagnosis of chronic osteomyelitis is suspected or made, orthopaedic and infectious disease referrals are indicated because the therapeutic recommendations may be complex, depending on the site, the infecting organism, and the extent and chronicity of infection. These factors help determine whether aggressive therapy with surgical debridement and with antibiotics are indicated.

SEPTIC ARTHRITIS

The diagnosis and treatment of bacterial arthritis are urgent because irreversible damage to articular cartilage may begin within a few days of the onset of symptoms. Additionally, sepsis with its attendant complications may supervene. *S. aureus* is the most common cause of septic arthritis, although a variety of bacterial and viral agents can involve one or several joints. Gonococcal arthritis classically presents as tenosynovitis in a woman who has neither a vaginal discharge nor a clinical picture suggestive of pelvic inflammatory disease. Other etiologies to be considered in the differential diagnosis include gout, acute rheumatoid arthritis, chondrocalcinosis, reactive polyarthritis associated with a systemic infection such as Yersinia, collagen vascular disease, sarcoidosis, Behçet's syndrome, and familial Mediterranean fever.

CLINICAL MANIFESTATIONS

Pain and limitation of movement of a single joint are the most common presenting complaints. The majority of patients have fever and visible joint swelling. In blood-borne infections, the knee and other large joints are most frequently affected. Ten percent of patients with infectious arthritis have polyarticular involvement, more commonly seen in patients with rheumatoid arthritis, diabetes, systemic lupus erythematosus, or those on corticosteroid therapy.

DIAGNOSIS

Prompt arthrocentesis is an important diagnostic and therapeutic procedure that should be performed without delay. Synovial fluid usually appears turbid or purulent and has a leukocyte count exceeding $50,000/\text{mm}^3$ with a neutrophil predominance. A Gram stain of joint fluid may identify the causative organism in up to 75% of cases, and a culture may be positive in as many as 90%. In addition to blood, any other suspicious sites, such as cerebrospinal fluid, skin lesions or ulcers, or genital swabs, should be cultured.

Radiographs have limited diagnostic value in early cases but may exclude other causes of joint pain, such as a tumor or fracture, and may provide a baseline for future comparisons. The ESR is elevated. Children tend to have an elevated white blood cell count with a predominance of neutrophils, whereas adults often do not manifest such an elevation.

TREATMENT

When possible, choice of antimicrobial therapy should be guided by the results of a Gram stain of synovial fluid. If this is not available, nonimmunocompromised hosts should initially be treated for infection caused by Gram-positive organisms. Cefazolin or nafcillin are excellent initial agents. If the patient is immunocompromised, treatment for Gram-negative organisms should be included. The recommended agent for gonococcal arthritis is ceftriaxone, 1 g/day, and for methicillin-resistant *S. aureus*, vancomycin is recommended. Daily aspiration of the joint should be performed as long as fluid is present. If response is slow or joint effusion persists beyond 7 days, consideration should be given to open drainage. All hip joint infections and most shoulder joint infections require open drainage. Intra-articular antibiotic injections are unnecessary and may result in chemical synovitis. The usual duration of antibiotic therapy is 2 to 3 weeks.

INFECTION OF PROSTHETIC JOINTS

Total joint replacement has become highly successful in restoring function in patients with disabling arthritic conditions. Despite meticulous attention to technique, infection complicates 1 to 5% of these procedures and is associated with significant morbidity, disability, and cost. Infection is more commonly seen in patients with diabetes mellitus, poor nutrition, extreme old age, obesity, rheumatoid arthritis, multiple prior operations, and concurrent corticosteroid therapy. Hematogenous seeding and local introduction of infection from wound sepsis or intraoperative contamination are the most common routes of infection. *S. aureus* and *S. epidermidis* account for one-half of all isolates; Gram-negative bacilli are causative in 10 to 20%; and streptococci, anaerobes, and other miscellaneous organisms are present in the remainder.

CLINICAL MANIFESTATIONS

The clinical manifestations are variable. Most patients present with a long history of joint pain without fever, swelling, or toxicity, making the major differential diagnosis that between infection and aseptic loosening of the appliance. Wound or sinus tract drainage is present in one-third of patients, whereas less than one-half of patients have fever, periarticular swelling, or signs of systemic toxicity.

DIAGNOSIS

Aspiration of the joint or adjacent bone and recovery of the causative organism in culture are required for definitive diagnosis. Elevated white blood cell count and ESR are suggestive of infection but are not diagnostic. Plain radiographs may reveal changes of osteomyelitis in surrounding bone, but it may take up to 6 months to manifest this change and is usually seen in less than one-half of cases. Radionuclide scans may be helpful but are usually nonspecific.

TREATMENT

Once the diagnosis is established, complete removal of all foreign material is essential to achieve a cure. This is usually accomplished by a two-stage surgical procedure that includes removal of the hardware and cement followed by a 6-week course of intravenous antibiotics. Re-implantation is then performed if all signs of infection have subsided. Management should always be tailored toward patient lifestyle and wishes. If the proposed surgery is prohibitive, suppression with oral antibiotics may be a reasonable approach.

If prosthetic joint infection is suspected, referral to an orthopaedic surgeon and to an infectious disease specialist are necessary. Treatment for this type of infection is complex and frequently involves surgical procedures.

PROPHYLAXIS TO PREVENT HEMATOGENOUS INFECTION

Hematogenous infection of a prosthetic joint implant can occur from a remote intercurrent bacterial infection or after a procedure associated with a transient bacteremia. Procedures associated with a transient bacteremia include dental work, such as having tooth extraction, and genitourinary manipulation, such as cytoscopy or gastrointestinal endoscopy. The consequences of infecting a prosthetic joint are devastating. A paucity of data exists regarding the risks with various procedures associated with a transient bacteremia. Cases of hematogenous seeding of a prosthetic joint have been associated with urinary tract sepsis. Urinary tract infections should be treated promptly, and it is important to minimize the duration of urinary catheterization to prevent a urinary tract infection. Any infection, such as cellulitis, should be treated promptly in a patient with a prosthetic joint.

The issue regarding antibiotic prophylaxis for dental or other procedures involving a manipulation associated with a transient bacteremia remains controversial. We would support using a single dose of an antibiotic for prophylaxis for a dental extraction, genitourinary procedures such as cytoscopy, or gastrointestinal endoscopy. However, any physician who fails to use prophylaxis in these settings should not be found at fault because no data exists regarding this issue.

SUGGESTED READINGS

Caputo GM, Cavanagh PR, Ulbrecht JS, Gibbons GW, Karchmer AW. Assessment and management of foot disease in patients with diabetes. N Engl J Med 1994;331:854–860.

Cunningham R, Cockayne A, Humphreys H. Clinical and molecular aspects of the pathogenesis of *Staphylococcus aureus* bone and joint infections. J Med Microbiol 1996;44:157–164.

Elgazzar AH, Abdel-Dayem HA, Clark JD, Maxon HR. Multimodality imaging of osteomyelitis. Eur J Nucl Med 1995;22:1043–1063.

Gold RG, Tong DJF, Crim JR, Seeger LL. Imaging the diabetic foot. Skeletal Radiol 1995;24:563–571.

Grayson ML. Diabetic foot infections. Infect Dis Clin North Am 1995;9:143–161.

Grayson ML, Gibbons GW, Balogh K, Levin E, Karchmer AW. Probing to bone in infected pedal ulcers. JAMA 1995;273:721–723.

Hass DW, McAndrew MP. Bacterial osteomyelitis in adults: evolving considerations in diagnosis and treatment. Amer J Med 1996;101:550–561.

Ozuna RM, Delamarter RB. Pyogenic vertebral osteomyelitis and postsurgical disc space infections. Orth Clin North Am 1996;27:87–94.

Pinals RS. Polyarthritis and fever. N Engl J Med 1994;330:769–774.

Rand JA, Fitzgerald RH. Diagnosis and management of the infected total Kenn Arthroplasty. Orth Clin North Am 1989;20:201–210.

Sapico FL. Microbiology and antimicrobial therapy of spinal infections. Ortho Clin North Am 1996;27:9–13.

Smith JW, Piercy EA. Infectious arthritis. Clin Infect Dis 1995;20:225–231.

Diseases of Bone

Daniel T. Baran, M.D.

The skeleton is the major reservoir of calcium in the body. Diseases of bone affect the strength of the bony skeleton as well as calcium homeostasis. Likewise, hormones or drugs that affect calcium homeostasis also alter skeletal integrity. Thus, the patient with Paget's disease of bone may present with hypercalcemia or hypercalciuria following immobilization. Similarly, the patient with primary hyperparathyroidism may present with osteopenia and fracture before the discovery of hypercalcemia and elevated parathyroid hormone levels.

This chapter will review the clinical characteristics, pathophysiology, and differential diagnosis of the metabolic bone diseases encountered by the primary physician: osteoporosis, Paget's disease of bone, and metastases to bone.

OSTEOPOROSIS

Osteoporosis is defined as a decrease in bone mass. Both the organic matrix (collagen) and mineral component (hydroxyapatite crystal) are diminished in the osteoporotic patient. Osteoporosis is a major health problem in the United States. Approximately 15 to 20 million women over the age of 45 have osteoporosis. Each year, 1.4 million fractures are attributed to osteoporosis, resulting in health expenditures of 14 billion dollars annually. Seventy percent of osteoporosis-related costs reflect the care of patients with hip a fracture.

CLINICAL CHARACTERISTICS

The woman at greatest risk for developing the disease is of Northern-European or Asian heritage, petite, a smoker, and sedentary, has a family history of osteoporosis (particularly in her mother), has a lifelong history of low dietary calcium intake, and has undergone an early menopause or an oophorectomy. Prolonged premenopausal amenorrhea caused by decreased body fat in elite female athletes is also a newly recognized risk factor for low bone mass. Men are less likely to develop osteoporosis because of greater initial bone mass, slower rate of bone loss, and shorter life span than women. Thirty-three percent of women and 16% of men who live to age 90 will suffer a hip fracture.

Osteoporosis is characterized by a decrease in bone substance and strength. The resulting diminution of bone tissue is expressed as a reduced bone mineral density. In the earliest stage, the patient is asymptomatic. However, as bone density decreases, spontaneous fracture occurs. These fractures most commonly involve the spine, hip, or distal radius. The morbidity and mortality associated with osteoporosis are most evident in relation to hip fractures, which occur in 300,000 women each year. Women who suffer hip fractures have a 12 to 20% greater risk of dying within the first year after the fracture. Vertebral fractures occur in 700,000 women each year causing loss of height, pain, and, if recurrent, deformity (dowager's hump).

PATHOPHYSIOLOGY OF OSTEOPOROSIS

Two general factors determine whether an individual will eventually develop osteoporosis. One factor is the peak bone mass attained at maturity and the other is the rate of bone loss as a function of age. Assume that two women lose bone density at the same yearly rate beginning at age 30. The individual with the lower initial bone density will cross the threshold of abnormally low density at an earlier age and be more prone to fracture.

The peak bone density reached in young adulthood is thought to depend on inheritance, hormonal factors, physical activity, and calcium intake. Genetic inheritance is considered to account for 70 to 75% of peak bone mass. Bone mass increases dramatically during puberty. Amenorrhea caused by weight loss in the elite female athlete is associated with a decrease in bone mass. Physical activity appears to be effective in maintaining and increasing normal bone mass. The exercise modality that optimally maintains or increases axial bone density has yet to be determined. However, positive correlations have been reported between bone mass and a variety of fitness and physical activity measurements, including maximal oxygen uptake, muscular strength, and lifetime physical activity. Similarly, a positive correlation between calcium intake and bone density has been noted in young women. This correlation is independent of physical activity. Likewise, calcium intake (1 to 1.5 g elemental calcium/day) in premenopausal women appears to reduce the rate of age-related bone loss. Thus, before menopause, estrogen levels, physical activity, and diet are important determinants of bone health.

Loss of ovarian function, whether caused by menopause or oophorectomy, is associated with an increase in the rate of bone loss for the ensuing 3 to 4 years. The premenopausal woman with low normal bone mass is therefore at greatest risk for the development of osteoporosis during the perimenopausal years. Recently, estrogen receptors have been demonstrated in osteoblasts and osteoclasts isolated from human bone. It appears that, in the absence of estrogen, the osteoblasts produce cytokines that stimulate osteoclastic bone resorption. The presence of estrogen also is associated with increased blood levels of the active vitamin D metabolite, 1,25-dihydroxyvitamin D, and enhanced intestinal calcium absorption. Therefore, loss of estrogen from either menopause or oophorectomy results in decreased intestinal calcium absorption and increased bone resorption.

Inactivity also augments the osteoporotic condition. The osteoporotic patient who fractures often immobilizes herself to reduce discomfort and the risk of additional fractures. Immobilization and lack of weightbearing decrease bone formation, resulting in greater bone loss.

DIAGNOSIS OF OSTEOPOROSIS

The osteoporotic skeleton is quantitatively diminished but histologically normal. The diagnosis of advanced or severe osteoporosis usually can be made by routine x-rays of the spine (Fig. 14.1) or femur. Characteristic x-ray features of the osteoporotic skeleton before fracture include cod-fish vertebrae, accentuation of the vertebral endplates, and accentua-

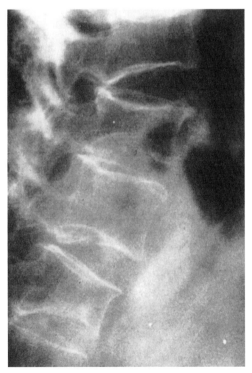

Figure 14.1. Lateral radiograph of the lumbar spine of an osteoporotic patient demonstrating anterior and central vertebral compression fractures and accentuation of the endplates.

tion of the vertical trabecular pattern in the vertebral bodies and the trabecular pattern in the femoral neck. It must be remembered, however, that a 30% loss of bone mineral is required before one can recognize these changes. Consequently, only the patient with severe osteoporosis can be diagnosed by these routine measures.

Awareness of osteoporosis has improved because of noninvasive techniques that quantify bone mass in vivo. Rather than relying on qualitative x-ray images of the axial skeleton, the physician can now obtain numeric values for bone mass in the spine and hip. Bone mass is an important predictor of fracture risk: as bone mass decreases, the incidence of vertebral and hip fractures increases. Techniques to measure bone mass of the spine and hip include dual photon absorptiometry, dual energy x-ray absorptiometry (DXA), and single and dual energy computed tomography. DXA has the advantage of speed (2 to 5 minutes for each scan), low radiation exposure (1 to 1.5 mrem), and reproducibility (a coefficient of variation of 1%) (Fig. 14.2). Other techniques such as single energy x-ray absorptiometry (SXA), peripheral DXA (pDXA), peripheral quantitative computed tomography (pQCT), and quantitative ultrasound (QUS) that measure bone mass at peripheral sites predict a patient's fracture risk as well as DXA. QUS is portable and is less expensive than DXA and quantitative computer tomography (QCT). The QUS is also radiation-free.

DXA can be used to confirm the diagnosis of osteoporosis, assess the severity of the disease, and determine the rate of bone loss or the efficacy of therapy by obtaining serial measurements. The clinical indications for bone mass measurement in patients seen in an orthopaedic practice include osteopenia on x-ray, "soft bones" during surgical repair, nontraumatic vertebral fracture, hip or Colles fracture, nonambulatory status, and glucocorticoid treatment (7.5 mg of prednisone or greater per day). In the older patient, bone mass assessment at the hip is preferred over a spine measurement because the spine measurement may be artifactually elevated in the older individual by degenerative changes or calcification of the great vessels. The data obtained on hip measurements of a normal and osteoporotic patient are shown in Figure 14.2. Bone mass is measured at the femoral neck, Ward's area, trochanter, shaft, and total hip. The bone mineral density (BMD) at the respective sites is reported as grams of bone mineral/cm^2. This measurement provides a quantitative assessment of bone mass. Additional data include the Young Adult Z-score (a comparison to premenopausal mean peak reference values) and the Age-Matched Z-score (a comparison to sex- and age-matched reference values). The Young Adult Z-score is the key clinical result. The World Health Organization defines osteoporosis as a Young Adult Z-score that is 2.5 SD or more below mean peak value. The DXA report (Fig. 14.2, Panel B) shows the patient to be osteoporotic with a Young Adult Z-score of −3.8 at the femoral neck. This represents a 46% decrease in bone mass. Thus, DXA offers the opportunity to detect low hip bone mass, assess its severity, and make the diagnosis of osteoporosis before fracture.

Because osteoporosis is asymptomatic before fracture, early detection is critical. Instruments using ultrasound to estimate bone mineral density at the calcaneus (Fig. 14.3) correlate closely with radiation-based techniques and predict fracture risk as well as DXA. Because of their lower cost, portability, and lack of radiation exposure, instruments using ultrasound are particularly suited for the office setting. Thus, patients at risk for osteoporosis may be more easily evaluated.

In addition to bone mass measurement, biochemical markers of bone remodeling are also helpful to the physician in the assessment of the osteoporotic patient. These markers reflect bone formation (bone-specific alkaline phosphatase and osteocalcin) or bone resorption (urinary collagen crosslinks). The collagen crosslinks hold the collagen molecules together (Fig. 14.4). As bone is resorbed during the osteoporotic process, the collagen in bone is degraded and the crosslinks are excreted in the urine. Although the level of these resorp-

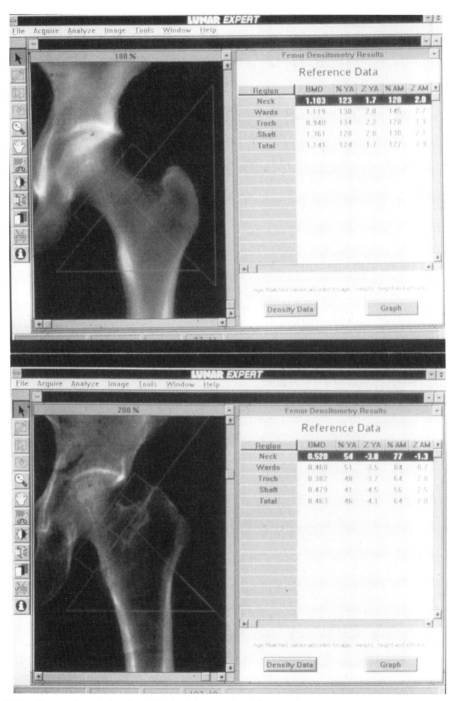

Figure 14.2. Bone mineral density (BMD) of the proximal femur of a normal patient (upper panel) and an osteoporotic patient (lower panel) measured by dual energy x-ray absorptiometry (DXA). The normal patient has a femoral neck density of 1.103 gm/cm^2. This is 1.7 SD above the average young normal and 2.0 SD above age-matched normals. The respective values for Ward's area, the trochanter, the shaft, and the total hip are also provided. The osteoporotic patient (lower panel) has a femoral neck density of 0.528 gm/cm^2. Based on the Young Adult Z-score of -3.8, the patient is osteoporotic at the femoral neck. Using World Health Organization criteria, the patient is also osteoporotic at Ward's area, the trochanter, the shaft, and the total hip.

tion markers in the urine cannot be used to identify the patient with low bone mass, they can be employed to assess the rate of bone turnover and to help to evaluate patient compliance. For example, consider a nonambula-

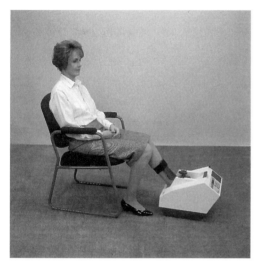

Figure 14.3. Estimated bone mineral density of the calcaneus can be rapidly determined in the office setting using quantitative ultrasound. (Reprinted with permission from Hologic, Inc., Waltham, MA.)

tory patient who has a BMD that is 1.9 SD below young normal. Although the BMD is not in the osteoporotic range, assessment of bone turnover using the crosslink assay shows that resorption is elevated. Therapy is indicated to prevent the development of osteoporosis. A repeat measurement of the marker after 2 to 3 months of therapy should show at least a 50% decrease in the level of the marker. This demonstrates not only the efficacy of therapy in preventing bone loss but also patient compliance. The combination of bone mass measurement and bone resorption markers is useful for the early diagnosis of osteoporosis and the rapid assessment of therapeutic efficacy. Recent studies suggest that the urine markers not only predict therapeutic effect, but also predict the response of bone mineral density to pharmacologic treatment.

DIFFERENTIAL DIAGNOSIS AND CLASSIFICATION

Idiopathic, postmenopausal osteoporosis is a diagnosis of exclusion. Osteomalacia, multiple myeloma, hyperparathyroidism, hyperthyroidism, carcinoma, malabsorption, and hy-

Location of Trivalent Hydroxypyridinium Cross-Links in Collagen Fibrils

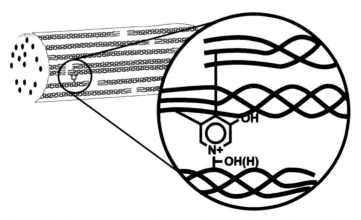

Figure 14.4. Location of trivalent hydroxypyridium crosslinks in collagen fibrils. Collagen molecules are held together by crosslinks. As collagen is broken down during the osteoporotic process, the crosslinks are excreted in the urine. Therefore, elevated levels of crosslinks indicate a higher rate of bone breakdown, whereas lower levels indicate decreased bone resorption. In response to therapy, e.g., estrogen or alendronate, crosslink excretion typically decreases by more than 40% within 2 to 3 months and can be used as an early indicator of therapeutic efficacy.

percortisolism must be considered. In the male, osteoporosis may be a manifestation of testicular failure, and in the young female, a presenting sign of Turner's syndrome.

Osteomalacia is a defect in collagen matrix mineralization. Because milk is supplemented with vitamin D in the United States, nutritional deficiency of the vitamin is rare in this country. Vitamin D deficiency in the elderly is more common because of decreased vitamin D intake and diminished skin synthesis of vitamin D from lessened sunlight exposure. Osteomalacia caused by abnormality in vitamin D metabolism may occur in renal failure (decreased 1,25-dihydroxyvitamin D production in the kidney), steatorrhea (loss of fat-soluble vitamins through the intestinal tract), or vitamin D-resistant rickets (decreased 1α-hydroxylase activity in renal mitochondria). Abnormalities in bone mineralization also occur in the severely hypophosphatemic patient (typically the result of excess ingestion of phosphate-binding antacid or phosphate diabetes).

Multiple myeloma, hyperthyroidism, hyperparathyroidism, and carcinoma can all present as osteopenia. Plasma cells are capable of producing a variety of substances termed osteoclast-activating factors or transforming growth factors that induce bone resorption. Similarly, parathyroid hormone and thyroid hormone in excess induce bone resorption. Recent studies suggest that chronic administration of suppressive doses of thyroid hormone is associated with decreased bone mass. Finally, certain tumors are capable of inducing bone resorption, resulting in hypercalcemia. The typical tumors that secrete these humoral factors are squamous, renal, bladder, and ovarian carcinomas.

Glucocorticoid excess, either intrinsic or iatrogenic, causes osteoporosis. The glucocorticoids inhibit intestinal calcium absorption and bone formation. Bone resorption is often increased to compensate for the decreased intestinal calcium absorption. Therapy for the osteoporosis requires treatment of glucocorticoid overproduction or reduction of steroid dose to the lowest effective level, preferably every-other-day steroid treatment.

Therefore, although idiopathic postmenopausal osteoporosis is the most common form of the disease that will be encountered by the practitioner, these other causes of diminished bone density need to be considered. With the exception of osteoporosis caused by humoral mechanisms associated with cancer and multiple myeloma, these entities may be treated by the practitioner.

TREATMENT OF OSTEOPOROSIS

General Measures

The patient with osteoporosis is asymptomatic unless a fracture has occurred. Fractures in osteoporotic patients heal properly, and the pain should be managed with the appropriate analgesics. Immobilization of the patient with fractures should be minimized, because lack of weightbearing can increase bone loss and increase the severity of the osteoporosis. Physical therapy and weightbearing exercises are beneficial because they strengthen lower extremity muscles and increase reflexes. Physical therapy makes falls less likely, and weightbearing exercises increase the likelihood that the individual will be able to maintain their balance. Many falls occur in the home, and attempts should be made to make the home safe: the use of a night light, elimination of throw rugs, handrails in the bath, etc.

The average calcium intake of postmenopausal women is 400 to 500 mg/day, well below the intake of the 1500 mg/day needed to maintain calcium balance. Increasing calcium intake in the immediate postmenopausal period does not appear to affect the rapid bone loss that occurs during early menopause. In contrast, increasing the calcium intake of 60-year-old women by 500 mg/day appears to reduce bone loss in the spine, femur, and radius.

Studies suggest that vitamin D deficiency in elderly women may contribute to bone loss and fracture risk. This is certainly true of women in nursing homes. The only source of vitamin D in the diet is milk. If the institutionalized patient does not drink milk and is not exposed to direct sunlight, vitamin D deficiency may occur. Treatment of older women in nursing homes with vitamin D, 800 U/day, and calcium, 1000 mg/day, decreases the incidence of hip fractures by 40%.

The most potent vitamin D metabolite is 1,25-dihydroxyvitamin D_3. It augments intestinal absorption of both calcium and phosphorus and prevents vertebral bone loss. The major side effects of 1,25-dihydroxyvitamin D_3 are the risk of hypercalciuria and hypercalcemia and, therefore, its administration requires constant monitoring. In one study, this metabolite increased bone density, but all of the patients developed hypercalciuria, and 89% manifested a serum calcium greater than 11 mg/dL at one time during the study. Reduction in the dose of 1,25-dihydroxyvitamin D_3 lessens the risk of hypercalciuria and hypercalcemia but does not appear to prevent bone loss. The therapeutic window between efficacy of the drug and side effects is narrow, making routine treatment difficult.

Pharmacologic Treatment

The Food and Drug Administration has approved estrogen, alendronate, and raloxifene for the prevention of osteoporosis, and estrogen, alendronate, and nasal calcitonin for the treatment of osteoporosis.

Estrogen

The main effect of estrogen is the prevention of bone loss, although estrogen does appear to increase bone mineral density of the spine by 4 to 5% and of the hip by 2% over 3 years. It's optimal use is in the perimenopausal woman to prevent the accelerated bone loss that occurs for the 3 to 4 years after menopause. Estrogen therapy prevents axial bone loss when administered either orally or transdermally. Estrogen is more effective in preventing vertebral bone loss at standard doses; virtually all women respond with at least a maintenance of vertebral bone mass, whereas 10 to 15% of treated women continue to lose hip bone mass. Numerous case control and cohort studies have documented that estrogen treatment decreases spine, wrist, and hip fracture risk. The risk of a hip fracture is decreased by 20 to 60%. Continued use of estrogen appears to be necessary to insure protection against fracture.

Candidates for estrogen therapy to prevent bone loss include women with a history of ovariectomy, women undergoing early menopause, women requiring prolonged glucocorticoid treatment, or women who are perimenopausal with a slight body build and a family history of osteoporosis. Because risk factors alone do not predict bone mass, the woman who is most likely to benefit from estrogen replacement therapy can best be determined by bone densitometry.

Alendronate

Alendronate, a member of a class of compounds called bisphosphonates, is approved for the prevention and treatment of osteoporosis. The biphosphonates possess a strong affinity for the hydroxyapatite crystal in bone. Their main effect is to inhibit bone resorption. The brief half-life of the compounds in the circulation plus the long half-life in bone explains their low systemic toxicity and the restriction of their effects to the skeleton.

Alendronate treatment of early postmenopausal women at a dose of 5 mg/day prevents bone loss at the spine and the hip. The effect is comparable to that observed with estrogen. In older women, alendronate at a dose of 10 mg/day increases spine density by 8 to 9% and hip density by 5 to 6% over 3 years while reducing vertebral fracture incidence by 50%. In 2027 women with a previous vertebral fracture, alendronate decreased the incidence of new vertebral fractures, wrist fractures, and hip fractures by 50%. The incidence of two or more new vertebral fractures was decreased by 90%.

The major side effect of alendronate is esophageal irritation, with heartburn and stomach upset being the most frequent complaints. The medication needs to be taken after an overnight fast with at least 8 oz of plain water. The patient must then wait 30 minutes before eating or taking any other beverages or medications. The patient may drink more water, but should not lie supine during the 30 minute period as this may increase the incidence of heartburn.

Candidates for alendronate therapy include women with low bone mass, women who cannot or will not take estrogen, women treated with glucocorticoids, and women with a previous vertebral compression fracture. Although 96 to 98% of women respond to alendronate with cessation of bone loss, efficacy of therapy is best determined by decreases in urinary markers of bone resorption or serial bone mass measurements.

Raloxifene

Raloxifene has recently been approved by the FDA for the prevention of osteoporosis. Like tamoxifen, raloxifene is a member of a class of drugs called SERMS, (Selective Estrogen Receptor Modulators). Raloxifene exerts estrogenlike activities at certain sites (bone, cardiovascular system) and estrogen-antagonistic effects in others (breast, uterus). The molecular basis of this antagonism may be caused by differences in the binding of estrogen and raloxifene to the estrogen receptor(s) and to alterations in receptor structure.

Raloxifene, 60 mg/day, increases spine and hip BMD by 1 to 2% after 2 years in early menopausal women (average 59 months postmenopause). Seventy-three percent of the women had an increase in their BMD, 7% had no change, and 20% had a decrease. Raloxifene also decreases LDL cholesterol, while having no effect on HDL cholesterol. A recent study indicates that raloxifene decreases vertebral fractures by 44%, but does not affect nonvertebral fractures (e.g., hip, wrist).

The 3-year studies showed no increase in breast or uterine cancer while on raloxifene. Although the initial evaluation suggests that the compound has protective effects at those sites, long-term studies (7 to 8 years) are required to assess effects on the breast and uterus. Raloxifene increases hot flashes, leg cramps, and the risk of venous thromboembolism. Although the hot flashes are described as being mild on raloxifene, an increase in this symptom may make it difficult to treat early menopausal women who frequently seek therapy to reduce hot flashes.

Calcitonin

Both injectable and nasal calcitonin are available for the treatment of osteoporosis. The drug is a potent inhibitor of osteoclastic bone resorption and possesses analgesic properties. Because of the analgesic properties, its use in the woman with an acute vertebral compression for 3 to 4 weeks may decrease her requirement for narcotics or nonsteroidal agents. The use of intranasal calcitonin (Miacalcin) is simple (one spray per day, alternating nostrils) with few side effects (10% incidence of rhinorrhea). The use of the medication is associated with a 2 to 4% increase in vertebral bone mineral density; however, it does not increase hip density. At present, no data exist to demonstrate its effect in reducing fractures. Pending fracture efficacy data, calcitonin should be considered for prolonged treatment only in the woman who cannot or will not take estrogen, alendronate, or raloxifene.

PAGET'S DISEASE OF BONE

Paget's disease is characterized by increased bone resorption and resultant increments in bone formation. The "turnover" of bone is increased greatly and results in a "mosaic" pattern of bone formation.

CLINICAL CHARACTERISTICS

Paget's disease occurs in 0.1 to 1% of elderly hospitalized patients in the United States, with equal frequency in men and women. The bones most commonly affected by Paget's disease, in order of decreasing frequency, are sacrum, spine, femur, skull, sternum, and pelvis. The bones of the axial skeleton are most frequently involved, but the disease may occur at any skeletal site and may involve one or many bones.

Pain is a common manifestation of Paget's disease, with some studies suggesting that prostaglandins may be the responsible agents.

The skin over the affected bone is often warm. This is thought to reflect the increased vascularity of the bone with resultant increased blood flow. Because of the chaotic turnover of bone, the size and shape of the bones often change, with the skull enlarging and long bones becoming deformed. Although the bone in Paget's disease may increase in size, the mosaic pattern of deposited lamellar bone makes it weaker. Hence, "bowing" deformities of the lower extremities and fractures are common occurrences. The treatment of fractures associated with Paget's disease is similar to treatment of fractures of normal bone; however, the practitioner must be aware that these bones are more vascular. Less than 1% of patients with Paget's disease progress to develop osteogenic sarcoma. This is heralded by increasing pain in a previously well-controlled patient, or rapidly increasing serum alkaline phosphatase.

The major complications of Paget's disease are spinal stenosis, degenerative arthritis, and nerve impingement caused by increasing bone size. Deafness is a common sequela of Paget's disease involving the skull. The deafness may result from damage to the auditory nerve as it passes through the auditory canal or from involvement of the bones of the inner ear with Paget's disease. Degenerative arthritis is a commonly associated finding when Paget's disease bridges a joint, e.g., pelvis and femur or femur and tibia.

PATHOPHYSIOLOGY OF PAGET'S DISEASE

The etiology of the disease remains unclear. Viral inclusion bodies have been reported in biopsies of Pagetic bone, but it is not certain that they are the causative agents. The observation that Paget's disease often occurs in several members of a family has led to speculation regarding genetic transmission. However, based on the known incidence of Paget's disease and the incidence of identical twin births, the paucity of Paget's disease in twin pairs makes genetic transmission unlikely.

DIAGNOSIS OF PAGET'S DISEASE

Paget's disease is characterized by increased bone resorption and, frequently, increased bone formation. The stages of Paget's disease may involve (*a*) increased resorption, (*b*) resorption plus formation, or (*c*) a sclerotic quiescent phase. The practitioner is referred to a textbook of radiology for a thorough description of the radiographic changes in bones affected by Paget's disease. A bone scan can differentiate between active and quiescent Paget's disease, and serum alkaline phosphatase is a marker for the activity of the disease. Although alkaline phosphatase is produced by osteoblasts, increased alkaline phosphatase may also reflect liver disease, ectopic pregnancy, a healing fracture, or any osteoblastic process in bone. Alkaline phosphatase from bone can be distinguished by fractionating the total alkaline phosphatase. The bone fraction is heat labile. Urinary hydroxyproline is increased in Paget's disease, reflecting increased collagen degradation. Although this is also an excellent marker for disease activity, the procedure requires the collection of a 24-hour urine sample, and the results may be affected by diet, e.g., gelatin, or skin disease, e.g., psoriasis. The urinary excretion of collagen cross-links is a better indicator of bone resorption than urinary hydroxyproline, because these molecules are more specific for bone collagen (Fig. 14.4). Acid phosphatase, most frequently considered a marker for prostatic malignancy, is also produced by bone cells and may be elevated in active Paget's disease. Because metastatic osteoblastic prostate malignancy is in the differential diagnosis of Paget's disease, increases in serum acid phosphatase must be further evaluated by measures of the prostatic fraction of acid phosphatase.

DIFFERENTIAL DIAGNOSIS

Any osteoblastic process, e.g., metastatic prostate cancer, may resemble Paget's disease roentgenographically, but appropriate testing should differentiate the conditions. Hereditary hyperphosphatasia may be similar to

Paget's disease, but the age of the patient and the involvement of the entire skeleton should easily differentiate the two.

TREATMENT OF PAGET'S DISEASE

The drugs most commonly employed to treat Paget's disease are bisphosphonates or calcitonin. Indications for treatment are increasing severity of symptoms and an elevated alkaline phosphatase (greater than threefold the upper limit of normal).

Bisphosphonates

Etidronate Disodium

Etidronate disodium (Didronel) is an oral medication effective in approximately 85% of patients with Paget's disease, decreasing both symptoms and activity of the disease as measured by alkaline phosphatase. The usual dosage is 400 mg/day for 6 months. Because food affects absorption of the drug, the drug should be given between meals or at bedtime. Sodium etidronate is an inhibitor of bone resorption and bone formation. At doses of 10 to 20 mg/kg body weight per day, the drug has been associated with increased incidence of fractures and the development of osteomalacia (impaired mineralization of the collagen matrix). Sodium etidronate may also cause a mild phosphaturia, and it is suggested that serum phosphorus as well as alkaline phosphatase be measured at 3-month intervals. In the patient on a normal diet, this mild phosphaturia is not clinically significant.

Alendronate

At a dose of 40 mg/day, alendronate normalizes biochemical markers of bone remodeling in 50% of patients with Paget's disease during 6 months of therapy. Based on the biochemical changes, alendronate is the most effective oral agent for the treatment of the disease. Alendronate does not cause a mineralization defect at this dose; however, 18% of patients experience upper gastrointestinal adverse experiences and 6% report musculoskeletal pain.

Pamidronate

The effectiveness of pamidronate has been demonstrated primarily in patients with moderate to severe Paget's disease (alkaline phosphatase more than 3 times the upper limit of normal). Because of gastrointestinal intolerance, pamidronate can only be administered intravenously. It appears to be effective in reducing the biochemical markers of bone remodeling in patients who no longer respond to other therapies. The recommended dose is 30 mg/day administered as a 4-hour infusion on 3 consecutive days for a total dose of 90 mg. A brief febrile response and mild flulike symptoms are common after the infusions. Headache and musculoskeletal pain occur in 10% of patients.

Calcitonin

Calcitonin is a polypeptide hormone produced by the C cells of the thyroid. Its major action is inhibition of osteoclastic bone resorption. Because bone resorption and formation appear to be "coupled," inhibition of bone resorption will ultimately inhibit bone formation. These effects result in decreased urinary hydroxyproline excretion and decreased serum alkaline phosphatase levels. Although the drug is effective in the treatment of hypercalcemia associated with malignancy, calcitonin treatment does not cause hypocalcemia in patients with Paget's disease.

Calcitonin is administered subcutaneously, usually 3 times a week. The dose of salmon calcitonin is 100 IU/day. The response rate ranges between 95 and 100%. The most common side effect is transient nausea. This can be minimized by administration of the calcitonin at bedtime.

Nonsteroidal Anti-Inflammatory Agents

Although these drugs do not specifically treat Paget's disease, they may be useful in the patient with arthritic changes associated with Paget's disease.

BONE METASTASIS

Tumors metastatic to bone may cause pain, hypercalcemia, and fractures. Osteolytic hypercalcemia results from bone resorption caused by tumors in direct contact with the bone cells. The tumors most likely to cause osteolytic hypercalcemia are breast cancers, multiple myelomas, and hematologic malignancies. In contrast, humoral hypercalcemia of malignancy in the absence of bone metastases is caused by osteoclastic resorption mediated by parathyroid hormonelike peptides. Tumors most commonly associated with humoral hypercalcemia are renal, squamous, bladder, and ovarian carcinomas. Although fractures occur in patients with hyperparathyroidism, the presence of hypercalcemia in a patient with a fracture should immediately raise concern regarding the possibility of a malignancy. A bone scan should be obtained to investigate potential skeletal involvement at other sites, and orthopaedic consultation should be requested. The bone scan may not show increased activity in patients with an osteolytic tumor, e.g., myeloma, who have not yet developed a pathologic fracture.

TREATMENT

The practitioner should consult an oncologist before treatment of the underlying tumor. Often, however, the hypercalcemia presents as a medical emergency with altered mental status and electrocardiographic changes, i.e., shortened QT interval. The goal of therapy is the rapid reduction in serum calcium to avoid cardiovascular and central nervous system complications. In the acute situation, this is initially accomplished by rehydrating the patient, thereby increasing renal calcium excretion. Intravenous fluids can be started quickly and can rapidly increase calcium excretion. The goal is to achieve a urine output of 3 to 5 L/24 hours. If the patient's cardiovascular system is compromised, care must be used to prevent congestive heart failure. Concomitant use of loop diuretics can help achieve the desired urinary output while minimizing the risk of fluid overload. Calcitonin is effective in the treatment of hypercalcemia. Up to 80% of hypercalcemic patients will respond to calcitonin with a decrease in serum calcium

levels within 4 to 6 hours. Unfortunately, tolerance to the calcitonin may develop within 6 to 10 days. Intravenous biphosphonates (etidronate disodium or pamidronate) may be a useful form of therapy. When administered along with intravenous fluids, calcium levels are normalized in 90% of patients. Glucocorticoids also may be beneficial in the treatment of hypercalcemia of malignancy caused by myeloma and other hematologic malignancies. Because a response to glucocorticoids usually is not seen for 7 to 10 days, they cannot be used to acutely lower serum calcium.

While the patient's serum calcium is being treated, the practitioner is urged to consult an oncologist so that diagnosis and therapy for the underlying malignancy may be initiated.

SUGGESTED READINGS

Black DM, Cummings SR, Karpf DB, et al. Randomized trial of effect of alendronate on risk of fracture in women with existing vertebral fractures. Lancet 1996;348:1535–1541.

Calvo MS, Eyre DR, Gundberg CM. Molecular basis and clinical application of biological markers of bone turnover. Endocr Rev 1996;17:333–368.

Chapuy MC, Arlot ME, Duboseu JF, et al. Vitamin D_3 and calcium to prevent hip fractures in elderly women. N Engl J Med 1992;327:1637–1642.

Chesnut CH III, Bell NH, Clark GS, et al. Hormone replacement therapy in postmenopausal women: urinary N-telopeptide of type I collagen monitors therapeutic effect and predicts response of bone mineral density Am J Med 1997;102:29–37.

Cummings SR, Nevitt MC, Browner WS, et al. Risk factors for hip fracture in white women. N Engl J Med 1995;332:767–773.

Delmas PD, Bjarnason NH, Mitlak B, et al. Effects of raloxifene on bone mineral density, serum cholesterol concentrations, and uterine endometrium in postmenopausal women. N Engl J Med 1997;337:1641–1647.

Delmas PD, Meunier PJ. The management of Paget's disease of bone. N Engl J Med 1997;36:558–566.

Ellerington MC, Hillard TC, Whitcroft SIJ, et al. Intranasal salmon calcitonin for the prevention and treatment of postmenopausal osteoporosis. Calcif Tissue Int 1996;59:6–11.

Favus MJ, ed. Primer on the Metabolic Bone Diseases and Disorders of Mineral Metabolism. Philadelphia: Lippincott-Raven, 1996.

Gallagher JC. Estrogen: Prevention and Treatment of Osteoporosis. In: Marcus R, Feldman D, Kelsey J, eds. Osteoporosis. San Diego: Academic Press, 1996:1191–1208.

Kanis JA, Melton LJ III, Christiansen C, et al. The diagnosis of osteoporosis. J Bone Miner Res 1994;9:1137–1141.

Liberman UA, Weiss SR, Broll J, et al. Effect of oral alendronate on bone mineral density and the incidence of fractures in postmenopausal osteoporosis. N Engl J Med 1995;333:1437–1443.

Orwoll ES, Klein RF. Osteoporosis in men. Endocr Rev 1995;16:87–116.

Overgaard K, Lindsay R, Christiansen C. Patient responsiveness to calcitonin salmon nasal spray: a subanalysis of a 2-year study. Clin Ther 1995;17:680–685.

Reid IR, Nicholson GC, Weinstein RS, et al. Biochemical and radiologic improvement in Paget's disease of bone treated with alendronate: a randomized, placebo-controlled trial. Am J Med 1996;171:341–348.

Stock JL, Bell NH, Chesnut CH III, et al. Increments in bone mineral density of the lumbar spine and hip and suppression of bone turnover are maintained after discontinuation of alendronate in postmenopausal women. Am J Med 1997;103:291–297.

Turner RT, Riggs BL, Spelsberg TC. Skeletal effects of estrogen. Endocr Rev 1994;15:275–300.

The Writing Group for the PEPI Trial. Effects of hormone therapy on bone mineral density: results from the postmenopausal estrogen/progestin intervention (PEPI) trial. JAMA 1996;276:1389–1396.

Orthopaedic Oncology for the Primary Care Physician

Henry DeGroot III, M.D.

INTRODUCTION

The primary care giver of today, more than ever before, is involved in the management and care of patients with primary and metastatic bone tumors. The primary care physician is often the first doctor that a patient with a bone or soft tissue tumor will encounter. Thus, today's primary care physician is often the manager of the process of patient evaluation, referral, and treatment. A systematic approach to the evaluation and workup of these patients can optimize management and facilitate early and appropriate referral. Once the diagnosis has been made, these patients are likely to require the services of a number of specialists that include the radiologist, pathologist, medical oncologist, radiation oncologist, and orthopaedic surgeon. In many settings, these care providers will be located in separate offices, or even in separate towns or cities, and they may not be willing or able to coordinate their treatment smoothly with those of the rest of the care team. The primary care provider needs the tools and knowledge to understand, coordinate, and optimize the diverse aspects of the care of a patient with a primary or metastatic bone tumor.

METASTATIC BONE DISEASE

In today's primary care practice, the most common bone tumor will be the metastatic lesion. In the United States, approximately 1 million new cases of malignancies occur each year, and about half of these are in primary sites that frequently metastasize to bone.

From 50 to 80% of all patients with carcinoma will develop bone metastases, as well as an estimated 85% of women with breast cancer. Most metastatic deposits in bone originate from tumors of the breast, prostate, lung, kidney, colon, and thyroid. Of these, the breast, prostate, and lung are the sites of origin of at least three-quarters of all metastatic lesions.

PATHOGENESIS

The ability of a given tumor to metastasize to a given site depends on intrinsic properties of the tumor and the properties of the site of metastasis. Malignant tumors most often metastasize via the blood stream, either by arterial or venous routes. Venous blood draining from a primary tumor normally enters the caval or portal venous systems. Tumor cells that enter the venous circulation are "filtered" and trapped in the lungs or the liver, making these two organs the most common sites of metastatic spread of tumors. Bone is the third most common site of metastatic deposits. The most common skeletal sites involved are the vertebral bodies, proximal femur, pelvis, ribs, sternum, and proximal humerus, in descending order of frequency (Fig. 15.1). These sites correspond to the locations of persistent hematopoietic marrow in the adult.

The anatomic distribution of the majority of metastatic deposits in the skeleton has a peculiar pattern that may be partially explained by Batson's plexus (Fig. 15.2). This system of low-pressure valveless veins connects the major organs that metastasize to bone with the spinal column, pelvis, ribs, and

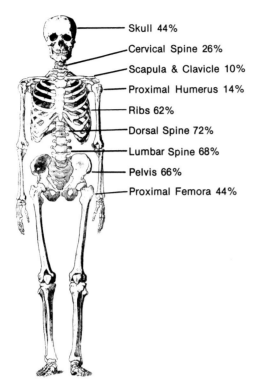

Skull 44%

Cervical Spine 26%

Scapula & Clavicle 10%

Proximal Humerus 14%

Ribs 62%

Dorsal Spine 72%

Lumbar Spine 68%

Pelvis 66%

Proximal Femora 44%

Figure 15.1. Common locations of metastatic deposits in bone.

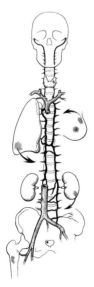

Figure 15.2. Diagrammatic representation of Batson's venous plexus. (Reprinted with permission from Sim FH. Diagnosis and Management of Metastatic Bone Disease. New York: Raven, 1988.)

proximal long bones. The direction of blood flow depends on the relative pressures in the thorax, the abdomen, and the retroperitoneum. Tumor cells that have broken free from the primary site can enter this venous system and be carried to the marrow of nearby bones by coughing, breathing, or Valsalva's maneuver. Tumors from the lung also may be disseminated by the arterial system. For this reason, metastases from lung tumors may be widely disseminated in distant locations such as the hand or foot. Normally, metastases from adenocarcinomas to bones below the knee and below the elbow are exceedingly rare. When a metastatic deposit in such a location is seen, a primary lung tumor should be suspected.

The presence of a rich blood supply alone does not completely explain the observed patterns of tumor metastasis to bone. Local factors that create a favorable environment for tumor growth are also required and may include cell surface and adhesion properties, as well as the presence of appropriate nutrients, growth factors, hormonal mediators, and oxygen tension.

Once the tumor cells have become implanted at the site of metastasis, they begin to multiply and permeate the trabecular spaces. This process may cause bone destruction and/or bone formation, depending on the type of tumor and rate of growth. Bone destruction may be mediated by osteoclasts that are activated by the tumor through prostaglandins, osteoclast-activating factors, parathyroid hormones, and cytokines. Some tumor cells are capable of direct destruction of bone without the mediation of osteoclasts. Significant bone formation is typically associated with metastatic prostate cancer. The consequences of metastatic bone disease include pathological fracture, severe pain caused by fracture or irritation of the periosteum, anemia as a result of marrow replacement, and hypercalcemia.

CLINICAL MANIFESTATIONS

The primary clinical symptom of metastatic bone disease is pain. Although many musculoskeletal conditions present with pain, the character and progression of metastatic cancer pain distinguishes it from the pain of muscle sprains, contusions, or tendonitis. The pain from bone cancer is normally insidious in onset and, at first, it may only bother the patient during weightbearing or certain activities. Active patients commonly relate the onset of the pain to a minor sports injury or household accident, but this is probably coincidental. The pain is usually characterized as a deep, dull, aching sensation. With time, there is a steady increase in the pain intensity that is no longer relieved by rest. Many patients report that the pain is more bothersome at night or that it will wake them from a sound sleep.

In many patients with degenerative arthritis of the spine and other joints, it may be difficult to isolate the true cause of the pain. Approximately one-third of patients with a primary carcinoma and back pain have a non-malignant cause for the pain. Patients with a known tumor should still have a careful history and physical examination to rule out common musculoskeletal problems before pain can be ascribed to a bone metastasis.

Eventually, the pain becomes severe enough to compel even the most reluctant to seek medical care. If the true diagnosis is missed at this point and the patient is given a prescription for narcotic analgesics, the patient may be able to tolerate the pain and disability for several additional weeks or months, or until a pathologic fracture occurs. Some patients will severely limit their activities to avoid the pain.

Other clinical manifestations of metastatic disease include burning pain, numbness, loss of continence, or weakness from nerve root or spinal cord compression. Pain from metastatic bone disease around the hip may be referred to the knee. Tumors of the lumbar spine, sacrum, or ilium may cause radicular symptoms that can lead to a misdiagnosis of herniated nucleus pulposus. In contrast to herniated nucleus pulposus, tumor pain is unremitting, progressive, and unrelieved by rest or positioning. Neurologic deficits are rarely the first symptoms of a metastatic deposit, but as many

as 70% of patients with tumors involving the spine will have clinical weakness by the time the correct diagnosis is made. As many as half of these patients will have bowel or bladder dysfunction.

CAUSES OF DIAGNOSTIC DELAY

Both patients and physicians can contribute to significant delays in the diagnosis and treatment of metastatic bone disease. In many cases, patients with a prior history of cancer will not volunteer their diagnosis on casual questioning because they were told by another physician that they needed no further cancer treatment and they consider themselves "cured." This situation is often compounded by a physician who does not take the time to question the patients carefully about their symptoms. A thorough history and physical examination can avoid delays in diagnosis.

Several "red flags" should alert the clinician to consider malignancy. The first is insidious and progressive pain in any patient over 40. The second is when the diagnosis does not adequately account for all the patient's symptoms. Finally, one should be concerned when expected improvement in a condition does not occur.

EVALUATION AND IMAGING

The first step in the evaluation of the patient should be a complete history. As noted previously, a prior history of cancer and cancer risk factors might not be volunteered by the patient. The most presenting complaint is pain. The patient may give a history of a minor injury, but careful questioning by the physician often reveals that the pain is far more serious and long lasting than would be expected after a minor sprain or contusion. The pain is often deep seated, not relieved completely by rest, and bothersome at night. Most patients do not notice a mass, and contrary to popular belief, only a small proportion will report any history of weight loss. If metastatic bone disease is suspected, the physician should ask questions specifically designed to cover the five major organ systems that are the most likely primary sites (breast, lung, prostate, kidney, and thyroid).

The next step is a thorough examination. Again, specific attention to the most likely primary sites is necessary. The thyroid can be directly palpated, the breasts examined, the lungs auscultated, the kidneys in some cases can be palpated by abdominal examination, and the prostate examined. These simple examination maneuvers will reveal the primary lesion in a surprising number of patients, eliminating many unnecessary and expensive tests. In many cases, the information gathered in the history and physical examination can lead to a differential diagnosis that includes only one entity. For example, a 67-year-old man who presents with severe, progressive pain in the hip and low back whose examination reveals a rock-hard mass in and around the prostate probably has metastatic prostate carcinoma. The doctor can proceed directly to specific tests and a treatment plan.

If the history and physical examination point to one specific entity, the only tests necessary are those that confirm the diagnosis. In other cases, there are no diagnostic findings on history or examination. For these, a systematic approach to the workup and biopsy of the bone lesion should be employed. Laboratory examination should include a complete blood count with a differential, erythrocyte sedimentation rate, serum electrolytes, liver function tests, calcium, phosphate, and serum protein electrophoresis. A serum prostatic specific antigen level should be obtained for males.

Plain radiographs of the entire length of the bone involved and a chest radiograph should be obtained. A whole body technetium-99m-phosphonate bone scan should be performed. In cases of probable metastatic disease with no apparent primary lesion, a computed tomography scan of the chest, abdomen, and pelvis should be planned. Additional imaging studies should only be performed if the results of the initial screening studies reveal a likely site of origin outside the chest, abdomen, or pelvis. Once all the required imaging studies are obtained, the most accessible lesion

should be selected for biopsy. For patients under the age of 40 and patients with a solitary bone lesion, the possibility of a primary tumor should be considered.

Many patients with a metastatic bone lesion have an established primary diagnosis at the time of presentation. The evaluation should then focus on determining the local extent of the metastatic lesion, detecting the presence or absence of other potentially significant bone lesions, and determining the proper course of treatment for each lesion. The best first test should be high-quality plain radiographs of the affected part. The radiographs should include good views of the whole bone to locate any other lesions that are present.

For patients presenting with their first bone metastasis before a bone scan has been done, full-length radiographs of both femurs and the pelvis as well as any other symptomatic site should be obtained. This enables a rapid assessment of the areas where a pathologic fracture has the potential to do the most harm to the patient's mobility and well-being. This also provides information needed to make decisions about the patient's overall risk and mobility level without having to wait for a bone scan. If weightbearing is to be limited on one leg because of the risk of a pathologic fracture, one needs to know if there are any potential problems with the other femur or the pelvis.

Occasionally, the patient had a radiograph of the area taken at a walk-in clinic or emergency room in the weeks or months before presentation. These recent radiographs represent a source of valuable information on the behavior and rate of progression of the lesion, and vigorous attempts should be made to locate and review them.

The presence of multiple metastatic lesions should be assessed by a whole body technetium bone scan. If the bone scan reveals any previously unknown lesions in the spine, pelvis, or the bones of the lower extremities, plain radiographs of these areas should be obtained and analyzed for fracture risk. Because the lytic lesions of multiple myeloma cannot be detected by a bone scan, a skeletal survey should be obtained in these patients.

BIOPSY

Biopsy of a bone lesion seems like a simple technical exercise, but is really a complex cognitive process. A biopsy is not part of the initial evaluation of a lesion and should be deferred until all the necessary information has been gathered and all the required imaging studies have been obtained. There are several reasons to defer the biopsy. A new lesion that is more accessible for the biopsy may be discovered during the workup. In a few cases, the results of the noninvasive portion of the workup will result in a definite diagnosis, making the biopsy unnecessary. In others once the full magnitude of the problem is appreciated by the patient and the family, a biopsy may become less useful because it might have no impact on the treatment plan. At other times, the biopsy can be combined with a stabilization procedure.

By far the most important reason to save the biopsy for last is to maximize the value of the information obtained and to minimize the possibility of a biopsy-related error or complication. The pathologist reviewing the specimen is better able to give the treatment team a definitive diagnosis when the workup has narrowed the differential down to one or a few entities, or if a likely primary organ has been identified. The workup can eliminate the important nonmalignant diagnoses, such as infection or stress fracture, that can be easily confused with a metastatic lesion. The biopsy is best used to confirm a diagnosis that is strongly suggested by other related findings from the workup.

Before a biopsy is planned, the case should be discussed with the surgeon who will be treating the patient, if surgery becomes necessary. If possible, the biopsy should be performed by the actual treating surgeon. This is particularly true when the lesion might represent a primary bone or soft tissue malignancy. A poorly planned biopsy can cause serious errors in diagnosis and treatment. Patients referred to musculoskeletal tumor centers after the biopsy have a significantly higher rate of errors in histologic diagnosis as well as complications requiring more extensive treatment or surgery.

The best location and method for the biopsy are selected based on the results of the staging workup and the experience and skills of the care team. In some centers, biopsies are performed via Tru-cut or other large bore needles using closed technique, with or without computed tomographic (CT) guidance. Other centers rely primarily on open biopsy. A sufficient volume of tissue is needed for conventional histologic diagnosis and tissue typing, special stains and studies, RNA and DNA analysis for chromosomal markers, determinations of DNA ploidy, and other special studies according to the protocols and preferences of the bone pathologist in charge.

ASSESSING FRACTURE RISK

No reliable method exists for assessing the risk of a pathologic fracture associated with any given lesion. Attempts to quantify the risk of fracture using a finite-element model generated from high-resolution computed tomography scan of the lesion and the surrounding bone have been encouraging but are not yet clinically useful. At the present time, the clinician should use a combination of an analysis of the plain films, the location and type of lesion, and evaluation of the patient's clinical complaints to assess the fracture risk. Lesions located in the area of the hip joint, in the spine, or in the long bones warrant prompt attention and referral because of the devastating consequences of a pathologic fracture at these sites. In addition, lesions from breast and renal cancer should be evaluated and referred promptly because of higher fracture rates in these lesions.

Patients with progressive pain or pain that returns after treatment of a lesion with radiation also should be referred promptly.

Plain radiographs should be reviewed to

assess the risk of fracture, but they may underestimate the actual amount of bone destruction. It is commonly believed that once a metastatic lesion is visible on a plain radiograph, at least 50% of the substance of the bone has already been lost. The fracture risk from any given lesion can be roughly estimated using two plain radiographs of the area taken at 90° to each other. Taken together, the two films show four portions of the cortex near the lesion. When two or more of the portions of cortex near the tumor are damaged or destroyed, the patient should be considered at high risk for pathologic fracture. In addition, lesions larger than 2.5 cm in diameter or that have destroyed more than 50% of the bone, lesions with widespread involvement of the metaphysis of a long bone, and any lesion in the proximal one-third of the femur should be considered at particular risk for fracture. Pathologic fracture may occur through blastic as well as lytic lesions.

The treating physician should closely monitor patients with adenocarcinomas for signs and symptoms of bone metastases. Patients should be encouraged to report any new ache or pain and should be carefully questioned for these symptoms by the nurse or doctor. A patient with a known cancer and a new problem of this type should be examined promptly and a plain radiograph of the area obtained. Due diligence will lead to the discovery of most metastases before causing a fracture. The lesions can then be electively and prophylactically stabilized by an orthopaedic surgeon with a minimum of morbidity and a significant cost savings.

INDICATIONS FOR OPERATIVE TREATMENT

Surgical stabilization is the treatment of choice for pathologic fractures and for lesions that pose a risk of impending fracture. Smaller lesions that do not require stabilization should be referred for treatment by a radiation oncologist. If a lesion in a long bone or a weight-bearing site progresses despite radiation, it should be stabilized. Surgical treatments are safer, easier for the patient and the surgeon, and more cost-effective if they can be done before a pathologic fracture occurs. Surgical treatment should be offered to patients who have a reasonable life expectancy, who can safely undergo the planned surgery, for whom the surgery can be accomplished in an expedient fashion, and whose expected outcome after surgery is thought to be better than that expected with nonoperative treatments such as splinting and radiation. A defeatist and fatalistic attitude should be avoided. Every patient deserves treatment if he or she will benefit from it, although there are clearly some patients for whom no operation should be considered. The operative treatment of metastatic bone lesions should be designed always to eliminate pain, often to preserve mobility, and rarely to prolong life.

Trying to predict the patient's remaining life span is difficult, and published statistics should be used as a general guide only. It is helpful to make a rough estimate of the patient's predicted survival, then double it, and plan any operative technique accordingly. In this way, poorly conceived stabilization procedures that fail during the patient's last weeks or months can be avoided. The first surgery should be done well enough to be the last.

Careful planning is necessary before surgical treatment is undertaken. For lesions in the spine and pelvis, a CT scan or MRI should be obtained. For large, highly vascularized lesions such as those caused by renal cell carcinoma, preoperative transarterial embolization of the lesion should be considered to reduce the risk of major blood loss. Most lesions are treated with some form of internal fixation with or without the addition of polymethylmethacrylate bone cement. Lesions in the diaphysis of a long bone are best treated by stabilization with an intramedullary rod, while lesions in the proximal and distal ends of the bone are often treated with a lateral plate and compression screw, or by resection and prosthetic replacement. Metastatic destruction of the acetabulum can be treated with total hip arthroplasty combined with a specialized acetabular insert augmented by polymethylmethacrylate bone cement and transilial stabilization with long screws or Kirschner wires. Large lesions involving virtually any length of the femur, tibia, or humerus can be treated with a massive prosthetic replacement comprised of modular segments that are assembled intraoperatively by the surgeon (Fig. 15.3). If a pathologic fracture occurs through an area of irradiated bone, prosthetic substitution may be preferable to internal fixation because of concerns about impaired fracture healing. Postoperative care of the patient with a metastatic lesion should focus on the specific risk factors presented.

The goal of surgery is to allow rapid mobilization of the patient. In most cases, this can be accomplished 1 or 2 days postoperatively. Prolonged recumbency exacerbates many of the physiologic derangements the patient with cancer is prone to, such as hypercalcemia, deep vein thrombosis, osteoporosis, and pressure sore breakdown. Patients with metastases are at increased risk of deep vein thrombosis and embolization, and effective prophylaxis should be instituted. If the surgical site was irradiated in the preoperative period, the sutures or staples used to close the skin should be left in for much longer than usual, sometimes as long as 6 weeks. For most lesions, surgery should be coupled with postoperative radiation to minimize the chance that the lesion will progress. If postoperative radiation is planned, it may begin 2 weeks after surgery provided the wound is benign. Skin staples do not interfere with radiation treatments. The orthopaedic surgeon should continue to monitor the lesion and the status of the stabilization of the patient as long as the patient survives and remains mobile.

HYPERCALCEMIA ASSOCIATED WITH SKELETAL METASTASES

Hypercalcemia is a relatively common and potentially life-threatening complication of skeletal metastases. Clinically, the patient may present with lethargy, confusion, or even coma; he or she may be weak, nauseated, or vomiting, and may have polyuria and dehydration. Myeloma and breast carcinoma most frequently are associated with hypercalcemia, but hypercalcemia can occur in the setting of other metastatic tumors.

Hypercalcemia is caused by specific factors that are secreted by the tumor that create local bone resorption and destruction. Tumor cells may elaborate a parathyroid hormone-related protein (PTHrP) and other osteoclast activating factors including cytokines. The secretion of PTHrP is common in squamous cell carcinoma, renal, ovarian, and bladder carcinoma. Treatment of hypercalcemia is outlined in Chapter 14.

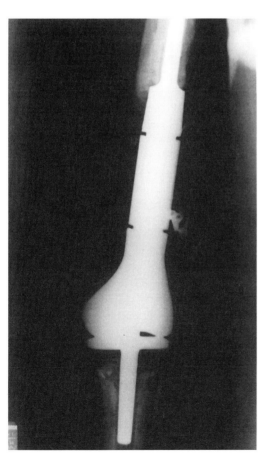

Figure 15.3. Radiograph of modular prosthesis with interchangeable components.

PRIMARY MALIGNANT BONE AND SOFT TISSUE TUMORS

Malignancies arising in mesenchymal tissues such as bone, muscle, and connective tissue are termed sarcomas. In contrast to the large number of metastatic tumors in bone, there are only 3000 new primary bone malignancies and 5000 new primary soft tissue malignancies in the United States each year. These tumors are so rare that they commonly are missed, misdiagnosed, or mistreated, because few physicians have any amount of experience with them. This is particularly true with soft tissue sarcomas.

The most common primary malignancy in bone is multiple myeloma (a marrow tumor), whereas the most common primary malignancy of bone tissue is osteogenic sarcoma. Conventional intramedullary osteosarcoma is the most common subtype. Other malignant bone tumors include malignant fibrous histiocytoma, chondrosarcoma, Ewing's sarcoma, and chordoma. The most common malignant primary soft tissue tumors are malignant fibrous histiocytoma, liposarcoma, synovial sarcoma, rhabdomyosarcoma, and neurofibrosarcoma (Table 15.1).

DIAGNOSIS AND WORKUP

As with any diagnostic strategy, the first step is a complete history and a thorough physical examination. Primary malignancies of bone and soft tissue can occur at any age in any location in the body. In the early stages of growth, the tumor is asymptomatic, and the pain only begins when the tumor starts to violate the periosteum of the bone or force its way out of a myofascial compartment. Initially, the symptoms and signs of a primary bone or soft tissue tumor may be interpreted by the patient or the doctor as a sprain, a case of tendonitis, a hematoma, or a ganglion. The patient may describe the insidious onset of pain or a mass that has been present for several weeks or a few months. A fall or blow may render an asymptomatic tumor mildly painful. Later, the pain persists independent of activities. The mass becomes too large to ignore. Local pressure on a nerve or a vessel may give rise to symptoms distal to the tumor, but these normally occur late. Patients with these tumors do not look ill when they present, which can result in a delay in the diagnosis.

Other than the nature and progression of the pain, little information can be obtained about a bone or soft tissue sarcoma from the patient's current complaint. One must be alert for a history of Paget's disease, a history of radiation treatments, or a chronic infection that can give rise to a secondary sarcoma or carcinoma. Asking about the family history may lead to the discovery of genetically linked syndromes such as neurofibromatosis, which is associated with a risk of neurofibrosarcoma. These key findings can lead to a strong working diagnosis based on the history alone.

On examination, a sarcoma usually presents as a deep, firm, fixed mass. Most are mildly tender and a few are pulsatile. Determine the mobility of the nearby joints and examine for signs of an effusion, which may indicate the tumor has invaded the synovial space. Check the status of nearby nerves and vessels. On the general examination, check for an abdominal

Table 15.1. Common Presentation and Location of Some Bone and Soft Tissue Sarcomas

Tumor Type	Typical Patient	Typical Location
Osteosarcoma	Teenager or young adult	Near the knee
Chondrosarcoma	Older adult	Pelvis and hip
Ewing's sarcoma	Child or teenager	Pelvis and leg
Synovial sarcoma	Young adult	Leg and foot
Epithelioid sarcoma	Adult	Hand or forearm

mass and once again look for neurofibromas and café-au-lait spots. Note any local, proximal, or central adenopathy. Metastasis to the local nodes is characteristic of synovial sarcoma and angiosarcoma, whereas most other sarcomas metastasize to the lungs and bones.

Certain types of bone and soft tissue sarcomas occur predominately in certain age groups and in certain locations on the body or within the bone. These unique features of sarcomas are extremely valuable in constructing the differential diagnosis.

After the primary care physician has done a careful history, a general examination, and a basic workup, he or she should rapidly initiate a referral to an orthopaedic oncologist, preferably by phone or by personal contact. The referring physician usually should not undertake an extensive workup until this contact has been made. The choice and sequence of imaging and diagnostic tests should be carefully coordinated between the two physicians. The best initial imaging modality for primary bone tumors is high-quality plain radiographs; for primary soft tissue tumors, magnetic resonance imaging is best. For a possible primary bone or soft tissue sarcoma, a complete workup generally includes a plain radiograph of the part, a complete blood count with differential and an erythrocyte sedimentation rate, a plain chest radiograph or computed tomography of the chest, and a magnetic resonance imaging scan of the entire extent of the tumor. More laboratory tests and imaging studies are indicated once the suspicion of a sarcoma is confirmed but are not a part of the initial evaluation of a suspected tumor. Evaluation of initial images by an experienced orthopaedic oncologist or musculoskeletal radiologist can confirm or deny the suspicion of a malignancy and can often narrow the differential diagnosis to one or two entities.

In some cases after early referral and the initial workup, the tumor may be found to be a benign or posttraumatic process, in which case multiple expensive tests may never be needed. Biopsy is not a part of the initial management of these lesions and is usually the last step in the workup. In the case of potential primary malignancies of bone or soft tissue, the biopsy should be performed by the surgeon who will be doing the definitive resection. Biopsy-related complications may result in an amputation, whereas the limb might otherwise have been salvaged. Prompt appropriate care in the first stages of the disease has an enormously positive impact on the overall patient satisfaction and outcome.

COMMON BONE SARCOMAS

Osteogenic sarcoma occurs most often in patients aged 10 to 20, and males somewhat outnumber females. The most common sites are the distal femur, the proximal tibia, and the proximal humerus (Fig. 15.4). Although no cause has been determined, chromosomal analysis has identified certain common alterations in the DNA of osteosarcoma cells that may have a role in the pathogenesis of the disease. Overall prognosis for survival is approximately 60% at 5 years; however, patients with low-grade tumors or high-grade tumors that respond well to treatment may have a 5-year survival of up to 85%.

Central medullary (or "conventional") osteosarcoma is the most common of several subtypes. Radiographically, it presents as a

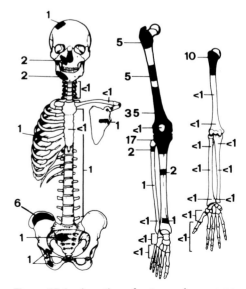

Figure 15.4.   Location of osteogenic sarcoma.

poorly defined lytic destructive lesion with amorphous ossification of neoplastic bone and an indistinct border, usually in the metaphyseal area of a long bone. A prominent periosteal reaction occurs (often appearing as "onion skin" layering or "hair on end" pattern, or showing a "Codman's triangle") (Fig 15.5) and occasionally an ossifying soft tissue mass is present.

Chondrosarcoma is a malignant tumor with cartilaginous features that affects patients in their 20s and 50s. Chondrosarcoma occurs in the bones of the pelvis, the proximal femur, and the shoulder girdle. Radiographically, the lesion has an aggressive appearance with a flocculent, popcornlike pattern of calcifications within the lesion, which is attributed to ossification of the outer portion of small nodules of cartilage within the tumor.

Malignant fibrous histiocytoma is a highly malignant tumor that is more common in patients over 50 and may arise in the setting of previous radiation treatment, long-standing Paget's disease, a loose total joint prosthesis, or an old bone infarct. It often presents as a pathologic fracture and appears on radiographs as an aggressive, destructive, poorly defined lesion lacking significant ossification or cartilaginous features.

Ewing's sarcoma is a highly malignant tumor of children aged 8 to 18 of both sexes often located in the diaphyseal area of the femur, pelvis, tibia, fibula, or humerus (Fig. 15.6). Ewing's sarcoma is the fourth most common bone sarcoma and is more likely to affect males. In contrast to other sarcomas that have no race-related differences in incidence, Ewing's sarcoma is rare in blacks. Patients may present with fever and leukocytosis, making osteomyelitis an important part of the differential diagnosis. The radiographic appearance is of a permeative lytic lesion with no ossification or calcification of cartilage (Fig. 15.7) that often has a striking onion-skinned periosteal reaction and a prominent soft tissue mass.

Chordoma is a tumor derived from primitive notochordal tissue that occurs exclusively in the sacrum, the lumbar spine, and the proximal cervical spine. Patients often complain

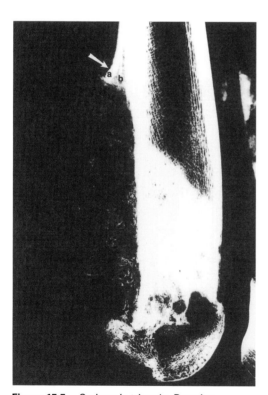

Figure 15.5. Codman's triangle. Reactive periosteal new bone formation that is suggestive of malignancy and is commonly seen in osteogenic sarcoma.

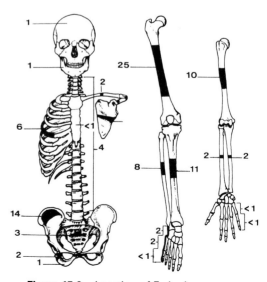

Figure 15.6. Location of Ewing's sarcoma.

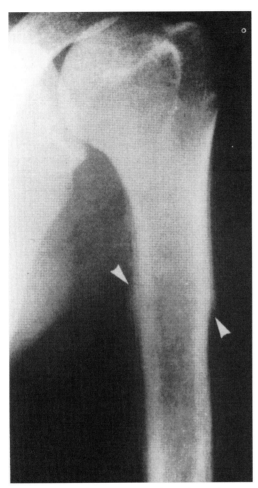

Figure 15.7. "Onion skin" periosteal reaction. Layered periosteal new bone formation that strongly suggests the lesion is malignant and is commonly seen in Ewing's sarcoma.

of low back pain or constipation for months before a rectal examination reveals a mass in the sacrum palpably obstructing the rectum. The tumor appears as a lytic, destructive mass centered in the spine and extending into adjacent bones and soft tissue structures.

COMMON SOFT TISSUE SARCOMAS

Malignant fibrous histiocytoma is the most common primary soft-tissue sarcoma. This tumor is an aggressive, high-grade sarcoma that is most common in older adults and occurs in the extremities and the retroperitoneum. A

number of subtypes have been described. Synovial cell sarcoma is the most common sarcoma of young adults in their teens and twenties. It often occurs in the region of the knee and lower leg but not in the joint itself. This tumor can sometimes present as a mass that has been present for several years. The physician seeing a patient with a long-standing mass that has begun to grow or change should proceed with extreme caution.

Liposarcoma is the second most common soft tissue malignancy in adults and is common in the proximal thigh, the retroperitoneum, and the trunk. Development of liposarcoma in a benign lipoma is rare. The tumor occurs in low-grade, well-differentiated forms with an excellent prognosis and in high-grade, pleomorphic forms with a poor prognosis.

Rhabdomyosarcoma is the most common soft tissue tumor in young children and is more common in boys. In infants, this tumor occurs in the head and neck; in children, it occurs in the pelvis and extremities.

TREATMENT OF SARCOMAS

After a workup, biopsy, and staging as outlined previously, patients with high-grade osteosarcoma, malignant fibrous histiocytoma, and Ewing's sarcoma are given multidrug cytotoxic chemotherapy. Chondrosarcoma and chordoma do not respond to chemotherapy. In many cases, the treatments begin before surgery. After several cycles of chemotherapy, the patient undergoes surgery intended to resect the lesion with a wide margin of normal surrounding tissue. Most patients are now treated with limb salvage surgery in which the tumor is removed without an amputation. The resected bone segment may be reconstructed with a variety of techniques, including a large prosthetic implant, a fresh-frozen allograft bone implant, or a combination of the two. A few patients cannot have a limb salvage procedure because of the large size of the tumor or a pathologic fracture, or because the remaining limb would not retain sufficient function. After surgery, additional cycles of chemotherapy may be given. Some tumors are better treated with radiation with 50 to 60 Gray (approximately 5000–6000 rads).

Soft tissue sarcomas are treated according to the size and grade. Small lesions and low-grade lesions are treated by surgical resection only, whereas large, high-grade lesions may be treated by combination preoperative and postoperative radiation and chemotherapy, as well as surgery. Most patients can be offered limb salvage surgery. Reconstruction of the surgical defect is less complicated because the nearby bone usually can be saved; however, grafting or substitution of a vessel, a nerve, or the surrounding soft tissue may be required.

FOLLOW-UP AND OUTCOMES OF TREATMENT

After treatment, patients will require regular follow-up to monitor the status and function of the reconstructed limb and the surgical site. Patients also need routine examinations of the surgical site and chest radiographs every 3 to 6 months for the first 2 years and every 6 to 12 months for 6 to 8 additional years to monitor for local or distant metastasis. Lung metastasis can be treated with surgical removal and reinduction chemotherapy with a definite survival benefit. Bone metastasis or local recurrence can be treated, but patient survival is poor. Routine follow-up MRI scans of the surgical site are not warranted as a screening study for recurrence. A baseline postsurgical magnetic resonance scan of the primary tumor site can be performed as a basis for comparison. Later, a new scan is ordered if the clinical examination reveals a possible local recurrence. Complications of limb salvage surgery are frequent, and reoperations and revisions to maintain the function of the limb are expected. Patients with amputations require ongoing prosthetic maintenance and periodic renewal. No significant overall quality of life or cost difference between treatment by amputation or limb salvage surgery has been demonstrated, but limb salvage patients have higher scores on functional outcome scales.

Survivors of sarcomas remain mildly impaired with respect to their functional capacity, ability to form intimate relationships, and ability to return to their previous occupation. They report a slight diminution in their overall quality of life as well as mild to moderate ongoing pain. These problems have been reported to be more severe in women. Functional status after treatment is more strongly related to the tumor grade and stage than to the type of treatment or surgery. Patients with strong psychosocial support networks recover better and remain less impaired in the long term.

SUGGESTED READINGS

Harrington KD. Orthopaedic Management of Metastatic Bone Disease. St. Louis: CV Mosby, 1988:16.
Higinbotham NL, Momore RC. The management of pathological fractures. J Trauma 1965;5:792–798.

CHAPTER 16

Orthopaedic Problems in the Pediatric Patient

Yvonne A. Shelton, M.D., and Errol Mortimer, M.D.

NONTRAUMATIC DISORDERS

The nontraumatic disorders of adulthood are typically degenerative, whereas the nontraumatic disorders of childhood are typically developmental. Therapy for adult disorders usually focuses on restoration of function and retardation of degeneration, while therapy for childhood disorders usually focuses on correction of distorted anatomy and prevention of accelerated degeneration.

CONGENITAL MUSCULAR TORTICOLLIS

Congenital muscular torticollis is a contracture of one of the sternocleidomastoid muscles, more commonly seen on the right side. The cause of this deformity is unknown, although it has recently been studied with MRI and appears to be related to an intrauterine compartment syndrome. The deformity is characterized by a "cock robin" position of the head in which the head is tilted toward the side of the shortened muscle and the chin rotated to the contralateral side. On pathologic section of excised specimens, the muscle appears to be replaced by fibrous tissue.

Clinical Characteristics

At birth, the torticollis may or may not be evident but usually is identified in the first 2 months of life. In children who are normal at birth, the deformity and mass in the sternocleidomastoid usually become obvious at 2 to 3 weeks. As the child grows, the abnormal posture progresses, and secondary structural changes occur in the face and skull, resulting in asymmetric molding of these structures. Palpation of the sternocleidomastoid may reveal a firm, nontender, fusiform "olive" within the substance of the muscle or replacing the muscle. When present at birth, the mass commonly enlarges over the subsequent several weeks. Regression of the "tumor" usually occurs over a period of 2 to 6 months. Without treatment, facial asymmetry, including changes in the levels of the ears, eyes, and skull, may develop. The superficial and deep muscular tissues of the neck may become shortened.

Because of an increased incidence of clubfeet, congenital hip dysplasia, and other congenital abnormalities in patients with torticollis, these infants should be carefully examined. Patients with torticollis often have a significant history of difficult delivery, and infants with such a history should be carefully checked for this deformity. Infants with congenital torticollis do not have any neurologic abnormality. Although pain may occur with passive stretching, it does not occur at rest.

X-ray studies are usually unremarkable in the muscular type of torticollis. However, x-rays are necessary because there may be congenital bony deformities of the cervical spine (Klippel-Feil syndrome and primary cervical synostosis) that need to be excluded. The differential diagnosis includes traumatic conditions such as fracture or rotatory subluxation, inflammation of the cervical lymph nodes, tumors of the spinal cord or brain, and Sprengel's deformity (congenital elevation of the scapula).

Treatment

Early recognition and treatment are important. Stretching of the involved sternocleidomastoid should be performed several times a day. A good stretching program is usually successful in completely correcting the deformity but must be closely supervised. The physician or an experienced physical therapist should instruct the parents in the technique of stretching. One hand is used to stabilize the chest and shoulders, while the other hand tilts the head away from the contracted muscle and rotates the chin toward the contracted side. Each stretching maneuver is best held to a count of 10 with 15 repetitions. The initial tenderness of the muscle mass with stretching subsides gradually, and a great majority of infants respond to these conservative measures.

If the deformity does not respond to passive stretching in 1 to 2 months, orthopaedic referral is indicated. If a child is over 1 year of age at initial presentation, the contracture and progressive deformity are probably best treated by surgical release of the sternocleidomastoid muscle.

KLIPPEL-FEIL SYNDROME

Klippel-Feil syndrome is a congenital fusion of two or more cervical vertebrae. Clinically, the neck is short, stiff, and webbed. The hairline is often low and horizontal. This syndrome is often associated with torticollis. These patients should be referred for orthopaedic evaluation.

ROTATORY SUBLUXATION OF C-1 ON C-2

Rotatory subluxation of the atlantoaxial joint is a relatively common problem in children. It may be the result of an injury or may present without a history of significant trauma. In these circumstances, this disorder often occurs in association with pharyngitis (Grisel's syndrome). It is thought that inflammation, edema, and hyperemia lead to weakening of the supportive ligaments at C-1/C-2, allowing spontaneous subluxation of the facet joints. This disorder also may be a consequence of an otherwise minor injury.

Clinical Characteristics

The diagnosis is based on a fixed, painful torticollis with muscle spasm. Cervical spine x-rays, particularly the open-mouth odontoid view, reveal the pathognomonic asymmetry of the C-1/C-2 joint with the odontoid deviated to one side. In some children, painful torticollis may be present without radiographic evidence of C1/C2 subluxation. In equivocal situations, the diagnosis can be confirmed using dynamic CT scanning with the head maximally rotated to each side.

Treatment

Treatment consists of bedrest, analgesics, and constant head-halter traction until painful spasms subside and the subluxation reduces. Children who have torticollis without subluxation can be treated with a closely supervised stretching program with a physical therapist. After reduction, the child's neck should be protected in a soft cervical collar (Fig. 16.1) until the neck is completely comfortable and stable with a full, painless cervical range of motion. If the subluxation does not respond to traction within 5 to 7 days, an orthopaedic surgeon should be consulted.

BIRTH INJURIES OF THE BRACHIAL PLEXUS

The two common types of brachial plexus injury, Erb's palsy and Klumpke's palsy, are caused by strong lateral flexion of the infant's head and neck, producing traction on the brachial plexus. These injuries typically occur during a difficult delivery in which there is cephalopelvic disproportion when the infant must be extracted quickly to ensure viability.

Clinical Characteristics

Erb's palsy is the more common of the two conditions. The infant presents with mixed sensory and motor defects of the upper nerve roots (C-5/C-6). These roots control shoulder abduction and external rotation, and elbow flexion. At birth, the arm is typically motionless and lies adducted and extended in internal rotation at the infant's side. The hand

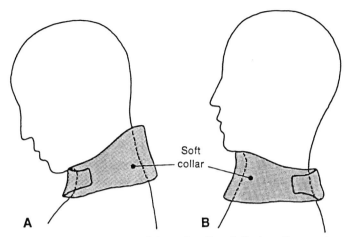

Figure 16.1. Applications of the soft collar. *A*, flexion. *B*, extension.

and wrist are usually functional. Although occasionally transient and reversible, the condition frequently results in residual paralysis and sensory deficits of the shoulder and upper arm. In contrast, "pseudoparalysis" may result from a perinatal fracture of the clavicle or humerus and can easily be confused with a brachial plexus injury. X-rays may be indicated to rule these out.

Klumpke's palsy is a rare condition. It involves the lower roots (C-8/T-1), resulting in a flail hand and wrist with atrophy of the forearm. The upper arm is functional. Spontaneous recovery is not likely.

Treatment

The initial treatment for both types of palsy is gentle passive range of motion exercises and splinting of the paralyzed muscle groups to prevent contractures. These exercises should be taught to the family by a skilled physical or occupational therapist so that the routine can be carried out several times each day. The prognosis depends on the severity of injury to the brachial plexus. If the root avulsion is adjacent to the spinal cord, the prognosis is poor, and nerve repair in the first year of life may be indicated. Return of biceps function by 3 to 6 months carries a good prognosis. Reconstructive orthopaedic surgery is sometimes useful to improve function of the impaired extremity. Orthopaedic consultation is necessary.

SCOLIOSIS

Scoliosis is an abnormal lateral curvature of the spine. When viewed from the front or back, the spine should be straight, centering the head over the sacrum. A number of conditions can produce an apparent scoliosis without a true, intrinsic spinal deformity. These conditions include a leg length discrepancy, muscular spasm, poor posture, or hysteria. We use the term "scoliosis" to describe a true, intrinsic spinal deformity.

Scoliosis may be secondary to congenital bone malformation, bony dysplasia, or metabolic or paralytic conditions. If no primary cause is obvious, it is designated as idiopathic scoliosis. Curvatures under 10°, as measured radiographically, that are not progressive do not require treatment or referral to an orthopaedist. Because scoliosis is often progressive, even the child with a mild degree of curvature greater than 10° should be referred to an orthopaedic surgeon for initial evaluation and possible treatment. Idiopathic scoliosis is the most common type of childhood scoliosis. This condition occurs in approximately 1% of the adolescent population and predominantly affects females.

With the advent of mandatory school screening programs, a large number of children with spinal asymmetries that do not represent true scoliosis are seen by the primary care physician. In this setting, the evaluation should define the exact nature of the condition. Abnormal posture, leg length discrepancy, or some painful condition producing an apparent spinal asymmetry must be ruled out. The presence of developmental, traumatic, or paralytic etiology must be evaluated. In the absence of these causes, the diagnosis of idiopathic scoliosis is confirmed. This is an inherited disorder characterized by a sex-linked or autosomal dominant genetic pattern with a variable expressivity and incomplete penetrance.

Clinical Characteristics

Idiopathic scoliosis is generally a painless disorder in the adolescent, although the onset of a deformity may be noticed at an earlier age. A complaint of back pain warrants thorough investigation to rule out other etiologies and should not be attributed to the underlying scoliosis. On physical examination, the patient presents with asymmetry in the levels of the shoulders and in the waist crease, prominence of one iliac crest, and a posterior rib hump prominence most obvious on forward bending. Leg length measurements will not show significant discrepancy, and neurologic examination is usually normal. If there is evidence of neuromuscular disease or metabolic abnormality, or if x-rays reveal a congenital basis, the scoliosis is not classified as idiopathic.

Radiographs of the spine are essential for the diagnosis and treatment of scoliosis. To diminish the radiation exposure of the breasts in adolescent girls, the frontal radiograph should be performed in an anterior to posterior projection and breast shields should be used. The radiograph will establish the extent and the severity of the curvature.

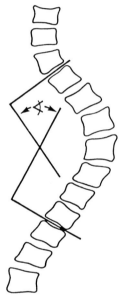

Figure 16.2. The Cobb method of measuring spinal curvature. (Copyright 1989. Novartis. Reprinted with permission from Clinical Symposia, Volume 41/4, Plate 12, illustrated by Frank H. Netter, MD. All rights reserved.)

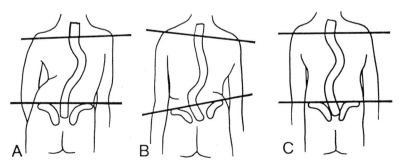

Figure 16.3. Examples of body contour with scoliosis. *A*, right thoracic curve. *B*, left lumbar curve. *C*, double major curve. (Copyright 1989. Novartis. Reprinted with permission from Clinical Symposia, Volume 41/4, Plate 3, illustrated by Frank H. Netter, MD. All rights reserved.)

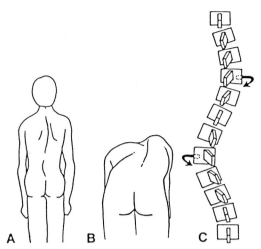

Figure 16.4. Right thoracic, left lumbar curve. *A*, patient standing upright. *B*, patient bending forward. *C*, the rotation accompanying lateral curvature. (Vertebral bodies rotate toward the convexity, hence clockwise rotation accompanies right thoracic curve, and counterclockwise rotation accompanies left lumbar curve, as viewed from overhead.) (Copyright 1989. Novartis. Reprinted with permission from Clinical Symposia, Volume 41/4, Plate 10, illustrated by Frank H. Netter, MD. All rights reserved.)

The amount of curvature is determined by the Cobb method (Fig. 16.2). Any number of combinations of curves may be encountered (Fig. 16.3). Lateral curvature is always accompanied by rotation of the vertebrae. The rotational component is an important determinant of clinical deformity and is most noticeable when the child bends forward and the examiner sites down the axis of the spine (Fig. 16.4).

Treatment

The treatment of idiopathic scoliosis is based on data obtained from long-term longitudinal studies of the natural history of scoliosis. A curvature of less than 30° at skeletal maturity appears to cause no prolonged disability as a person matures in later life. However, curves that have reached 50° at the time of skeletal maturity tend to progress later in life and may cause restrictive pulmonary disease, cor pulmonale, and severe back pain. Therefore, the treatment of idiopathic scoliosis in the adolescent attempts to prevent the

curve from progressing to 50°. A curvature of greater than 10° in a skeletally immature patient needs to be followed by periodic clinical and radiographic examinations until skeletal maturity has been reached. An interval of 4 to 6 months between each visit is an acceptable follow-up program. After initial orthopaedic consultation, the primary care physician may monitor children in this early stage. However, while under observation if the curve progresses more than 5°, or on presentation if the curve is greater than 20°, referral to an orthopaedic surgeon for follow-up and treatment is recommended.

At this degree of deformity, brace therapy is initiated. The spinal orthosis, or brace, consists of a polypropylene shell that is contoured to provide a corrective force to the spine while the child grows. It is necessary that the child wear the brace for at least 16 hours a day until skeletal maturity is reached. The Charleston Bending brace is a new design that uses overcorrection of the spine to prevent further progression. This brace can be used in a nighttime only program. A bracing program usually involves treatment for approximately 3 to 4 years. This is difficult for the adolescent patient to accept, and the primary care physician is very helpful in providing guidance, direction, and emotional support to the patient and family. A scoliosis clinic where other similarly affected adolescents are treated can provide a supportive treatment environment.

If the curvature progresses to a point of 45 to 50°, the patient is at high risk for further progression in adulthood. Therefore, surgical stabilization of the spine with corrective instrumentation is performed to correct the curvature and prevent further progression.

ADOLESCENT KYPHOSIS (SCHEUERMANN'S DISEASE)

Adolescent kyphosis, also known as Scheuermann's disease, is thought to be secondary to repetitive trauma and stress fractures of the anterior aspect of the vertebral endplates in the growing adolescent. Untreated, the disease causes permanent kyphosis of a variable degree, which will be established at the end of the adolescent growth period. Nonoperative treatment is effective only when applied before the cessation of skeletal growth.

Clinical Characteristics

The patient presents in early adolescence with thoracic or lumbar back pain or a kyphotic postural deformity. The child is often taller and heavier than other children of his or her age. Girls are affected as often as boys. When the disease process is in the thoracic area, there is an increased thoracic kyphosis; however, in a few children, the disease affects the lumbar region, causing that portion of the spine to look abnormally flat. The pain usually is aggravated by prolonged activity or standing for long periods of time and is relieved by rest. There may be local tenderness. The sensory and motor examinations are normal. The diagnosis is confirmed by a lateral radiograph of the spine that should be obtained while the patient is standing. The normal thoracic kyphosis measured from T4 to T12 by the Cobb method is between 20 and 40°. An increase in the amount of kyphosis of at least 5° in three or more consecutive vertebral bodies associated with anterior wedging of the vertebral body establishes the diagnosis. Concave osteolytic defects at the endplates, known as Schmorl's nodes, may be noted. These represent herniation of disc material into the weakly ossified vertebral endplate (Fig. 16.5).

Treatment

The primary care physician should refer children to the orthopaedist if the radiographic findings of Scheuermann's disease are present. The treatment of Scheuermann's disease in a skeletally immature patient incorporates the use of a thoracolumbar brace and active physical therapy programs. Such treatment may decrease the amount of inevitable deformity. For severe deformity, however, surgical treatment may be necessary. Corrective spinal fusion with instrumentation can be performed in cases resistant to the aforementioned modalities. In the absence of radio-

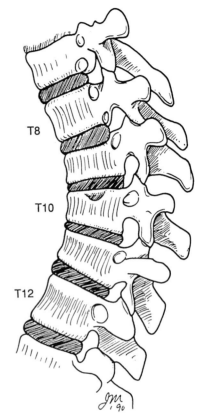

Figure 16.5. Juvenile kyphosis. Anterior vertebral body wedging on three or more consecutive vertebrae.

graphic findings of Scheuermann's disease, the "round back" deformity simply represents a postural habit. In these children, physical therapy is helpful in strengthening the thoracic extensor muscles and flattening the accentuated lumbar lordosis, which is commonly present. The therapy regimen should emphasize antilordotic lumbar exercises and thoracic extension exercises.

SPONDYLOLYSIS AND SPONDYLOLISTHESIS

The term spondylolysis refers to a bony defect in the pars interarticularis of the posterior elements of the vertebral body (Fig. 16.6B). Spondylolysis is thought to be the result of nonunion of a stress fracture in the

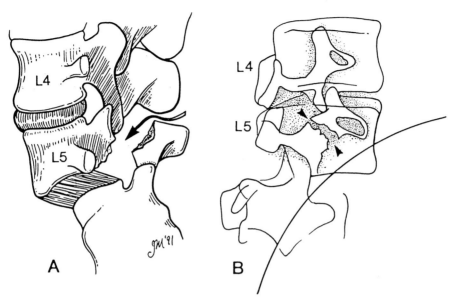

Figure 16.6. *A,* lateral view of spondylolytic spondylolisthesis. *B,* spondylolysis. A 45° oblique view of the lumbar space will show a defect in the pars interarticularis.

posterior elements. Defects of the pars interarticularis may be due to infection, trauma, tumor, congenital or developmental defects. The condition most commonly occurs at the L-5 lamina but has been seen throughout the spine. A high incidence of spondylolysis occurs in athletes who undergo constant hyperextension activity of the lumbar spine, such as gymnasts and football linemen. Spondylolisthesis refers to an anterior displacement of the vertebral column on a lower vertebra, most commonly an anterior slippage of L-5 on S-1 (Fig. 16.6A). This may be the result of spondylolysis, articular process malformation, or elongation of the pars interarticularis. Moderate or severe degrees of spondylolisthesis may cause nerve root impingement, and may consequently present with signs and symptoms of nerve root irritation.

Clinical Characteristics

Spondylolysis typically occurs in preadolescent and adolescent children. The initial symptom is an aching pain in the lumbar region, which is associated with activity. It may radiate into the buttock and thigh on the affected side. The pain typically is relieved by rest or limiting the aggravating activity. Spondylolysis is often associated with a feeling of stiffness. This is particularly true for gymnasts or ballerinas, who complain that they are unable to perform their usual routine. This may be difficult to detect on clinical examination because these children are so flexible that even with a decrease in their flexibility they still appear to be within normal standards. The physical examination reveals spasm in the paravertebral muscles, and a flattening of the normal lumbar lordosis may be present during the acute presentation with back pain. The child with long-standing and severe spondylolisthesis may have a kyphotic deformity at the lumbosacral junction with a compensatory hyperlordosis in the lumbar region. Hamstring tightness is common. This presents as diminished straight leg raising, increased popliteal angle, and diminished stride length on walking or running. The neurologic examination is usually normal except in those infrequent cases in which there is nerve root irritation. The diagnosis is confirmed by radiographs of the lumbar spine (Fig. 16.6B). A lumbosacral series should consist of standing lateral and anteroposterior (AP) views, as well as 45° oblique views of the lumbar spine. Occasionally, back pain will be the presenting symptom in a child before the plain film radiographs show the bony defect. In these cases, a bone scan will be helpful.

Treatment

The goals of treatment in a child with spondylolisthesis or spondylolysis are (*a*) pain relief, (*b*) return to activity, and (*c*) prevention of deformity. It is necessary to monitor children with spondylolysis until they reach skeletal maturity. A child with spondylolysis may be treated by the primary care physician with a conservative program consisting of nonsteroidal anti-inflammatory medications, limiting activity below the pain threshold, and a physical therapy regimen. The physical therapy regimen emphasizes antilordotic exercises for the lumbar spine, such as pelvic tilts and modified situps, with stretching exercises for the hamstrings. Patients who do not respond to this therapy should be referred to an orthopaedic surgeon. Any patient who has pain associated with spondylolisthesis should be referred to an orthopaedic surgeon for evaluation. In the adolescent years, a spondylolysis may progress to spondylolisthesis, or a spondylolisthesis may increase in severity; however, this is unlikely to be true for the adult population. For children who do not respond to conservative treatment, a brace may be helpful to control their pain level and allow them to participate in activities. Surgical repair of the spondylolysis or posterolateral fusion of the involved vertebrae are indicated when the patient is unresponsive to conservative treatment, shows progression of a spondylolisthesis, or presents with a severe degree of spondylolisthesis. Surgical fusion is effective in controlling the pain and progression of the disease under these circumstances.

DEVELOPMENTAL DYSPLASIA OF THE HIP

Developmental dysplasia of the hip is the most common disorder of the hip presenting during the first 3 years of life. The term developmental dysplasia is commonly applied to the full spectrum of congenital and developmental hip diseases, which includes dysplasia without subluxation, the subluxatable hip, and the dislocated hip. The current terminology has gained acceptance as a result of the understanding that occasionally a hip that is clinically normal at birth will become dysplastic in the early months of life. The incidence of true congenital dislocation of the hip is approximately l.2 in 1,000 live births. Developmental dysplasia of the hip is more commonly associated with intrauterine crowding, breech presentation, and ligamentous laxity. It is much more common in females, is most often unilateral with predilection for the left hip, and has a familial pattern. Other associated features include torticollis, hyperextension of the knee, and abnormalities of the feet. Because the development of the acetabulum and femoral head depend on normal physiologic stress, untreated dysplasia or dislocation may result in secondary developmental changes of both the acetabulum and femoral head, further compounding the initial deformity.

The pathology of developmental dysplasia of the hip is variable, depending on the severity of the condition. Infants may be born with minimal dysplasia in which some deformity of the acetabulum is evident, but the hip is not actually dislocated. In other infants, the hip may be dislocatable or dislocated; in the most severe form, there is obvious teratologic deformity of the joint and soft tissue with complete dislocation. Teratologic hip dislocation refers to a particular subset of hips associated with a syndrome in which the dislocation occurred earlier in intrauterine life. This type of dislocation is usually more difficult to treat.

The initial suspicion of hip instability or dislocation is clinical, requiring careful examination of the newborn and infant at the "well baby visits." Any child with a significantly abnormal walking gait requires x-rays of the hips. This does not usually include the common problems such as isolated in-toeing or out-toeing, or the expected variations of a newly walking child.

Clinical Characteristics

The clinical presentation of developmental dysplasia varies according to the age of presentation and the pathologic state of the joint. In infants, the most common findings are a positive Barlow test and Ortolani test. With the Barlow test, the hip can be felt subluxing posteriorly with an adduction-axial loading maneuver. With the Ortolani test, the dislocated hip can be felt reducing with an abduction maneuver that is often accompanied by an audible or palpable "clunk" (Fig. 16.7). This should be distinguished from the distinctive "click" that often is seen in normal hips and is related to myofascial motion in the hip or knee. Asymmetry of the gluteal, inguinal, and thigh skin folds may exist. In most infants older than 3 to 4 months, abduction will be limited, and the Barlow and Ortolani tests may no longer be positive. The affected extremity may appear short in comparison with the normal side.

When an infant presents at age 3 to 6 months and the femoral head has been dislocated for several months, it may not be possible to relocate the hip during examination. The hip appears more adducted. This is secondary to contracture of the adductor musculature, which can be demonstrated by palpation of the adductor tendon at the pubic tubercle. Significant asymmetry of skin folds is more common at this stage. Slight proximal migration of the hip also may be observed. Palpation of the greater trochanter will indicate that the involved hip is higher than the opposite hip. This abnormality can be confirmed by leg length measurement.

When a child presents after walking has begun, the chief complaint may be a limp. This gait pattern is the result of ipsilateral hip abductor weakness.

When congenital dysplasia of the hip is suspected in the infant, ultrasonography of the hips should be obtained. This should be performed by an experienced radiologist because this is the most sensitive method of making the proper diagnosis. In the child older than 3 or 4 months, x-rays should be obtained (Fig. 16.8). When the hip is subluxed or dislocated, Shenton's line (the continuous curve of the inner margin of the femoral neck and the inner margin of the obturator foramen) is broken. Ossification of the capital femoral epiphysis often is delayed; therefore, the bony portion of the epiphysis may be absent or appear smaller in the dysplastic hip. When the femur is laterally subluxed, its malposition may be demonstrated relative to a vertical line (Perkins line) drawn from the lateral lip of the acetabulum perpendicular to a line drawn through the triradiate cartilage of the two hips (Hilgenreiner line). The beak of the medial metaphysis of the normally articulating femur lies well medially to this line, while the beak of the neck of the dislocated femur lies closer to or laterally to this line. When the acetabulum is dysplastic, the slope of its superior margin is increased.

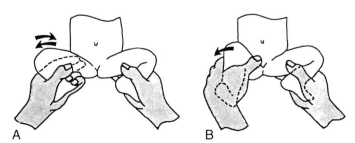

Figure 16.7. Infant hip examination for instability. *A,* Barlow sign. Adduction causes posterior subluxation or dislocation of the reduced hip. *B,* Ortolani sign. Abduction causes reduction of the subluxed or dislocated hip.

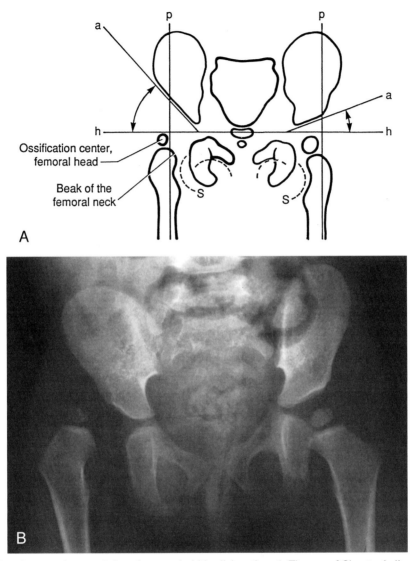

Figure 16.8. *A,* x-ray characteristics of congenital hip dislocation. 1. The arc of Shenton's line (*S*) is discontinuous on the dislocated side. 2. The beak of the femoral neck and the ossification center of the femoral head are displaced laterally and upward toward or beyond the Perkins line (*p*) and the Hilgenreiner line (*h*). 3. The angle between the acetabular line (*a*) and the Hilgenreiner line (*h*) is increased. *B,* plain x-ray of a 12-month-old female shows changes analogous to those in part *A.*

Treatment

Once the diagnosis of developmental dysplasia of the hip is made, referral to the orthopaedist is indicated. The principle in treatment of the dysplastic hip is to obtain or maintain reduction to allow for normal development. For patients who present from birth to 6 months, successful treatment can be achieved with a Pavlik harness. This is successful in up to 90% of cases. Failure is more commonly associated with bilaterality, "Ortolani negative" hips, and older infants. If treatment with the harness is unsuccessful, further measures are required including traction, closed reduction under anesthesia, and possible surgical intervention. In a child presenting older than 6 months, treatment is more difficult. Success of the abduction device is less predictable, and the need for closed reduction under anesthesia or surgical treatment is more likely.

TRANSIENT OR TOXIC SYNOVITIS OF THE HIP

This is a self-limited synovitis of the hip joint most commonly seen in children between the ages of 3 and 5 years. The etiology is unclear, but unrecognized injuries and viral infections have been considered. This condition must be differentiated from pyogenic arthritis and from avascular necrosis of the hip (Legg-Calvé-Perthes disease). When suspicion of pyogenic arthritis exists, the joint must be aspirated. The distinction from aseptic necrosis is made by clinical follow-up and x-ray.

Clinical Characteristics

The child presents with complaints of pain in the groin, anteromedial thigh, or knee. Also the child has an associated limp. Duration of pain is from several days to 2 weeks. Low-grade fever may be present with slight leukocytosis and slight increase in the sedimentation rate. The affected hip is maintained in a flexed and externally rotated position. The child resists efforts to move the hip rapidly or to the extremes of motion. This contrasts with septic arthritis in which the pain is usually more severe and the fever, white blood count, and sedimentation rate are more elevated. X-rays are unremarkable in both conditions except for evidence of soft tissue swelling and an effusion, which may be subtle.

Treatment

Initial treatment should consist of bed rest. If septic arthritis cannot be ruled out on the basis of the physical examination and hematology, hospital admission for close observation should be considered. Crutches should be used with nonweightbearing gait. Acetaminophen or ibuprofen may be given on a symptomatic basis. If simple bed rest is not adequate, a few days of Buck's traction (Chapter 10) will almost always produce symptomatic relief. This can be done at home with orthopaedic consultation. Patients may begin full weightbearing when they have regained full, painless range of motion and can ambulate without pain and without a limp. They may then return to normal activity as tolerated. If pain is persistent or recurrent, or if pyogenic arthritis or aseptic necrosis is suspected, orthopaedic consultation should be obtained promptly. Even if the child becomes asymptomatic and returns to normal activity without restriction, a follow-up visit at 8 to 12 weeks is recommended. At that time, a repeat x-ray should be obtained to rule out aseptic necrosis.

AVASCULAR NECROSIS OF THE FEMORAL HEAD (LEGG-CALVÉ-PERTHES DISEASE)

This condition affects children between the ages of 2 and 11 years old. The cause of the interruption of the blood supply to the femoral head is not known. After infarction, reparative tissue grows into the necrosed head, and healing occurs by a process of creeping substitution with resorption of dead bone and deposition of new bone. The process of necrosis and reconstitution can take 2½ years. Deformity of the femoral head and acetabulum may occur if the disease is extensive and exceeds the remodeling capacity of the developing epiphysis. Younger children have a better prognosis as do those children with smaller areas of involvement of the femoral head.

Clinical Characteristics

Although the disease may occur in children between the ages of 2 and 11 years, the incidence is highest in children between 5 and 9 years of age. Pain is usually in the groin, anterior thigh, and sometimes the knee. Some children present without pain, but almost all limp. The onset is usually insidious, and the patient has frequently been symptomatic for several months before presentation. Limping increases with activity and may be intermittent. The condition frequently presents with synovitis, which is associated with muscle spasm and restricted hip abduction and rotation. X-ray changes are variable depending on the stage of the disease. The first bony change noted may be a subtle subchondral crescent-shaped radiolucency of the femoral head. This is followed by more diffuse sclerosis and later, an irregular mottled appearance as the head undergoes fragmentation (Fig. 16.9). Patients with a poorer prognosis are older and have more extensive involvement of the femoral head. They are at risk of developing early osteoarthritis. The condition is bilateral in 15 to 20% of cases.

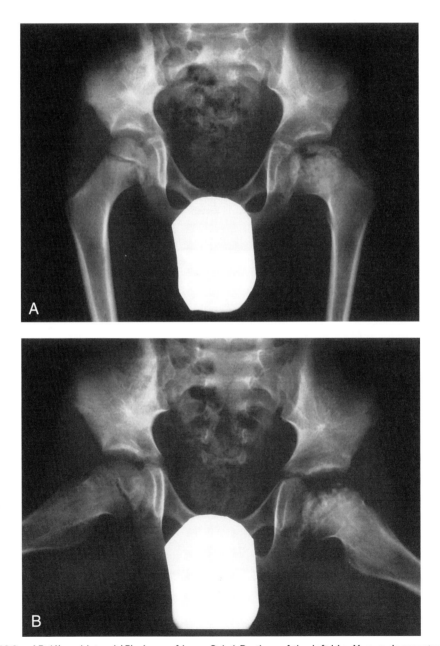

Figure 16.9.   AP *(A)* and lateral *(B)* views of Legg-Calvé-Perthes of the left hip. X-rays demonstrate partial collapse, lateral subluxation, and irregular, mottled appearance as a result of advanced fragmentation and early repair.

Treatment

Orthopaedic referral should be made. Treatment is based on the principle that hip mobility and containment of the femoral head within the acetabulum will lead to the best healing and remodeling of the infarcted femoral head. Patients who are young (4 to 6 years old) and who have involvement of less than 50% of the head simply may be observed without active treatment. For patients with a less optimistic prognosis, containment of the femoral head within the acetabulum can be achieved with physical therapy, home traction, and sometimes an external brace or cast. For some patients, osteotomy of the femur or pelvis is necessary.

One of the problems for the primary practitioner is distinguishing the child with avascular necrosis from the child with toxic synovitis of the hip. X-rays are most important in making this distinction. Orthopaedic consultation is indicated if avascular necrosis is suspected. It also is important to re-examine patients who present with symptoms of "nonspecific synovitis" to make certain that the diagnosis is correct.

SLIPPED CAPITAL FEMORAL EPIPHYSIS

During the period of rapid growth during adolescence, the capital femoral epiphyseal plate is relatively weak. The exact cause of this condition remains unknown. Various etiologies have been suggested including hormonal dysfunction. Whatever the cause, it appears that the stresses of normal activity exceed the strength of the growth plate through the zone of cartilage hypertrophy. This results in progressive slippage of the capital femoral epiphysis in a posterior and medial direction. In most patients, the condition has an insidious onset; however, in some there is an acute presentation associated with injury. Many patients report some preinjury pain and have an acute slip superimposed on a chronic condition.

Clinical Characteristics

A child between the ages of 10 and 16 years presents with a history of insidious hip, thigh,

or knee pain associated with a limp. The patient may also present with acute pain after an injury, superimposed on a history of intermittent pain. Males are more commonly affected, and the patient is often obese with somewhat delayed development of secondary sexual characteristics. The condition may be bilateral and the opposite hip must be examined. A "silent slip" on the contralateral side should always be sought when the diagnosis is made on one side. In the acute phase, there is significant muscle spasm and synovitis with restricted range of motion; internal rotation usually is significantly limited. Because of the limitation in internal rotation, the extremity tends to externally rotate when the hip is flexed. X-rays demonstrate posterior and medial displacement of the epiphysis (Fig. 16.10). The change may be subtle and often apparent only on the lateral view of the hip.

Treatment

Once the diagnosis is made, orthopaedic referral and treatment should be obtained. The treatment is surgical (Fig. 16.11), unless the diagnosis is late and the growth plate is already closed. With small or moderate degrees of slip, fixation of the epiphysis may be performed in situ with a single screw. This results in fusion of the epiphysis and long-term stability. Shortening of the extremity usually is not a problem. In slips of a greater degree, more extensive surgical reconstruction may be necessary.

ANTERIOR KNEE PAIN

Knee pain is a common complaint in childhood, especially among rapidly growing adolescents. The differential diagnosis includes a variety of disorders that often can be identified by careful physical examination. Fortunately, the most worrisome diagnoses are seen infrequently and include juvenile rheumatoid arthritis, osteochondritis dissecans of the lateral femoral condyle, infection, and tumor. Conversely, the most common diagnoses are usually self-limiting and may resolve with analgesics and physical therapy. These include

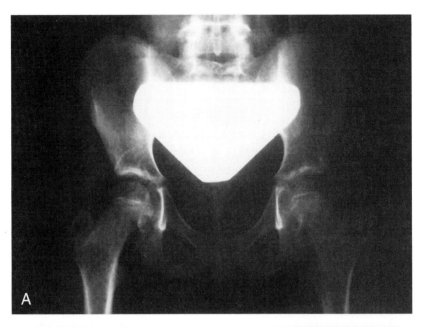

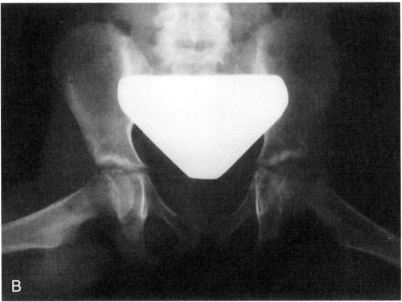

Figure 16.10. AP and lateral views of a low-grade slipped capital femoral epiphysis. *A*, normal appearing AP view of both hips. *B*, note the subtle loss of the contour of the femoral neck and head on the lateral view.

Osgood-Schlatter disease (tibial tubercle apophysitis), Sinding-Larsen-Johansson disease (apophysitis of the distal patella), abnormalities of patellar tracking, bursitis, and tendinitis.

Chondromalacia patella is a pathological term that has been grossly overused in the diagnosis of anterior knee pain in adolescents. It describes gross histologic abnormalities of the patellar articular cartilage, which is infrequently present. The preferred terminology is patellofemoral disorder if symptoms arise from this articulation, or simply adolescent

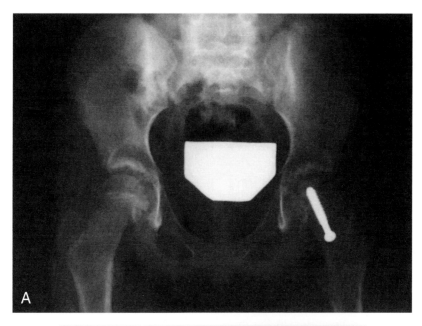

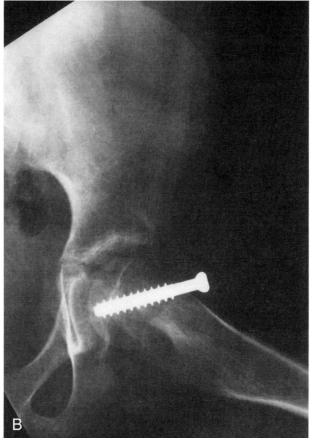

Figure 16.11. Postoperative views of the same patient seen in Figure 16.10. The close-up of the lateral x-ray shows the true magnitude of the slip.

anterior knee pain if a more precise diagnosis cannot be made. (For a more detailed discussion of several of these topics, see Chapter 7.)

TIBIAL APOPHYSITIS (OSGOOD-SCHLATTER DISEASE)

Apophysitis of the tibial tubercle occurs at the time the apophysis undergoes the transition from cartilage to bone. This disease commonly occurs between 12 and 14 years of age. Traction of the patellar ligament on the apophysis may result in microfractures.

Clinical Characteristics

Pain in the region of the tibial tubercle is related to activity, and it may be relieved by rest. Swelling and tenderness are present over the tibial tubercle and along the patellar ligament. A lateral x-ray may or may not show irregular ossification or fragmentation of the tibial tubercle. Although this is not evident early in the disease, irregular ossification or fragmentation may persist long after the disease has become asymptomatic.

Treatment

Instruct the child to avoid all activity that requires resisted knee extension, such as climbing, running, or kicking, until pain and tenderness have fully remitted. This restriction usually applies for 6 to 8 weeks. In addition, a program of gentle quadriceps and hamstring stretching may be combined with a mild analgesic and application of ice when symptoms are acute. This treatment applies to many of the common knee pain syndromes and is likely to be more effective than strengthening programs. Prolonged restriction of activity is not appropriate. Although activity may exacerbate symptoms, it does not cause long-term morbidity.

When pain is severe and recurrent, casting in a walking cylinder for 2 to 3 weeks lessens symptoms. When pain persists, the usual cause is the presence of ossicles within the tuberosity or tendon, which can be seen on x-ray. Surgical excision of the loose ossicles, although

rarely necessary, will relieve symptoms. This procedure may be indicated either before or after skeletal maturity.

NECROSIS WITHIN THE POLES OF THE PATELLA (SINDING-LARSEN-JOHANSSON DISEASE)

This condition occurs in children 8 to 13 years of age. Its presentation is similar to Osgood-Schlatter disease except that maximal tenderness is localized to the distal pole of the patella. The initiating event is unknown. Clinical characteristics include pain that occurs during resisted extension of the knee and during kneeling. Onset is insidious and activity related. Swelling and tenderness also is present over the inferior pole of the patella. X-rays may or may not show fragmentation of bone near the affected pole. Treatment and prognosis are the same as those presented for Osgood-Schlatter disease.

NECROSIS WITHIN THE CONDYLAR EPIPHYSES OF THE FEMUR (OSTEOCHONDRITIS DISSECANS)

Osteochondritis dissecans (OCD) is the result of avascular necrosis in the area of subchondral bone. The lateral aspect of the medial femoral condyle is involved in 75% of cases, but the lateral condyle or patella may be affected (Fig. 16.12). The result is a small area of bone, usually around 1 cm, which is biologically separated from the remaining bone by an area of necrosis. These lesions may heal, particularly if the growth plates are open. The etiology is probably traumatic from impingement of the tibial spine on the femoral condyle.

Clinical Characteristics

OCD is characterized by aching pain in the knee at rest that worsens with weightbearing, causing the patient to limp. The onset is insidious. Physical examination may demonstrate a restricted range of motion, but it is usually normal. Rarely, an effusion will be evident. If the fragment detaches, it may produce locking or symptoms of a loose body. AP, lateral, and

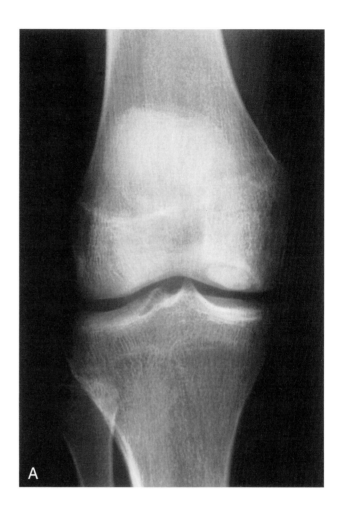

Figure 16.12. AP *(A)* and lateral *(B)* views of the knee of a 14-year-old female with anterior knee pain show the typical location of osteochondritis dissecans in the lateral aspect of the medial femoral condyle.

tunnel x-rays of the knee will usually demonstrate a characteristic lesion that appears as a half-moon defect or irregularity of the subchondral bone. The physician should always obtain bilateral x-rays, because physiologic irregular ossification of the femoral condyles can easily be confused with OCD, although the former is almost always bilateral and the latter, less commonly.

Treatment

Because the prognosis is unpredictable, at the outset the patient should be referred to an orthopaedist. A decrease or elimination of weightbearing with immobilization may be prescribed until the lesion heals. This treatment may be prolonged, and its efficacy has not been confirmed. If the fragment separates

completely, it can become a loose body that may have to be removed. The remaining defect can be drilled to promote revascularization and healing, or if the fragment is large, it can be fixed by screws. Most recent technology allows cartilage grafting for large defects in the weightbearing area, although this is experimental.

ABNORMALITIES OF PATELLAR TRACKING

Anterior knee pain may be a manifestation of abnormal patellar tracking. This is more common in females, especially near the adolescent growth spurt. The spectrum of abnormality ranges from subtle deviation of the patella from the center of the femoral condyles to frank dislocation. Predisposing factors

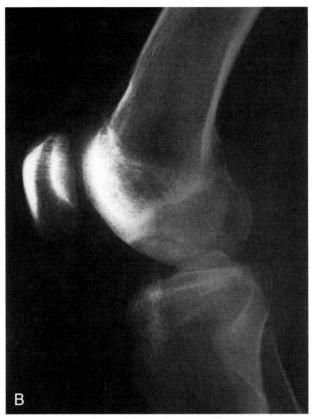

Figure 16.12. (*continued*)

include relative weakness of the vastus medialis muscle, ligamentous laxity, and valgus alignment of the tibio-femoral "Q-angle." Observing the position of the patella as the straight knee is flexed will demonstrate lateral deviation in a "J" pattern. In addition, it may be possible to markedly translate the patella laterally, and the patient may experience pain or apprehension of the patella dislocating if the examiner attempts to translate it too far. For maltracking without dislocation, strengthening the quadriceps muscle, especially the vastus medialis, is indicated. Acute treatment of patellar dislocation should include a 4- to 6-week period of immobilization in a knee immobilizer, or a cylinder cast. This should be followed by a period of vigorous quadriceps strengthening. Recurrent dislocation may require surgical realignment of the extensor mechanism.

ALIGNMENT PROBLEMS

Angular and rotational problems are among the most common reasons for referrals to a pediatric orthopaedic surgeon. Among these, bowlegs and in-toeing are by far the most frequently seen. The bones of the lower extremities remodel rapidly until 6 to 8 years of age, and most physiologic deformities will completely resolve without treatment by this time. The challenge is to identify the small subset of children who are at risk of progressive deformity.

Angular Deformities

Angular deformities may occur in the coronal plane or in the sagittal plane. They are named according to the apex of the angle. In the coronal plane, these include bowlegs (genu vara) and knock-knees (genu valga). Either of these may be physiologic or pathologic. In the sagittal plane, the deformities are usually posteromedial or anterolateral—these are always pathologic.

Physiologic tibia vara usually is noted from infancy to approximately 24 months of age. This is replaced by a variable amount of valgus from 24 months through the age of 5 to 6 years. By then, the knee will usually have assumed the normal adult value of 5 to 8° of knee valgus. In contrast, pathologic tibia vara does not follow the aforementioned pattern of growth and becomes progressively worse. Initially, it may be impossible to distinguish between physiologic and pathologic bowlegs by clinical evaluation alone, and x-rays of the entire limb from hips to ankles are often indicated. These x-rays may show that the deformity represents Blount's Disease (Fig. 16.13) in which an abnormality of the medial tibial growth plate is present or a metabolic bone disease is present in which the epiphysis, physis, or metaphysis is affected. If it is impossible to determine with certainty whether bowing is physiologic or pathologic, a child with a significant deformity should be referred to an orthopaedic surgeon. Surgery is limited to severe or progressive deformities.

Valgus deformity of the lower extremities is less common than varus deformity. Like bowlegs, this valgus deformity is usually a physiologic alignment that will remodel. Valgus deformity can be associated with certain pathologic states such as juvenile rheumatoid arthritis or hypoplasia of the lateral femoral condyle. Bracing is not usually effective or indicated. As in bowlegs, surgical treatment is only indicated in severe cases. Early arthritis is not usually a problem.

Angular deformities in the sagittal plane are much less common and include anterior and posterior angulation. These are usually noted at birth and invariably require specialized treatment by an orthopaedic surgeon.

Posteromedial Angulation

In posteromedial bowing, the angle of the bow is almost always directed posteriorly and medially, but rarely may be purely posterior.

The etiology is unknown but it may be caused by intrauterine positioning of the infant, resulting in tight anterior compartment musculature and limited plantar flexion of the ankle.

Treatment

Treatment is initially nonoperative. Passive stretching of the tight musculature is required and occasionally a total contact orthosis is used. The angular deformity usually corrects by about 4 years of age, but a residual limb length discrepancy usually remains and may require a limb length equalization procedure at the appropriate time. Osteotomies of the tibia and fibula are not indicated in this deformity.

Anterolateral Angulation

This direction of angulation is more serious, and the deformity may be caused by congenital deficiency of the fibula, congenital pseudarthrosis of the tibia, or fibrous dysplasia.

In fibular hemimelia, the fibula may be short or completely absent. It is usually associated with abnormalities of the foot and often the femur as well. Treatment may range from limb length equalization procedures to an amputation of the foot. Congenital pseudarthrosis of the tibia is a condition in which a portion of the diaphysis of the tibia fails to develop normally and is partially or completely replaced by fibrous tissue. This condition is associated with neurofibromatosis over 50% of the time and is infrequently seen with polyostotic fibrous dysplasia. In either case, management is extremely complex and involves making the correct diagnosis, correcting the angular deformity, and achieving bony union and maintaining it through adulthood.

Rotational Problems

In-Toeing

In-toeing is a common pediatric lower extremity disorder. Most cases can be evaluated and definitively treated by the primary care physician.

Although in-toeing frequently needs no

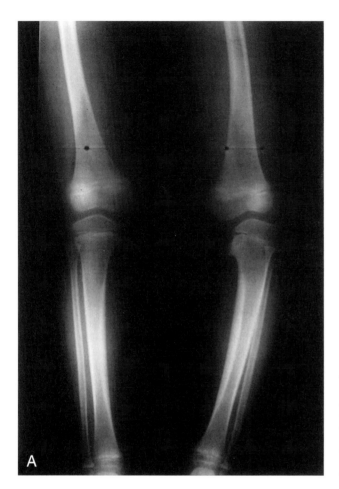

Figure 16.13.   *A*, a 3½-year-old female with a 1-year history of progressive bowing of the left knee. X-rays show genu varum with sloping of the medial proximal tibial epiphysis and metaphysis consistent with Blount's disease. The tibia is subluxed on the femoral condyles. Surgery is indicated in this child with advanced disease. *B*, close-up of the left knee.

specific treatment, the physician must understand the causes and explain the natural history of the deformity to the patient's parents. The foot progression angle is used to document the presence and magnitude of in-toeing (Fig. 16.14). The foot progression angle has a wide range of normal, from 5° of turning in to 20° of turning out. Although the patient will present with a chief complaint of turning in of the feet, it is important to remember that the etiology may be abnormal rotation of the femur, the tibia, or the foot. In-toeing may be caused by one or more of the following: (*a*) increased femoral anteversion (Fig. 16.15), (*b*) increased internal tibial torsion (Fig. 16.16), or (*c*) metatarsus adductus. Each of these entities has specific physical findings, natural history, and treatment options, and each will be

discussed separately. It is important to be aware that the natural history of these deformities is spontaneous resolution in over 90% of cases. Those individuals with residual anatomical deformities can almost always overcome their problem by consciously altering the gait, leaving few children who actually require active treatment.

Femoral Anteversion

Femoral anteversion is the angle of the femoral neck relative to the femoral condyles in the sagittal plane (Fig. 16.15). In the average adult standing with the femoral condyles directed straight ahead, the femoral necks will angle forward about 15° to enter the acetabula. Normal infants may have up to 45° of anteversion, which gradually decreases to an average

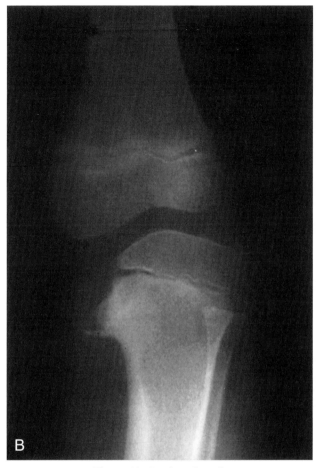

Figure 16.13. (*continued*)

of 15° during adolescence. If the amount of anteversion is increased, the hip will have more internal rotation and less external rotation. This will allow increased internal rotation of the entire leg during gait, thus causing in-toeing. Because of soft tissue contracture, normal infants may have much more external rotation of the hips than internal rotation. Normally, an older child will have slightly more external rotation than internal rotation of the hips, measured with the child in the prone position and the knees flexed (Fig. 16.17). If a patient is found to have more than 70° of internal rotation of the hips and less than 30° of external rotation of the hips, then femoral anteversion is causing or contributing to the in-toeing.

Treatment Various devices such as twister cables, external rotation (Denis Browne) splints, and shoe wedges have been used in the past to treat femoral anteversion. However, these are either ineffective or may cause secondary deformities such as excessive external tibial torsion or foot deformities and are rarely indicated. The parents can be reassured that most femoral anteversion resolves by adolescence and that the use of braces has not been shown to be any more effective than no treatment at all. The physician should explain to the parents that femoral anteversion has not been shown to cause back pain, hip pain or hip arthritis, flatfeet, or any problems with sports participation. Femoral anteversion plus abnormal external tibial torsion, however,

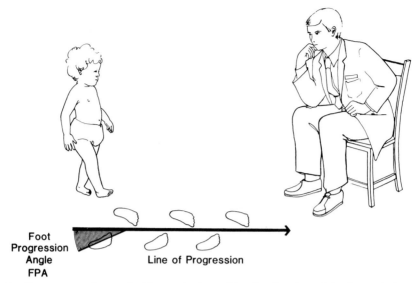

Figure 16.14. Foot progression angle. The angle formed by the direction of the foot relative to the line of progression of gait.

may cause patellar malalignment and subsequent knee symptoms. In the rare case of severe femoral anteversion persisting in late childhood, only derotational osteotomies of the femurs will change the anteversion and correct the in-toeing, and orthopaedic referral will be necessary.

Internal Tibial Torsion

Tibial torsion is the angular relationship of the medial and lateral malleoli to the coronal plane of the knee. This is best measured as the thigh-foot angle with the child prone (Figs. 16.16 C and D). If the transmalleolar axis and, therefore, the foot are internally rotated compared with the thigh, then internal tibial torsion is present. If the foot and ankle are externally rotated to the thigh, then external tibial torsion is present. Tibial torsion may be associated with physiologic genu vara, and the combination of the two deformities can be striking. The range of normal tibial torsion is variable, and up to 20° of internal tibial torsion is normal in infants. The transmalleolar axis normally becomes more externally rotated during childhood, resulting in 15 to 20° of external tibial torsion by adolescence. If internal tibial torsion persists, the ankle joint

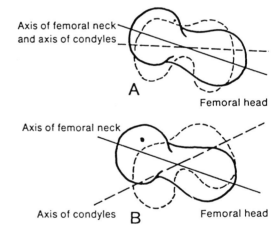

Figure 16.15. Anteversion of the femur. *A*, normal axis. *B*, the axial twist of anteversion.

will be internally rotated compared with the knee, and in-toeing will result. During gait, the child with in-toeing secondary to femoral anteversion will be noted to have both patellae turned inward toward each other (because the inward rotation occurs at the level of the hips), whereas in a child with internal tibial torsion, the feet will turn in, but the patellae will not (because the inward rotation occurs below the knees).

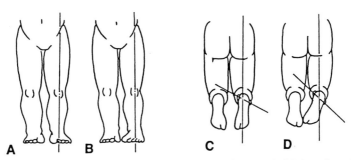

Figure 16.16.   Tibial torsion. *A*, normal axis. *B*, the axial twist of internal tibial torsion. *C*, normal thigh-foot angle. *D*, thigh-foot angle in internal tibial torsion.

Treatment   Internal tibial torsion, like femoral anteversion, improves spontaneously with growth, and usually only reassurance is needed rather than active treatment. Special shoes, shoe wedges, and casts are ineffective in treating internal tibial torsion, but in severe cases, an external rotation splint may be recommended. The indications for this device and its efficacy are questionable, and many clinicians will prefer to simply observe the child. If severe internal tibial torsion persists, orthopaedic referral is indicated for possible tibial osteotomies near skeletal maturity.

FOOT DEFORMITIES

Metatarsus Adductus

The final cause of in-toeing is metatarsus adductus, a deformity of the foot itself. In patients with metatarsus adductus, the alignment of the legs will be normal from the hips down to and including the hindfoot. However, the forefoot will be adducted or turned inward relative to the hindfoot (Fig. 16.18E). This is best seen when the foot is examined from the bottom. Normally, the lateral border of the foot will form a straight line from the heel to the fifth toe. In metatarsus adductus, there will be a break or curve at the midfoot such that, even with the entire leg and hindfoot directed straight ahead, the forefoot will turn in toward the midline of the body.

Treatment

Metatarsus adductus is a common positional deformity of the newborn and, unless

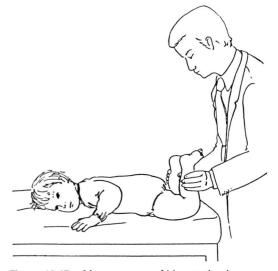

Figure 16.17.   Measurement of hip rotation in prone position.

associated with a deformity of the hindfoot (such as a true clubfoot), it usually corrects with growth and stretching. Parents should be instructed to perform passive stretching exercises with each diaper change. If the metatarsus adductus is rigid at birth, serial casting may be instituted to assist in rapidly correcting the deformity. When the infant is 1 to 3 months old, the metatarsus adductus is evaluated again to determine severity and also flexibility, which is measured by how easily the foot can be passively overcorrected by the examiner. If significant metatarsus adductus persists to the age of 4 to 6 months, it can usually be well-corrected by manipulation and serial

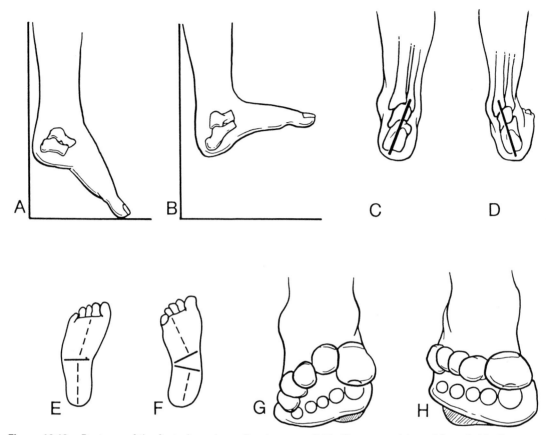

Figure 16.18. Postures of the foot. *A,* equinus. *B,* calcaneus. *C,* hindfoot varus (viewed from behind). *D,* hindfoot valgus (viewed from behind). *E,* metatarsus adductus (viewed from sole of foot). *F,* metatarsus abductus (viewed from sole of foot). *G,* forefoot supination (varus). *H,* forefoot pronation.

corrective casts. The proper molding of these corrective casts is difficult to perform, and because of potential skin problems, the authors recommend that these children be referred to the orthopaedic surgeon for cast treatment of persistent metatarsus adductus. A variety of shoes with modifications are available to assist in obtaining or maintaining the correction.

Flatfeet

Flatfeet, or pes planus, is divided into the common and rarely symptomatic flexible flatfoot and the uncommon but symptomatic rigid flatfoot. The differentiation between a flexible and rigid flatfoot is made by physical examination. In both types of pes planus, there is loss of the normal plantar arch when the child stands. However, in a flexible flatfoot, there will be a normal arch when the patient is sitting with the feet hanging over the side of the examination table as well as when the patient stands on tiptoes. Also, a flexible flatfoot will have normal motion of the subtalar joint. The patient with flexible flatfeet often will have other findings of increased ligamentous laxity, e.g., hyperextension of the knee or elbow, or a history of being "double-jointed." In children up to the age of 2, the fat pad on the medial side of the foot may give a false appearance of a flatfoot when the toddler is standing. Flexible pes planus is usually bilateral, often hereditary, and as mentioned previously, usually asymptomatic.

Longitudinal studies of large groups of children have shown that some flexible flatfeet will gradually develop a plantar arch without treatment. No study has shown any significant difference in arch development in children with flexible flatfeet treated with orthoses versus simple observation. Therefore, orthotic treatment of asymptomatic flexible flatfeet is not usually recommended. However, orthotics may decrease symptoms in an older child with flexible flatfeet who has discomfort in the legs or feet.

In contrast to flexible pes planus, the rigid flatfoot is usually symptomatic. The rigid flatfoot will be flat with loss of the arch even when the child is nonweightbearing or standing on tiptoes. The rigid flatfoot has limited or absent motion of the subtalar joint. Peroneal muscle spasm also is frequently noted on physical examination, and hence the term "peroneal spastic flatfoot" is sometimes used interchangeably with rigid flatfoot. The most common cause of a rigid flatfoot is a tarsal coalition or fusion between the calcaneus and either the talus or navicular. The radiographic diagnosis of tarsal coalition is sometimes difficult and may require conventional tomography, CT scanning, or MRI evaluation, in addition to routine x-rays. However, any pathology involving the subtalar joint, such as arthritis, infection, or trauma, may result in a rigid flatfoot and must be considered in the differential diagnosis.

Treatment

If symptoms of a tarsal coalition persist after conservative treatment with immobilization, orthoses, and anti-inflammatory medication, surgery is often indicated. Therefore, patients with rigid flatfeet should be referred to the orthopaedist for evaluation.

NEWBORN FOOT DEFORMITIES

Significant foot deformities in the newborn usually will be referred to the orthopaedic surgeon, but these congenital deformities must first be recognized by the primary care physician. These include talipes equinovarus (clubfoot), calcaneovalgus foot deformity, and congenital vertical talus.

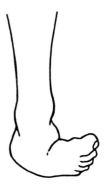

Figure 16.19.   Talipes equinovarus (clubfoot).

Talipes Equinovarus (Clubfoot)

Talipes equinovarus is a congenital foot deformity in which the heel is in equinus (plantar flexed) and varus, and the forefoot is adducted (Fig. 16.19). The initial treatment is stretching combined with corrective casting. This manipulative treatment of clubfoot is much more effective when started immediately. Therefore, the orthopaedic surgeon should be consulted promptly so that treatment can begin within the first days of life. The foot is then treated by serial manipulation and casting, often for several months. If manipulation and casting are not successful in completely correcting the foot, surgery may be necessary. Surgery may be performed as early as 3 or 4 months of age, but in some cases can be delayed until the child is 1 to 2 years old.

Calcaneovalgus

The calcaneovalgus foot presents with dorsiflexion of the ankle and eversion and abduction of the forefoot (Figs. 16.18 B and F). In severe cases, the dorsal surface of the foot will be resting on the anterolateral aspect of the lower leg. Although this deformity may initially look as severe as a clubfoot, its prognosis is much better. A calcaneovalgus foot usually will respond within 1 to 3 months with simple passive stretching exercises. The parents are taught to stretch the foot down out of the dorsiflexed position and inward toward the midline of the body with each diaper change. In a severe case that does not correct well by the age of 2 to 3 months with passive stretch-

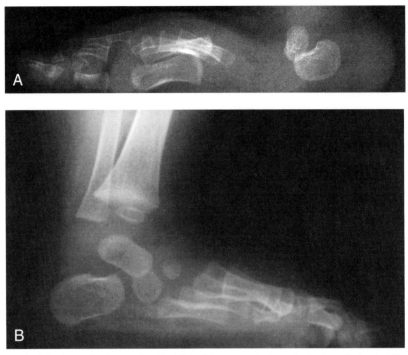

Figure 16.20. *A,* right foot of a 2-month-old child with congenital vertical talus. Note that the talus is nearly parallel to the axis of the tibia and is perpendicular to the axis of the calcaneus. *B,* comparison to a normal foot shows the talus at almost 90° to the tibia and the calcaneus at approximately 45° to the talus.

ing exercises, manipulation by the orthopaedic surgeon and a corrective cast may be necessary. Surgery is almost never required for a calcaneovalgus deformity of the foot. Because calcaneovalgus foot is the result of an intrauterine "packaging problem," there is a strong association with hip dysplasia, thus the hips should be carefully and repeatedly examined to rule this out.

Vertical Talus

A rare but severe congenital foot deformity is a congenital vertical talus (Fig. 16.20). In this deformity, the navicular is dislocated onto the dorsal surface of the talus, forcing the talar head down into a plantar-flexed position. The Achilles tendon is tight, pulling the calcaneus into a plantar-flexed position also. This results in a rigid flatfoot with a rounded "rocker bottom" appearance on the sole of the foot caused by the displaced head of the talus. This uncommon deformity should be referred to the orthopaedic surgeon immediately. This deformity is usually a manifestation of an underlying neurologic problem that should be carefully investigated. Manipulation may partially correct the deformity, but surgery usually is necessary to gain a satisfactory correction of this foot deformity.

Cavus Foot

The foot with a high arch and a plantarflexed forefoot is called a cavus foot (Fig. 16.21). This foot deformity is frequently associated with hammertoes or claw toes and may or may not be symptomatic. A cavus foot should alert the physician to the possibility of an underlying neurologic disorder. Neurologic causes of a cavus foot include Charcot-Marie-Tooth disease, diastematomyelia, myelomeningocele, and polio. Therefore, examination of the spine, a careful neurologic examination, as well as a family history are necessary in the evaluation of a patient with

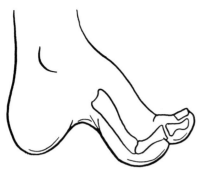

Figure 16.21. Cavus (high arch) foot. This deformity may be caused by calcaneus position of hindfoot (Fig. 16.18B) and/or equinus position of forefoot.

a cavus foot. Because of the plantar-flexed forefoot and the claw toes, there is frequently pain in the plantar aspect of the metatarsal heads. This pain may be relieved with orthoses and metatarsal pads or shoe modifications. Children with cavus feet should be referred to the orthopaedist for global evaluation, which may include consideration of surgical correction of the foot deformity.

TRAUMATIC DISORDERS

Developing bones and joints respond to injuries differently in several respects from fully developed and deteriorating bones and joints. The greater remodeling potential of growing bones and its effect on treatment plans were summarized under "General Principles of Treatment of Forearm Fractures" in Chapter 3. This ability of growing bones to remodel allows acceptance of positions that would not be acceptable in adult injuries. Growing joint capsules, ligaments, and muscles are more tolerant to prolonged immobilization than mature joint capsules, ligaments, and muscles. Thus, the need for prolonged immobilization does not commonly contraindicate closed methods of treatment in children as it does in adults. This is often important in the treatment of fractures of the radius, ulna, femur, and tibia in a child. Unfortunately, application of these principles is difficult to teach in a text. Consequently, until experience is

gained, it is recommended that orthopaedic consultation be obtained when questions of this sort are problematic in the care of a specific injury.

Fracture patterns that involve the articular surface of a joint are much less common in children than they are in adults. Fractures in children that do involve the articular surface share the same risk involved in articular fractures in adults. Any fracture involving the articular surface in either a child or an adult should be referred to an orthopaedist.

PHYSEAL FRACTURES

Physeal fractures of the long bones usually do not interfere with the growth of the injured bone. These fractures occur through the zone of provisional calcification in the physis. The growth potential of the physis usually is not disturbed. However, if the fracture extends through the zone of proliferation into the epiphysis, there is a significant risk of interfering with the growth of the injured bone (Fig. 16.22). Fractures involving the growth plate have been classified into five groups, each of which presents different diagnostic and prognostic characteristics.

Salter I fractures are transverse fractures of the growth plate without injury to the bony metaphysis or epiphysis. When these fractures are undisplaced, they are not radiologically

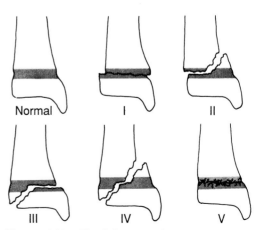

Figure 16.22. The Salter classifications of epiphyseal fractures.

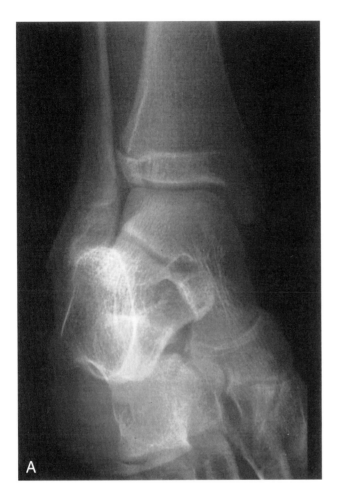

Figure 16.23.   *A,* plain x-ray shows minimal displacement of the anterolateral corner of the distal tibial physis. *B,* CT scan more accurately demonstrates the degree of displacement. *C,* postoperative plain x-ray after percutaneous screw fixation.

evident at the time of injury. Tenderness over the level of the growth plate of a long bone and a normal x-ray imply a Salter I fracture until developments prove otherwise. Stress views may be diagnostic. Repeat x-rays after 2 weeks usually will show bone response characteristic of fracture healing if the Salter I fracture has actually occurred. Salter I fractures must be reduced and immobilized until clinical union is evident. In the upper extremity, union usually requires 3 to 4 weeks of immobilization, whereas in the lower extremity, clinical union is usually present by 6 weeks after the injury. In most cases, nondisplaced Salter I fractures do not interfere with growth (refer to Salter V fractures).

Salter II fractures are transverse fractures of the growth plate that extend obliquely into the bony metaphysis. This fracture and the Salter I fracture are by far the most common physeal fractures. The fracture separation of the distal radial epiphysis discussed in Chapter 3 in "Fractures of Both Bones of the Forearm" is an example. Since the fracture into the metaphysis is radiologically evident, a Salter II fracture is rarely missed at the time of injury. Treatment and prognosis are identical to those of the Salter I fracture. Special attention must be paid to injuries in the distal femoral physis. Growth inhibition after Salter I fractures has been reported. Salter II fractures of the distal physis are more likely to result in a complete or partial growth arrest than similar injuries at other growth plates. Therefore, children who have an injury to the distal femoral physis should be followed by clinical and

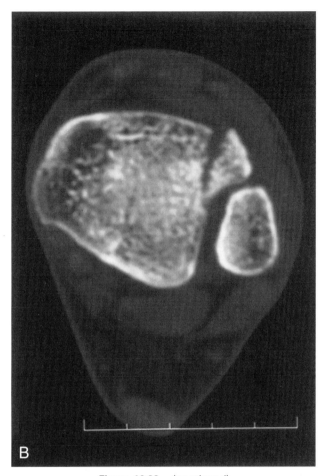

Figure 16.23. (*continued*)

radiographic examination for at least 2 years after their injury.

Salter III fractures are transverse fractures of the growth plate that have involved the bony epiphysis. The Salter III fracture occurs in adolescence and is commonly seen in the distal tibia (Fig. 16.23). When the physis is in the process of closing, the fracture pattern extends through the remaining open part of the physis, through the epiphysis, and into the nearby joint. Because this is an intra-articular fracture, reduction must be anatomic. This injury should be referred to an orthopaedist.

Salter IV fractures extend axially into the bony metaphysis and into the bony epiphysis. The fracture may appear to extend axially from the bony epiphysis to the bony metaphy-

sis directly through the growth plate, or it may appear to extend axially through the bony epiphysis, transversely across part of the growth plate, then axially into the bony metaphysis. The danger of growth arrest is greatest in these fractures. Reduction must be anatomic, and close follow-up of leg length discrepancies and angular deformities is required. The injury must be referred to an orthopaedist.

Salter V fractures are compression injuries of the growth plate. The initial clinical characteristics are usually indistinguishable from those of the undisplaced Salter I fracture: no radiologic visibility, tenderness at the region of the growth plate, and eventual appearance of radiologic signs of bone healing (usually

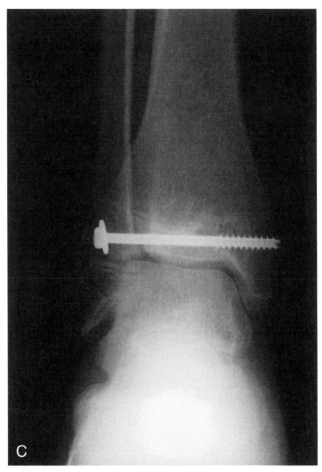

Figure 16.23. (*continued*)

within 2 to 3 weeks). The distinction occurs much later when it becomes evident that the injured physis is either no longer growing or is growing in an asymmetric fashion. Asymmetric closure of a physis can be recognized on a roentgenogram by a bridge of sclerotic bone spanning the normal lucency of the physis. The growth arrest line may be asymmetric as well, which would be indicative of a Salter injury. Even if the injury had been recognized on the first day, nothing could have been done to prevent the outcome. When the undisplaced Salter I/Salter V clinical presentation appears, parents must be warned of the poor prognosis of the Salter V fracture while the injury is treated as a Salter I fracture.

The prognosis of epiphyseal fractures differs not only among the types but among the locations as well. Epiphyseal fractures in the upper extremity are rarely followed by growth failure except after Salter V injuries. In the lower extremity, any epiphyseal fracture can be followed by growth failure, and the Salter III, IV, and V fractures carry a particularly guarded prognosis.

SUGGESTED READINGS

Atar D, Lehman WB, Tenenbaum Y, et al. Pavlik harness versus Frejka splint in treatment of developmental dysplasia of the hip: bicenter study. J Pediatr Orthop 1993;13:311–313.

Bennett JT, MacEwen JD. Congenital dislocation of the hip: recent advances and current problems. Clin Orthop 1989;247:15–21.

Canale ST, Barr JS Jr, eds. Problems and complications of slipped capital femoral epiphysis. Instr Course Lect 1989;38:281–290.

Canale ST, King RE. Pelvic and Hip Fractures. In: Rockwood CA Jr, Wilkins K, King RE, eds. Fractures in Children. Philadelphia: JB Lippincott Co, 1984: 733–844.

Coleman SS. Diagnosis of congenital dysplasia of the hip in the newborn infant. Clin Orthop 1989;247:312.

Haueisen DC, Weiner TS, Weiner SD, et al. The characterization of transient synovitis of the hip in children. J Pediatr Orthop 1986;6:11–17.

Herring JA, Barr JS Jr, eds. Legg-Calves-Perthes disease. A review of current knowledge. Instr Course Lect 1989;38:309–315.

Lovell WW, Winter RB, eds. Pediatric Orthopedics. Philadelphia: JB Lippincott Co, 1990.

Ogden JA. The Uniqueness of Growing Bones. In: Rockwood CA Jr, Wilkins KE, King RE, eds. Fractures in Children. Philadelphia: JB Lippincott Co, 1984:1–86.

Ponseti IV. Growth and development of the acetabulum in the normal child: anatomical, histological and roentgenographic studies. J Bone Joint Surg [Am] 1978;60-A:575–585.

Tachdjian MO. Pediatric Orthopedics. Philadelphia: WB Saunders Co, 1990.

Evaluation of the Injured Patient and Basic Principles of Management

Walter J. Leclair, M.D.

INTRODUCTION

Injury is the leading cause of death in the 1- to 34-year age group and the third most common cause of death in the 35- to 54-year age group. Approximately 150,000 deaths occur per year as a result of injury. Although there are many subcategories of specific types of injury, motor vehicle accidents (MVAs) continue to be one of the leading causes. More than 43,000 people lose their lives in MVAs alone each year, which translates into one MVA fatality every 12 minutes. The total dollar cost to society is difficult to measure accurately. Recent estimates place the cost to society from MVAs alone at approximately $150 billion per year. Safety improvements over the past 10 years have dramatically improved the survivability of an automobile crash. The combination of a safety belt and an air bag can reduce the risk of serious head and upper body injury by 75%. However, with more than 200 million automobiles on the road, there are still 4 to 5 million injuries and more than 500,000 hospitalizations yearly caused by motor vehicle accidents.

In response to this "trauma epidemic," trauma subspecialists have been developed in the fields of surgery, orthopaedics, plastic surgery, and neurosurgery. However, the first encounter with the trauma patient is often not by the trauma subspecialist but by the primary care practitioner. During this first encounter, appropriate evaluation and treatment can pro-

long the patient's life and minimize eventual disability. In this chapter, we will review the principles and techniques of the early management of the trauma patient.

The American College of Surgeons Committee on Trauma has made great strides in establishing standards for the care of the trauma patient. The committee has been instrumental in the establishment of standardized care in designated trauma centers and in the development of the Advanced Trauma Life Support (ATLS) Course for Physicians. The ATLS course is designed to teach physicians life-saving skills and a standardized approach to trauma care. It is in the best interest of every physician in a position to treat trauma to become certified in ATLS, and many principles outlined in this chapter adhere to these standards.

TRIAGE

Fifty percent of trauma deaths occur before hospitalization. Sixty-two percent of the remaining deaths occur within the first 4 hours of hospitalization. Delays in the recognition and transportation of the trauma patient to a facility with the appropriate level of trauma care can reduce survival rates.

Triage is the route by which trauma patients with severe and life-threatening injuries can be transported to facilities with staff and equipment immediately available to treat these patients in an aggressive and timely fash-

Table 17.1. Glasgow Coma Scale

Response	Points		
Verbal			
Oriented	5		
Confused	4		
Inappropriate	3		
Incomprehensible	2		
None	1		
Eye opening			
Spontaneous	4		
To voice	3		
To pain	2		
None	1		
Motor			
Obeys command	6		
Localizes pain	5		
Withdraws to pain	4		
Flexion to pain	3		
Extension to pain	2		
None	1		
	14–15	5	
Total	11–13	4	GCS
Points	8–10	3	Score
	5–7	2	
	3–4	1	

Table 17.2. Trauma Score

Parameter	Points
Respiratory rate	
≥36/min	2
25–35/min	3
10–24/min	4
0–9/min	1
None	0
Respiratory expansion	
Normal	1
Shallow	0
Retractive	0
Blood pressure (systolic)	
≥90 mm Hg	4
70–90 mm Hg	3
50–69 mm Hg	2
0–49 mm Hg	1
Pulseless	0
Capillary return	
Normal	2
Delayed	1
None	0
Glasgow Coma Scale	
14–15	5
11–13	4
8–10	3
5–7	2
3–4	1
Total	1–16

ion. Patients with less severe injuries should be transported to other appropriate facilities, avoiding the expense and burden placed on the patient and the trauma center.

The use of an injury severity score in some form is essential to the consistent estimation of injury. The Trauma Score, which has found widespread use for trauma triage, is an index composed of the Glasgow Coma Score (Table 17.1), cardiac function, and respiratory function (Table 17.2). Patients with trauma scores less than 14 benefit from expedient transport to a regional trauma center. Transporting these patients to the nearest hospital wastes precious minutes if the institution is not equipped to handle a particular patient. In a rural setting where transport time to a trauma facility may exceed 1 hour, transport to the nearest hospital may be indicated. In this case, the hospital should be notified as to the severity of the injuries so they may begin to mobilize their services appropriately.

In areas where an injury severity scale is not in common usage, a patient should be considered a multitrauma patient if the blood pressure is less than 90 mm Hg; respiratory distress or airway compromise is evident; the patient has a penetrating injury to chest, abdomen, head or neck; and the patient has suffered a high-energy injury (MVA at 20 mph or more, falls from greater than 20 feet, etc.).

ASSESSMENT AND RESUSCITATION ABCs (AIRWAY, BREATHING, CIRCULATION)

As in a cardiac arrest, a single physician with the most trauma training (ATLS) or experience should be in charge. An organized response is the best method to avoid missing important injuries or allowing attention to stray toward obvious but not life-threatening injuries, i.e., open fractures (Fig. 17.1).

AIRWAY

The establishment of an adequate airway is the first priority and must be the initial step, because adequate ventilation of the patient is

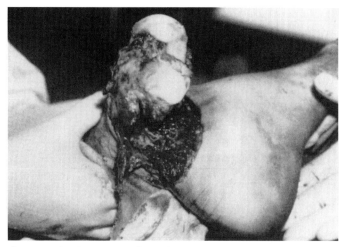

Figure 17.1. Attention must be drawn away from the systematic evaluation of the patient by obvious but not life-threatening injuries.

impossible without a clear airway. One must assume that the patient has sustained a cervical spine injury until proven otherwise and must take precautions to prevent unprotected manipulation of the neck with possible spinal cord injury. The cervical spine should be secured with "in-line" traction, a semirigid cervical collar, or a spine board with sandbags and tape.

The oropharynx should be cleared of secretions, loose teeth, and foreign material. The airway may be maintained with the chin-lift or jaw-thrust maneuver, plastic oral airway, or tracheal intubation via oral or nasal route. If facilities are available for endotracheal intubation, the use of an esophageal obturator airway should be avoided, because the obturator airway can result in esophageal damage, is substantially inferior in ventilatory efficiency, and does not protect the airway against nasopharynx bleeding or secretions. Endotracheal intubation is the preferable airway in patients needing assistance with ventilation. Intubation will eventually be necessary in patients who are unconscious, have maxillofacial injuries, require anesthesia, are otherwise unable to protect their own airway, or need respiratory support. In patients with proven or suspected cervical spine injuries, nasotracheal intubation rather than endotracheal intubation may be necessary.

If the patient cannot be successfully intubated in two attempts, then one must establish an airway surgically. Emergency surgical access to the airway may be obtained with either a cricothyroidotomy or a tracheostomy (Fig. 17.2). Tracheostomy is not particularly suited for the emergency situation because it can be time-consuming and is often accompanied by significant bleeding. This procedure is best left for a more controlled and elective environment.

A surgical cricothyroidotomy can be performed in the adult patient (more than 12 years of age) by making a midline skin incision extending through the cricothyroid membrane into the trachea. The incision is then dilated and held open with a hemostat while a small-bore (5 to 7 mm) endotracheal tube or tracheostomy tube is inserted into the trachea and secured with tape or ties.

A needle cricothyroidotomy is preferred in patients under 12 years of age. This technique uses a 12- to 14-gauge IV cannula that is inserted through the cricothyroid membrane. The adaptor from a 3.5 mm pediatric endotracheal tube fits onto the hub of the cannula and allows connection to a ventilation bag.

Surgical cricothyroidotomy and needle cricothyroidotomy are temporary emergency measures and should be replaced by a surgical tracheostomy or endotracheal intubation.

The needle cricothyroidotomy in particular can only support adequate ventilation for 45 minutes.

BREATHING

Adequate air exchange is achieved when a secure airway is obtained and 12 to 15 mL/kg of oxygen-enriched air is delivered to the lungs. If this cannot be achieved, the physician must quickly identify and correct the problem.

The most common reason for failure of ventilation is intubation of the esophagus; thus, the airway should be checked first. Three other common reasons for failure of ventilation are pneumothorax, tension pneumothorax, and flail chest.

Pneumothorax and tension pneumothorax can be managed by the insertion of a chest tube and assisted ventilation. The chest tube is inserted into the pleural space through the fifth intercostal space in the midaxillary line.

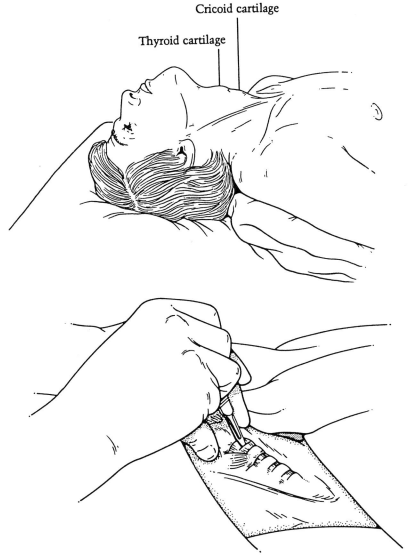

Cricoid cartilage

Thyroid cartilage

Figure 17.2. In the emergency situation, a cricothyroidotomy has many advantages over a tracheostomy.

The chest tube is then connected to a 20- to 30-cm water seal suction. A flail chest can be managed with positive pressure, manual ventilation, or volume cycled ventilator.

The physician should be aware that patient agitation may be a sign of hypoxia or shock. Auscultation of the chest should confirm equal movement of air within each lung.

CIRCULATION

Once satisfactory ventilation has been established, the evaluation and management of hemorrhage should be addressed. A pulse should be palpable in the carotid or femoral arteries. If a pulse is not palpable, cardiopulmonary resuscitation should be begun accompanied by volume replacement. When a pulse is palpable in the carotid or femoral arteries, the patient's systolic blood pressure is generally greater than 70 mm Hg.

Shock is defined as inadequate perfusion of body tissues with oxygenated blood. In the setting of the multiple trauma patient, the most likely cause of shock is hypovolemia. Unless other evidence presents itself, one should assume hypovolemia. A patient with pelvic and long bone fractures, abdominal organ injury, or injury to major vessels in the chest or abdomen can rapidly lose a large percentage of their total blood volume from the circulatory system to the third space. Because this does not present as external hemorrhage, a patient may be acutely hypovolemic without any outward signs of bleeding.

Once a pulse has been established, the physician should perform a brief examination for significant bleeding. Direct pressure should be applied to the bleeding wound. Pneumatic splints or pneumatic antishock garment may be useful in controlling multiple areas of profuse hemorrhage. Small wounds with little bleeding should be ignored at this point; however, one must be aware that these smaller wounds can become a significant source of blood loss once volume has been replaced and blood pressure is corrected. Do not attempt to blindly ligate or clamp bleeding vessels in the depths of a wound. Bleeding from large vessels can be controlled with direct digital pressure. The use of a tourniquet for bleeding control is usually avoidable.

Two large-bore IV catheters should be started (#16 in the adult). A subclavian line or a saphenous vein cutdown should be used when peripheral venous access is limited. In patients who have penetrating abdominal injuries, one should avoid starting all IV lines in the lower extremities, because an injury to the superior vena cava would allow extravasation of infused crystalloid or blood products. At least one large-bore catheter should be started proximal to the region of injury. Once IV access has been established, volume replacement should begin.

Normal circulating blood volume is approximately 7% of ideal body weight in the adult and 8 to 9% body weight in the child. The American College of Surgeons has divided hemorrhagic shock into the following four categories:

1. Class 1: up to 15% of blood volume is lost and minimal clinical symptoms exist.
2. Class 2: 15 to 30% of blood volume is lost. Clinical symptoms present as tachycardia, tachypnea, decreased pulse pressure, central nervous system changes, and reduced capillary refill. Blood pressure can remain unchanged.
3. Class 3: 30 to 40% of blood volume is lost. In addition to a worsening of previous signs, the patient with this amount of blood loss shows a deterioration in systolic blood pressure.
4. Class 4: greater than 40% of blood volume is lost.

One should assume that any patient with cool extremities, flat neck veins, and tachycardia is suffering from hypovolemic shock. The hematocrit will not accurately reflect acute blood loss because it takes up to 6 hours to equilibrate. A fluid challenge should be given to the patient with signs of shock in the form of warmed lactated Ringer's solution. Warming the crystalloid solution will help avoid problems with hypothermia. An initial bolus of 2 L in the adult or 20 mL/kg in the child should be rapidly administered. The response to the fluid challenge should be noted and a decision made as to the continued administration of crystalloid solutions and blood products. A failure to improve blood pressure, pulse rate, urine output, respiratory rate, and central nervous system status would constitute an unfavorable response to the fluid challenge, indicate more severe blood loss, and signify the need for crystalloids and blood products. In general, class 1 or class 2 shock will require crystalloid replacement, whereas class 3 or class 4 will require both crystalloid and blood administration. In class 3 or class 4 shock in which replacement cannot keep up with loss, immediate surgical intervention may be necessary to stop the source of bleeding. Continued need for volume replacement in less severe blood loss should alert the physician to an unrecognized source of bleeding. Third space (internal) blood loss may collect within the chest, retroperitoneal space, abdomen, or extremity fracture sites (Table 17.3). Chest, pelvic, and extremity radiographs should aid the physician in the diagnosis of these potential third space losses.

The physician should keep in mind that myocardial infarction may precede or follow a trauma and result in an alteration of vital signs. Spinal cord injury and head injury may also result in hypotension; however, one should not assume these to be the cause of shock. In cases in which blood products are needed immediately, type O or type-specific blood may be used; however, this should be avoided under almost all circumstances. Type O or type-specific blood should be used only when life-threatening shock occurs and the

physician is unable to wait for crossmatched blood products. This problem stresses the need to anticipate blood loss in the trauma setting and to draw blood for type and crossmatch upon arrival. Fresh-frozen plasma and platelet transfusions are necessary to avoid coagulopathy in patients who require large amounts of blood products.

SECONDARY SURVEY

Once the initial assessment and resuscitation have been completed, a more complete secondary survey should be performed. The medical history should be obtained to determine medical problems, allergies, medications, and mechanisms of injury. Much of the history must be obtained from family and emergency personnel on the scene.

This step is imperative because a change in neurologic status may trigger operative intervention. It is helpful to draw sensory levels or abnormalities in ink directly on the patient as well as recording them in the medical record. The Glasgow Coma Score and Trauma Score should be recorded at this time.

EMERGENCY ROOM DIAGNOSTICS

Upon arrival in the emergency ward, the trauma patient should have diagnostic blood work drawn. This should include a hematocrit, prothrombin time (PT), partial thromboplastin time (PTT), arterial blood gas, BUN, blood sugar, electrolytes, and a crossmatch specimen. An extra red-top tube of blood drawn at this time and set aside may be used later for diagnostic testing.

Initial x-ray studies should include a lateral cervical spine, an anteroposterior (AP) chest film, and an AP pelvis. Additional x-ray studies should await stabilization. One must understand that a single negative cervical spine x-ray does not exclude a cervical spine injury, and cervical spine and intubation precautions must be maintained. The cervical spine series, including AP, lateral, obliques, and open mouth odontoid films should be completed before discontinuation of cervical spine precautions.

Table 17.3. Potential Third Space Blood Loss from Circulating Volume with Closed Injuries

Bleeding Site	Potential Blood Loss
Chest	3000 mL/side
Abdomen	Variable
Retroperitoneum	3000 mL
Extremity fracture	1500 mL/femur if closed
	500 mL/humerus or tibia if closed

A Foley catheter should be inserted. If urinary tract damage is suspected (certain pelvic fractures, genital or peroneal hematoma, meatal blood), a urethrogram and cystogram should be considered before insertion of a Foley catheter. Difficulty inserting the Foley catheter can be a sign of urethral tear, and repeated attempts at Foley insertion may worsen the injury. A nasogastric tube should be placed if no contraindications exist. Nasogastric tubes should be avoided in patients suspected of having fractures of the cribriform plate or penetrating trauma to the esophagus.

A systematic examination of the entire patient should be performed to include the head, neck, chest, abdomen, pelvis, and extremities. All bandages and splints not applied by the examiner should be removed, the wounds inspected, and dressings re-applied. Difficult to reach areas, such as the back and buttocks, should not be ignored during this phase.

Head

Facial bones are palpated for evidence of instability. All wounds are palpated for evidence of open skull and facial fracture. The ear and nasal passages are examined for evidence of cerebrospinal fluid. Cerebrospinal fluid is often difficult to detect when mixed with blood. A drop of suspect fluid can be placed onto filter paper and a "ring sign" will develop, as the blood components remain in the center while a clear ring of cerebrospinal fluid forms around it. At this time, repeat and record any changes in the neurologic examination and Glasgow Coma Score. An increase in intracranial pressure can cause a slowing of the respiratory rate, an elevation in blood pressure, and a change in pulse rate. If any evidence of central nervous system damage is noted, then immediate neurosurgical consultation should be obtained. Decisions for CT scan, steroids, diuretics, and operative intervention should be made by the neurosurgeon. For spinal cord injuries, high-dose steroid administration (such as methylprednisolone) is recommended by many surgeons. More detailed information on the use of steroids may be found in Chapter 1.

Neck

The cervical collar should be removed with manual stabilization of the patient's cervical spine to inspect for penetrating neck wounds, subcutaneous emphysema, tracheal deviation, and hematoma, which may signal a vascular injury and endanger the airway. A penetrating neck wound will require surgical exploration. Evidence of trauma above the level of the clavicle should heighten the physician's suspicion of cervical spine injury. The cervical collar and spine precautions should not be discontinued until a full set of cervical spine x-rays are completed. All seven cervical vertebrae must be visualized on x-ray. A patient with pain and cervical muscle spasm may have a ligamentous injury not apparent on the cervical spine x-rays. In this case, supervised lateral flexion and extension x-rays are needed to rule out injury. These may be postponed until the patient is fully stabilized (Fig. 17.3).

Chest

Chest injuries immediately threatening the airway or breathing (flail chest, hemothorax, pneumothorax, tension pneumothorax, and cardiac tamponade) should have been treated during the primary survey. The chest should now be reassessed for these injuries. The chest x-ray should be carefully examined for widening of the mediastinum and obscuring of the aortic knob, which may signal a tear of the great vessels (Fig. 17.4). An angiogram should be obtained when hypovolemia does not necessitate immediate surgical intervention. The electrocardiogram (ECG) should be monitored carefully for cardiac arrhythmias resulting from cardiac contusions. Although more than 60% of trauma patients sustain some degree of cardiac contusion, only a small percentage will develop cardiac arrhythmia or decreased cardiac output. Cardiac enzymes are not useful in the early evaluation and treatment phase. Cardiac enzymes can be sent with the initial blood draw, but it is unlikely that the results will be available in time to aid in the resuscitation phase. Pulmonary contusions are also common. Early, diffuse infiltrates on chest x-ray should raise suspicion of pulmo-

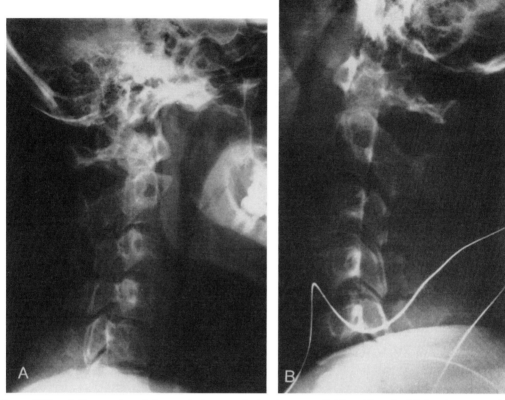

Figure 17.3. *A*, ligamentous injury noted on cervical spine x-ray (C4-5 subluxation) following a negative initial film (*B*). Ligamentous injury must be suspected in any patient with cervical pain and spasm.

nary contusion. These usually cause more problems at 12 to 24 hours. Management may include fluid restriction and intubation with volume-cycled ventilation and positive end-expiratory pressure.

An elevated hemidiaphragm on chest x-ray, especially on the left, may signal a rupture of the diaphragm with herniation of abdominal organs into the chest cavity. This is a commonly missed injury, and any malposition of the chest tube (such as traversing the diaphragm) or persistent elevation of the hemidiaphragm should be investigated with an abdominal and chest CT scan.

Abdomen

The abdomen is examined for evidence of penetrating trauma. One must assume that the penetrating knife or gunshot wound has penetrated abdominal organs and, frequently,

the diaphragm and chest organs as well. These injuries will require surgical exploration. Contusions, abrasions, and a mechanism of injury involving deceleration forces cause blunt abdominal trauma. A firm abdomen with either tenderness to palpation or rebound tenderness should be investigated. A rectal examination must be performed. In the stable patient, CT scan may be used to evaluate blunt abdominal injury; however, even under the best of circumstances, CT consumes a great deal of time. Peritoneal lavage may be quickly performed and is beneficial in evaluating intra-abdominal bleeding but less valuable in the detection of retroperitoneal organ injuries. Peritoneal lavage is a surgical procedure with potential iatrogenic complications and should be performed only by the surgeon who will perform the laparotomy. Diagnosing significant abdominal injury is difficult in the

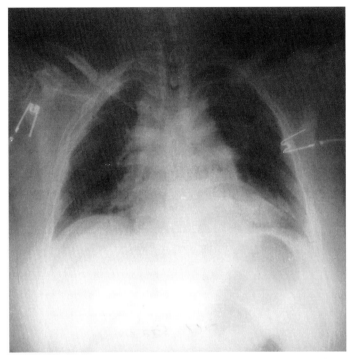

Figure 17.4. Widening of the mediastinum on chest x-ray may indicate injury to the aorta or pulmonary vasculature.

unconscious patient or patient with spinal cord injury. Abdominal CT and peritoneal lavage are particularly important in these patients.

Pelvis

Tremendous force is necessary to produce pelvic ring fractures or dislocations. This force, often transmitted from the lower extremity through the pelvis and to the spine, may produce damage to the lower extremity, spine, and pelvic contents (Table 17.4). There is a high association between pelvic fractures and genitourinary injury (Fig. 17.5).

The pelvis is a well-vascularized structure, and a disruption of its architecture can produce massive hemorrhage with third space loss of circulating volume in the retroperitoneum and abdominal cavity (Fig. 17.6). The bony pelvis itself need not fracture to produce this bleeding. A ligamentous injury to the sacroiliac joints or the symphysis pubis will produce similar results. Pelvic instability can often be

Table 17.4. Commonly Associated Fractures with Similar Mechanism of Injury

Found	Look
Knee	Hip, spine
Wrist	Elbow
Skull	Cervical spine
Calcaneus	Knee, spine

diagnosed by compression and distraction of the iliac wings noting abnormal movement. An AP pelvic x-ray will disclose injuries not apparent on examination. Pelvic ring disruptions should alert the physician to expect major blood loss, and fluid replacement should be instituted accordingly (Fig. 17.7). In many cases, pelvic bleeding will tamponade and stabilize. If pelvic blood loss continues and the patient manifests signs of hypovolemia, orthopaedic stabilization of the pelvis with an external fixator is indicated in an unstable pelvic injury. Angiographic identification of the bleeding vessels and embolization or surgical ligation of those vessels also may be required. The use of a pneumatic antishock garment may help temporarily in this situation. Open pelvic fractures represent an especially difficult problem because of the loss of the tam-

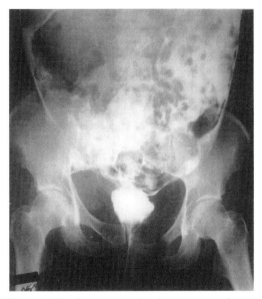

Figure 17.5. Cystogram showing extravasation of contrast into the peritoneum with rupture of the bladder.

ponading effect of third space hematoma. Open pelvic fractures also result in a high infection and mortality rate.

Extremities

Injuries to the extremities are often apparent. Sometimes these obvious injuries tend to misdirect the attention of the examiner away from the more life-threatening problems reviewed earlier. At times an extremity injury is a threat to life, usually because of an associated vascular injury. Fortunately, even profuse bleeding from a vascular injury usually can be controlled by direct pressure. When all other methods have failed, a tourniquet should be used only as a life-saving measure because its application may sacrifice the limb. A closed fracture of a long bone may produce a hematoma containing 2 to 3 units of blood and contribute to hypovolemic shock.

Although limb injuries are rarely life-threatening, they are often limb-threatening. Limb-threatening injuries include the following: dislocations of the elbow, knee, and hip (with or without immediate vascular compromise); open fractures; crush injuries; and fractures with circulatory compromise.

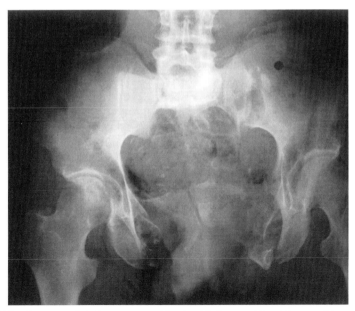

Figure 17.6. Severe pelvic fracture resulting in third space blood loss and hypovolemia.

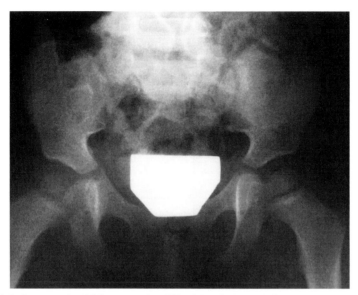

Figure 17.7. Pelvic fractures in children may be difficult to distinguish from normal growth plates. Comparison to normal pelvic films may be helpful.

All splints and dressings are removed, limbs inspected, and dressings re-applied. All joints and long bones should be palpated for swelling, tenderness, deformity, and crepitation. However, if these signs are present, range of motion examination should not be performed before x-ray to rule out fracture or dislocation. If these signs are absent, the joints may be placed through a range of motion looking for tenderness and crepitation. The joints are also gently stressed to detect instability. A thorough assessment of vascular and neurologic function is performed for all four limbs. X-rays are obtained of all limbs where fracture or dislocation is suspected, and these extremities must be splinted. It is important to record the neurovascular examination because the deterioration might signal the development of a compartment syndrome or subsequent vascular insufficiency. The presence of palpable pulses does not rule out all vascular injuries. Prompt orthopaedic consultation should be obtained for injuries to the extremities. Patients with open fractures should be started on broad-spectrum antibiotics and their tetanus status established. Dislocations of major joints will require immediate reduction, and open fractures will require debridement and stabilization by the orthopaedic surgeon.

Definitive Care

After the primary and secondary survey and the evaluation and control of the emergency situation, a definitive care plan should be developed. The more urgent problems will take priority over the less urgent. The definitive care plan may include immediate surgical intervention, additional x-ray, CT, and angiographic evaluation or transfer to another facility where the necessary specialized care can be administered. This is the time for reassessment and monitoring of the patient for early changes and complications.

SUGGESTED READINGS

Amato JJ, Rheinlander HF, Cleveland RJ. Post-traumatic adult respiratory distress syndrome. Orthop Clin North Am 1978;9:693–713.

Baker SP, O'Neill B, Haddon W Jr, et al. The injury severity score: a method for describing patients with multiple injuries and evaluating emergency care. J Trauma 1974;14:187–196.

Baker SP, O'Neill B, Karpf RS. The Injury Fact Book. Lexington, MA: Lexington Books, 1984.

Baker SP, Whitfield RA, O'Neill B. Geographic variations in mortality from motor vehicle crashes. N Engl J Med 1987;317:1601–1602.

Berger JJ, Britt LD. Pelvic fracture hemorrhage: current strategies in diagnosis and management. Surg Ann 1995;27:107–112.

Dabezies EJ, D'Ambrosia RD. Treatment of the multiply injured patient: plans for treatment and problems of major trauma. Instr Course Lect 1984;33:242–252.

Groen GS, Leit ME, Gruen RJ, Peitzman AB. The acute management of hemodynamically unstable multiple trauma patients with pelvic ring fractures. J Trauma 1994;36:706–711.

Levy PS, Goldberg J, Hui S, et al. Severity measurement in multiple trauma by use of ICDA conditions. Stat Med 1982;1:145–152.

Lowe DK. Management of multiple trauma. Surg Rounds 1989;3:75–84.

Morris JA Jr, Auerbach PS, Marshall GA, et al. The trauma score as a triage tool in the prehospital setting. JAMA 1886;256:1319–1325.

Murat JE, Huten N, Mesny J. The use of standardized assessment procedures in the evaluation of patients with multiple injuries. Arch Emerg Med 1985; 2:11–15.

O'Donnell TF Jr, Belkin SC. The pathophysiology, monitoring, and treatment of shock. Orthop Clin North Am 1978;9:589–610.

Index

Page numbers in italics followed by f denote figures; those in italics followed by t denote tables.

A

Abdominal injuries, 419–420
Abductor sway, 179, 184, 185
Achilles tendinitis, 252, 253–254, 342
Acid phosphatase, 365
Acute cervical myalgia (muscular wryneck), 16–17
Acute disc herniation, 11–16
Acute osteomyelitis, 350–353
Acute subacromial bursitis, 45
Adhesive capsulitis, 49
Adolescents. *See* Children
Adrenaline, 326
Adson maneuvers, 20, 21
Adson's test, 8
Adults
    avascular (aseptic) necrosis of the adult hip, 189–190
    compression fractures in older, 166–167
    fractures of both bones of the forearm in, 88
    hip fractures in older, 199–201
    nontraumatic foot conditions in adulthood, 278, 280–292
    nontraumatic hip and pelvis conditions in adulthood, 184–194
    nontraumatic knee conditions in adulthood, 218–222
    nontraumatic and traumatic cervical spine conditions in adulthood, 11–28
Advanced Trauma Life Support (ATLS) Course for Physicians, 412
Age-Matched Z-score, 359
Airway, establishing an adequate, 413–415, *415f*
Alendronate, 363–364, 366
Alkaline phosphatase, 153, 365
Allopurinol, 345–346

American College of Surgeons Committee on Trauma, 412, 416
Amputations
    digital tip, 122–123, *122f*
    guidelines for the care of amputation of digits or the hand, 124
    and surgical treatment for sarcomas, 380
Anastomosis, 181
Animal bites, human and, 110–111
Ankle. *See* Leg and ankle
Ankylosing hyperostosis, 335
Ankylosing spondylitis, 147, 153–154, 163–164, 333, 341–342
Anserine bursitis, 220–221
Anterior drawer test, 216
Anterolisthesis, 154
Antibiotics
    antibiotic therapy for septic arthritis, 354–355
    for human and animal bite injuries, 110
    IV antistaphylococcus, 158
    for spinal infections, 158
Apley's test, 218, 219
Arthritis
    degenerative arthritis of the hip, 184–188
    degenerative arthritis and metastatic bone disease, 371
    degenerative arthritis and Paget's disease, 365
    inflammatory arthritis of the hip, 188
    Lyme disease and, 347
    septic, 354–355
    septic arthritis of the hip, 188, 391
    See also Rheumatoid arthritis
Arthroscopy, glenohumeral, 43
Aspiration and injection techniques, 321–322, *322f*

local anesthesia, 322–324
local anesthetics—drugs, agents, adjuncts, 324–326
local infiltration of fracture sites, 332
needle insertion, *322f, 323f, 324f, 325f*
prevention of toxic reactions, 326–327
regional blocks, 327–332, *328f, 329f, 330f, 331f*
Avascular necrosis
    of the femoral head, 391–393
    in the hip, 180–181, 188, 189–190
    in the knee, 218–219
Axial joint disease, 342

B

Back pain, evaluating patients with
    herniated discs, 160–163
    history, 146–148
    inflammatory back pain, 163–164
    laboratory studies, 151–154
    miscellaneous causes of low back pain, 167–169
    pain diagrams, 147–148, *148f*
    physical examination, 149–150
    Waddell signs, 149, 150–151, 168
Baker's cyst, 221
Barton's fracture, 128, *128f*
Batson's plexus, 145, 369, 370
Behçet's syndrome, 354
Bell's palsy, 347
Bennett fractures, 131, *132f*
Betadine, 258
Bicipital tendinitis, 44, 45, 47–48
Biopsy, bone lesion, 373
Biphosphonates, 363–364, 366
Blocks
    extraforaminal nerve block, 162
    use of regional, 327–332, *328f, 329f, 330f, 331f*